The Australian Home Guide to Medication

Dr Warwick Carter
MBBS, FRACGP

For Vern

This book is intended as a reference volume only, not as a manual for self treatment. If you suspect that you have a medical problem, please seek competent medical care. The information here is designed to help you make informed choices about your health. It is not intended as a substitute for any treatment described by your doctor.

Published in 2006 by Hinkler Books Pty Ltd
17–23 Redwood Drive
Dingley VIC 3172 Australia
www.hinklerbooks.com

© Warwick Carter 2004
Cover design © Hinkler Books Pty Ltd 2006
First Printed in 2004

Cover design: Hinkler Design Studio
Cover prepress: Splitting Image

ISBN-13: 978 1 7415 7581 1
ISBN-10: 1 7415 7581 8

2 4 6 8 10 9 7 5 3
07 09 11 10 08

All rights reserved. No part of this publication may be reproduced, stored in a retrieval system, or transmitted in any way or by any means, electronic, mechanical, photocopying, recording or otherwise, without the prior written permission of the copyright holders.

Every effort has been made to ensure this book is free from error or omissions. However, the Publisher, the Editor or their respective employees or agents, shall not accept responsibility for injury, loss or damage occasioned to any person acting or refraining from action as a result of material in this book whether or not such injury, loss or damage is in any way due to any negligent act or omission, breach of duty or default on part of the Publisher, the Editor or their respective employees or agents.

Printed and bound in Australia

CONTENTS

INTRODUCTION
    Preface 4
    Format 6
    Pregnancy Risk Categorisation 8
    Pharmaceutical Benefits Scheme (PBS) 9
    Generic Prescribing 12
    Safe Storage of Medication 13
    Home Medicine Chest 14

EMERGENCIES
    Allergy Reaction 15
    Anaphylactic Reaction 16
    Choking 16
    Diarrhoea 17
    Overdose 18
    Poisoning 19
    Vomiting 20

MEDICATIONS – An Alphabetical Listing
    A 21
    B 81
    C 111
    D 165
    E 205
    F 223
    G 250
    H 269
    I 288
    J 307
    K 308
    L 314
    M 333
    N 376
    O 399
    P 420
    Q 480
    R 483
    S 498
    T 538
    U 582
    V 586
    W 595
    X 597
    Y 598
    Z 600

INDEX 609

Home Guide to Medication

INTRODUCTION

Preface

Australians are prescribed medications by their doctors and dentists at the rate of five prescriptions per person every year. These prescriptions are expensive, but in many cases the government subsidises them through the Pharmaceutical Benefits Scheme (PBS). Even so, it is you — the taxpayer — who eventually pays the bill.

All medications on the Australian market have been extensively tested for effectiveness and lack of serious side effects. Nevertheless, every medication has potential problems, interactions, adverse reactions and correct methods of use. For these reasons it is important for everyone who takes any medication that they know as much as possible about its uses and actions.

This book is designed to educate users of medication in simple language about the medications they are taking. If you have any concerns, discuss them further with your general practitioner.

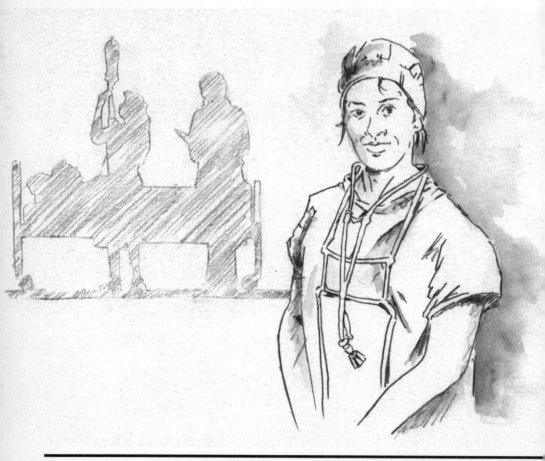

Introduction

Every entry has a standard format, and entries are extensively cross referenced. Every prescription medication available in the country (with the exception of general anaesthetics and some injections used in operating theatres and for exotic cancer treatments) is explained, as well as many non-prescription pharmacy only medicines.

The terminology of medications can be confusing. Every medication has at least three names – a chemical name which is used only by scientists, a generic (common) name that is specific to that medication, and a trade name (or several trade names) that is given to the medication by the various manufacturers. For example:

Chemical name: Acetyl salicylic acid

Generic name: Aspirin

Trade names: Aspro, Astrix, Cartia, Disprin etc.

Every medication also belongs to a class of similar medications (some belong to two or more classes). Aspirin belongs to the Analgesic, Salicylate and Nonsteroidal Anti-inflammatory Drug (NSAID) classes. Common drug classes are listed with the drug generic names in the main part of the book.

The main entries are either under the medication's generic name or its drug class. It will depend on the complexity of the listing if all medications in one drug class can be listed together (eg. all Proton Pump Inhibitors are listed together) or separately (eg. the various forms of Penicillin are listed separately). These entries are listed in alphabetical order in the body of the book and are cross-referenced between generic drug name and drug class so that looking up either will lead you to the required entry.

If you wish to find a medication by its trade name, consult the index, where you will be directed to the appropriate entry.

If you wish to find different medications that treat the same condition (eg. epilepsy), look up one medication that treats the condition, see which drug class it is in (eg. Anticonvulsant), and under that drug class you will find listed other medications that will treat that condition.

Some illegal drugs (cocaine, marijuana and heroin) and commonly used herbs are also covered in this book.

New medications are introduced into the Australian market at the rate of about a dozen every month, while others are removed because they have been superseded, are found to have unacceptable complications or they are not profitable. Other medications are added to, or withdrawn from, the PBS, have additional uses or side effects determined, are found to interact with other medications, or may become more readily available without prescription. This fifth edition of *The Complete Home Guide to Medication* therefore contains thousands of alterations and additions that reflect these changes. More than 90% of the entries have been modified for this edition.

Understanding the medications they are using by referring to this book will help patients cope with their condition, and enable them to understand why their doctor has chosen a particular course of action.

Dr Warwick Carter MBBS, FRACGP, FAMA.
Brisbane
April 2003

Introduction

Format

Generic Name or
DRUG GROUP NAME
(Alternative Name)

TRADE NAMES, or
TRADE and GENERIC NAMES:

Trade Names of medication listed above, or **Trade Name** followed by generic names within a drug group. The specific ingredient that is being discussed in this entry is <u>underlined</u> when there is any possibility of confusion.

DRUG CLASS:
Class of drug to which medication belongs. Only common drug classes are mentioned, as not all medications can be put into a drug class that has any meaning outside university laboratories.

USES:
The conditions that can be treated by the medication.

DOSAGE:

The way in which the medication should be taken.
Normal adult dose shown.

FORMS:
The ways in which the medication is presented, eg. capsules, mixture, injection (colour and storage precautions in brackets).

Aerosol spray | Atomiser spray, Inhaler | Capsule Rotacap | Cream, Gel, Lotion Ointment, Paste | Drops

Elixer, Liquid, Gargle, Infusion, Mixture, Solution, Suspension | Lozenge, Pessary, Supository | Nasal spray | Paint, Tincture | Powder

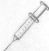

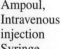

Ampoul, Intravenous injection Syringe, Injection | Flimtabs, Tablets | Syrup
1 Teaspoon = 5ml
1 Desertspoon = 10ml
1 Tablespoon = 15ml

Home Guide to Medication

PRECAUTIONS:
The precautions that a doctor or pharmacist should warn a patient about if taking this medication, including its use in pregnancy (with pregnancy risk categorisation in brackets after the word 'pregnancy' – see below), breast feeding and children.

Do not take if:

 suffering from certain conditions

- under other circumstances

SIDE EFFECTS:
Common: Unwanted problems that many patients may experience.
Unusual: Less common problems that fewer than 3% of patients may experience.
Severe but rare (stop medication, consult doctor): Rare and serious complications.

INTERACTIONS:
Other drugs:
- Drug name that may interact with medication. This interaction may affect the medication unfavourably, increase or decrease its action or side effects, or increase or decrease its excretion from the body. Some interactions may improve the effects of the drug. Discuss any possible interaction with your doctor or pharmacist.

Herbs:
- Herbs and other natural substances that may cause an interaction.

Other substances:
- Reactions with substances such as alcohol, caffeine, foods, exercise etc.

PRESCRIPTION:
Whether a prescription is required for the medication.

PBS:
Is the medication available at a subsidised price on the Pharmaceutical Benefits Scheme (restrictions listed in brackets)? See Introduction for explanation of this scheme.

PERMITTED IN SPORT:
Can the medication be taken legally while competing in high levels of sport?

OVERDOSE:
The effects of an overdose, and the first aid treatment of an overdose. See section on 'Overdose' and 'Poisoning' in Introduction for further information.

OTHER INFORMATION:
Other relevant and interesting information about the medication, including problems with addiction and long term use.
See also Other Related Medication.

DRUG GROUP NAME

DISCUSSION:
An explanation of drug group action and discussion on its effects.
See Generic Name(s).

Generic Name
See DRUG GROUP NAME.

Pregnancy Risk Categorisation

Most medications in Australia have been given a category depending on the risk they pose to the unborn child of a pregnant woman. The risk category is shown in the **PRECAUTIONS** section of most entries in brackets after the word 'pregnancy'. The definitions of the categories are:

A	No proven direct or indirect harmful effects to the foetus.
B1	Studies in animals have shown no evidence of increased foetal damage.
B2	Studies in animals are inadequate, but available data shows no evidence of increased foetal damage.
B3	Studies in animals have shown evidence of increased foetal damage, but the significance of this in humans is uncertain.
C	May cause harmful effects to the foetus but not malformations. These effects may be reversible.
D	Cause an increased incidence of foetal malformations, other irreversible damage and/or adverse pharmacological effects on the foetus.
X	High risk of permanent damage to the foetus. Should not be used if pregnancy is even a possibility.

Pharmaceutical Benefits Scheme (PBS)

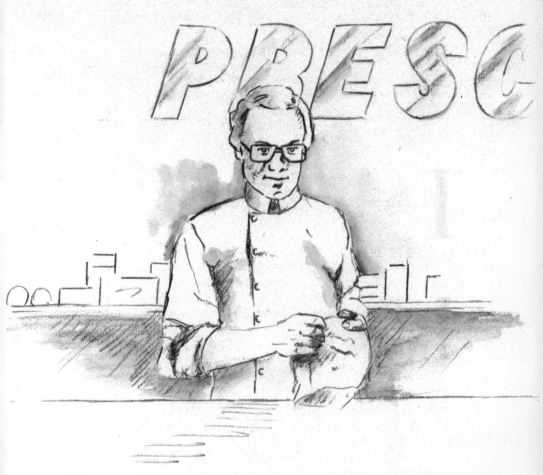

Australia has a national subsidised Pharmaceutical Benefits Scheme (PBS) that was started after the Second World War to provide essential medications to all Australians at a reasonable price. The definition of what medications are essential has changed significantly over the years. There are about 3000 different trade name medications available on the market in this country, but only one fifth of them are listed on the PBS.

A doctor can write a private prescription for any medication s/he wishes, in any quantity, with any number of repeats (with some restrictions for narcotics and stimulants), but the patient must pay the full cost.

If the patient is to benefit from the PBS, a considerable number of requirements must be fulfilled by the doctor when writing the prescription.

A large book is published every four months by the Commonwealth Department of Health to list the regulations regarding the medications on the PBS.

In order to write a prescription for a PBS medication a doctor first needs to know if the patient is a Health Care or Health Benefits card holder (about 30% of the population). Cards are issued in various categories for pensioners, unemployed, chronically ill, single parents, low income earners and war veterans.

War veterans are entitled to a larger range of medications on the Veteran Affairs Pharmaceutical Benefits Scheme than on the PBS, and less stringent limits on what can be prescribed.

Once the patient's status is established the doctor can decide if they can afford a private script (eg. for Digesic which is not PBS listed) or of their pain will have to be treated with Paracetamol (which is one of the few analgesics on the PBS list).

When writing a PBS prescription, the maximum number of tablets (amount of elixir etc.) and the maximum number of repeats is determined by government regulation and cannot be exceeded unless special application is made to the appropriate government department. If a mistake is made with these numbers, the script must be rejected by the pharmacist.

Provided the doctor writes a generic prescription (or a brand name of a medication that is priced at the generic price – see Brand Name Premiums below) a card-holder will pay $3.30 for the script, while a non-card-holder will pay a maximum $20.60 (prices as at February 2001).

BRAND NAME PREMIUMS

The manufacturers of many popular trade name medications are not prepared to lower their price to that of their generic competitors, so if the doctor prescribes the Amoxil brand of amoxycillin 500mg instead of the Moxacin brand, the patient will pay an extra 72¢. These premiums are usually quite small, but may be several dollars for some more unusual medications.

The companies that charge a premium for their medications are usually those who originally spent millions of dollars developing the product and establishing it on the market. About 100 brands of medication carry a premium, but in all cases there is a generic equivalent that has no premium.

See 'Generic Prescribing' below.

SAFETY NET

Once a non-card holding family has spent a certain amount in one calendar year on PBS medications (according to a complex formula – approximately 52 prescriptions), they are issued a card that gives them further medications at the lower rate of $3.50 for the rest of that year. Card holding families, under the same formula, receive free prescriptions after they have spent the required amount in a calendar year. Regulations limit the number of repeats that can be filled in any month to prevent stockpiling of drugs at the cheap rate.

AUTHORITY MEDICATIONS

About 200 medications are further restricted, not usually because of any inherent risk, but because of their cost. These medications must be prescribed (in quadruplicate) on a special 'Authority to Prescribe' form, and doctors must obtain phone or mail approval from a government clerk before issuing the script. Medications such as Noroxin (for urinary infections), Neurontin (for epilepsy), Imigran (for migraine) and Valtrex (for herpes and shingles) are included on this list. The aim is to reduce the cost to government by making it harder for the doctor to prescribe.

Authority medications must be certified to be used for an approved purpose (eg. Valtrex for shingles). Doctors who falsely certify in order to benefit their patients can be heavily fined.

THERAPEUTIC GROUP PRICING

Australian doctors, pharmacists and their patients also have to cope with an additional piece of bureaucracy (none ever seems to be taken away) in the form of Therapeutic Group Pricing.

In simple terms, a number of drug groups have been chosen, and every brand and generic (copies of original medications by companies that undertake no research or development) medication in each class has been priced at the level of the cheapest drug in that class. The doctor can prescribe, and the chemist can dispense, any medication, but if the pharmaceutical company has priced its product at a level higher than the cheapest product, then the patient must pay the difference or the chemist will be out of pocket.

Under the Therapeutic Group Pricing scheme, the largest gap between the cheapest and most expensive product in a group is about $5 for one month's supply at the normal recommended dose, but most have a gap of about $2. For someone already paying over $23 for the medication, these gaps are not likely to be onerous, but for those paying the heavily subsidised $3.50, or those who use large doses of medication regularly, the gap may become significant.

As with all restrictions, there is an appeal mechanism. If the doctor feels that his/her patient absolutely must have a more expensive brand, the doctor can fill in a form, phone or post it to the bureaucrats, and have it rubber stamped, so the patient can obtain the medication at the base price.

The criteria for exemption are:
- Adverse effects and/or drug interactions occur, or are expected to occur with all base priced drugs.
- The transfer to a base priced drug would cause patient confusion resulting in problems with compliance.

If any patient feels that they are having problems with the cost of their medication, or believes they may be eligible for an exemption, they should discuss the matter with their doctor.

There are innumerable other minor rules and regulations that regulate PBS prescribing, and the situation is so complex that some doctors issue private scripts for PBS items when the patient is privately insured, as the patient can claim back most of the cost from their health insurance fund.

NB: PBS regulations, inclusions and entitlements change every four months. Please check with your pharmacist or doctor for the latest information.

Introduction

Generic Prescribing

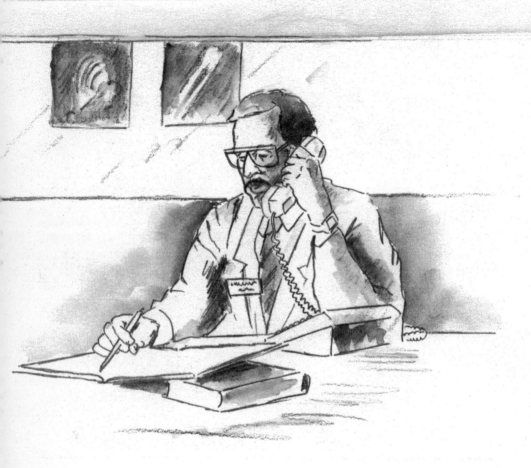

Generic substitution of prescription medications was introduced by the Commonwealth Government in Australia in December 1994. This means that if the doctor prescribes a particular brand (trade name) of a medication, the pharmacist may substitute another equivalent brand unless the doctor specifically endorses the prescription that substitution is not allowed.

There are many arguments for and against this procedure.

The reasons in favour of generic prescribing are:
- The cost of medication to the patient is kept as low as possible.
- Australian companies are given a better chance to compete against international drug companies.
- The cost to government (and taxpayers) of medication is minimised.

The reasons against generic prescribing are:
- Price differentials between the brand medications and the generic substitutes are usually less than a dollar.
- Australian drugs are already very cheap (although most patients will disagree) at 60% of average price in western countries.
- Low prices may delay the introduction of new drugs to the Australian market.
- Research into new medications is carried out by companies with more expensive drugs. Less use of brand name drugs means less research.
- The reputation of a manufacturer is at stake when brand names are used, and if there are any problems the patient has a major company to support them, which has a worldwide reputation to defend.
- Changes in tablet or capsule shape and colour can cause confusion. One month you may receive pink tablets, the next month yellow ones and the month after white ones. Some patients may start taking incorrect doses leading to significant medical problems.
- Variations in bioavailability (effectiveness) of up to 20%. This may seem a small amount, but in some medications such variation can be critical for the correct control of the patient's condition.
- Less pleasant flavours of mixtures. Brand name mixtures tend to have more sophisticated (and expensive) methods of disguising unpleasant flavours.
- Less effective and reliable delivery systems. Creams may have different bases that affect their absorption into the skin, and tablets may disintegrate in the stomach at different rates.
- Less patient information in packaging.
- Using generic substitutes is equivalent to using 'No Name' brands from the supermarket.
- Doctors may be blamed if a generic substitute does not work.

You should discuss this matter further
with your own doctor if you have any queries.

Safe Storage of Medication

Accidental overdoses of medications, even common ones like Paracetamol (eg. Panadol) can kill young children. Many tablets and capsules are brightly coloured and naturally attractive to little people who want to find out what they are like.

A safe storage area for all medications is absolutely essential.
A high, locked cupboard with a child-proof latch is best.

Introduction

Home Medicine Chest

A comprehensive home medical chest should contain the following items:

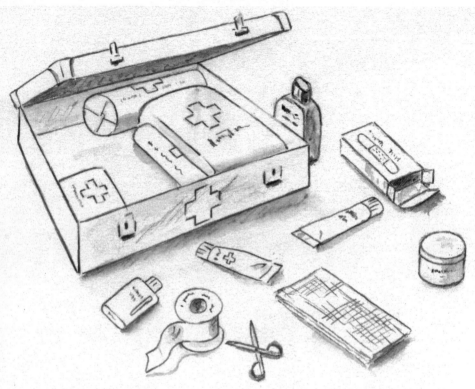

Paracetamol Tablets
Paracetamol Liquid
Charcoal Tablets or Solution
(for overdose)
Lotion for bites and stings
Anti-itch Cream
Antiseptic Cream
Antiseptic Liquid
Pseudoephedrine Tablets and/or Liquid
(for nasal congestion)
Oxymetazoline Nose Drops
Menthol Inhalant

Cough Syrup
Antiseptic Ear Drops
Antiseptic Eye Drops
Sunscreen Lotion or Cream.
Splinter Forceps
Scissors
Triangular Bandage (sling)
Adhesive Dressing
(various sizes)
Elastic Bandages (wide)
Cotton Gauze (NOT cotton wool)
Adhesive Tape

EMERGENCIES

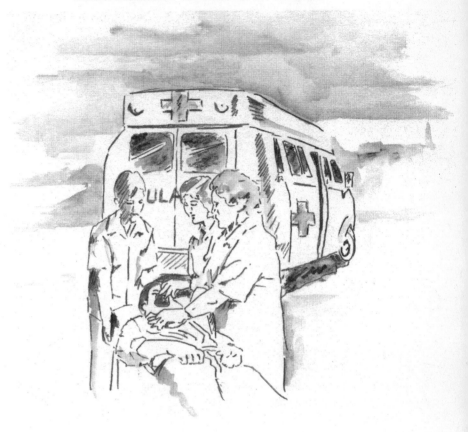

Allergy reaction

An allergy is excess sensitivity to a substance that produces a reaction in the body.

Allergies may occur on exposure to almost any type of chemical. As well as medications, animal hair, dust, milk, eggs, pollen, fish, fruit, insect bites, moulds and parasites are just a few of the thousands of possible allergies.

An allergen is a substance (such as a medication) that causes an allergic reaction. When the body first encounters an allergen, the defence mechanisms of the body are triggered, but there is usually no detectable effect. On the second and subsequent occasions of exposure to the allergen, the defence mechanism over-reacts, causing effects that may be merely a nuisance, or severe and life threatening (see Anaphylactic Reaction below), in different areas of the body.

In an allergic reaction, a substance called histamine is released. It causes rapid swelling of the tissue, which in the nose or lungs then secretes copious amounts of watery phlegm, and becomes intensely itchy.

The body gradually breaks down the histamine itself, and the reaction disappears, but this process can be sped up by the use of antihistamine drugs that are taken by mouth or injection to destroy the histamine that is causing the allergy reaction.

In an emergency, anyone exposed to a medication or substance to which they have an allergic reaction should be given antihistamines by mouth and then taken to a doctor. Antihistamines are available without prescription from chemists.

Tests may be performed to determine whether or not you are allergic to a particular medication, but because there are so many possibilities, you must have some idea of which medication is causing the problem before the tests are commenced. The tests may take the form of skin pricks with a number of suspected substances, or blood tests that can detect the body's reaction to an allergen.

If someone is found to be highly allergic to a specific substance, they can be desensitised so that they do not react as strongly, or sometimes do not react at all. This process is often long and involved, and unfortunately does not always work, but many people have had life threatening and disabling allergies cured or reduced by this procedure.

Allergies are usually annoying rather than serious, but in a small number of people, they may become a life threatening anaphylactic reaction (see below). Those who know they may have a life threatening allergy should always carry adrenaline with them, to be self-injected if they have an attack.

Anaphylactic reaction

An anaphylactic reaction is an immediate, severe, life-threatening allergic reaction. Death may occur within minutes if medical help is not immediately available.

The patient becomes rapidly sweaty, develops widespread pins and needles, swelling develops in one or more parts of the body (possibly including the tongue and throat), starts wheezing, becomes blue around the lips, may become incontinent of urine, loses consciousness, convulses and stops breathing.

Swelling of the tongue and throat alone may be enough to cause death if air is unable to pass into the lungs. The terrified victim suffocates.

First aid can give only limited assistance. The patient must be placed on their back with the neck extended to give the best possible airway, and mouth to mouth resuscitation, and external cardiac massage may be necessary.

Medical treatment must be sought urgently, as an injection of drugs such as adrenaline, aminophylline, hydrocortisone or an antihistamine will reverse the allergic reaction rapidly, and save the patient's life.

Patients who are aware that they may have an anaphylactic reaction usually carry an injectable form of adrenaline with them at all times to be used in an emergency.

Insect stings (eg. bees, hornets, wasps and ants) and injected drugs are the most likely substances to produce acute anaphylaxis. It is rare for inhaled, touched or eaten substances to cause this reaction.

Choking

If a piece of food or other foreign body is caught in the windpipe, the person may die from asphyxiation in a few minutes. It is essential to dislodge the blockage as rapidly as possible.

In a child, turn him upside down, and while holding him by the feet, bang firmly on the back.

In an older child or adult, with the patient sitting or standing, place your arms around them from behind, and cross your wrists over the breast bone. Firmly compress the chest by pressure on the breast bone to force the air out of the lungs, and hopefully the foreign body out of the windpipe.

Alternatively, lie the patient in the coma position on their side on the floor, give several sharp blows between the shoulder blades, and then if necessary, give several firm quick pushes on the side of the chest wall below the arm pit.

If unsuccessful, lie the victim on a table or bed, with the body above the waist hanging over the edge, and bang on the back several times before repeating the chest compression. These manoeuvres are successful in the vast majority of cases.

If you fail to dislodge the food blocking the windpipe, and the patient is turning blue, mouth to mouth resuscitation should be started, in an attempt to force some air past the blockage and into the lungs.

Diarrhoea

Diarrhoea has causes that vary from the serious (cancer, ulcerative colitis), to the annoying (food poisoning, drug reactions), but the most common type of diarrhoea in Australians is that caused by a viral infection of the gut.

A virus may infect your bowel to cause diarrhoea, in the same way that another may cause a cold by infecting your nose and throat. The virus particles enter the gut on food or droplets of breath, they are swallowed, and immediately start multiplying into incredibly large numbers. Billions upon trillions of them will eventually be present.

Once in the stomach in these vast numbers, viruses irritate the tissue around them. This in turn causes the lining of the gut to secrete large amounts of fluid, and it also interferes with the normal absorption of food from the intestine, so anything eaten passes straight through.

The third effect is an irritation of the gut, causing it to go into repeated spasms. This causes severe, colic-like pain, and anything that is inside the gut is pushed out through the nearest appropriate orifice (mouth or anus) by these strong contractions.

The upper part of the gut is normally attacked first, causing six to 12 hours of vomiting. This settles as the virus moves down the intestine, and the lower gut becomes inflamed, causing diarrhoea that may last from one to three days.

Because the infection is caused by a virus, antibiotics have no effect on the disease – they may in fact, make the diarrhoea worse.

It is not desirable in most circumstances to use drugs to stop the diarrhoea either, as all this does is hold the virus in the body, and allow it to reproduce further. The body is cleaning the infection from the gastrointestinal system with the diarrhoea, and within reason, it is best to allow this process to proceed.

The treatment of viral gastroenteritis is therefore primarily rest and diet. Fluids and food should be taken in small amounts frequently, not large amounts occasionally.

For the first 24 hours, only clear fluids should be taken by mouth. Commercial preparations that contain salts and sugars are ideal, but clear soups, cordial and very dilute cordials with a pinch of salt added may also be used as a short term substitute. Freezing the liquid and allowing the child to lick the resultant block is an excellent way to get fluids into a vomiting child.

Emergencies

Plain water should not be drunk, as the body requires the salts and sugars for the absorption of fluids from the gut.

On the second and subsequent days, food should be gradually introduced. Cereals, bread, rice and dry biscuits are the first foods to be tried, and if they cause no problems, boiled vegetables, fruit and white meat can be added.

It is important to avoid all dairy products, eggs, fatty and fried foods until you are completely better.

Only if the vomiting lasts more than 12 hours, or the diarrhoea is excessively severe or prolonged, is further medical attention and medication required.

Extra care must be observed with young children, as severe diarrhoea may cause dehydration in less than a day.

Overdose

Excessive doses of medication can be taken by accident (eg. children finding a bottle of pills, confused elderly people) or deliberately (eg. suicide attempt). The appropriate first aid by the person discovering the overdose may be lifesaving.

Some medications are far more dangerous than others when taken in excess. These relative dangers are discussed in the 'Overdose' section in the section on each medication in the main part of this book.

For virtually all medication overdosages, the first aid treatment is to administer charcoal to neutralise the medication. Activated charcoal solutions are readily available from chemists without a prescription, and should be included in any home medicine chest.

If activated charcoal is not available, and there will be some delay in obtaining medical attention it is preferable to induce vomiting rather than allow the medication to be absorbed. Vomiting should NOT be induced if the patient is unconscious or otherwise liable to inhale any vomitus.

Activated charcoal should be given at any time after the overdose has been taken. Induction of vomiting is most beneficial within 30 minutes of the overdose having been taken, but even up to two hours later it may be beneficial. Many medications cause vomiting as part of their overdose effects, but by this time, the drug has already been absorbed and the vomiting is unlikely to reduce the effects of the drug significantly.

Vomiting can be induced by giving Ipecacuanha syrup and water, by giving soapy water to drink, by applying pressure to the upper belly or by putting a finger down the back of the person's throat (be careful not to be bitten, particularly if the patient is likely to convulse). The patient should be lying on their side with the neck extended, or sitting up and leaning over to avoid inhaling vomitus.

Carers should seek medical advice as soon as possible, and sometimes urgent medical attention must be obtained.

Advice is available from your own general practitioner, local hospital or the Poisons Information Centre (phone 13 11 26 from any phone in Australia).

See also 'Poisoning' on page 19.

Poisoning

Innumerable substances in our environment can poison the human body. A brief summary of common poisons and their treatment follows, but if in doubt, contact your general practitioner, local hospital or Poisons Information Centre (phone 13 11 26 from any phone in Australia).

CHEMICAL/DRUG	EFFECT OF POISON	FIRST AID TREATMENT
Alkalis (household bleaches)	Burning, vomiting, shock, difficult breathing.	Dilute with milk, allow vomiting, give vinegar.
Aspirin (Aspro, Disprin etc.)	Rapid breathing, brain disturbance, coma, kidney failure.	Give activated charcoal or induce vomiting.
Barbiturates	Drowsiness, confusion, coma, breathing difficulty.	Give activated charcoal or induce vomiting, black coffee, assist breathing.
Codeine (in painkillers, cough mixtures, antidiarrhoeals)	Constipation, reduced breathing, stupor, coma, heart attack.	Give activated charcoal or induce, assist breathing.
Digoxin (Lanoxin)	Vomiting, irregular pulse, heart failure.	Dilute with milk or water then give activated charcoal or induce vomiting.
Insecticides	Vomiting, diarrhoea, difficult breathing, convulsions.	Dilute with large amount of milk, give activated charcoal or induce vomiting, assist breathing.
Lysol and creosote	Burning of throat, vomiting, shock, breathing difficulty.	Dilute with large amount of milk. Do NOT induce vomiting.
Mushrooms	Varies depending on type.	Dilute with water, give activated charcoal or induce vomiting, assist breathing.
Narcotics (Morphine, heroin)	Headache, nausea, excitement, weak pulse, shock, coma.	Give activated charcoal or induce vomiting if narcotic swallowed, assist breathing.
Paracetamol (Panadol, Dymadon, Panamax etc.)	Vomiting, low blood pressure, liver damage, death [>50 tabs].	Give activated charcoal or induce vomiting.
Petroleum products (petrol, kerosene, etc.)	Liver damage, lung damage.	Do NOT induce vomiting, dilute with milk.
Tranquillisers (Phenothiazines)	Drowsiness, low blood pressure, rapid pulse, convulsions, coma.	Give activated charcoal or induce vomiting.
Tricyclic antidepressants (Sinequan, Tofranil, Prothiaden, Tryptanol etc.).	Coma, muscle spasm, convulsions, death.	Give activated charcoal or induce vomiting, assist breathing.

Emergencies

Vomiting

The stomach, and sometimes the upper part of the small gut, will go into spasm and discharge their contents via the gullet and mouth for a very wide variety of reasons. Some causes of vomiting are common and innocuous, but others may indicate serious disease.

By far the most common reason to vomit is a toxin irritating the gut. This is food poisoning, and a contaminated prawn, sausage or other foodstuff is usually responsible. The vomiting occurs two to eight hours after eating the food, and is usually sudden, violent and short-lived. It is unusual for the problem to persist for more than a few hours, and is only occasionally accompanied by diarrhoea.

Gastroenteritis is the other very common cause of vomiting. In this, a virus enters the stomach, causing it to become inflamed. In this state it secretes excess amounts of digestive juices and can go into spasm very easily, particularly if any further food is eaten. Initially the upper part of the gut is affected, and as the virus moves down through the alimentary canal, the large bowel is involved. When the gut goes into spasm, its contents are expelled causing vomiting and/or diarrhoea, and may be associated with painful abdominal cramps.

The virus can easily spread from one person to another, and so one member of the family after another may become infected. Spread is avoided by hand washing, especially after toilet and before eating. Fortunately, the disease is self limiting, and a strict diet for a few days is all that is normally required for treatment.

Nausea (the feeling that you want to be sick) and vomiting often accompany migraine-type headaches. Some patients find that their migraine actually eases after vomiting.

Overindulgence in food and alcohol is another common cause of this distressing condition. Even today, sympathy for a self-induced condition is not often forthcoming, but 2000 years ago, the Romans sometimes left a feast to vomit so that they could consume even greater amounts of the delicacies being offered.

Other people who may induce vomiting in themselves are those suffering from bulimia and anorexia nervosa. They have a compulsive desire to be thin, and may appear to eat normally, but later regurgitate their food. They steadily loose weight, and may become extremely ill as a result.

Vomiting after a head injury is a sign that there may be some brain damage. One or two vomits are not unusual, but if it becomes prolonged, urgent medical attention should be sought.

Sinusitis and colds may be associated with nausea and vomiting because of the large amounts of infected phlegm that are swallowed. Medications are available to dry up the phlegm and control the sinus infection.

Many rarer diseases from meningitis and stomach cancer to liver disease and pregnancy may be associated with vomiting. If you suffer from this condition, and it does not settle rapidly, have the cause diagnosed and treated by your family doctor.

MEDICATIONS

Abacavir

TRADE NAMES:
Ziagen.
Trizivir (with lamivudine and zidovudine).

DRUG CLASS:
Antiviral.

USES:
Treatment of AIDS and HIV infection.

DOSAGE:
 One tablet or 15mLs solution twice a day.

FORMS:
Tablet of 300mg (yellow), solution

PRECAUTIONS:
Intolerance to fructose in solution.

SIDE EFFECTS:
Common: Liver damage, diarrhoea, tiredness, sensitivity reactions, fever, loss of appetite.
Severe but rare (stop medication, consult doctor): Allergy reaction (cease immediately and never use again).

INTERACTIONS:
Other drugs: Retinoids.

PRESCRIPTION:
Yes.

PBS:
Yes (very restricted).

PERMITTED IN SPORT:
Yes.

OVERDOSE:
Effects not known.

OTHER INFORMATION:
Released in 1999 as one of numerous medications that may be beneficial in slowing the progress of AIDS.
See also Delavirdine, Didanosine, Efavirenz, Indinavir, Lamivudine, Nelfinavir, Nevirapine, Ritonavir, Saquinavir, Stavudine, Tenofovir, Zalcitabine, Zidovudine.

Abciximab

TRADE NAME:
Reopro.

DRUG CLASS:
Anticoagulant

USES:
Prevents blood clots during heart and artery surgery.

DOSAGE:
 Given by injection via a drip only.

FORMS:
Injection vial.

PRECAUTIONS:
Used only under strict supervision in hospital. May cause abnormal and excessive bleeding.

Home Guide to Medication   **21**

SIDE EFFECTS:
Common: Unwanted bleeding.
Unusual: Development of antibodies to the medication.

INTERACTIONS:
None serious.

PRESCRIPTION:
Yes.

PBS:
No.

PERMITTED IN SPORT:
Yes.

OVERDOSE:
May cause excessive bleeding.

OTHER INFORMATION:
Drug introduced in 1996 for prevention of complications of surgery on heart and arteries.
See also Heparin, Ticlopidine.

Acamprosate

TRADE NAME:
Campral.

USES:
Reduces desire for alcohol in alcoholics.

DOSAGE:
 One or two tablets three times a day.

FORMS:
Tablets of 333mg

PRECAUTIONS:
Reduce dose in elderly and small body weight patients.
Use with caution in pregnancy (B2) and breast feeding.
Not to be used until completely withdrawn from alcohol.
Do not take if:
 suffering from severe kidney disease, severe liver disease.

SIDE EFFECTS:
Common: Diarrhoea.
Unusual: Itch, red skin.

INTERACTIONS:
Other drugs:
• Psychotropic drugs.

PRESCRIPTION:
Yes.

PBS:
Yes (authority required).

PERMITTED IN SPORT:
Yes.

OVERDOSE:
Serious effects unlikely.

OTHER INFORMATION:
Introduced in 1999. Manufactured and developed in Australia.
See also Disulfiram, Naltrexone.

Acarbose

TRADE NAME:
Glucobay.

DRUG CLASS:
Hypoglycaemic.

USES:
Maturity onset diabetes type 2.

DOSAGE:
 50 to 200mg two to three times a day.

FORMS:
Tablets of 50mg and 100mg (white).

PRECAUTIONS:
Use with caution in pregnancy (B3) breast feeding and children. Regular blood tests to check sugar levels and liver function.

SIDE EFFECTS:
Common: Low blood sugar, nausea, diarrhoea.
Unusual: Liver abnormalities.

INTERACTIONS:
Other drugs:
- Other hypoglycaemics (medications that lower blood sugar levels), neomycin, cholestyramine.

Herbs:
- Alfalfa, celery, eucalyptus, fenugreek, garlic, ginger.

PRESCRIPTION:
Yes.

PBS:
Yes (authority required).

PERMITTED IN SPORT:
Yes.

OVERDOSE:
May cause coma due to excessively low blood sugar levels. Give activated charcoal or induce vomiting if medication taken recently. Seek medical assistance.

OTHER INFORMATION:
Introduced in 1998 as an additional form of treatment for difficult to control maturity onset diabetes.
See also Glibenclamide, Gliclazide, Glimepride, Glipizide, INSULINS, Metformin, Repaglinide, Rosiglitazone, Tolbutamide.

ACE INHIBITORS
(Angiotensin Converting Enzyme Inhibitors)

TRADE and GENERIC NAMES:
Accupril, Asig (Quinapril).
Accuretic (Quinapril, hydrochlorothiazide).
Acenorm, Capoten, Captohexal, Captopril (numerous generic brands), **Enzace** (Captopril).
Alphapril, Amprace, Auspril, Enahexal, GenRx Enalapril, Renitec (Enalapril).
Coversyl (Perindopril).
Coversyl Plus (Perindopril, indapamide).
Gopten, Odrik (Trandolapril).
Monopril (Fosinopril).
Monoplus (Hydrochlorothiazide, fosinopril).
Fibsol, GenRx Lisinopril, Liprace, Lisodur, Prinivil, Zestril (Lisinopril).
Ramace, Tritace (Ramipril).
Renitec Plus (Enalapril, hydrochlorothiazide).

DRUG CLASS:
Antihypertensive.

USES:
High blood pressure, heart failure, improves survival after heart attack.

DOSAGE:
 Different forms are longer acting than others. Follow doctor's instructions.
Dosage varies from one capsule or tablet a day, to two capsules or tablets three times a day.
Do not vary dosage without medical advice.

FORMS:
Tablets, capsules. Capoten available as injection and mixture.

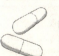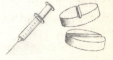

Medications

PRECAUTIONS:
Should not be used in pregnancy (D). Should be used only if specifically medically indicated and with caution in children and while breast feeding.

Do not take if:
suffering from severe kidney disease, reduced blood supply to brain or taking immunosuppressive drugs.

SIDE EFFECTS:
Common: Dry cough, swelling of ankles and other tissue, rash.
Unusual: Stomach upsets, abnormal taste.
Severe but rare (stop medication, consult doctor): Abnormal bleeding.

INTERACTIONS:
Other drugs:
- Interacts with diuretics, and some arthritis drugs, but often carefully used with these drugs.
- Reacts with lithium, potassium increasing drugs, tetracycline, vasodilators.

Herbs:
- Goldenseal, guarana, hawthorn, Korean ginseng, liquorice.

PRESCRIPTION:
Yes.

PBS:
Yes.

PERMITTED IN SPORT:
Yes.

OVERDOSE:
May cause low blood pressure. First aid involves giving activated charcoal or induction of vomiting and seeking medical attention.

OTHER INFORMATION:
A group of drugs that are rapidly becoming the first choice in the treatment of high blood pressure and heart failure. First released early 1980s, but many new forms came onto the market in the mid 1990s. Angiotensin is a hormone that naturally increases blood pressure. ACE Inhibitors reduce the amount of angiotensin produced in the body to reduce blood pressure by preventing the contraction of the tiny muscles that circle around small arteries.

See also Angiotensin II Receptor Antagonists.

Acetazolamide

TRADE NAME:
Diamox.

USES:
Glaucoma, retention of fluid, swelling, petit mal and some other forms of epilepsy.

DOSAGE:
 Complex. Depends on condition being treated, its severity and weight of patient. Must be individually determined for each patient by doctor.

FORMS:
Tablets (white) of 250mg, injection.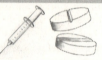

PRECAUTIONS:
Not to be used in pregnancy (B3). Use with caution in breast feeding and children.
Care must be used in long term use. Regular blood tests to check blood chemistry advisable.
Use with caution in emphysema.
Do not exceed recommended dose.

Do not take if:
 suffering from disorders of blood chemistry, liver disease, kidney disease, adrenal gland disease.

SIDE EFFECTS:
Common: Pins and needles, frequent passing of urine, loss of appetite.
Unusual: Biochemical imbalances in blood.

Home Guide to Medication

Medications

INTERACTIONS:
Other drugs:
- Aspirin, hypoglycaemics, anticoagulants, phenytoin, digoxin.

Herbs:
- Willow bark.

PRESCRIPTION:
Yes.

PBS:
Yes.

PERMITTED IN SPORT:
No.

OVERDOSE:
Significant abnormalities in blood chemistry may occur. Give activated charcoal or induce vomiting if medication taken recently. Seek medical assistance.

OTHER INFORMATION:
In glaucoma, usually taken in combination with eye drops.

See also Apraclonidine, Betaxolol, Bimatoprost, Brimonidine tartratel, Brinzolamide, Carbachol, Dipivefrine hydrochloride, Dorzolamide hydrochloride, Latanoprost, Levobunolol, Phenylephrine, Pilocarpine, Timolol, Travoprost.

Acetic acid

TRADE NAMES:
Aci-Jel (with ricinoleic acid, hydroxyquinolone).
Aquaear, Ear Clear for Swimmer's Ear (with isopropyl alcohol).

USES:
Ear drops – drying water in ears to prevent swimmer's ear.
Gel – restoring vaginal acidity.

DOSAGE:

Ear drops – four to six drops in each ear after swimming.
Gel – one applicator full of gel twice a day.

FORMS:
Ear drops, vaginal gel.

PRECAUTIONS:
Ear drops – safe in pregnancy.
Gel – not for use in pregnancy.
Do not use ear drops if:
 suffering from ear infection, ear discharge, blocked ear canals, perforated ear drum.
- grommets inserted.

SIDE EFFECTS:
Ear drops – ear canal irritation
Gel – minimal.

INTERACTIONS:
None.

PRESCRIPTION:
No.

PBS:
Ear drops: No.
Gel: Available to Veteran Affairs card holders.

PERMITTED IN SPORT:
Yes.

OVERDOSE:
Not likely to be harmful if swallowed.

Acetaminophen

See Paracetamol.

Acetylcholine chloride

TRADE NAME:
Miochol.

DRUG CLASS:
Miotic.

USES:
Rapid contraction of the pupil in the eye.

DOSAGE:
 As determined by doctor.

FORMS:
Eye drops.

PRECAUTIONS:
Use with caution in pregnancy (B2). Drops must be prepared immediately before use.

SIDE EFFECTS:
Reduced vision in dull light.

INTERACTIONS:
None significant.

PRESCRIPTION:
Yes.

PBS:
No.

PERMITTED IN SPORT:
Yes.

OVERDOSE:
Unlikely to have adverse effects if swallowed.

OTHER INFORMATION:
Introduced in 1999. Used only by ophthalmologists (eye doctors) in their rooms or hospital.
See also Carbachol.

Acetylcysteine

TRADE NAMES:
Mucomyst, Parvolex.

USES:
Inhaler: Breaks up mucus in lungs and airways in bronchiectasis and cystic fibrosis. Also used in general anaesthesia to clear mucus.
Injection: Paracetamol overdose.

DOSAGE:
 Inhaler: Directly sprayed into throat or inhaled with aid of nebuliser.
Injection: As determined by doctor.

FORMS:
Inhaler, injection.
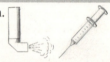

PRECAUTIONS:
Use with caution in pregnancy (B2), worsening asthma.
Do not take if:
 suffering from severe liver or kidney disease.

SIDE EFFECTS:
Inhaler: Mouth inflammation and ulcers, diarrhoea, fever, drowsiness, runny nose, asthma.
Injection: Asthma.

INTERACTIONS:
None significant.

PRESCRIPTION:
Yes.

PBS:
Mucomyst: Yes.
Parvolex: No.

PERMITTED IN SPORT:
Yes.

OTHER:
Should be used within 10 hours of paracetamol overdose. Minimal benefit after 15 hours.

Aciclovir

TRADE NAMES:
Acihexal, Acyclo-V, GenRx Aciclovir, Lovir, Zolaten, Zovirax, Zyclir.
Numerous other brands of locally produced aciclovir.

DRUG CLASS:
Antiviral.

USES:
Treatment of genital herpes, shingles, cold sores, chickenpox and herpes eye infections.

DOSAGE:

Tablets: 200mg to 800mg every four to eight hours.
Cream: Apply five times a day starting as soon as possible after onset of symptoms.
Eye ointment: Insert five times a day for 14 days.

FORMS:
Tablets of 200mg, 400mg and 800mg; eye ointment; skin cream; injection.

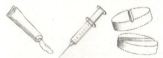

PRECAUTIONS:
Use in pregnancy (B3) and breast feeding only when medically essential. May be used in children.
Lower doses necessary in elderly.
Use tablets with caution in serious kidney disease, dehydration, brain disorders.

SIDE EFFECTS:
Common: Minimal.
Unusual: Tablets – Nausea, vomiting, headache.

INTERACTIONS:
Other drugs:
- Probenecid, diuretics (fluid tablets), interferon, methotrexate.

PRESCRIPTION:
Tablets, eye ointment: Yes.
Skin cream: No.

PBS:
Tablets, eye ointment: Yes (authority restricted to eye infections, shingles and genital herpes only).
Skin cream, injection: No.

PERMITTED IN SPORT:
Yes.

OVERDOSE:
Exacerbation of side effects likely.

OTHER INFORMATION:
Very safe and effective medication that has a very high success rate in treating Herpes infections. Chickenpox and shingles are caused by Herpes zoster, and cold sores and genital herpes by Herpes simplex. It is vital that any patient who suspects they have shingles must see their doctor immediately as Aciclovir only works if started within 72 hours of onset of rash. Chickenpox and cold sores are normally only treated under special circumstances as the medication is quite expensive. Eye infections with Herpes may cause blindness if not treated rapidly and effectively. Cream effective against cold sores only if started as soon as symptoms appear.

ACIDS

See **Eicosapentaenoic acid, Lactic acid, Salicylic acid.**

Acitretin

TRADE NAME:
Neotigason.

DRUG CLASS:
Keratolytic.

USES:
Severe psoriasis.

DOSAGE:
 Determined individually for each patient. 25 to 50mg a day.

FORMS:
Capsules of 10mg (brown/cream) and 25mg (brown/yellow).

PRECAUTIONS:
Absolutely forbidden in pregnancy (X) and breast feeding. Use with caution in children and adolescents. Use with great caution in liver and kidney disease.

SIDE EFFECTS:
Common: Dry skin, itchy skin, rashes, fragile skin.
Unusual: Kidney and liver abnormalities, eye irritation, increased blood fat and cholesterol levels, bone and brain growths.
Severe but rare (stop medication, consult doctor): Rare and serious complications.

INTERACTIONS:
Other drugs:
- Mini-contraceptive pill, tetracycline antibiotics, phenytoin.

Other substances:
- Vitamin A, alcohol.

PRESCRIPTION:
Yes. Additional state-based restrictions may limit its use to specialists only.

PBS:
Yes (authority required. Restricted to severe intractable psoriasis).

PERMITTED IN SPORT:
Yes.

OVERDOSE:
May cause headache, vomiting, flushing, mouth soreness and dryness, abdominal pain, flushing and incoordination. Seek medical assistance.

OTHER INFORMATION:
First introduced in 1997 to replace Etretinate. A very potent and potentially dangerous drug, but if used correctly can dramatically and often permanently cure severe chronic psoriasis. Use in pregnancy will always cause severe damage to foetus. Vitamin A derivative.

Acriflavine

TRADE NAME:
Acriflavine.

DRUG CLASS:
Antiseptic.

USES:
Minor skin abrasions.

DOSAGE:
 Apply once or twice.

FORMS:
Solution.

PRECAUTIONS:
Do not mix with detergents or other chemicals.
Safe in pregnancy.

SIDE EFFECTS:
Minor skin irritation.

INTERACTIONS:
None significant on the skin.

PRESCRIPTION:
No.

PBS:
No.

PERMITTED IN SPORT:
Yes.

OVERDOSE:
May cause vomiting and diarrhoea if swallowed.

OTHER INFORMATION:
Old-fashioned skin antiseptic.

Activated Charcoal
See Charcoal.

Adapalene

TRADE NAME:
Differin.

USES:
Severe acne.

DOSAGE:

Apply thinly once a day at bedtime to clean dry skin.

FORMS:
Gel, cream.

PRECAUTIONS:
Do not use if pregnant (D).
Use with caution in children and breast feeding.
Avoid eyes, lips, mouth, nostrils.
Do not apply to broken skin, moist skin, moist tissues, eczema, dermatitis.
Avoid sun exposure.

SIDE EFFECTS:
Common: Red skin, dry skin.
Unusual: Itch, burning, scaly skin.

INTERACTIONS:
Other drugs:
• Retinoids, astringents, drying agents.
Other substances:
• Abrasive cleansers.

PRESCRIPTION:
Yes.

PBS:
No. Expensive.

PERMITTED IN SPORT:
Yes.

OVERDOSE:
Wash affected area thoroughly.

Adenosine

TRADE NAMES:
Adenocor, Adenoscan

DRUG CLASS:
Antiarrhythmic.

USES:
Control of some types of irregular heartbeat starting in the upper chambers of the heart (the atria).
Dilates arteries of heart to allow adequate x-ray pictures to be taken.

DOSAGE:

Given rapidly by injection into a vein.

FORMS:
Injection.

PRECAUTIONS:
Use with caution in pregnancy (B2), children and breast feeding.
Must only be used if type of irregular heart rhythm has been definitely established.

SIDE EFFECTS:

Common: Flushed face, headache.
Unusual: Shortness of breath, pressure in chest, light headedness, nausea, very slow heart rate.

INTERACTIONS:

Other drugs:
- Carbamazepine, xanthines, dipyridamole.

PRESCRIPTION:

Yes. Used in hospital only.

PBS:

No.

PERMITTED IN SPORT:

Yes.

OVERDOSE:

Serious. Always given under close medical supervision

Adrenaline

TRADE NAMES:

Adrenaline, Epipen.
Citanest Dental (with prilocaine).
Lignospan, Xylocaine (with lignocaine)
Marcain (with bupivacaine).
Rectinol (with benzocaine and zinc oxide).
Scandonest (with mepivacaine).

DRUG CLASS:

Vasoconstrictor, Mydriatic.

USES:

Constriction of blood vessels to prolong effect of medication (eg. local anaesthetics).
Control of very severe allergy reactions and asthma.
Dilates the size of the pupil in eye surgery and examination.
Treatment of certain type of glaucoma (chronic simple glaucoma).
Emergency treatment of some forms of heart disease.

DOSAGE:

 Rectinol: Anal ointment or suppository used once or twice a day.
Eye drops: One drop in affected eye once or twice a day.
Injection: Self inject for severe allergic reaction.

FORMS:

Injection, injection pen, eye drops. In combination with other ingredients as anal ointment and suppository.

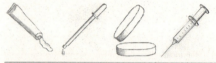

PRECAUTIONS:

May be used in pregnancy, breast feeding and children.
Very safe to use as anal suppository or cream.
Eye drops should not be used for prolonged periods.
Injections only used by doctors in emergency situations. Never inject into ear, fingers, toes or penis. Never inject into artery or vein.
Use with caution if suffering from overactive thyroid gland, heart disease, high blood pressure, psychiatric conditions or diabetes.

SIDE EFFECTS:

Common: Eye drops – Eye pain, headache, brow ache, red eye.
Ointment and suppository – No problems.
Injection – Rapid heart rate, reduced circulation at site of injection, difficulty in breathing, dizziness, weakness, tremor, headache, irritability, anxiety, fear.

INTERACTIONS:

Other drugs:
- Injection may interact with tricyclic antidepressants, thyroxine and some antihistamines.

Other substances:
- Do not use alcohol or caffeine, or undertake vigorous exercise.

PRESCRIPTION:
Rectinol: No.
Other forms: Yes.

PBS:
Eye drops and injections: Yes.
Other forms: No.

PERMITTED IN SPORT:
Eye drops, ointment, suppository: Yes.
Injection: No.

OVERDOSE:
Ointment and suppository: No problems.
Eye drops: Flush eye with water.
Injection: Very serious. May result in stroke, heart attack and death. Extremely urgent medical attention required to administer counter acting drugs.

OTHER INFORMATION:
Widely used to prolong effect of local anaesthetics and reduce bleeding at operation site. Effective in extreme cases of severe allergy to reduce effects of swelling.
See also Isoprenaline.

AIDS (HIV) TREATMENTS

See Abacavir, Delavirdine, Didanosine, Efavirenz, Indinavir, Lamivudine, Nelfinavir, Nevirapine, Ritonavir, Saquinavir, Stavudine, Tenofovir, Zalcitabine, Zidovudine.

Albendazole

TRADE NAMES:
Eskazole, Zentel.

DRUG CLASS:
Anthelmintics.

USES:
Treatment of hydatid worms and cysts.

DOSAGE:

As determined by doctor for each patient.

FORMS:
Tablets of 200mg (chewable, white) and 400mg (chewable, pale orange).

PRECAUTIONS:
Must not be used in pregnancy (D) or within one month of conception. Use with caution under six years of age and while breast feeding.
Ensure adequate contraception in all women.
Use with caution in liver disease.
Close monitoring by a doctor and regular blood tests essential while taking medication.

SIDE EFFECTS:
Common: Liver abnormalities, white blood cell abnormalities, nausea, diarrhoea, dizziness.
Unusual: Temporary hair loss.

INTERACTIONS:
Other drugs:
• Cimetidine, praziquantel, dexamethasone.

PRESCRIPTION:
Yes.

PBS:
Yes (authority required).

PERMITTED IN SPORT:
Yes.

OVERDOSE:
Serious. Seek urgent medical attention. Induce vomiting.

OTHER INFORMATION:
Rarely used in Australia as hydatid disease usually occurs in Africa and Asia.

Alclometasone

TRADE NAMES:
Logoderm.

DRUG CLASS:
Corticosteroid.

USES:
Eczema, dermatitis.

DOSAGE:
 Apply thinly two or three times a day.

FORMS:
Cream, ointment.

PRECAUTIONS:
Should be used with caution in pregnancy and breast feeding. Safe for use in children.
Avoid eyes.
Use for shortest period of time possible.
Do not use if:
 suffering from any form of skin infection, skin ulcers, acne or cracked lips.

SIDE EFFECTS:
Minimal.

INTERACTIONS:
None significant.

PRESCRIPTION:
Yes.

PBS:
No.

PERMITTED IN SPORT:
Yes.

OTHER INFORMATION:
Removed from market 2002.

ALCOHOLS

See Ethanol, Isopropyl alcohol.

Aldioxa

TRADE NAME:
Zeasorb (with chloroxylenol).

USES:
Intertrigo, excessive sweating, prevention of athlete's foot (tinea pedis).

DOSAGE:
 Smooth powder over dry skin.

FORMS:
Powder (keep dry).

PRECAUTIONS:
Do not apply to broken skin.
Avoid eyes.

SIDE EFFECTS:
Minimal.

INTERACTIONS:
Nil.

PRESCRIPTION:
No.

PBS:
No.

PERMITTED IN SPORT:
Yes.

Medications

Alendronate

TRADE NAME:
Fosamax.

USES:
Osteoporosis, Paget's disease.

DOSAGE:
Up to 10mg a day – Complex. Take one tablet a day 30 minutes before eating or drinking after waking in morning. Remain erect until after eating. 70mg tablets – Take one tablet a week 30 minutes before first food or drink of day with full glass of water, Do not lie down for 30 minutes and until after first food.

FORMS:
Tablet 5mg, 10mg and 70mg (white).

PRECAUTIONS:
Use with great caution in pregnancy (B3), breast feeding and children.
Use with caution with recent peptic ulcer and kidney damage.
Calcium and vitamin D levels must be monitored.
Do not take any other medications within two hours.

Do not take if:
 suffering from peptic ulcer.

- under other circumstances.

SIDE EFFECTS:
Common: Nausea, vomiting, indigestion.
Unusual: Ulceration of oesophagus and stomach, mouth ulcers, peptic ulcers, muscle pain, headaches.
Severe but rare (stop medication, consult doctor): Vomiting blood, black motions.

INTERACTIONS:
Other drugs:
- Calcium supplements, antacids, biphosphonates, aspirin.
- May affect almost any medication taken by mouth.

PRESCRIPTION:
Yes.

PBS:
Yes (authority required).

PERMITTED IN SPORT:
Yes.

OVERDOSE:
Very low blood levels of calcium may occur. This may interfere with the function of nerves and other tissues. Other symptoms may include indigestion and vomiting. Induce vomiting if medication taken recently, or drink large amounts of milk.

OTHER INFORMATION:
Potent and effective medication for osteoporosis introduced in 1996. Once a week dose (70mg) introduced in 2001 has dramatically increased ease of use.
See also Resedronate.

Alfentanil

TRADE NAME:
Rapifen.

DRUG CLASS:
Narcotic.

USES:
Pain relief while under anaesthesia.

DOSAGE:
 Calculated by anaesthetist for each individual patient.

FORMS:
Injection.

PRECAUTIONS:
Must not be used in pregnancy (C) or children under 12 years.
Use with caution in head injuries, obesity and elderly.

Medications

Do not take if:
 suffering from liver failure, underactive thyroid gland.

SIDE EFFECTS:
Unusual: Reduced ability to breathe, muscle rigidity, slow heart rate, low blood pressure, throat spasm.

INTERACTIONS:
Other drugs:
- Some anaesthetics, erythromycin, cimetidine, MAOI, medications that depress brain function.

PRESCRIPTION:
Yes (restricted).

PBS:
No.

PERMITTED IN SPORT:
No.

See also Buprenorphine, Codeine Phosphate, Dextromoramide, Dextropropoxyphene, Fentanyl, Heroin, Hydromorphone, Methadone, Morphine, Oxycodone, Pentazocine, Pethidine.

Alginic acid
See ANTACIDS.

ALKYLATERS
See CANCER-TREATING DRUGS.

Allantoin

TRADE NAMES:
Available in Australia only in combination with other medications.
Alphosyl (with tar).
Blistex Lip Ointment and **Balm** (with camphor and other ingredients).
Chemists' Own Soothing Lotion (with titanium dioxide, zinc oxide, calamine, camphor and other ingredients).
Curacel Acne and Pimple Gel (with sulfur).
ER Cream, Macro Natural Vitamin E Cream, SoloSite, VR Gel (with multiple ingredients).
Hemocane (with lignocaine and zinc oxide).
Medi Creme (with chlorhexidine, cetrimide, lignocaine, hexamidine isethionate).
Medi Pulv (with hexamidine isethionate and chlorhexidine).
Paxyl (with lignocaine and benzalkonium).
Solyptol Cream (with benzalkonium).

USES:
Repairs damaged skin, minor burns, grazes, acne, psoriasis.

DOSAGE:
 Apply several times a day.

FORMS:
Powder, cream, ointment, lotion.

PRECAUTIONS:
Safe to use in pregnancy, breast feeding and children.
Avoid eye contact.

SIDE EFFECTS:
Minimal.

INTERACTIONS:
None significant.

PRESCRIPTION:
No.

PBS:
No. Some forms available to Veterans Affairs pensioners.

PERMITTED IN SPORT:
Yes.

ALLERGEN EXTRACTS

TRADE NAMES:

Albay, Allypral and other brands. Allergens against a wide range of plants, foods, animals, moulds, insects etc. available.

DRUG CLASS:

Antiallergen.

USES:

Reduction of allergy reaction to specific substances.

DOSAGE:

 Complex. Series of injections over many months in very slowly increasing concentrations and doses as determined by doctor.

FORMS:

Injection.

PRECAUTIONS:

Patient must wait in surgery for 30 minutes after injection given in case of serious allergy reaction.
Injection must be given subcutaneously (just under the skin) and not into muscle or a vein.
Should not be used in pregnancy, but unlikely to be serious consequences if administered inadvertently.

Do not take if:

 allergy reaction at time of planned injection.

SIDE EFFECTS:

Common: Local redness of skin at site of injection.
Unusual: Widespread redness and itching of skin around site of injection.
Severe but rare: Generalised severe anaphylactic (allergy) reaction that may be life threatening unless treated promptly.

INTERACTIONS:

None.

PRESCRIPTION:

Yes.

PBS:

No.

PERMITTED IN SPORT:

Yes.

OVERDOSE:

Very severe, life threatening anaphylactic (allergy) reaction may occur. Adrenaline should be injected subcutaneously every few minutes to counteract anaphylaxis. Doctor may need to give oxygen and cardiopulmonary resuscitation.

Allopurinol

TRADE NAMES:

Allohexal, Allorin, Capurate, Progout, Zyloprim.

DRUG CLASS:

Uricosuric.

USES:

Prevention of gout and its complications.

DOSAGE:

 One or two tablets once a day.

FORMS:

Tablets of 100mg and 300mg

PRECAUTIONS:

Use with caution in pregnancy (B2) and breast feeding. Not for use in children. Use with caution in kidney and liver disease, and haemochromatosis.

Do not take if:

 suffering from acute gout

SIDE EFFECTS:
Common: Minimal.
Unusual: Fever, arthritis, nausea, drowsiness.
Severe but rare (stop medication, consult doctor): Rash.

INTERACTIONS:
Other drugs:
- Azathioprine, mercaptopurine, sulfinpyrazone, probenecid, aspirin.

Other substances:
- Alcohol may aggravate gout.

PRESCRIPTION:
Yes.

PBS:
Yes.

PERMITTED IN SPORT:
Yes.

OVERDOSE:
May cause vomiting, diarrhoea and dizziness.

OTHER INFORMATION:
Widely used, very safe and effective medication for the prevention of gout. Not to be used for treatment of acute gout. Does not cause dependence or addiction.
See also Probenecid.

ALPHA BLOCKERS

DISCUSSION:
Alpha receptor blockers are drugs that block the reception of certain nerve signals to the arteries, and if these signals are not received, the artery relaxes, allowing more blood to flow through at a lower pressure, thus easing high blood pressure. These drugs have undergone considerable refinement over the years, and most of the earlier ones that had significant side effects are no longer used.
See Labetalol, Prazosin, Tamsulosin.

Alpha tocopherols
See Tocopherols

Alprazolam

TRADE NAMES:
Alprax, Kalma, Xanax.

DRUG CLASS:
Benzodiazepine (Anxiolytic).

USES:
Relief of anxiety and panic attacks.

DOSAGE:
 Usually 0.5 to 4mg a day. Maximum 10mg a day. Do not exceed dose directed by doctor.

FORMS:
Tablets of 0.25mg (white), 0.5mg (pink), 1mg (lilac) and 2mg (white).

PRECAUTIONS:
Should be used with caution in pregnancy (C), but not at all if delivery of infant imminent as it may decrease desire to breathe in newborn infant. Should be used with caution in breast feeding. Not for use in children.
Lower dose required in elderly.
Dependency may develop.
Use with caution in glaucoma, myasthenia gravis, heart disease, kidney or liver disease, psychiatric conditions, schizophrenia, depression and epilepsy.
Do not take if:
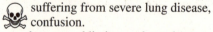 suffering from severe lung disease, confusion.
- tendency to addiction or dependence.
- operating machinery, driving a vehicle or undertaking tasks that require concentration and alertness.

SIDE EFFECTS:
Common: Reduced alertness, dependence.
Unusual: Incoordination, tremor,

confusion, increased risk of falls in elderly, rash, low blood pressure, nausea, muscle weakness,
Severe but rare (stop medication, consult doctor): Jaundice (yellow skin).

INTERACTIONS:
Other drugs:
- Sedatives, other anxiolytics, disulfiram, cimetidine, anticonvulsants, anticholinergics.

Herbs:
- Guarana, kava kava, passionflower, St John's wort, valerian.

Other substances:
- Reacts with alcohol to cause sedation and confusion.

PRESCRIPTION:
Yes.

PBS:
Yes (authority required).

PERMITTED IN SPORT:
Most sports: Yes.
Some sports: No.
Check with organising committee of sport involved.

OVERDOSE:
Seldom life threatening. May cause drowsiness, confusion and coma. Induce vomiting if tablets taken recently. Seek medical assistance.

OTHER INFORMATION:
Very useful drug for the control of severe anxiety and panic attacks, but dependency a problem.
See also Bromazepam, Buspirone, Clobazam, Diazepam, Lorazepam, Oxazepam.

Alprostadil
(Prostaglandin E1)

TRADE NAMES:
Caverject, Muse, Prostin VR.

USES:
Caverject, Muse: inability to obtain an erection in the male penis.
Prostin VR: to keep arteries open in newborn babies with heart defects.

DOSAGE:
Caverject: inject into shaft of penis as directed by doctor.
Muse: insert pellet with applicator into urethral opening at end of penis.
Prostin: as determined by doctor.

FORMS:
Injection, pellet.

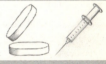

PRECAUTIONS:
Do not use for erection if:
- suffering from blood borne diseases.
- partner pregnant
- suffering from curvature or deformity of penis
- penile implant inserted

SIDE EFFECTS:
Common: Pain during injection and erection, bruising.
Unusual: Prolonged erection, scarring and curvature of penis.

INTERACTIONS:
Other drugs:
- Warfarin, heparin.

Other substances:
- Reactions with substances such as alcohol, caffeine, foods, exercise etc.

PRESCRIPTION:
Yes.

PBS:
No.

PERMITTED IN SPORT:
Yes.

OVERDOSE:
Prolonged painful erection, diarrhoea, depression, rapid breathing. Medical attention essential for any penile erection lasting longer than four hours.

OTHER INFORMATION:
Caverject introduced in 1996 as a safe and effective form of treatment for impotence. Muse introduced in 1998 as an alternative to injected form.
See also Sildenafil, Tadalafil

Alteplase
See FIBRINOLYTICS.

Altretamine
(Hexamethylmelamine)

TRADE NAME:
Hexalen.

DRUG CLASS:
Antineoplastic.

USES:
Advanced cancer of the ovary.

DOSAGE:
 As determined by doctor.

FORMS:
Capsule of 50mg (clear).

PRECAUTIONS:
Not to be used in pregnancy (D) or breast feeding.
Regular blood tests essential. Regular checks on nerve function required.
Do not take if:
 suffering from bone marrow or nerve disease.

SIDE EFFECTS:
Common: Abnormal stimulation or loss of function of nerves, nausea, vomiting.
Unusual: Bone marrow damage, kidney damage.

INTERACTIONS:
Other drugs: Monoamine oxidase inhibitors (used for severe depression), cimetidine, pyridoxine.

PRESCRIPTION:
Yes.

PBS:
Yes.

PERMITTED IN SPORT:
Yes.

OVERDOSE:
Serious damage to bone marrow, nerves and kidneys possible.

OTHER INFORMATION:
Introduced in 1998, usually for use when other treatments have failed.

Aluminium chloride

TRADE NAME:
Driclor.

USES:
Excessive sweating from arm pits, hands and feet.

DOSAGE:

Apply nightly initially, reducing to once or twice a week depending on response.

FORMS:
Solution.

PRECAUTIONS:
Safe to use in pregnancy, breast feeding and children over six years.
Avoid contact with eyes.
Do not use on broken or damaged skin.
Do not shave arm pit within 24 hours of use.
Do not bathe immediately before use.

SIDE EFFECTS:
None significant.

INTERACTIONS:
None.

PRESCRIPTION:
No.

PBS:
No.

PERMITTED IN SPORT:
Yes.

OVERDOSE:
Seek medical attention if swallowed.

OTHER INFORMATION:
One of the more useful treatments for the distressing condition of hyperhidrosis (excess sweating).

Aluminium hydroxide

See ANTACIDS.

Aluminium oxide

TRADE NAME:
Brasivol

DRUG CLASS:
Keratolytic.

USES:
Acne.

DOSAGE:

Apply once a day to dry skin. Rub into affected area then rinse skin. Start with strength 1, progress to strength 2 after several weeks if necessary.

FORMS:
Suspension in two strengths.

PRECAUTIONS:
Safe in pregnancy. Not for use in children.
Avoid eye contact.
Do not use for rosacea and superficial veins.

SIDE EFFECTS:
Common: Skin irritation.

INTERACTIONS:
None significant.

PRESCRIPTION:
No.

PBS:
No.

PERMITTED IN SPORT:
Yes.

See also KERATOLYTICS.

Aluminium sulfate

TRADE NAME:
Stingose.
Widely used in other skin preparations and cosmetics at far lower concentrations.

USES:
Relief of stings caused by marine stingers, insects and plants.

DOSAGE:
 Apply promptly and liberally to affected area. Remove any jellyfish tentacles with gloves or forceps before use.

FORMS:
Solution, gel.

PRECAUTIONS:
Safe to use in pregnancy, breast feeding and children.
Avoid eye contact.
Do not apply alcohol to sting site.

SIDE EFFECTS:
Minimal.

INTERACTIONS:
Other drugs:
- Alcohol on skin.

PRESCRIPTION:
No.

PBS:
No.

PERMITTED IN SPORT:
Yes.

OVERDOSE:
No serious effects expected.

OTHER INFORMATION:
Widely and effectively used, particularly on beaches by Surf Lifesaving clubs.

Alverine Citrate

TRADE NAME:
Alvercol (with sterculia).

DRUG CLASS:
Antispasmodic.

USES:
Irritable bowel syndrome, bowel spasms.

DOSAGE:
 One or two heaped teaspoons once or twice a day.

FORMS:
Granules.

PRECAUTIONS:
Ensure adequate fluid intake. Use with caution in pregnancy. Safe in breast feeding.
Do not take if:
 obstructed bowel, bowel cancer

SIDE EFFECTS:
Common: Mild feeling of belly distension.

INTERACTIONS:
Other drugs:
- May interfere with the absorption of many medications.

PRESCRIPTION:
No.

PBS:
No.

PERMITTED IN SPORT:
Yes.

OVERDOSE:
Take additional water. Belly discomfort and passing excess wind only effects.
See also Dicyclomine, Mebeverine.

Amantadine

TRADE NAME:
Symmetrel.

DRUG CLASS:
Antiparkinsonian.

USES:
Parkinson's disease, prevention of influenza type A.

DOSAGE:

Parkinson's disease: Increase slowly over several weeks under doctor's instructions.
Influenza A prevention: One capsule twice a day.

FORMS:
Capsule of 100mg (brown).

PRECAUTIONS:
Use in pregnancy (B3) only if medically essential. Use in breast feeding with considerable caution. Not for use in children under 9 years.
Use with caution in glaucoma, enlarged prostate gland, confused or psychiatrically disturbed patients, heart failure, low blood pressure, liver and kidney disease.

 Do not stop suddenly, but reduce dose slowly.

Lower dose required in elderly.

SIDE EFFECTS:
Common: Indigestion, excitement, dizziness, poor concentration, dry mouth, blurred vision, constipation, anxiety, confusion, swelling of ankles and feet.
Unusual: Tremor, headache, slurred speech, incoordination, sleeplessness, palpitations, difficulty in passing urine.
Severe but rare (stop medication, consult doctor): Unable to pass urine, convulsions, irrational behaviour.

INTERACTIONS:
Other drugs:
- Other antiparkinsonians, L-Dopa.

Other substances:
- Reacts adversely with alcohol and caffeine.

PRESCRIPTION:
Yes.

PBS:
Yes (Parkinson's disease only).

PERMITTED IN SPORT:
Yes.

OVERDOSE:
May cause confusion, hallucinations, delirium, rapid heart rate, rapid breathing, vomiting, dry mouth and retention of urine. Deaths have not been reported. Induce vomiting if medication taken recently. Seek medical attention.

OTHER INFORMATION:
Widely used for decades to help Parkinsonism, but has the additional benefit of protecting against one form (the less common form) of influenza, which may be useful during an epidemic.

Amethocaine

See ANAESTHETICS, LOCAL.

Amfebutamone

See Bupropion.

Amifostine

TRADE NAME:
Ethyol.

USES:
Decreases damage to white blood cells and kidneys in patients having chemotherapy for cancer.

DOSAGE:

Complex. As determined for each patient by doctor.

FORMS:
Injection.

PRECAUTIONS:
Use with caution in pregnancy (B3), elderly and children.
Blood pressure and blood calcium levels must be checked regularly.
Use with caution in kidney, liver, heart and brain disease.

SIDE EFFECTS:
Common: Low blood pressure, nausea, vomiting, flushing, chills, dizziness, tiredness.
Unusual: Hiccups, sneezing.

INTERACTIONS:
Other drugs: Drugs that lower blood pressure and blood calcium levels.

PRESCRIPTION:
Yes.

PBS:
No.

PERMITTED IN SPORT:
Yes.

Amikacin

TRADE NAMES:
Amikin.

DRUG CLASS:
Aminoglycoside antibiotic.

USES:
Short term treatment of serious infections.

DOSAGE:

As determined by doctor.

FORMS:
Injection.

PRECAUTIONS:
Must not be used in pregnancy (D). Use with caution in elderly, children and during breast feeding.
Not designed for long term use as it may accumulate in body.
Adequate fluid intake essential.

Do not take if:

suffering from severe kidney disease.

SIDE EFFECTS:
Unusual: Adverse effects on ears, kidneys and brain.

INTERACTIONS:
Other drugs: Other antibiotics, fluid removing medications (diuretics), anaesthetics and muscle relaxants.

PRESCRIPTION:
Yes.

PBS:
No (expensive).

PERMITTED IN SPORT:
Yes.

OVERDOSE:

Causes ringing in ears, dizziness, deafness which may be permanent, rash, fever, headache, pins and needles sensation and kidney failure. Seek urgent medical attention so that blood dialysis can be performed.

See Gatifloxacin, Gentamicin, Neomycin, Tobramycin.

Amiloride

TRADE NAMES:

Kaluril, Midamor.
Amizide, Moduretic (with hydrochlorothiazide).

DRUG CLASS:

Potassium sparing diuretic (removes fluid from body through kidneys without excess loss of potassium).

USES:

High blood pressure, conserving potassium within body, excess fluid in body.

DOSAGE:

 One to four tablets in morning

FORMS:

Tablets.

PRECAUTIONS:

Should only be used in pregnancy (C) and breast feeding if medically essential.
Should not be used in children.
Should be used with caution in diabetes or liver disease.

Do not take if:

 suffering from kidney disease.

SIDE EFFECTS:

Common: Minimal.
Unusual: Nausea, loss of appetite, belly discomfort, rash, excess wind.

INTERACTIONS:

Other drugs:
- Lithium.
- Do not use with potassium supplements or triamterene.

Herbs:
- Celery, dandelion, uva ursi.

PRESCRIPTION:

Yes.

PBS:

Yes.

PERMITTED IN SPORT:

No (acts as a masking agent for other illegal drugs).

OVERDOSE:

Dehydration may occur. Induce vomiting if tablets taken recently. Give extra fluids.

See also Bumetanide, Ethacrynic Acid, Frusemide, Indapamide, Spironolactone, THIAZIDE DIURETICS.

Aminacrine hydrochloride

TRADE NAME:

Medijel (with lignocaine).

DRUG CLASS:

Antiseptic.

USES:

Minor eye infections, minor burns, mouth ulcers, sore gums.

DOSAGE:

 Apply as needed every 20 minutes.

FORMS:

Gel.

PRECAUTIONS:

Safe to use in pregnancy, breast feeding and children.

Seek medical advice if failure to heal. Not designed for prolonged use.

SIDE EFFECTS:
Minimal.

INTERACTIONS:
None significant.

PRESCRIPTION:
No.

PBS:
No.

PERMITTED IN SPORT:
Yes.

Aminocaproic Acid

TRADE NAME:
Amicar.

DRUG CLASS:
Haemostatic.

USES:
To stop excessive bleeding caused by loss of fibrin in blood.

DOSAGE:

As determined by doctor.

FORMS:
Injection.

PRECAUTIONS:
Use with caution in pregnancy (B3) and children.
Must only be used to treat exact form of excessive bleeding for which they are designed.
Use with caution in heart disease.
Patients must be carefully monitored by doctor.

SIDE EFFECTS:
Unusual: Muscle damage.

PRESCRIPTION:
Yes.

PBS:
No.

PERMITTED IN SPORT:
Yes.

OVERDOSE:
Serious. Seek urgent medical attention.
See also HAEMOSTATIC AGENTS.

Aminoglutethamide

TRADE NAME:
Cytadren.

USES:
Breast cancer, Cushing syndrome.

DOSAGE:

Must be individualised for each patient by doctor depending on disease.

FORMS:
Tablets (white) of 250mg

PRECAUTIONS:
Must not be used in pregnancy (D) unless the mother's life is at risk. Breast feeding must be ceased before use. May be used with caution in children.
Regular checking of blood pressure essential.
Regular blood tests to check thyroid gland and blood chemistry essential.
Do not take if:
 suffering from porphyria.

SIDE EFFECTS:
Common: Tiredness, incoordination, dizziness, rash, nausea.
Unusual: Confusion, vomiting, fever.

INTERACTIONS:
Other drugs: Dexamethasone, anticoagulants, hypoglycaemics (used for diabetes).

PRESCRIPTION:
Yes.

PBS:
Yes.

OVERDOSE:
May cause incoordination, sedation, difficulty in breathing and coma. Death unlikely. Induce vomiting if medication taken recently. Seek urgent medical assistance.

AMINOGLYCOSIDES

DISCUSSION:
Aminoglycosides are a group of less commonly used antibiotics that can destroy certain types of bacteria causing infections in the urinary tract, skin and bloodstream.

See Amikacin, Gatifloxacin, Gentamicin, Neomycin, Tobramycin.

Aminophylline
See THEOPHYLLINES.

Amiodarone

TRADE NAMES:
Aratac, Cardinorm, Cordarone X.

DRUG CLASS:
Antiarrhythmic.

USES:
Severe rapid irregular heartbeat.

DOSAGE:

One tablet, one to three times a day. Should be started in hospital.

FORMS:
Tablet of 100mg and 200mg (white), injection.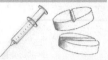

PRECAUTIONS:
Should not be used in pregnancy (C) unless medically essential. Not to be used in breast feeding or children.
Regular cardiograph (ECG) and blood test monitoring may be required.
Should be used with caution in heart failure and liver disease.

Do not take if:
 suffering from slow heart rate, thyroid disease or iodine sensitivity.

SIDE EFFECTS:
Common: Serious heart irregularities, slow heart rate, sensitivity to sunburn increased, nausea.
Unusual: Grey skin pigmentation, rashes, vomiting, loss of appetite, metallic taste, constipation, tremor, sleeplessness, headache, dizziness, anxiety, shortness of breath.
Severe but rare (stop medication, consult doctor): Angina, weight loss, restlessness.

INTERACTIONS:
Other drugs:
- Beta blockers, calcium channel blockers, digoxin, anticoagulants (eg. warfarin).
- Other drugs for treatment of irregular heartbeat.

Herbs:
- Echinacea.

Other substances:
- Alcohol use should be restricted.
- Smoking should be ceased.
- Caffeine intake should be restricted.

PRESCRIPTION:
Yes.

PBS:
Yes.

PERMITTED IN SPORT:
Yes.

OVERDOSE:
Exaggerated side effects only response. If tablets taken recently, give activated charcoal or induce vomiting.
Seek medical advice.

OTHER INFORMATION:
Medication reserved for the most serious forms of heart arrhythmia.
See also Disopyramide, Flecainide, Mexiletine, Procainamide, Quinidine, Sotalol, Verapamil.

Amisulpride

TRADE NAME:
Solian.

DRUG CLASS:
Antipsychotic.

USES:
Schizophrenia and similar psychoses.

DOSAGE:

Acute episodes: 400 to 800 mg a day.
Maintenance: 50 to 300mg a day.

FORMS:
Tablets of 100mg, 200mg and 400mg (white).

PRECAUTIONS:
Use in pregnancy (B3) and breast feeding only if essential. Not for use in children.
Use with caution in kidney disease, epilepsy, Parkinson's disease, slow heart rate, low potassium levels in blood, abnormal heart rhythm.
Do not take if:
 suffering from prolactin dependent tumours, phaeochromocytoma.

SIDE EFFECTS:
Common: Inability to sleep, cessation of menstrual periods.
Unusual: Abnormal heart rhythm, incoordination, production of breast milk.
Severe but rare (stop medication, consult doctor): High fever (neuroleptic malignant syndrome).

INTERACTIONS:
Other drugs:
- Quinidine, disopyramide, amiodarone, sotalol, cisapride, erythromycin, pentamidine, levodopa, lithium, calcium channel blockers, beta blockers, clonidine, digoxin, diuretics, amphotericin, steroids and some antidepressants and blood pressure medications.

Herbs:
- Evening primrose (linoleic acid).

Other substances:
- Alcohol.

PRESCRIPTION:
Yes.

PBS:
Yes (authority required).

PERMITTED IN SPORT:
Yes.

OVERDOSE:
Very serious. Seek urgent medical attention.

OTHER INFORMATION:
Introduced in 2002 to treat more difficult cases of schizophrenia.
See also Droperidol, Flupenthixol, Haloperidol, Lithium Carbonate, Olanzapine, PHENOTHIAZINES, Pimozide, Quetiapine, Risperidone, Thiothixene, Zuclopenthixol.

Amitriptyline

See TRICYCLICS.

Amlodipine

TRADE NAME:
Norvasc.

DRUG CLASS:
Calcium channel blocker (calcium antagonist).

USES:
High blood pressure, angina.

DOSAGE:

2.5 to 10mg a day.

FORMS:
Tablets (white) of 5mg.

PRECAUTIONS:
Should only be used in pregnancy (C) and breast feeding if medically essential. Not designed for use in children.
Do not take if:
 suffering from severe heart failure, low blood pressure, atrial flutter or fibrillation.

SIDE EFFECTS:
Common: Constipation, tiredness, headache, dizziness, indigestion, swelling of feet and ankles.
Unusual: Flushing, palpitations, slow heart rate, scalp irritation, depression, flushes, nightmares, excess wind.
Severe but rare (stop medication, consult doctor): Fainting.

INTERACTIONS:
Other drugs:
- Beta blockers (eg. propranolol), cyclosporin, digoxin, cimetidine, diazepam, amiodarone, quinidine, rifampicin, phenytoin, cisapride, theophylline, terbutaline, salbutamol, diltiazem.
- Additive effect with other medications for high blood pressure.

Herbs:
- Goldenseal, guarana, hawthorn, Korean ginseng, liquorice.

Other substances:
- Smoking may aggravate conditions that these medications are treating.
- Grapefruit juice.

PRESCRIPTION:
Yes.

PBS:
Yes.

PERMITTED IN SPORT:
Yes.

OVERDOSE:
May continue to be absorbed for up to 48 hours after overdose. Administer activated charcoal or induce vomiting. Purging should be encouraged to eliminate drug from gut. Overdose may cause low blood pressure, irregular heart rhythm, difficulty in breathing, heart attack and death. Obtain urgent medical attention.

OTHER INFORMATION:
Commonly used as a first line medication in high blood pressure and to prevent angina.
See also Diltiazem, Felodipine, Nifedipine, Nimodipine, Verapamil.

Ammonium bicarbonate

TRADE NAME:
Senegar (with senega).

DRUG CLASS:
Expectorant.

USES:
Cough.

OTHER INFORMATION:
See entry for senega for further information.

Ammonium chloride

TRADE NAMES:
Ammonium Chloride.
Avil Decongestant (with pheniramine and menthol).
Benadryl Original (with diphenhydramine and other ingredients).

DRUG CLASS:
Urinary acidifier, cough suppressant.

USES:
Maintains acid urine, increases urine production, eases coughs.

DOSAGE:

One to four tablets a day.
Take mixture every four hours.

FORMS:
Tablets (white) of 500mg, mixtures.

PRECAUTIONS:
Safe for use in pregnancy (A), breast feeding and children.
Blood tests to check level of potassium recommended if used long term.
Do not take if:
 suffering from kidney or liver disease.

SIDE EFFECTS:
Common: Nausea.
Unusual: Vomiting, belly pains, low blood potassium.

INTERACTIONS:
None significant.

PRESCRIPTION:
No.

PBS:
Tablets: Yes.
Mixtures: No.

PERMITTED IN SPORT:
Yes.

OVERDOSE:
Exacerbation of side effects likely.
See also Codeine Phosphate, Dextromethorphan, Dihydrocodeine, EXPECTORANTS, Pentoxyverine citrate, Pholcodine.

Amorolfine

TRADE NAME:
Loceryl.

DRUG CLASS:
Antifungal.

USES:
Fungal infections of the nails.

DOSAGE:

Apply paint to affected nails once or twice a week for three to six months.

FORMS:
Nail lacquer.

PRECAUTIONS:
Should not be used in pregnancy (B3).
Use with caution in children.
Do not apply to skin.

SIDE EFFECTS:
Common: Temporary burning sensation, itching.
Unusual: Redness, nail discolouration, scaling of nail.

INTERACTIONS:
Nil.

PRESCRIPTION:
Yes.

PBS:
No (expensive).

PERMITTED IN SPORT:
Yes.

OVERDOSE:
Serious effects if swallowed. Seek urgent medical attention.

OTHER INFORMATION:
Introduced in 1996 as a very effective way of treating severe fungal infections of nails that caused disfigurement.

Amoxycillin

TRADE NAMES:
Alphamox, Amohexal, Amoxil, Amoxil Duo, Ampexin, Bgramin, Cilamox, Fisamox, Maxamox, Moxacin.
Augmentin, Augmentin Duo, Ausclav, Ausclav Duo, Clamoxyl, Clamoxyl Duo, Clavulin, Clavulin Duo
(with clavulanic acid).
Klacid HP7, Losec HP7, Pylorid KA
(with omeprazole and clarithromycin).
Numerous other locally produced and labelled brands.

DRUG CLASS:
Penicillin antibiotic.

USES:
Treatment of infections caused by susceptible bacteria.
Klacid HP7, Losec HP7, Pylorid KA used to destroy Helicobacter pylori, a bacteria that may be responsible for peptic ulcers.

DOSAGE:

Most forms: One or two capsules every eight hours before food.
Augmentin Duo, Ausclav Duo, Clamoxyl Duo, Maxamox: One capsule twice a day.
Klacid HP7, Losec HP7, Pylorid KA: Complex dosage schedule of multiple capsules taken three times a day.
Course (usually five to seven days) should be completed.

FORMS:
Tablets, capsules, mixture (store in door of refrigerator), injection.

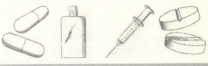

PRECAUTIONS:
Safe in pregnancy (A), children and breast feeding.
Use with caution in kidney failure and leukaemia.
Do not take if:
 allergic to penicillin.

- suffering from glandular fever.

SIDE EFFECTS:
Common: Mild diarrhoea, nausea, vomiting.
Unusual: Genital itch or rash, headache, dizziness, hot flushes, tiredness.
Severe but rare (stop medication, consult doctor): Itchy rash, hives, severe diarrhoea, jaundice, muscle pains, throat tightness.

INTERACTIONS:
Other drugs:
- Allopurinol.

Other substances:
- Alcohol should be avoided.
- May cause false positive results for glucose in urine.

PRESCRIPTION:
Yes.

PBS:
Yes.

PERMITTED IN SPORT:
Yes.

OVERDOSE:
Not life threatening unless allergic to penicillin. Vomiting and diarrhoea likely.

OTHER INFORMATION:
Australia's most commonly used antibiotic. Does not cause dependence or addiction.

See also Ampicillin, Benzathine penicillin, Benzylpenicillin, Dicloxacillin, Flucloxacillin, Phenoxymethyl penicillin, Piperacillin, Procaine penicillin, Ticarcillin sodium.

AMPHETAMINES
See Dexamphetamine.

Amphotericin

TRADE NAMES:
Abelcet, AmBisome, Amphocil, Fungilin, Fungizone.

DRUG CLASS:
Antifungal.

USES:
Injection: Severe internal fungal infections.
Other forms: Fungal infections of gut and mouth.

DOSAGE:

Suspension: 1mL four times a day with meals.
Lozenges: Suck one four times a day.

FORMS:
Lozenges, suspension, injection.

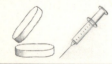

PRECAUTIONS:
Must be used with caution in pregnancy (B2). May be used in breast feeding and children.
Use medication without a break for full course or until infection resolves.

SIDE EFFECTS:
Suspension and lozenges: Nil.
Injection: Causes significant and varied effects in most patients.

INTERACTIONS:
Other drugs:
- Flucytosine.

PRESCRIPTION:
Yes.

PBS:
No.

PERMITTED IN SPORT:
Yes.

OVERDOSE:
Unlikely to be serious.

OTHER INFORMATION:
Amphotericin is very well tolerated and effective when taken by mouth as it is not absorbed from the gut, but when given by injection for severe life threatening fungal infections it can cause significant side effects which must be balanced against the severity of the infection.

See also Fluconazole, Griseofulvin, Itraconazole, Ketoconazole, Terbinafine.

Ampicillin

TRADE NAMES:
Alphacin, Ampicyn, Austrapen.

DRUG CLASS:
Penicillin antibiotic.

USES:
Treatment of infections caused by susceptible bacteria.

DOSAGE:

One or two capsules every eight hours before food. Course (usually seven days) should be completed.

FORMS:
Capsule, injection.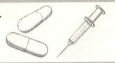

PRECAUTIONS:
Safe in pregnancy (A), children and breast feeding.
Use with caution in leukaemia.
Do not take if:
 allergic to penicillin.
- suffering from glandular fever.

SIDE EFFECTS:
Common: Mild diarrhoea, nausea, vomiting.
Unusual: Headache, dizziness, black tongue, tiredness.
Severe but rare (stop medication, consult doctor): Itchy rash, hives, severe diarrhoea, yellow skin (jaundice), throat tightness.

INTERACTIONS:
Other drugs:
- Allopurinol.

Other substances:
- Alcohol should be avoided.
- May cause false positive results for glucose in urine.

PRESCRIPTION:
Yes.

PBS:
Yes.

PERMITTED IN SPORT:
Yes.

OVERDOSE:
Vomiting and diarrhoea only likely effects.

OTHER INFORMATION:
Widely used in the 1970s, but has now been superseded by Amoxycillin. Does not cause dependence or addiction.

See also Amoxycillin, Benzathine penicillin, Benzylpenicillin, Dicloxacillin, Flucloxacillin, Phenoxymethyl penicillin, Piperacillin, Procaine penicillin, Ticarcillin sodium.

Amsacrine

TRADE NAME:
Amsidyl.

DRUG CLASS:
Antineoplastic.

USES:
Leukaemia not responding to other treatment.

DOSAGE:
 As determined by doctor.

FORMS:
Intravenous infusion.

PRECAUTIONS:
Must not be used in pregnancy (D) or breast feeding.
Must be given by a drip into a centrally located vein.
Regular blood tests to monitor blood cells necessary.
Use with caution in heart disease.
Adequate fluids must be given through drip or by mouth.
Do not take if:
 suffering from bone marrow depression or significant infection.

SIDE EFFECTS:
Common: Multiple including diarrhoea, vomiting, mouth ulcers, hair loss and heart rhythm irregularities.
Unusual: Liver and kidney damage, rash.
Severe but rare (stop medication, consult doctor): Brain function disturbances.

INTERACTIONS:
None significant.

PRESCRIPTION:
Yes.

PBS:
No.

PERMITTED IN SPORT:
Yes.

OVERDOSE:
Very serious. Seek urgent medical attention.

OTHER INFORMATION:
Introduced in 1998 for very serious forms of leukaemia.
See also CANCER-TREATING DRUGS, VINCA ALKALOIDS.

Amylmetacresol

TRADE NAMES:
Strepsils, Strepsils Sugar-Free (with dichlorobenzyl alcohol).
Strepsils Plus (with lignocaine).

DRUG CLASS:
Antiseptic

USES:
Minor mouth and throat infections.

DOSAGE:
 One lozenge dissolved in mouth every two or three hours.

FORMS:
Lozenges.

PRECAUTIONS:
Safe in pregnancy and children.
Do not take if:
 suffering from diabetes.

SIDE EFFECTS:
Nil.

INTERACTIONS:
Nil.

PRESCRIPTION:
No.

PBS:
No.

PERMITTED IN SPORT:
Yes.

OVERDOSE:
Diarrhoea only likely result.

Amylobarbitone

See BARBITURATES.

ANABOLIC STEROIDS

DISCUSSION:
Anabolic steroids are drugs that repair and build up body tissue. They are used illegally by athletes and body builders to increase muscle mass, and are available as tablets and injections. There are many serious side effects and problems associated with their long term use, including liver disease and damage, the development of male characteristics and cessation of periods in women, stunting of growth and early onset of puberty in children, swelling of tissue, water retention, infertility, personality disorders and voice changes.

See Methenolone, Nandrolone decanoate.

ANAESTHETICS, LOCAL

TRADE and GENERIC NAMES:

Abbott Cold Sore Balm (Lignocaine, nitromersol).
Alcaine, Ophthetic (Proxymetacaine).
Applicaine Drops (Benzocaine, cetylpyridinium and other ingredients).
Auralgan Otic (Benzocaine, phenazone).
Bupivacaine, Marcain (Bupivacaine).
Carbocaine (Mepivacaine).
Cepacaine (Benzocaine, cetylpyridinium chloride).
Cepacol Lozenges (Benzocaine, dextromethorphan, cetylpyridinium chloride).
Citanest (Prilocaine).
Cophenylcaine Forte (Lignocaine, phenylephrine).
Cornkil (Benzocaine, salicylic acid, lactic acid).
SOOV Bite, SOOV Burn (Lignocaine, cetrimide and other ingredients).
EMLA (Lignocaine, Prilocaine).
Hemocane, Paraderm Plus, Seda-Gel Lotion (Lignocaine, chlorhexidine and other ingredients).
Lignocaine, Lignospan Special, Nurocain, Xylocaine (Lignocaine with or without Adrenaline).
Lignocaine Gel, Stud 100 Spray, Xylocard (Lignocaine).
Logicin Rapid Relief (Lignocaine, benzydamine and other ingredients).
Medijel (Lignocaine, aminacrine).
Minims Local Anaesthetic (Amethocaine, or lignocaine, or oxybuprocaine).
Naropin (Ropivacaine).
Naropin with Fentanyl (Fentanyl, ropivacaine).
Paraderm Plus (Lignocaine, chlorhexidine, bufexamac).
Paxyl (Lignocaine and other ingredients).
Proctosedyl, Rectinol HC (Cinchocaine, hydrocortisone).
Rectinol (Benzocaine, adrenaline, zinc Oxide).
Scandonest (Mepivacaine, adrenaline).
Scheriproct (Cinchocaine, prednisolone, clemizole).
SM-33 (Lignocaine, salicylic acid and other ingredients).
SOOV Cream (Lignocaine, chlorhexidine and cetrimide).
Strepsils Plus (Lignocaine and amylmetacresol)
Ultraproct (Cinchocaine, corticosteroids and other ingredients).
Virasolve (Lignocaine, idoxuridine, benzalkonium Chloride).
Xylocaine Jelly with Chlorhexidine (Lignocaine, chlorhexidine).
Xyloproct (Lignocaine, hydrocortisone, zinc oxide, aluminium acetate).
NB: Generic medications with the suffix '-caine' and underlined are local anaesthetics.

USES:

Relief of superficial pain of skin, mouth, lips, vagina, penis, anus and other areas. Lignocaine injection may relieve migraine and irregular heartbeat.

DOSAGE:

Skin preparations: Apply three to four times a day.
Mouth and lip preparations: Apply or use every two to four hours.
Anal and vaginal preparations: Apply or use three or four times a day
Eye drops and injections used by doctors only.

FORMS:

Cream, eye drop, gel, injection, lozenge, ointment, paint, paste, patch, spray, suppository.

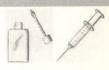

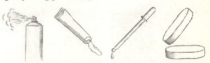

PRECAUTIONS:

Safe in pregnancy (A), breast feeding and children.
Use skin preparations with care on thin skin, genitals, broken skin, eczema or infected skin.

Medications

Elderly may need lower doses.
Special precautions apply to eye preparations and injections. Eye must be protected after use.
Drops should not be used for prolonged periods.
Area injected must be protected from inadvertent injury.

Advise doctor before injection if:

 suffering from heart disease, over-active thyroid gland.

SIDE EFFECTS:

Common: Injections: nervousness, dizziness, blurred vision, tremor, drowsiness, ringing in ears, numbness, nausea, vomiting, low blood pressure, slow heart rate.
Eye preparations: eye irritation, stinging.
Other preparations: Adverse reactions rare.
Unusual: Injections: Convulsions, allergy.
Severe but rare: Injection: Unconsciousness, cessation of breathing.

INTERACTIONS:

Other drugs:
- Creams: Other local anaesthetics, sulfonamides.
- Injection: Drugs acting on heart, cimetidine, anticonvulsants.

PRESCRIPTION:

Most creams, ointments, gels, lozenges, anal preparations etc.: No.
Eye drops, injections: Yes.

PBS:

Injections, eye drops: Yes.
Other forms: No.

PERMITTED IN SPORT:

Yes.

OVERDOSE:

No serious effects except from injection. Effects of injection overdose are very serious and include irregular heartbeat, cessation of breathing, heart attack and death.

OTHER INFORMATION:

All local anaesthetics are derived from cocaine, but are not addictive. Widely used in many forms for relief of pain and discomfort, and generally very safe. Poorly absorbed through skin, but well absorbed through mucous membranes of mouth, anus, vagina etc.

See also Cocaine, Hexylresorcinol

Anagrelide

TRADE NAME:

Agrylin.

DRUG CLASS:

Antineoplastic.

USES:

Essential thrombocythemia (excessive numbers of platelets in blood).

DOSAGE:

 As determined by doctor for each patient individually.

FORMS:

Capsules of 0.5mg (white).

PRECAUTIONS:

Use with caution in pregnancy (B3), breast feeding and children.
Use with caution in heart disease, liver and kidney disease.
Comprehensive neurological examination necessary before commencement.

 Do not stop suddenly, but reduce dose gradually.

Regular blood tests to check cell levels and liver function essential.

SIDE EFFECTS:

Common: Headache, tiredness, chest pain, nausea, diarrhoea, loss of appetite.
Unusual: Heart failure, liver damage, anaemia, joint pain, dizziness, shortness of breath.

Medications

INTERACTIONS:
Other drugs:
- Heparin, sucralfate.

PRESCRIPTION:
Yes.

PBS:
No.

PERMITTED IN SPORT:
Yes.

OVERDOSE:
Very serious. Seek urgent medical attention. Induce vomiting or give activated charcoal if swallowed recently.

ANALGESICS

DISCUSSION:
Drugs that reduce the sensation of pain are called analgesics. There are three main types – narcotics, salicylates (see also NSAIDs) and paracetamol. Many analgesic preparations are combinations of two or more different medications.

See Aspirin, Buprenorphine, Capsaicin, Codeine Phosphate, Dextromoramide, Dextropropoxyphene, Dihydrocodeine, Fentanyl, Heroin, Methadone, Morphine, NSAIDs, Oxycodone, Paracetamol, Pentazocine, Pethidine, SALICYLATES, Tramadol.

Anastrozole

TRADE NAME:
Arimidex.

DRUG CLASS:
Antineoplastic.

USES:
Treatment of advanced breast cancer.

DOSAGE:

One tablet a day.

FORMS:
Tablet of 1mg (white).

PRECAUTIONS:
Must not be used in pregnancy (C), breast feeding or children.
Caution with use before the menopause, liver and kidney disease.

SIDE EFFECTS:
Common: Hot flushes, dry vagina, nausea, thinning of hair.
Unusual: Vaginal bleeding, tiredness, headache, rash, vomiting, diarrhoea, increase in blood cholesterol.
Severe but rare (stop medication, consult doctor): Liver or kidney failure.

INTERACTIONS:
Other drugs:
- Oestrogen.

PRESCRIPTION:
Yes.

PBS:
Yes (restricted to specific types of serious breast cancer).

PERMITTED IN SPORT:
Yes.

OVERDOSE:
Very serious. Seek urgent medical attention. Induce vomiting or administer activated charcoal.

OTHER INFORMATION:
Introduced in 1996. Acts to destroy oestrogen-producing cells in the body.

ANGINA MEDICATIONS

DISCUSSION:
These medications are used to treat angina (chest pain caused by a poor blood supply to the heart).
See Glyceryl Trinitrate, Isosorbide nitrate, Nicorandil, Perhexiline.

ANGIOTENSIN CONVERTING ENZYME INHIBITORS
See ACE Inhibitors.

ANGIOTENSIN II RECEPTOR ANTAGONISTS

TRADE and GENERIC NAMES:
Atacand (Candesartan).
Atacand Plus (Candesartan with hydrochlorothiazide).
Avapro HCT, Karvezide (Irbesartan with hydrochlorothiazide).
Avapro, Karvea (Irbesartan).
Cozaar (Losartan).
Micardis, Pritor (Telmisartan).
Micardis Plus (Telmisartan with hydrochlorothiazide).
Teveten (Eprosartan).
Teveten Plus (Eprosartan with hydrochlorothiazide).

DRUG CLASS:
Antihypertensives.

USES:
High blood pressure (hypertension), congestive heart failure.

DOSAGE:

Usually one tablet a day, but may be increased to two a day.

FORMS:
Tablets.

PRECAUTIONS:
Not to be used in pregnancy (D) or breast feeding. No trials on use in children have been performed.
Use with caution in heart failure, primary hyperaldosteronism, dehydration, heart valve disease and kidney transplant.
Do not take if:

Severe kidney, liver or bile duct disease.

SIDE EFFECTS:
Common: Minimal.
Unusual: Diarrhoea, back and muscle pain.
Severe but rare (stop medication, consult doctor): Liver damage.

INTERACTIONS:
Other drugs:
• Potassium supplements.
Herbs:
• Goldenseal.

PRESCRIPTION:
Yes.

PBS:
Yes.

PERMITTED IN SPORT:
Yes.

OVERDOSE:
Low blood pressure most likely effect. Take activated charcoal to reduce absorption. Seek medical attention.

OTHER INFORMATION:
Very similar in action to ACE Inhibitors (see separate entry) but with fewer side effects. Some forms combined with a

thiazide diuretic (fluid tablet – hydrochlorothiazide) to increase effectiveness. Initially released on to market between 1998 and 2000.
See also ACE Inhibitors.

ANORECTICS

DISCUSSION:

Anorectic drugs are used to reduce appetite. These drugs do NOT reduce weight but act as an aid to controlling appetite while the patient complies with a strictly controlled diet. They are available in tablet and capsule form only. Anorectics should not be used for long periods, as dependence can occur. Some are stimulants, which may cause insomnia if used in the evening, and are used illegally by long-distance drivers and other who wish to remain awake for long periods of time. Many drugs in this class have been removed from the market in recent years because of abuse, interactions and side effects (eg. Adifax, Ponderax, Sanorex).
See Diethylpropion hydrochloride, Orlistat, Phentermine, Silbutramine.

ANTACIDS

TRADE and GENERIC NAMES:

Alu-Tab (Aluminium hydroxide).
Andrews Tums (Calcium carbonate).
Degas Extra (Calcium carbonate, magnesium carbonate, sodium bicarbonate, simethicone).
DeWitt's Antacid, Gastrogel Suspension (Aluminium hydroxide, calcium carbonate, Magnesium salts, potassium bicarbonate and other ingredients).
Dexsal (Sodium bicarbonate, sodium citrotartrate, tartaric acid).
Eno (Sodium bicarbonate and sodium carbonate, citric acid).
Gastrogel Tablets, Gelusil, Mylanta Original, Mylanta Double Strength, Sigma Liquid Antacid (Aluminium hydroxide, magnesium carbonate, simethicone).
Gaviscon, Meracote (Aluminium salts, magnesium salts, bicarbonates, alginic acid)
Gaviscon Double Strength (Potassium bicarbonate, calcium carbonate, sodium alginate).
Infant Gaviscon (Magnesium alginate, sodium alginate).
Mucaine (Aluminium salts, magnesium salts, oxethazine).
Mucaine 2 in 1 (Aluminium salts, magnesium salts, simethicone).
Mylanta Heartburn Relief (Aluminium hydroxide, magnesium hydroxide, calcium carbonate and other ingredients)
Mylanta Rolltabs (Calcium carbonate, magnesium hydroxide).
Rennie (Calcium carbonate, magnesium salts).
Salvital (Bicarbonates, magnesium salts, tartaric acid).
Sodibic (Sodium bicarbonate).
Titralac (Calcium carbonate, glycine).
Titralac SIL (Calcium carbonate, simethicone).

USES:

All forms: Heartburn, acid reflux, peptic ulcer, gastritis, hiatus hernia, reduce stomach acid.
Aluminium salts: Drying agent on skin, diarrhoea.
Sodium bicarbonate: Acidosis of kidney.

DOSAGE:

Multiple presentations. Follow instructions on packaging, or from doctor or pharmacist. Take immediately before meals or one hour after meals.

FORMS:

Mixture, tablets, capsules, granules, powder, chewable tablets, lotion.

  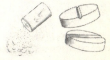

PRECAUTIONS:
Safe in pregnancy (A), children and breast feeding.
Care required in patients with kidney disease, bleeding from stomach, irregular bowels.
Should not be taken for prolonged period without medical advice.

Do not take if:
- ☠ suffering from severe belly pain.
- you have recently had kidney or bladder stones.

SIDE EFFECTS:
Common: Mild.
Unusual: Constipation, loss of appetite.
Severe but rare (stop medication, consult doctor): Severe abdominal pain, muscle weakness, bone pain.

INTERACTIONS:
Other drugs:
- Tetracycline antibiotics, beta blockers, digoxin

Herbs:
- Ginger, garlic, parsley, senega, ginkgo biloba, alfalfa, capsicum, eucalyptus.

Other substances:
- Food and alcohol reduce antacid effect.

PRESCRIPTION:
No.

PBS:
Gastrogel, Gelusil, Mylanta Original: Yes. Mylanta Double Strength, Sodibic: Available for Veteran Affairs card holders. Others: No.

PERMITTED IN SPORT:
Yes.

OVERDOSE:
Very unlikely to be life threatening but may cause weakness, dizziness, tiredness and confusion.

OTHER INFORMATION:
Widely used preparations for minor stomach upsets, antacids are drugs that neutralise acid in the stomach. A very large number of these medications are available without prescription as both mixtures and tablets. Sometimes they cause problems with the absorption of other medications if taken at the same time. They often contain multiple ingredients.

See also Cimetidine, Cisapride, Famotidine, Misoprostol, Nizatadine, PROTON PUMP INHIBITORS, Ranitidine, Simethicone, Sucralfate.

Antazoline
See Naphazoline and Antazoline.

ANTHELMINTICS

DISCUSSION:
Helminths are different types of worms that infect the gut. The drugs that destroy these unwanted internal worms are called anthelmintics. There are many different types of helminths, including threadworms, hookworms, roundworms, and a number of rarer worms that are not normally found in Australia. Most common anthelmintics can be purchased without prescription in mixture, tablet and granule formulations. It is important to treat all family members, and to carefully wash clothing and bedding at the time of treatment. A number of prescription drugs are available for the treatment of resistant cases or rarer types of infection.

See Albendazole, Ivermectin, Mebendazole, Praziquantel, Pyrantel embonate.

Anthralin
See Dithranol.

ANTIALLERGEN

DISCUSSION:

Medications that reduce allergy reactions.
See Allergen extracts.

ANTIANDROGEN

DISCUSSION:

Medications that act against the male hormone, testosterone.
See Cyproterone Acetase, Flutamide, Nilutamide.

ANTIANGINALS

DISCUSSION:

Medications that relieve or prevent angina (heart pain).
See BETA BLOCKERS, CALCIUM CHANNEL BLOCKERS, Glyceryl trinitrate, Isosorbide nitrate, Nicorandil, Perhexiline.

ANTIARRHYTHMICS

DISCUSSION:

Antiarrhythmics are the drugs that keep the heartbeating regularly. If the heart rhythm is uneven, beats are being missed, or extra beats are causing palpitations, doctors will prescribe an antiarrhythmic. There is a wide range of medications in this class that work in different ways depending on the type of heart rhythm irregularity
See Adenosine, Amiodarone, Disopyramide, Flecainide, Mexiletine, Procainamide, Quinidine bisulphate, Sotalol, Verapamil.

ANTIBIOTICS

DISCUSSION:

Every sixth prescription written by doctors in Australia is for an antibiotic. They are thus the most widely prescribed group of drugs, but most patients understand very little about them. Although there were chemical compounds used against infection before the Second World War, the isolation of penicillin from a mould grown in a laboratory represented the first real exploitation of a purified natural substance that could kill bacteria. The very first supplies of penicillin came from the mould grown, due to wartime exigencies, in large numbers of bedpans. Most antibiotics today are produced as the result of chemical reactions (i.e. synthesised) as opposed to harvesting the drug from primitive life forms grown in bulk in areas that resembled mushroom farms.

Antibiotics are only effective against bacteria, and not against viral infections. Most of the infections seen by a general practitioner are caused by viruses, and there is no need for antibiotics in these cases. Antibiotics are used by doctors in several situations:

- If the infection appears to be bacterial, the appropriate antibiotic will be selected to cure it. Samples or swabs may be taken so that the infecting bacteria and the correct antibiotic to kill it can be identified in a laboratory.
- If the problem is not clear-cut, or if there is some doubt as to the cause of a problem, an antibiotic may be prescribed to cover one of the possibilities. This may be the case with a severely sore throat.
- If a person has reduced immunity, is elderly, frail, liable to recurrent infections or due for an operation, an antibiotic may be used to prevent a bacterial infection. Women with recurrent bladder infections are one example.

Major problems can occur with the overuse of antibiotics. Cost is the first one, and as the government (ie. you the taxpayer) pays part of the cost of everyone's antibiotics, this is a problem affecting you. Side effects are another problem, including stopping the oral contraceptive pill from working. The most important problem is the development of resistance which can enable bacteria to change in a way that makes them able to resist the actions of an antibiotic that was previously very effective. The need for new antibiotic agents is therefore always with us. Their development is a long and costly process involving huge investments by the drug companies. A good antibiotic deserves a long and effective life, and the needs of the public will be best served by the prescribing of antibiotics only when they are really needed, thus reducing the rate at which resistant strains develop.

See Amoxycillin, Ampicillin, Azithromycin, Aztreonam, Bacitracin, Benzylpenicillin, CEPHALOSPORINS, Chloramphenicol, Cilastatin and Imipenem, Ciprofloxacin, Clarithromycin, Clindamycin, Demeclocycline, Dicloxacillin, Doxycycline, Erythromycin, Flucloxacillin, Framycetin, Gentamicin, Gramicidin, Lincomycin, Linezolid, Meropenem, Metronidazole, Minocycline, Mupirocin, Neomycin, Netilmicin, Nitrofurantoin, Norfloxacin, Ofloxacin, Phenoxymethyl penicillin, Piperacillin, Polymyxin B, Potassium clavulanate, Procaine penicillin, Roxithromycin, Silver sulfadiazine, Sodium fusidate, Spectinomycin, Sulfamethoxazole, Sulfasalazine, SULFONAMIDES, Tazobactam, Telcoplanin, Tetracycline, Ticarcillin sodium, Tinidazole, Tobramycin, Trimethoprim, Vancomycin.

ANTICANCER DRUGS

See CANCER-TREATING DRUGS.

ANTICHOLINERGICS

DISCUSSION:

A group of drugs that act as drying agents, relieve spasm of gut and other hollow organs, and dilate the pupil of the eye.

See Atropine, Dicyclomine, Diphemanil methylsulfate, Hyoscine and Hyoscyamine, Ipratropium bromide, MYDRIATICS, Oxybutynin, Propantheline, Tiotropium.

ANTICHOLINESTERASES

DISCUSSION:

A group of drugs used to treat difficulty in passing urine and myasthenia gravis.

See Donepezil, Neostigmine, Pyridostigmine.

ANTICOAGULANTS

DISCUSSION:

Anticoagulants are drugs that stop blood from clotting at the normal speed. They are used in patients who have had strokes due to blood clots, clots in leg veins and clots in heart and lung arteries. Aspirin is also a mild anticoagulant and can be used in small doses to prevent strokes. All anticoagulants should be stopped before any surgical procedure.

Patients on the stronger anticoagulants listed below must be monitored carefully by their doctors and have blood tests regularly to ensure that the clotting factors in their blood are kept at the desirable level. Patients using anticoagulants will bruise and bleed more easily than normal, and care must be taken when using some antiarthritic medications, as they may cause bleeding into the gut while the patient is on anticoagulants. There are many precautions necessary with these drugs that make compliance with a doctor's instructions vital.

See Abciximab, Aspirin, Clopidogrel, Dalteparin, Danaparoid, Dipyridamole, Enoxaparin, Heparin, Phenindione, Ticlopidine, Warfarin.

ANTICONVULSANTS

DISCUSSION:

This large group of drugs is used to control and prevent fits and convulsions caused by epilepsy and other diseases. Barbiturates (see separate entry) and benzodiazepines (see separate entry) are also used for this purpose. Patients must sometimes take quite large quantities of anticonvulsants, or combinations of several drugs to control their problem, and blood levels are usually checked to arrive at the correct dosage. Side effects from anticonvulsants vary widely from one person to another and between drugs. They are usually worst when treatment is first started, and wear off as time passes. All these drugs have a tendency to interact with other drugs, and the doctor must be made aware of all medications being taken and any other diseases (eg. diabetes) that may be present.

See BARBITURATES, BENZODIAZEPINES, Carbamazepine, Clonazepam, Ethosuximide, Gabapentin, Lamotrigine, Levetiracetam, Oxcarbazepine, Phenytoin, Primidone, Sodium valproate, Sulthiame, Tiagabine, Topiramate, Vigabatrin.

ANTIDEPRESSANTS

DISCUSSION:

Antidepressants are used to control depression. This is as much a disease as diabetes or high blood pressure but is often thought to be a mental disorder that patients can 'pull themselves out of'. Nothing could be further than the truth. Depression is caused by a biochemical imbalance in the brain, and requires appropriate medication to correct it before a tragedy occurs. There are many sub-classes of antidepressants including MAOI, RIMA, SNRI, SSRI, tetracyclics and tricyclics.

See Citalopram, Fluoxetine, Fluvoxamine, MAOI, Mianserin, Mirtazapine, Moclobemide, Nefazodone, Paroxetine, Reboxetine, Sertraline, TRICYCLIC ANTIDEPRESSANTS, Venlafaxine.

ANTIDIARRHOEALS

DISCUSSION:

Antidiarrhoeals are one of the most popular drug groups with patients. When you just have to go and go and go — and you want to stop — antidiarrhoeals are just the thing to help. There are some types of diarrhoea that they are not suitable for, including those associated with jaundice (yellow skin), bacterial gut infections and diarrhoea during pregnancy. Diarrhoea has a vast number of causes, and the exact treatment chosen will depend on that cause. Many types of diarrhoea require no medication but a correct diet.

See Atropine, Attapulgite, Codeine Phosphate, Diphenoxylate Hydrochloride, Kaolin, Loperamide, Pectin.

ANTIDIURETICS

DISCUSSION:

The antidiuretics are used to reduce the amount of urine produced by the kidneys in bed wetting, diabetes insipidus and in some other even rarer conditions. They are unusual in that some forms are given routinely as a nasal spray or injection.

See Desmopressin acetate, Vasopressin.

ANTIDOTES

DISCUSSION:

Medications that counteract poisons or a drug overdose.

See Charcoal, Methionine, Naloxone.

ANTIEMETICS

DISCUSSION:

Antiemetics are medicines that stop vomiting. They are often difficult to give in tablet or mixture form, so many of them are also available as an injection or suppository (for insertion into the back passage). There are many different drugs in this category, from the mild over-the-counter travel sickness pills, to the more effective and potent prescription drugs such as prochlorperazine, domperidone and metoclopramide. These are also available as injections.

See ANTIHISTAMINES, SEDATING, Dimenhydrinate, Domperidone, Hyoscine and Hyoscyamine, Metoclopramide, Ondansetron, PHENOTHIAZINES, Prochlorperazine.

ANTIFUNGALS

DISCUSSION:

Antifungals treat fungal infections. Fungi are members of the plant kingdom and are one of the types of microscopic life that can infect human beings in many diverse ways. The most common site of infection is the skin, where they cause an infection that is commonly known as tinea. Fungi are also

Medications

responsible for many gut infections, particularly in the mouth and around the anus. It is a rare infant that escapes without an attack of oral thrush. Around the anus, the fungus can cause an extremely itchy rash, but in women it may spread forward from the anus to the vagina to cause the white discharge and intense itch of vaginal thrush or candidiasis. The most serious diseases develop when fungal infections occur deep inside the body in organs such as the lungs, brain and sinuses. These diseases are very difficult to treat and it may take many months with potent antifungal drugs to bring them under control. Fortunately, this type of condition is relatively rare.

See Amorolfine, Amphotericin, Atovaquone, Bifonazole, Chlorphenesin, Fluconazole, Flucytosine, Griseofulvin, IMIDAZOLES, IODINE, Itraconazole, Ketoconazole, Nystatin, Pyrithione zinc, Selenium sulfide, Sodium propionate, Terbinafine, Tolnaftate, Undecenoic acid, Undecylenamide.

ANTIHISTAMINES, NON-SEDATING

TRADE and GENERIC NAMES:

Claratyne, Lorastyne (Loratadine).
Clarinase, Sinease Repetabs (Loratadine with pseudoephedrine).
Telfast (Fexofenadine).
Telfast Decongestant (Fexofenadine with pseudoephedrine).

USES:

Allergy reactions, hay fever, urticaria (hives).

DOSAGE:

 One or two tablets or capsules a day.

FORMS:

Capsules, tablets, mixture.

PRECAUTIONS:

Should be used with caution in pregnancy (B1). Fexofenadine (B2). Should not be used in breast feeding.

Do not take if:

 suffering from severe liver disease.

SIDE EFFECTS:

Common: Nil.
Unusual: Increase in appetite, fainting, dry mouth, gastric upset, blurred vision, muscle pains, tremor, sweating, rash.

INTERACTIONS:

Other drugs:
- Fexofenadine may react with ketoconazole (antifungal) and erythromycin (antibiotic) to cause heart problems.

PRESCRIPTION:

No.

PBS:

No. Some available to Veteran Affairs Pensioners.

PERMITTED IN SPORT:

Yes.

OVERDOSE:

Mild effects only. Possible heartbeat irregularities. First aid involves induction of vomiting and then observing in hospital for a day.

OTHER INFORMATION:

Antihistamines are divided into two broad groups – those that cause sedation and those that do not. In an allergy reaction, a substance called histamine is released from special cells (mast cells) to cause swelling, itching and increase in secretions. Antihistamines counteract this reaction. The non-sedating antihistamines will not have any effect on excessive secretions from causes other than allergy (eg. they have no effect on runny noses caused by the common cold).

See also **ANTIHISTAMINES, SEDATING.**

Medications

ANTIHISTAMINES, SEDATING

TRADE and GENERIC NAMES:

Actifed (Triprolidine, pseudoephedrine).
Action Cold and Flu (Chlorpheniramine, phenylephrine, aspirin).
Avil Decongestant (Pheniramine, ammonium chloride).
Avil, Fenamine (Pheniramine).
Benadryl Family Dry (Diphenhydramine, pseudoephedrine, dextromethorphan).
Benadryl Family Original, Chemists' Own Difenacol Cough (Diphenhydramine, ammonium chloride, sodium citrate).
Biotech Cold & Flu (Chlorpheniramine, codeine, pseudoephedrine, paracetamol, belladonna)
Chemists' Own Cold & Flu Night, Codral 4 Flu (Chlorpheniramine, pseudoephedrine, codeine, paracetamol).
Chemists' Own Coldeze Chlorpheniramine, paracetamol).
Chemists' Own Dry Raspy Cough (Chlorpheniramine, pseudoephedrine, dextromethorphan).
Chemists' Own Hayfever Sinus Relief, Logicin Flu Strength Night, Logicin hay Fever, Panadol Allergy Sinus, Panadol Children's Cold Relief Elixir, Sinutab Sinus Allergy and Pain Relief (Chlorpheniramine, paracetamol, pseudoephedrine).
Chemists' Own Infant's Cold & Allergy Drops, Demazin Syrup, Duro-Tuss Cold & Allergy (Chlorpheniramine, phenylephrine).
Chemists' Own Kiddicol (Chlorpheniramine, phenylephrine, pholcodine and other ingredients).
Chemists' Own Peetalix, Vallergan (Trimeprazine).
Chemists' Own Promethazine, Gold Cross Antihistamine, Phenergan (Promethazine).
Codalgin Plus, Dolased Analgesic Relaxant, Dolased Night Pain, Fiorinal, Mersyndol, Mersyndol Forte, Panalgesic (Doxylamine, codeine, paracetamol).
Codral Cough Cold & Flu Night, Orthoxicol Night Cold & Flu, Parke-Davis Night Cold & Flu (Chlorpheniramine, paracetamol, dextromethorphan).
Codral Night Time, Sudafed Nightime Relief, Sudafed Sinus Pain and Allergy Relief (Triprolidine, paracetamol, pseudoephedrine).
Demazin Cold & Flu, Logicin Flu Night (Chlorpheniramine, pseudoephedrine, paracetamol).
Demazin Repetabs, Demazin Day/Night Relief (Dexchlorpheniramine, pseudoephedrine).
Demazin Tablets (Chlorpheniramine, pseudoephedrine).
Dilosyn (Methdilazine).
Dimetapp Cold Cough & Flu Night (Doxylamine, pseudoephedrine, paracetamol).
Dimetapp Elixir, Dimetapp Drops (Brompheniramine, phenylephrine).
Dimetapp DM (Brompheniramine, phenylephrine, dextromethorphan).
Dozile, Restavit (Doxylamine).
Ergodryl (Diphenhydramine, ergotamine, caffeine).
Euky Bear Cough Syrup (Chlorpheniramine, dextromethorphan, sodium citrate).
Lemsip Pharmacy Flu Strength Nightime, Tylenol Cold & Flu (Chlorpheniramine, dextromethorphan, pseudoephedrine, paracetamol).
Naphcon-A, Visine Allergy with Antihistamine (Pheniramine with naphazoline).
Paedamin (Diphenhydramine, phenylephrine).
Painstop (Promethazine, paracetamol, codeine).
Panadol Allergy Sinus, Panadol Children's Cold Elixir, Tylenol Allergy Sinus (Chlorpheniramine, pseudoephedrine, paracetamol).
Panadol Night (Diphenhydramine, paracetamol).
Panadol Sinus Night, Orthoxicol Night Cold & Flu (Chlorpheniramine,

Home Guide to Medication

pseudoephedrine, paracetamol).
Panquil (<u>Promethazine</u>, paracetamol).
Periactin (<u>Cyproheptadine</u>).
Phensedyl Dry Family Cough Syrup (<u>Promethazine</u>, pseudoephedrine, pholcodine).
Polaramine (<u>Dexchlorpheniramine</u>).
Relaxa-Tabs (<u>Mepyramine</u>).
Tixylix Nightime Linctus (<u>Promethazine</u>, pholcodine).
Tussinol Cough & Cold Infant, Tussinol Night-Time Cough & Cold (<u>Chlorpheniramine</u>, dextromethorphan, pseudoephedrine).
Unisom Sleepgels (<u>Diphenhydramine</u>).
Zadine (<u>Azatadine</u>).
Zyrtec (<u>Cetirizine</u>).
NB: Antihistamines are <u>underlined</u>. Numerous locally produced and marketed antihistamine products also exist.

USES:
Allergies (eg. hay fever, hives, urticaria), drug allergies, drying of secretions.
PLUS Meclozine, pheniramine and promethazine: Nausea, vomiting, motion sickness, Ménière's disease.
Diphenhydramine and doxylamine: Spasms of Parkinson's disease, migraine, muscle spasms.
Methdiazine and cyproheptadine: Prevention of migraine.
Diphenhydramine, doxylamine, promethazine, mepyramine and trimeprazine: Sedation.

DOSAGE:
Follow directions on packaging. Some antihistamines are far longer acting than others. Dose will vary from once a day to four times a day.

FORMS:
Tablets, capsules, mixture, oral drops, injection, eye drops.

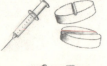
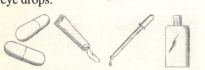

PRECAUTIONS:
Promethazine and Trimeprazine should only be used in pregnancy (C) and breast feeding on medical advice.
Diphenylpyramine, and Azatadine should be used with caution in pregnancy (B2) and breast feeding.
All other sedating antihistamines are safe in pregnancy (A) and breast feeding. All are safe in children over two years. Seek medical advice if using in younger children. All should be used with caution in patients with liver disease, heart disease, glaucoma, chronic lung disease, enlarged prostate or severe peptic ulcer.

Do not take if:
 operating machinery or undertaking tasks that require concentration and coordination.
- Drinking alcohol.

SIDE EFFECTS:
Common: Drowsiness, dry mouth, constipation, restlessness in children, incoordination, blurred vision.
Unusual: Upper belly discomfort, loss of appetite, nausea, diarrhoea, irritability.
Severe but rare (stop medication, consult doctor): Unusual bleeding.

INTERACTIONS:
Other drugs:
- May interfere with Anticoagulants, MAOI (monoamine oxidase inhibitors), sedatives and relaxants.
- Skin preparations have no significant interactions.

Other substances:
- Do not use alcohol with sedating antihistamines.

PRESCRIPTION:
No.
Some combination products require a prescription.

PBS:
No.
Some forms are available to Veteran Affairs Pensioners.

PERMITTED IN SPORT:
Yes.

OVERDOSE:
May result in convulsions, hallucinations, delirium, anxiety, muscle spasms, rapid heart rate, flushing, dry skin, dry mouth and coma. First aid involved inducing vomiting and seeking urgent medical attention.

OTHER INFORMATION:
Antihistamines are widely used to dry the excessive secretions of hay fever and common colds. Taken in the correct dosage, they are very safe, but care must be taken with drowsiness.

Antihistamines are divided into two broad groups – those that cause sedation and those that do not. In an allergy reaction, a substance called histamine is released from special cells (mast cells) to cause swelling, itching and increase in secretions. Antihistamines counteract this reaction. The non-sedating antihistamines will not have any effect on excessive secretions from causes other than allergy (eg. they have no effect on runny noses caused by the common cold). Sedating antihistamines are available in a huge range of cold and flu remedies. They are added to painkillers to relax muscles and tension.

See also ANTIHISTAMINES NON-SEDATING, Azelastine, Dimenhydrinate, Levocabastine, Metoclopramide, Prochlorperazine.

ANTIHYPERTENSIVES

DISCUSSION:
A very mixed bag of medications that treat high blood pressure in many different ways.

See ACE INHIBITORS, ANGIOTENSIN II RECEPTOR ANTAGONISTS, BETA BLOCKERS, CALCIUM CHANNEL BLOCKERS, Clonidine, Diazoxide, Hydralazine, Indapamide, Labetalol, Lercanidipine, Methyldopa, Minoxidil, Prazosin, THIAZIDE DIURETICS.

ANTIMALARIALS

DISCUSSION:
Antimalarials treat and prevent malaria. Malaria is becoming an increasing problem in the world, as many forms of the disease are becoming resistant to the commonly used medications. Millions of people die of malaria in tropical countries every year, and the most resistant and virulent form in the world can be found in our nearest neighbour country, Papua New Guinea. It is essential for travellers to any tropical country to discuss with their doctor, at least a month before their departure, the appropriate medications necessary to prevent malaria. Because it is spread by mosquitoes, insect repellents, protective clothing and mosquito nets also play an important part in preventing malaria. Generally speaking, the same drugs are used for both prevention and treatment of malaria, but they are given in much higher dosages for treatment.

See Artemether and Lumefantrine, Atovaquone, Chloroquine, Doxycycline, Hydroxychloroquine, Mefloquine, Primaquine, Proguanil, Pyrimethamine, Quinine, Sulfadoxine.

ANTIMETABOLITES
See CANCER-TREATING DRUGS.

ANTIMIGRAINE

DISCUSSION:
Medications that prevent and treat migraine.
See ANALGESICS, BETA BLOCKERS, Clonidine, Dihydroergotamine, Ergotamine, Methysergide, Naratriptan, NSAIDs, Pizotifen, Sumatriptan, Zolmitriptan.

ANTINEOPLASTICS
See CANCER-TREATING DRUGS

ANTIPARASITICS

DISCUSSION:

Medications that kill skin parasites.

See Benzyl benzoate, Bioallethrin, Crotamiton, Maldison, Permethrin, Piperonyl butoxide, Pyrethrins.

ANTIPARKINSONIANS

DISCUSSION:

Medications that treat and slow the progression of Parkinson's disease.

See Amantadine, Apomorphine hydrochloride, Benzhexol, Benztropine, Biperiden, Bromocriptine, Entacapone, LEVODOPA COMPOUNDS, Orphenadrine, Pergolide, Selegiline.

ANTIPSYCHOTICS

DISCUSSION:

A psychosis is a serious mental disorder, in which the patients normally have no idea that there is anything wrong with them. There are a large number of specific mental diseases that fit into this category, and different antipsychotic drugs are known to be more useful in treating some types of psychoses. Psychoses are often characterised by agitation, anxiety, tension, personality changes and emotional disturbances. Common psychotic diseases include mania, some types of depression, and schizophrenia. Nearly all of the drugs that can correct these problems are available as tablets, and some as mixtures and injections. The main class of antipsychotics is the phenothiazines.

See Amisulpride, Droperidol, Flupenthixol, Haloperidol, Lithium Carbonate, Olanzapine, PHENOTHIAZINES, Pimozide, Quetiapine, Risperidone, Thiothixene, Zuclopenthixol.

ANTIPYRETICS

DISCUSSION:

These medications reduce fevers as well as easing pain.

See Aspirin, Paracetamol.

ANTIRHEUMATICS

DISCUSSION:

An amazingly diverse range of drugs can be placed in the category of relieving rheumatoid arthritis and other rheumatic conditions. Most of them have found their place here serendipitously, when patients being treated for other diseases found that their rheumatoid arthritis was improved. There is no cure for rheumatoid arthritis, but by the use of painkillers, physiotherapy, NSAIDs (see separate entry) and the antirheumatic drugs, control is normally possible.

See Chloroquine, CORTICOSTEROIDS, Hydroxychloroquine, Methotrexate, NSAIDs, Penicillamine, Sulfasalazine.

ANTISEPTICS

DISCUSSION:

Antiseptics are drugs that kill bacteria and other infecting organisms on the skin, in the mouth or other areas, without being absorbed into the body or blood. They may also be used to sterilise medical instruments and equipment. Something that is 'septic' is infected, so antiseptics act against infection.

See Acriflavine, Aminacrine hydrochloride, Amylmetacresol, Azelaic acid, Benzalkonium chloride, Cetrimide, Cetylpyridinium, Chlorhexidine, Chloroxylenol, Clioquinol, Crotamiton, IODINE, Nitromersol, Pyrithione zinc, Sodium perborate, Triclosan.

ANTISEPTIC, URINARY

DISCUSSION:
Medications that can be used on a long term basis to prevent urine infections.
See Hexamine hippurate.

ANTISPASMODICS

DISCUSSION:
Antispasmodics prevent or treat painful muscular spasm of hollow tubes within the body, such as the gut. If the gut goes into spasm, severe intermittent pains can develop in the abdomen. Irritable bowel syndrome, infantile colic, gastroenteritis and gut infections are just a few of the diseases that can cause this problem. There are a large number of antispasmodic drugs for the gut that vary from mild over-the-counter tablet and mixture preparations to potent prescription tablets such as dicyclomine, mebeverine, hyoscine and propantheline. Some of these are also available as injections.
See Alverine citrate, Atropine, Dicyclomine, Hyoscine and Hyoscyamine, Mebeverine, Peppermint Oil, Propantheline.

ANTITHYROIDS

DISCUSSION:
An overactive thyroid gland can cause a multiplicity of serious problems. The excess production of thyroxine hormone by the gland must be reduced before serious damage occurs to other organs in the body. The antithyroid drugs that act against the thyroid gland are carbimazole and propylthiouracil. Because of their significant side effects, these tablets are used only in the acute situation, until a cure by means of surgery or irradiation is undertaken.
See Carbimazole, Propylthiouracil.

ANTIVENOMS

GENERIC NAMES:
Antivenoms against box jellyfish, funnel web spider, red back spider, sea snake, numerous snakes, stonefish and ticks are available.

USES:
Treatment of bites by specific toxic animal.

DOSAGE:

As determined by doctor depending on patient's condition and weight.

FORMS:
Injection.

PRECAUTIONS:
May be used in pregnancy, breast feeding and children if medically indicated.
All patients must be carefully monitored and any signs of allergy reaction treated early.
Use with caution in asthma, eczema and previous history of allergy.
Use with caution if antivenom used previously.

SIDE EFFECTS:
Common: Minimal.
Unusual: Allergy reaction, generalised illness.

INTERACTIONS:
None significant.

PRESCRIPTION:
Yes.

PBS:
No. Usually only available in hospitals.

PERMITTED IN SPORT:
Yes.

OVERDOSE:
May cause serious allergy reaction.

Medications

OTHER INFORMATION:

Life saving, but must be given as soon as possible after any bite. Most venoms are large compounds and spread very slowly from the site of the bite. The spread of venom can be prevented by applying a firm bandage (not too tight to cut off circulation) while arranging urgent medical care. Keep any dressing or material contaminated by the venom as it can be used to identify the type of animal responsible.

ANTIVIRALS

DISCUSSION:

Medications that can be used to treat a limited number of viral infections (mainly HIV AIDS and Herpes infections such as shingles and genital herpes).

See Abacavir, Aciclovir, Amantadine, Delavirdine, Didanosine, Efavirenz, Ganciclovir, Idoxuridine, Indinavir, Lamivudine, Nelfinavir, Nevirapine, Oseltamivir, Ribavirin, Ritonavir, Saquinavir, Stavudine, Tenofovir, Valaciclovir, Valganciclovir, Zanamivir, Zidovudine.

ANXIOLYTICS

DISCUSSION:

Medications that relieve both anxiety and muscle spasm.

See Alprazolam, Bromazepam, Buspirone, Clobazam, Diazepam, Lorazepam, Oxazepam.

Apormorphine hydrochloride

TRADE NAME:

Apomine.

DRUG CLASS:

Antiparkinsonian.

USES:

Severe Parkinson's disease.

DOSAGE:

As determined by doctor for each individual patient.

FORMS:

Injection.

PRECAUTIONS:

Use with great caution in pregnancy (B3), during breast feeding and in elderly.

Do not take if:

suffering from dementia and some psychiatric disorders, liver disease, kidney disease, angina and other unstable heart diseases, poor blood circulation to brain or poor brain function.
- sensitive to morphine or levodopa.

SIDE EFFECTS:

Common: Nausea, diarrhoea, drowsiness.
Unusual: Vomiting, nodule at injection site, allergy reaction.

INTERACTIONS:

Other drugs:
- Some drugs affecting brain function.

PRESCRIPTION:

Yes.

PBS:

Yes (authority required).

PERMITTED IN SPORT:

Yes.

Apraclonidine

TRADE NAME:
Iopidine.

USES:
Certain forms of severe glaucoma.

DOSAGE:

One drop to affected eye three times a day. Apply pressure to tear duct at inside corner of eye following application.

FORMS:
Eye drops.

PRECAUTIONS:
Use with caution in pregnancy (B3), children and breast feeding.
Benefits may decrease after more than 60 days.
Use with caution in high blood pressure, severe heart disease, depression, liver disease, kidney disease.

SIDE EFFECTS:
Common: Eye irritation.
Unusual: Excessive response.

INTERACTIONS:
Other drugs:
- MAOI, sympathomimetics, tricyclic antidepressants, beta blockers, digoxin, clonidine, antihypertensives, brain depressants.

PRESCRIPTION:
Yes.

PBS:
Yes (restricted to patients already on maximum doses of other glaucoma medications, and for short term use only).

PERMITTED IN SPORT:
Yes.
See also Acetazolamide, Betaxolol, Bimatoprost, Brimonidine tartrate, Brinzolamide, Carbachol, Dipivefrine hydrochloride, Dorzolamide hydrochloride, Latanoprost, Levobunolol, Phenylephrine, Pilocarpine, Timolol, Travoprost.

Aprotinin

TRADE NAME:
Trasylol.

DRUG CLASS:
Fibrinolytic.

USES:
Prevention of excessive blood loss during heart surgery, and after serious injury.

DOSAGE:

As determined by doctor for individual patient. Test dose must be given initially.

FORMS:
Injection.

PRECAUTIONS:
Relatively safe in pregnancy (B1) and children.
May cause severe allergy reaction if used a second time.

SIDE EFFECTS:
Common: Excessive sensitivity.

INTERACTIONS:
Other drugs: Thrombolytics.

PRESCRIPTION:
Yes.

PBS:
No (expensive).

PERMITTED IN SPORT:
Yes.

OVERDOSE:
Very serious. Always given under strict medical supervision.

Arachis Oil

TRADE NAMES:

Cerumol Ear Drops (with chlorbutol and other ingredients).
Medevac Solution (with sorbitol).
Polytar Medicated Bar (with coal tar and other ingredients).

USES:

Softens ear wax, bile and dry skin.

DOSAGE:

Ear drops: Two drops daily for three days.
Bar: Use daily as soap
Solution: Single dose of 500mLs to assist in emptying bile from gall bladder during x-rays and surgery.

FORMS:

Ear drops,
soap bar,
solution.

PRECAUTIONS:

Safe in pregnancy and breast feeding.
No significant precautions.

SIDE EFFECTS:

None significant.

INTERACTIONS:

None significant.

PRESCRIPTION:

No.

PBS:

No.

PERMITTED IN SPORT:

Yes.

OVERDOSE:

Diarrhoea only likely effect if swallowed.

Artemether and Lumefantrine

TRADE NAME:

Riamet.

DRUG CLASS:

Antimalarial.

USES:

Treatment of malaria.

DOSAGE:

Four tablets at once then at intervals of 8, 24, 36, 48 and 60 hours.

FORMS:

Tablets (yellow).

PRECAUTIONS:

Use with caution in pregnancy (B3) and children under 12 years.
Not for use if breast feeding.
Use with caution if suffering from irregular heart rhythm, heart disease, electrolyte (blood chemistry) disturbances, anorexia nervosa, liver and kidney disease.

SIDE EFFECTS:

Common: Headache, loss of appetite, muscle pains.
Unusual: Fever, tiredness.
Severe but rare (stop medication, consult doctor): Irregular heart rhythm.

INTERACTIONS:

Other drugs:
- Severe interaction with erythromycin, ketoconazole, metoprolol, itraconazole, cimetidine, flecainide, imipramine, amitriptyline, clomipramine.
- Other antimalarials.

PRESCRIPTION:

Yes.

PBS:

No.

PERMITTED IN SPORT:
Yes.

OVERDOSE:
Very serious. Heart rhythm abnormalities may cause sudden death. Induce vomiting or give activated charcoal if taken recently. Seek urgent medical attention.

OTHER INFORMATION:
Released in 2003. These medications are only available in this combination in Australia.

See also Atovaquone, Chloroquine, Doxycycline, Hydroxychloroquine, Mefloquine, Primaquine, Proguanil, Pyrimethamine, Quinine bisulphate, Sulfadoxine.

Ascorbic acid
(Sodium ascorbate, Vitamin C)

TRADE NAMES:
A large number of preparations include ascorbic acid (vitamin C) alone or in combination with other medications.

DRUG CLASS:
Vitamin.

USES:
Scurvy, vitamin deficiency, convalescence.

DOSAGE:

Recommended daily allowance: Males – 40mg, Females – 30mg.

FORMS:
Tablets, capsules, mixture, drops, injection.

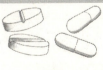

PRECAUTIONS:
Safe in pregnancy, breast feeding and children.
Do not take in high doses or for prolonged periods of time.
Use with caution in kidney disease.

SIDE EFFECTS:
Common: Minimal.
Unusual: Kidney stones if taken in excessive doses.

INTERACTIONS:
None significant.

PRESCRIPTION:
No.

PBS:
No.

PERMITTED IN SPORT:
Yes.

OVERDOSE:
May cause kidney damage if taken in high doses long term.

OTHER INFORMATION:
Ascorbic acid is a water soluble vitamin found in citrus fruit, tomatoes and greens. Its level in food is reduced by mincing, grating and contact with copper utensils. It is essential for the formation and maintenance of bone, cartilage and teeth. Remember, vitamins are merely chemicals that are essential for the functioning of the body, and if taken to excess, act as a drug. There is unfortunately, no evidence that it helps the common cold.

Aspirin
(Acetylsalicylic Acid)

TRADE NAMES:

Aspro, Astrix, Bayer Aspirin, Bex, Cardiprin, Cartia, DBL Aspirin, Disprin, Ecotrin, Herron Aspirin, Solprin, Spren, Vincents.
Action Cold & Flu Effervescent (with chlorpheniramine, phenylephrine).
Alka-Seltzer (with sodium bicarbonate and other ingredients).
Asasantin SR (with dipyridamole)
Aspalgin, Codiphen, Codis, Codral Forte, Disprin Forte, Veganin (with codeine).
Codox (with dihydrocodeine).
Morphalgin (with morphine).

DRUG CLASS:

Analgesic (painkiller), NSAID (anti-inflammatory), Anticoagulant (stops blood clotting), Antipyretic (reduces fever).

USES:

Relief of pain, reduction of fever, reduction of inflammation, prevention of blood clots and strokes.

DOSAGE:

Prevention of blood clots and strokes: 75mg to 150mg once a day.
Other uses: 600mg (usually two tablets) every four hours. Maximum 4500mg a day.

FORMS:

Tablets, capsules, soluble tablets, powders.

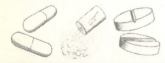

PRECAUTIONS:

Aspirin should not be used in pregnancy (C) unless medically essential. Should be used with caution in breast feeding and children. Not for use in infants, or children under 15 years with a fever.

Do not take if:

☠ suffering from bleeding disorders, peptic ulcer, fluid retention.
• surgery planned in next few days, or recent surgery performed.

SIDE EFFECTS:

Common: Gut irritation, heartburn, nausea.
Unusual: Vomiting, blood in faeces, rash, aggravation of asthma, hay fever, ringing in ears.
Severe but rare (stop medication, consult doctor): Unusual bleeding, asthma.

INTERACTIONS:

Other drugs:
• Anticoagulants, NSAIDs, phenytoin, allopurinol, sodium valproate, sulfonamides, methotrexate, spironolactone.
Herbs:
• Garlic, tamarind.
Other substances:
• Reacts adversely with alcohol.

PRESCRIPTION:

Most forms: No.
Combined with high dose codeine or morphine: Yes.

PBS:

Astrix, Cardiprin, Cartia, Solprin, Spren: Yes.
Asasantin SR: Yes (restricted).
Other forms: No

PERMITTED IN SPORT:

Yes

OVERDOSE:

Adult lethal dose is over 25000mg (about 85 tablets). Symptoms include dizziness, ear noises, deafness, sweating, nausea, vomiting, headache, confusion, fever, rapid breathing, restlessness and coma. If tablets swallowed recently, induce vomiting. Seek medical assistance.

OTHER INFORMATION:

First synthesised in 1899, Aspirin is now one of the most widely used medications in the world.

Atenolol

TRADE NAMES:
Anselol, Antehexal, Atenolol, GenRx Atenolol, Noten, Tenormin, Tensig. Numerous locally produced brands also exist.

DRUG CLASS:
Beta-Blocker.

USES:
High blood pressure, angina, rapid heart rate, irregular heartbeat, paroxysmal atrial tachycardia, heart attack.

DOSAGE:
 One to three tablets a day.

FORMS:
Tablets of 50mg, injection.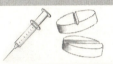

PRECAUTIONS:
Should be used in pregnancy (C) only if medically essential.
Safe to use in breast feeding.
May be used with caution in children.
Use with care if suffering from alcoholism, liver or kidney failure or about to have surgery.

Do not take if:
 suffering from diabetes, asthma, or allergic conditions.
- suffering from heart failure, shock, slow heart rate, or enlarged right heart.
- if undertaking prolonged fast.

SIDE EFFECTS:
Common: Low blood pressure, slow heart rate, cold hands and feet, asthma.
Unusual: Loss of appetite, nausea, diarrhoea, impotence, tiredness, sleeplessness, nightmares, rash, loss of libido, hair loss, noises in ears.
Severe but rare (stop medication, consult doctor): Severe asthma.

INTERACTIONS:
Other drugs:
- Calcium channel blockers, disopyramide, clonidine, adrenaline, other medications for irregular heartbeat, lignocaine, ergotamine, indomethacin, chlorpromazine.

Herbs:
- Goldenseal, guarana, hawthorn, Korean ginseng, liquorice.

PRESCRIPTION:
Yes.

PBS:
Yes.

PERMITTED IN SPORT:
No.

OVERDOSE:
Slow heart rate, low blood pressure, asthma and heart failure may result. Administer activated charcoal or induce vomiting if tablets taken recently. Use Salbutamol or other asthma sprays for difficulty in breathing. Seek medical assistance.

OTHER INFORMATION:
Except for asthmatics, very safe and effective. First developed in 1960s.

See also Carvedilol, Esmolol, Labetalol, Metoprolol, Oxprenolol, Pindolol, Propranolol, Sotalol.

Atorvastatin

TRADE NAME:
Lipitor.

DRUG CLASS:
Hypolipidaemic.

USES:
Lowers blood cholesterol level.

DOSAGE:
 10mg to 40mg once a day.

FORMS:
Tablets (white) of 10mg, 20mg and 40mg.

PRECAUTIONS:
Not to be used in pregnancy, breast feeding or children.
Use with caution in liver and kidney disease.
Regular blood tests to check cholesterol level and liver function advisable.

Do not take if:
 suffering from active liver disease.
- previous adverse effects (eg. muscle pain or weakness) experienced from other medication used to lower cholesterol.

SIDE EFFECTS:
Common: Altered bowel habits (diarrhoea or constipation), indigestion, heartburn, nausea, headache.
Unusual: Belly pain, sleeplessness, rash, itch, muscle and joint pain.
Severe but rare (stop medication, consult doctor): Swelling of face or lips, muscle pain, tingling in hands and feet.

INTERACTIONS:
Other drugs:
- Digoxin, erythromycin, rifampicin, phenytoin, oral contraceptives, immunosuppressives, antifungals, other medications used to lower cholesterol levels.

Herbs:
- Alfalfa, fenugreek, garlic, ginger.

Other substances:
- Alcohol.

PRESCRIPTION:
Yes.

PBS:
Yes.

PERMITTED IN SPORT:
Yes.

OVERDOSE:
Liver and muscle damage possible. Induce vomiting or give activated charcoal if taken recently. Seek medical assistance.

OTHER INFORMATION:
Introduced in 1998 as an additional version of similar drugs. Very effective in lowering cholesterol levels in blood, and may have fewer side effects than other hypolipidaemics. Designed for long term use as it controls high cholesterol but does not cure the problem. Stopping the medication without advice from a doctor may lead to a rapid increase in cholesterol to the pre-treatment level. High cholesterol levels increase the risk of heart attack and stroke.

See also Cholestyramine, Colestipol, Fluvastatin, Gemfibrizol, Nicotinic acid, Pravastatin, Probucol, Simvastatin.

Atovaquone

TRADE NAMES:
Wellvone.
Malarone (with proguanil).

DRUG CLASS:
Antifungal and antimalarial.

USES:
Wellvone: Treatment of specific fungal infections caused by *Pneumocystis carinii* in AIDS patients.
Malarone: Treatment of malaria.

DOSAGE:

Wellvone: Three tablets three times a day.
Malarone: Once a day with food.

FORMS:
Wellvone: Tablets of 250mg – pale yellow.
Malarone: Tablets – pink

PRECAUTIONS:
Use with caution in pregnancy (B2), breast feeding and children.
Use with caution in patients with lung and intestinal diseases.
Malarone must be used with caution if malaria affects brain and in other complicated cases.

SIDE EFFECTS:
Common: Loss of appetite, diarrhoea, nausea, rash, headache, belly pain.
Unusual: Vomiting, fever, sleeplessness, dizziness, muscle pains.

INTERACTIONS:
Other drugs: Metoclopramide, rifampicin, paracetamol, benzodiazepines, aciclovir, morphine, pethidine, codeine, cephalosporins, antidiarrhoeals, laxatives, many other drugs.

PRESCRIPTION:
Yes.

PBS:
Wellvone: Yes (authority required – restricted to certain categories of patients).
Malarone: No (expensive).

PERMITTED IN SPORT:
Yes.

OVERDOSE:
Severe intestinal effects. Seek urgent medical treatment. Vomiting will probably occur spontaneously.

OTHER INFORMATION:
Wellvone introduced in 1997 for treatment of severe complication of AIDS infection. Malarone introduced in 1999.

See also Artemether and Lumefantrine, Chloroquine, Doxycycline, Hydroxychloroquine, Mefloquine, Primaquine, Proguanil, Pyrimethamine, Quinine, Sulfadoxine.

Atropine

TRADE NAMES:
Atropine, Atropt, Minims Atropine.
Atrobel, Donnalix, Donnatab (with hyoscine).
Donnagel (with multiple other medications).
Lomotil, Lofenoxal (with diphenoxylate hydrochloride).

DRUG CLASS:
Mydriatic, Anticholinergic.

USES:
Tablets: Diarrhoea, intestinal cramps, drying of secretions.
Eye drops: Enlargement of pupil.
Injection: Drying of secretions and saliva.

DOSAGE:

Depends on usage. Follow directions on pack or doctor's advice.
Lomotil: One or two tablets four times a day as required for diarrhoea.

FORMS:

Tablets, capsule, mixture, eye drops, injection.

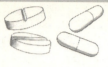

PRECAUTIONS:

Safe in pregnancy and children. Injection and tablets should be used with caution in elderly or debilitated patients.

Do not take:

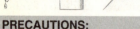 as eye drops if suffering from glaucoma.
- in other forms if suffering from rapid heart rate, heart failure, lung failure or over-active thyroid gland.

SIDE EFFECTS:

Common: Dry mouth, dilated pupils, dry eyes, difficulty in passing urine, rapid heart rate.
Unusual: Flushing, palpitations, constipation, dry skin, rash, drowsiness, vomiting, mood changes.

INTERACTIONS:

Other drugs:
- Additive effect with antihistamines, phenothiazines, and tricyclic antidepressants.

PRESCRIPTION:

Eye drops: No.
Injection: Yes.
Tablets and capsules: Varies with formulation.

PBS:

Eye drops and injections: Yes.
Tablets and capsules: Lomotil, Lofenoxal yes, others no.

PERMITTED IN SPORT:

Yes.

OVERDOSE:

Eye drops: No problem.
Other forms: May be very serious, depending upon dose and form. Seek urgent medical advice.

OTHER INFORMATION:

Widely used for over a century to dry secretions before an operation, to dilate the pupil to aid examination of the eye, and to ease intestinal cramps and diarrhoea. Occurs naturally in certain herbal extracts.

Attapulgite

TRADE NAME:

Diareze (Tablets – with aluminium hydrochloride, pectin; suspension – with simethicone, pectin).

DRUG CLASS:

Antidiarrhoeal.

USES:

Mild diarrhoea.

DOSAGE:

 Adults – 30mLs initially, then 15mLs after each bowel movement.

FORMS:

Tablets, suspension.

PRECAUTIONS:

Probably safe in pregnancy, breast feeding and children over 6 years.

SIDE EFFECTS:

Common: Intestinal discomfort.

INTERACTIONS:

Other drugs:
- May interfere with the absorption of many medications.

PRESCRIPTION:
No.

PBS:
No.

PERMITTED IN SPORT:
Yes.

OVERDOSE:
Constipation and intestinal colic only likely effects.
See also Loperamide.

Auranofin
(Gold)

TRADE NAME:
Ridaura.

DRUG CLASS:
Antirheumatic.

USES:
Rheumatoid arthritis.

DOSAGE:
 One tablet two or three times a day with food.

FORMS:
Tablets of 3mg (yellow).

PRECAUTIONS:
Should be used with caution in pregnancy (B3), breast feeding and children.
Use with caution in liver and kidney disease, inflammatory bowel disease. Lower doses required in elderly.
Regular blood and urine tests required to assess kidney and liver function, blood cells and effectiveness of treatment.

Do not take if:
 suffering from severe diabetes, severe kidney or liver disease, severe high blood pressure, heart failure, severe dermatitis, bone marrow damage, systemic lupus erythematosus, Sjögren syndrome, eczema, blood diseases or colitis.

SIDE EFFECTS:
Common: Dermatitis, itch, mouth ulcers, flushing, fainting.
Unusual: Sweating, dizziness, weakness, feeling unwell, nausea, diarrhoea, light sensitive skin, eye damage.
Severe but rare (stop medication, consult doctor): Severe rash, unusual bleeding or bruising.

INTERACTIONS:
Other drugs:
- Phenylbutazone, hydroxychloroquine, immunosuppressives, warfarin, dextropropoxyphene, clonidine, penicillamine, antimalarials, cytotoxics, phenylbutazone, oxphenbutazone, levamisole, high dose steroids.

PRESCRIPTION:
Yes.

PBS:
Yes.

PERMITTED IN SPORT:
Yes.

OTHER INFORMATION:
An unusual but remarkably effective treatment that has been used for over 30 years. Careful monitoring of blood tests and skin reactions essential. Gold is not addictive when swallowed or injected, only when collected!
See also Sodium aurothiomalate.

Aurothiomalate
See Sodium aurothiomalate.

Azatadine
See ANTIHISTAMINES, SEDATING.

Azathioprine

TRADE NAMES:
Azahexal, Azamun, GenRx Azathioprine, Imuran, Thioprine.

DRUG CLASS:
Immunomodifier.

USES:
Prevents rejection of transplanted organ, autoimmune diseases.

DOSAGE:
 Complex. Must be determined individually for each patient by doctor.

FORMS:
Tablets of 25mg and 50mg, injection.

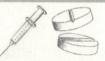

PRECAUTIONS:
Not to be used in pregnancy (D) unless mother's life at risk. Breast feeding must be ceased before use. May be used with caution in children.
Regular blood tests to monitor response essential.
Use with caution in liver and kidney disease.
Do not take if:
 undertaking dental procedures without consulting doctor.
- having live virus vaccine (eg. Sabin for polio).

SIDE EFFECTS:
Very complex. Wide range of side effects may occur, and must be discussed with doctor before use of medication. Report any unusual effects to doctor.

INTERACTIONS:
Other drugs:
- Allopurinol, oxypurinol, thiopurinol, cancer-treating medications, captopril, many others.

Other substances:
- Reacts with alcohol.

PRESCRIPTION:
Yes.

PBS:
Yes.

PERMITTED IN SPORT:
Yes.

OVERDOSE:
May cause damage to immune system which leads to multiple infections, ulceration of mouth and throat, bruising and bleeding. Seek medical assistance.

OTHER INFORMATION:
Potent medication that must be finely balanced to prevent rejection of donated organ but allow protection of body against infection.

Azelaic acid
See KERATOLYTICS.

Azelastine

TRADE NAME:
Azep.

DRUG CLASS:
Antihistamine.

USES:
Hay fever.

DOSAGE:
 One spray into each nostril twice a day.

FORMS:
Nasal spray.

PRECAUTIONS:
May be used with caution in pregnancy (B3), breast feeding and and children under 5 years.
Use with caution in elderly.

SIDE EFFECTS:
Common: Bad taste in mouth (bend head forward when spraying to reduce this effect).
Unusual: Nose irritation.

INTERACTIONS:
Other drugs:
- Sedatives.

Other substances:
- Alcohol is theoretically (but probably not practically) a problem.

PRESCRIPTION:
No.

PBS:
No.

PERMITTED IN SPORT:
Yes.

OVERDOSE:
May cause convulsions, hallucinations, delirium, anxiety, muscle spasms, rapid heart rate, flushing, dry skin, dry mouth and coma if contents of bottle drunk. First aid involves inducing vomiting and seeking urgent medical attention.

OTHER INFORMATION:
Introduced in 2000 as a way of controlling hay fever with minimal side effects as occurs with other antihistamines that are usually swallowed.
See also **ANTIHISTAMINES, SEDATING**.

Azidothymidine
See Zidovudine.

Azithromycin

TRADE NAME:
Zithromax.

DRUG CLASS:
Macrolide antibiotic.

USES:
Infections caused by susceptible bacteria (eg. bronchitis, sinusitis, throat infection), genital or eye Chlamydia infections.

DOSAGE:

1000mg taken once, away from meals. Longer courses sometimes necessary.

FORMS:
Tablets (white) of 500mg and 600mg, suspension.

PRECAUTIONS:
Use with care in pregnancy (B1) and breast feeding. Safe for children.
Lower doses necessary in elderly and debilitated.
Use with caution in severe pneumonia, liver and kidney disease.

SIDE EFFECTS:
Common: Nausea, diarrhoea, belly pains.
Unusual: Vomiting, palpitations, dizziness, vaginal thrush, rash, headache.

INTERACTIONS:
Other drugs:
- Theophylline, antacids, cyclosporin, digoxin, zidovudine, astemizole, warfarin.

PRESCRIPTION:
Yes.

PBS:
Yes (restricted).

PERMITTED IN SPORT:
Yes.

OVERDOSE:
Exacerbation of side effects likely. Induce vomiting if medication taken recently. Seek medical assistance.

OTHER INFORMATION:
Introduced in 1995 to treat difficult infections.

AZT
See Zidovudine.

Aztreonam

TRADE NAME:
Azactam.

DRUG CLASS:
Antibiotic.

USES:
Severe bacterial infections.

DOSAGE:

As determined by doctor for each individual patient.

FORMS:
Injection.

PRECAUTIONS:
Relatively safe in pregnancy (B1), breast feeding and children.
Use caution in use with severe kidney and liver disease.
Use caution in use with premature infants and elderly.
Must be used with caution in gynaecological infections.

SIDE EFFECTS:
Common: Minimal.
Unusual: Development of resistant infections.
Severe but rare (stop medication, consult doctor): Bowel inflammation (pseudomembranous colitis).

INTERACTIONS:
Other drugs:
- Frusemide.

PRESCRIPTION:
Yes.

PBS:
No (expensive).

PERMITTED IN SPORT:
Yes.

OVERDOSE:
Always given by infusion or injection under strict medical supervision.

OTHER INFORMATION:
Only used after other antibiotics have been proved to be ineffective.

Medications

Bacitracin

TRADE NAMES:
Available in Australia only in combination with other medications.
Cicatrin, Nemdyn (with neomycin).
Neosporin (with neomycin and polymyxin B).

DRUG CLASS:
Antibiotic.

USES:
Infections of skin and ear.

DOSAGE:
 Apply three or four times a day.

FORMS:
Ointment, powder, ear ointment, eye ointment.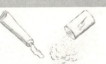

PRECAUTIONS:
Bacitracin used on the skin or in the ear is safe in pregnancy, breast feeding and children, but the medications with which it is combined must not be taken internally during pregnancy.
Do not use on large areas that are weeping or lacking in good quality skin.
Not designed for long term use.

SIDE EFFECTS:
Common: Skin irritation.

INTERACTIONS:
None significant.

PRESCRIPTION:
Yes.

PBS:
Neosporin eye ointment: Yes.
Others: No.

PERMITTED IN SPORT:
Yes.

Baclofen

TRADE NAMES:
Baclo, Baclohexal, Clofen, DBL Baclofen, GenRx Baclofen, Lioresal.

DRUG CLASS:
Muscle relaxant.

USES:
Muscle spasm in multiple sclerosis, muscle spasm in spinal injury, muscle spasm in cerebral palsy, bladder spasm.

DOSAGE:
 5mg to 25mg three times a day.

FORMS:
Tablets of 10mg and 25mg,
spinal injection.
Injection for use
in spinal cord.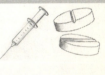

PRECAUTIONS:
Use in pregnancy (B3) only if medically essential. Use with caution in breast feeding and children.
Use with caution in psychiatric disorders, peptic ulcer, heart disease, stroke, lung disease, liver or kidney disease, diabetes, difficulty in passing urine.
Lower doses required in elderly.
Do not stop suddenly, but reduce dosage slowly.

Medications

Do not take if:
 suffering from epilepsy or brain injury.

SIDE EFFECTS:
Common: Dose related. Sedation, drowsiness, nausea
Unusual: Dry mouth, vomiting, confusion, dizziness, headache, sleeplessness, mood changes.
Severe but rare (stop medication, consult doctor): Convulsions.

INTERACTIONS:
Other drugs:
- Tricyclics, sedatives, medications for lowering blood pressure, L-dopa, diazepam.

Other substances:
- Reacts with alcohol to increase sedation.

PRESCRIPTION:
Yes.

PBS:
Yes.

PERMITTED IN SPORT:
Yes.

OVERDOSE:
Drowsiness, difficulty in breathing, confusion, hallucinations, slow heart rate, coma and rarely death may occur. Administer or induce vomiting if medication taken recently and patient alert. Seek urgent medical attention.

OTHER INFORMATION:
Used successfully in a number of difficult conditions that cause distressing muscle spasms.

BARBITURATES

TRADE and GENERIC NAMES:
Amytal Sodium, Neur-Amyl (Amylobarbitone).
Phenobarb (Phenobarbitone).
Prominal (Methylphenobarbitone).

DRUG CLASS:
Sedative/Hypnotic, Anticonvulsant.

USES:
Sedation, insomnia (sleeplessness), epilepsy (phenobarbitone).

DOSAGE:
 One or two tablets one to three times a day.

FORMS:
Tablets, injection.
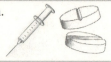

PRECAUTIONS:
Should not be taken in pregnancy (D), particularly early pregnancy, unless medically essential (eg. for uncontrolled epilepsy). May be used in breast feeding and children.
Lower doses required in elderly.
Should not be stopped suddenly if used for long period constantly, but dose should be reduced gradually. Use intermittently if possible.

Do not take if:
 suffering from poor lung function, porphyria, severe liver or kidney disease, uncontrolled pain.
- likely to develop a drug dependency.
- history of alcohol or drug abuse.
- operating machinery, driving a vehicle, or undertaking tasks that require concentration and alertness.

SIDE EFFECTS:
Common: Drowsiness, incoordination, slow breathing, hangover sensation, slow heart rate, low blood pressure, nausea,

diarrhoea, dependence on drug.
Unusual: Memory defects, dizziness, paradoxical excitement, nightmares, hallucinations, constipation, vomiting, headache.
Severe but rare (stop medication, consult doctor): Loss of consciousness.

INTERACTIONS:
Other drugs:
- Griseofulvin, folic acid, pethidine, morphine, phenytoin, rifampicin, oral contraceptives, chlorpromazine, tricyclic antidepressants, warfarin, antihistamines, MAOI.

Herbs:
- Valerian, kava kava, goldenseal, valerian, St John's wort.

Other substances:
- Reacts with alcohol to cause sedation.

PRESCRIPTION:
Yes.

PBS:
Yes (restricted to use in epilepsy).

PERMITTED IN SPORT:
Yes.

OVERDOSE:
Very serious. Low blood pressure, coma, cessation of breathing and death may occur. Induce vomiting if tablets taken recently. Seek urgent medical assistance.

OTHER INFORMATION:
Used for many decades to sedate, calm and ease sleeplessness. Dependency problem limits its use today mainly to the control of some forms of epilepsy.

See also BENZODIAZEPINES, Carbamazepine, Clonazepam, Ethosuximide, Gabapentin, Lamotrigine, Levetiracetam, Oxcarbazepine, Phenytoin, Primidone, Sodium valproate, Sulthiame, Tiagabine, Topiramate, Vigabatrin.

BCG vaccine
(Tuberculosis vaccine)

TRADE NAMES:
BCG Vaccine, Immucyst, Oncotice.

DRUG CLASS:
Vaccine.

USES:
BCG Vaccine: Prevention of tuberculosis (TB).
Immucyst, Oncotice: Treatment of bladder cancer.

DOSAGE:

Single vaccination (skin scratch, not injection).
Intravenous infusion for bladder cancer.

FORMS:
Injection.

PRECAUTIONS:
Vaccination during pregnancy (B2) is not recommended, but unintentional or necessary vaccination is unlikely to have any adverse effects. May be used safely in breast feeding, children and infants. Prevent vaccination fluid from being inhaled.
Use with caution near any skin disorder.
Do not take if:
 suffering from significant illness or reduced immunity.

SIDE EFFECTS:
Common: Skin irritation at site of vaccination.

INTERACTIONS:
Other drugs:
- Other vaccines.

PRESCRIPTION:
Yes.

Medications

PBS:
Vaccine: Available only through authorised State Government offices and doctors.
For bladder cancer: Yes.

PERMITTED IN SPORT:
Yes.

OTHER INFORMATION:
Routine vaccine use in Australia is restricted to immigrants and Aboriginal communities. Widely used in poorer countries. Recently found to also assist in the treatment of bladder cancer, and used in a different concentration for this purpose.

Beclomethasone dipropionate

TRADE NAMES:
Aldecin, Becloforte, Beconase, Becotide, Qvar, Respocort.

DRUG CLASS:
Corticosteroid.

USES:
Prevention of asthma, prevention of hay fever.

DOSAGE:

Asthma: One or two inhalations, two to four times a day.
Nasal spray: One spray in each nostril twice a day.

FORMS:
Inhaler, autohaler, rotacaps, nebuliser solution, nasal spray.

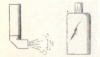

PRECAUTIONS:
Use with caution in pregnancy (B3), breast feeding and children.
Use with caution in lung, nose or throat infection and tuberculosis.
Lung function should be checked regularly to ensure adequate dose is received.

SIDE EFFECTS:
Common: Fungal (thrush) infections of mouth, sore throat and mouth, dry mouth.
Unusual: Hoarseness, unusual bleeding and bruising, slowed growth.

INTERACTIONS:
None significant

PRESCRIPTION:
Asthma sprays: Yes.
Nose sprays: Depends on concentration of solution.

PBS:
Asthma sprays: Yes.
Nose sprays: No.

PERMITTED IN SPORT:
Yes.

OVERDOSE:
Unlikely to have any serious effects.

OTHER INFORMATION:
Beclomethasone is the main medication used to prevent asthma and is designed for long term use. Very safe and effective. Does not cause dependence or addiction. Qvar is in the form of microfine aerosol that penetrates further into the lungs, so lower doses can be used.
See also Budesonide, Fluticasone propianate.

Bendrofluazide
See THIAZIDE DIURETICS.

Benserazide
See LEVODOPA COMPOUNDS.

Benzalkonium chloride

TRADE NAMES:
Bepanthen, Dettol Antiseptic Spray, Ionil Rinse.
Mycil Healthy Feet (with tolnaftate).
Oilatum Plus, QV Flare Up Oil (with triclosan and paraffin).
Ora-Sed Jel (with choline salicylate).
Paxyl (with lignocaine).
Solyptol Cream (with allantoin).
Virasolve (with idoxuridine and lignocaine).

DRUG CLASS:
Antiseptic.

USES:
Minor skin and mouth infections.

DOSAGE:
 Apply several times a day as required.

FORMS:
Cream, gel, liquid, ointment, shampoo, powder, spray.

PRECAUTIONS:
Safe to use in pregnancy, breast feeding and children.
Not to be swallowed. Causes eye irritation.

SIDE EFFECTS:
Minimal.

INTERACTIONS:
None significant.

PRESCRIPTION:
No.

PBS:
No.

PERMITTED IN SPORT:
Yes.

OVERDOSE:
Nausea, stomach cramps and diarrhoea may occur.

OTHER INFORMATION:
Safe and effective antiseptic that is widely used.

Benzathine penicillin

TRADE NAME:
Bicillin L-A.

DRUG CLASS:
Penicillin antibiotic.

USES:
Treatment of infections caused by susceptible bacteria.

DOSAGE:
 One injection every six to 12 hours.

FORMS:
Injection.

PRECAUTIONS:
Safe in pregnancy (A), children and breast feeding.
Use with caution in kidney failure and heart failure.

Do not take if:
 allergic to penicillin.

- suffering from glandular fever.

SIDE EFFECTS:
Common: Minimal.
Unusual: Rash, convulsions.

INTERACTIONS:
Nil.

Medications

PRESCRIPTION:
Yes.

PBS:.
Yes

PERMITTED IN SPORT:
Yes.

OVERDOSE:
No serious effects expected.

See also Amoxycillin, Ampicillin, Benzylpenicillin, Dicloxacillin, Flucloxacillin, Phenoxymethyl penicillin, Procaine penicillin, Ticarcillin.

Benzhexol

TRADE NAME:
Artane.

DRUG CLASS:
Antiparkinsonian.

USES:
Parkinson's disease, some other movement disorders.

DOSAGE:
 Slowly increase dosage under medical supervision until adequate response obtained.

FORMS:
Tablets (white) of 2mg and 5mg.

PRECAUTIONS:
Use with caution in pregnancy (B1) and breast feeding.
Use with caution in glaucoma, heart disease, kidney or liver disease, high blood pressure, enlarged prostate gland.
Use with caution in elderly.
Eye pressure should be checked before use.

SIDE EFFECTS:
Common: Dry mouth, blurred vision, nausea, dizziness, rapid heart rate, constipation.
Unusual: Salivary gland disease, rash, constipation, hallucinations.

INTERACTIONS:
None significant.

PRESCRIPTION:
Yes.

PBS:
Yes.

PERMITTED IN SPORT:
Yes.

OVERDOSE:
Serious. Seek urgent medical attention. Induce vomiting or give activated charcoal if swallowed recently.

Benzocaine

See ANAESTHETICS, LOCAL.

BENZODIAZEPINES

DISCUSSION:
Benzodiazepines all sedate and may cause dependency, and they also relieve anxiety, but the degree of sedation and dependency varies dramatically from one drug to another and one patient to another. Dependency should not be a problem unless the drugs are used inappropriately. Some of these drugs (eg. diazepam) can also be used to relax muscle spasm and control convulsions. They should be stopped slowly, with a gradual reduction in dosage if they have been used for a long time. They will increase the effects of alcohol, and care should be taken with driving and using machinery while taking them.

See Alprazolam, Bromazepam, Buspirone, Clobazam, Diazepam, Lorazepam, Oxazepam.

Benzoic acid
See KERATOLYTICS.

Benzoyl peroxide
See KERATOLYTICS.

Benztropine

TRADE NAMES:
Benztrop, Cogentin.

DRUG CLASS:
Antiparkinsonian.

USES:
Parkinsonism.

DOSAGE:

Individualised dose depending on response. Must be closely monitored by doctor.

FORMS:
Tablets (white) of 0.5mg and 2mg, injection.
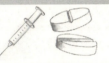

PRECAUTIONS:
Use with caution in pregnancy (B2) and breast feeding. Not for use in children under 3 years.
Use with caution with enlarged prostate gland, rapid heart rate, psychiatric conditions, glaucoma.

SIDE EFFECTS:
Common: Rapid heart rate, constipation, dry mouth, nausea, confusion, blurred vision.
Unusual: Vomiting, hallucinations, difficulty passing urine, rash.

INTERACTIONS:
Other drugs:
- Phenothiazines, tricyclic antidepressants, haloperidol.

PRESCRIPTION:
Yes.

PBS:
Yes.

PERMITTED IN SPORT:
Yes.

OVERDOSE:
Confusion, nervousness, psychiatric disturbances, dizziness, weakness, rapid heart rate, incoordination, palpitations and vomiting may occur. Administer activated charcoal or induce vomiting if medication taken recently. Seek medical assistance.

Benzydamine hydrochloride

TRADE NAMES:
Difflam Solution, Difflam Anti-inflammatory Throat Spray, Difflam Cream, Difflam Gel.
Difflam Mouth Gel, Difflam Anti-inflammatory Lozenges, Difflam Sugar-free Lozenges (with cetylpyridinium).
Difflam Anti-inflammatory Cough Lozenges (with pholcodine, cetylpyridinium, menthol).
Difflam-C Anti-inflammatory Antiseptic Solution (with chlorhexidine).
Logicin Rapid Relief Lozenges (with lignocaine and other ingredients).

DRUG CLASS:
Topical anti-inflammatory.

USES:
Reduces inflammation and pain.

DOSAGE:

Varies with form. Follow directions on packaging.

FORMS:
Lozenges, gel, cream, gargle, spray, solution.

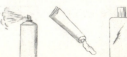

PRECAUTIONS:
Safe in pregnancy, breast feeding and children.
Avoid eyes with all preparations.
Cream and gel should not be used in mouth, nose, anus and vagina.
Use with caution in severe liver disease.

SIDE EFFECTS:
Common: Minimal.
Unusual: Skin reaction.

INTERACTIONS:
None significant.

PRESCRIPTION:
No.

PBS:
No.

PERMITTED IN SPORT:
Yes.

OVERDOSE:
Unlikely to be a problem.

OTHER INFORMATION:
Does not cause addiction or dependence.

Benzyl benzoate

TRADE NAMES:
Ascabiol, Benzemul.

DRUG CLASS:
Antiparasitic.

USES:
Scabies, head and body lice.

DOSAGE:

Apply to small area of skin for 10 minutes before using to test for sensitivity.
Apply to whole body from neck down after a hot bath. Remove by washing after one day. Repeat after five days. More applications may be necessary for lice.

FORMS:
Lotion.

PRECAUTIONS:
Use with caution in pregnancy (B2). Safe for use in breast feeding. Dilute for use in children.
Avoid use on face, head and around vagina, head of penis and anus.

SIDE EFFECTS:
Common: Skin irritation.
Unusual: Skin burning.

INTERACTIONS:
None significant.

PRESCRIPTION:
No.

PBS:
Ascabiol: No
Benzemul: Yes.

PERMITTED IN SPORT:
Yes.

OVERDOSE:
If swallowed, administer activated charcoal or induce vomiting if medication taken recently. May cause convulsions. Seek urgent medical advice.

OTHER INFORMATION:
Commonly used and effective treatment. All members of family must be treated at same time. Change and wash all bed linen and clothing in hot water with each treatment.

See also Maldison, Permethrin, Pyrethrins.

Benzylpenicillin

TRADE NAMES:
BenPen.

DRUG CLASS:
Penicillin antibiotic.

USES:
Treatment of infections caused by susceptible bacteria.

DOSAGE:

One injection every six hours or by continuous drip infusion.

FORMS:
Injection.

PRECAUTIONS:
Safe in pregnancy (A), children and breast feeding.
Use with caution in kidney failure and heart failure.
Do not take if:
 allergic to penicillin.
- suffering from glandular fever.

SIDE EFFECTS:
Common: Minimal.
Unusual: Rash, convulsions.

INTERACTIONS:
None significant.

PRESCRIPTION:
Yes.

PBS:
Yes.

PERMITTED IN SPORT:
Yes.

OVERDOSE:
No serious effects expected.

See Amoxycillin, Ampicillin, Benzathine penicillin, Dicloxacillin, Flucloxacillin, Phenoxymethyl penicillin, Piperacillin, Procaine penicillin, Ticarcillin.

Berberine hydrochloride

TRADE NAME:
Murine.

USES:
Eye irritation.

DOSAGE:

One or two drops as necessary.

FORMS:
Eye drops.

PRECAUTIONS:
Safe in pregnancy and breast feeding.
Do not use if:
wearing soft contact lenses.

SIDE EFFECTS:
None significant.

INTERACTIONS:
None significant.

PRESCRIPTION:
No.

PBS:
No.

PERMITTED IN SPORT:
Yes.

OVERDOSE:
Not serious.

BETA-2 AGONISTS
(ß2 AGONISTS)

DISCUSSION:
The bronchi are the tubes in the lung that contain air. Bronchodilators open these tubes to their maximum extent to allow more air to enter and leave the lungs. The most common bronchodilators are the beta-2 agonists. They are available as pressure pack sprays, nebuliser additives, various inhalers, mixtures, tablets and injections. They act very rapidly if inhaled or injected but more slowly, and with more side effects, if taken as a mixture or tablet. Some forms have a very long action and can act effectively as both a preventer and a treatment.

See Fenoterol, Salbutamol, Salmeterol, Terbutaline.

BETA BLOCKERS
(ß ADRENERGIC BLOCKING AGENTS)

DISCUSSION:
High blood pressure, migraine, irregular heartbeat, stage fright, prevention of heart attack, exam nerves, angina, over-active thyroid gland, tremors and glaucoma – all these diseases can be controlled, or treated, by the amazingly versatile group of drugs called beta blockers. Some beta blockers are very specific for particular diseases (eg. timolol is used only in eye drop form for glaucoma; atenolol acts mainly on the heart), but others (eg. propranolol) can act in virtually all areas.

Beta receptors are present on certain nerves in the body, and blocking the action of these nerves with beta blockers produces the desired effects. Because they can control a fine tremor and anxiety over performance, these drugs are banned in the Olympic and Commonwealth Games, as they would give athletes such as archers and shooters an unfair advantage. Beta blockers are generally very safe medications but cannot be used in asthmatics, and must be used with care in diabetics.

See Atenolol, Betaxolol, Bisoprolol, Carvedilol, Esmolol, Labetalol, Levobunolol, Metoprolol, Oxprenolol, Pindolol, Propranolol, Sotalol, Timolol.

Betacarotene
(Vitamin A)

TRADE NAMES:
A form of vitamin A (retinol is another form) found in numerous vitamin and mineral preparations, as well as soothing and healing creams and lotions.

DRUG CLASS:
Vitamin.

USES:
Vitamin A deficiency, malnutrition, poor diet, soothing agent in creams for minor burns.

DOSAGE:

Recommended daily allowance: 2500 International Units a day.

FORMS:
Capsules, tablets, mixture, lotion, cream.

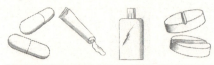

PRECAUTIONS:
Must not be used in pregnancy (D) as high doses may cause birth defects. May be used in breast feeding and with caution in children. Skin preparations safe in pregnancy.
Do not exceed recommended dose.
Use with caution in Vitamin K deficiency.

SIDE EFFECTS:
Common: Minimal.
Severe but rare (stop medication, consult doctor): Yellow skin, particularly of palms and soles.

INTERACTIONS:
None significant.

PRESCRIPTION:
No.

PBS:
No.

PERMITTED IN SPORT:
Yes.

OVERDOSE:
Chronic overdosage will lead to carotenaemia in which excess Betacarotene is deposited in skin (causes it to turn yellow) and may cause damage to organs.

OTHER INFORMATION:
Fat soluble vitamin. Dangerous in pregnancy and overdose. Remember, vitamins are merely chemicals that are essential for the functioning of the body, and if taken to excess, act as a drug.
See also Cod liver oil, Retinols.

Betahistine

TRADE NAME:
Serc.

DRUG CLASS:
Vasodilator.

USES:
Ménière's syndrome (dizziness, nausea, vomiting, noises in ears), some forms of poor hearing.

DOSAGE:

Two tablets three or four times a day.

FORMS:
Tablet of 4mg (white).

PRECAUTIONS:
Should not be used in pregnancy, breast feeding or children.

Do not take if:
 suffering from phaeochromocytoma, asthma, peptic ulcer.

SIDE EFFECTS:
Common: Minimal
Unusual: Rash, diarrhoea, dizziness, headache, nausea, sleeplessness.

INTERACTIONS:
None significant.

PRESCRIPTION:
Yes.

PBS:
No.

PERMITTED IN SPORT:
Yes.

OVERDOSE:
No serious effects

See also Diazoxide, Guanethidine, Nicotinic Acid, Phenoxybenzamine.

Betaine

TRADE NAME:
Cystadane.

DRUG CLASS:
Detoxifying agent.

USES:
Treatment of the rare metabolic condition homocystinuria.

DOSAGE:

3 grams twice daily dissolved in 150mLs water.

FORMS:
Powder.

PRECAUTIONS:
Not to be used in pregnancy (C) or breast feeding.
SIDE EFFECTS:
Common: Nausea, diarrhoea.
INTERACTIONS:
Other drugs:
- Affects the absorption of all other medications taken at the same time.
PRESCRIPTION:
No.
PBS:
No.
PERMITTED IN SPORT:
Yes.
OVERDOSE:
Significant diarrhoea only likely effect.

Betamethasone
TRADE NAMES:
Antroquoril, Betnovate, Celestone-V, Celestone-M (Betamethasone valerate).
Celestone Chronodose (Betamethasone acetate and betamethasone sodium phosphate).
Celestone-VG (Betamethasone valerate with gentamicin).
Diprosone, Eleuphrat (Betamethasone dipropionate).
DRUG CLASS:
Corticosteroid.
USES:
Creams and lotions: Severe inflammation of skin (eczema, dermatitis etc.).
Injection: Severe asthma, rheumatoid and other forms of severe arthritis, autoimmune diseases (eg. Sjögren Syndrome), severe allergy reactions, and other severe and chronic inflammatory diseases.

DOSAGE:

Creams, ointments: Apply two or three times a day.
Lotions: Apply once or twice a day.
FORMS:
Cream, ointment, gel, lotion, injection.

PRECAUTIONS:
Injection should be used in pregnancy (C), breast feeding and children only on specific medical advice.
Skin preparations safe in pregnancy (A), breast feeding and children over 3 years.
Use injections with caution if under stress, and in patients with under-active thyroid gland, liver disease, diverticulitis, high blood pressure, myasthenia gravis or kidney disease.
Avoid eyes with all forms.
Use for shortest period of time possible.
Do not use if:
 suffering from any form of infection, peptic ulcer, or osteoporosis.
- having a vaccination
SIDE EFFECTS:
Common: Skin preparations – minimal. Injection may cause bloating, weight gain, rashes and intestinal disturbanccs.
Unusual: Skin preparations – thinning of skin, premature ageing, itching, scarring of skin.
Injection – Biochemical disturbances of blood, muscle weakness, bone weakness, impaired wound healing, skin thinning, tendon weakness, peptic ulcers, gullet ulcers, bruising, increased sweating, loss of fat under skin, premature ageing, excess facial hair growth in women, pigmentation of skin and nails, acne, convulsions, headaches, dizziness, growth suppression in children, aggravation of diabetes, worsening of infections, cataracts, aggravation of glaucoma, blood

clots in veins and sleeplessness.
Most significant side effects occur only with prolonged use of injections.
Severe but rare (stop medication, consult doctor): Any significant side effect should be reported to a doctor immediately.

INTERACTIONS:
Other drugs:
- Injections may be affected by oral contraceptives, barbiturates, phenytoin and rifampicin.

PRESCRIPTION:
Yes.

PBS:
Yes.

PERMITTED IN SPORT:
Yes.

OVERDOSE:
Medical treatment is required. Serious effects and death rare.

OTHER INFORMATION:
Extremely effective and useful medication if used correctly. Lowest dose and shortest possible course should be used. Not addictive.

See also Desonide, Hydrocortisone, Methylprednisolone, Mometasone, Triamcinolone.

Betaxolol

TRADE NAMES:
Betoptic, Betoquin.

DRUG CLASS:
Beta blocker.

USES:
Glaucoma.

DOSAGE:

One drop twice a day.

FORMS:
Eye drops.

PRECAUTIONS:
Should be used with caution in pregnancy (C), but eye drops unlikely to cause problems.
Safe to use in breast feeding.
May be used with caution in children.
Use with care if suffering from alcoholism, liver or kidney failure or about to have surgery.
Use with caution with enlarged right heart, diabetes, asthma, or allergic conditions.

Do not take if:
 suffering from heart failure, slow heart rate.

SIDE EFFECTS:
Common: Low blood pressure, slow heart rate, burning eyes, stinging, asthma.
Severe but rare (stop medication, consult doctor): Severe asthma.

INTERACTIONS:
Other drugs:
- Calcium channel blockers, disopyramide, clonidine, adrenaline, other medications for irregular heartbeat, lignocaine, ergotamine, indomethacin, chlorpromazine, beta blocker tablets.

PRESCRIPTION:
Yes.

PBS:
Yes.

PERMITTED IN SPORT:
Yes.

OVERDOSE:
Unlikely to be serious effects if eye drops swallowed.

See also Bimatoprost, Levobunolol, Timolol.

Bethanechol

TRADE NAMES:
Urocarb.

USES:
Inability to pass urine, reflux of stomach contents in children.

DOSAGE:

One to five tablets, three or four times a day.

FORMS:
Tablets of 10mg (pink).

PRECAUTIONS:
Not for use in pregnancy (B2).
Use with caution if taking blood pressure medication.
Do not take if:
suffering from bowel obstruction, over-active thyroid gland, asthma, peptic ulcer, epilepsy, slow heart rate, low blood pressure, heart failure or urinary tract infection.

SIDE EFFECTS:
Common: Discomfort in the belly, excess production of saliva, flushing of skin, sweating.
Unusual: Tiredness, headache, diarrhoea, nausea, belching.
Severe but rare (stop medication, consult doctor): Severe belly pain, asthma attack.

INTERACTIONS:
None significant.

PRESCRIPTION:
Yes.

PBS:
Yes.

PERMITTED IN SPORT:
Yes.

Bicalutamide

OVERDOSE:
Atropine is a specific antidote. Seek medical assistance.

TRADE NAME:
Cosudex.

DRUG CLASS:
Antineoplastic.

USES:
Severe cancer of the prostate gland.

DOSAGE:

One tablet a day.

FORMS:
Tablets of 50mg (white).

PRECAUTIONS:
Not to be used in women or children.
Use with caution in liver disease.

SIDE EFFECTS:
Common: Hot flushes, itchy skin, breast enlargement and tenderness, nausea, diarrhoea, tiredness.
Unusual: Liver damage, vomiting, depression, hair loss, poor libido, blood in urine.

INTERACTIONS:
Other drugs:
- Warfarin, astemizole, cisapride, midazolam, calcium channel blockers, cyclosporin, antivirals, carbamazepine, quinidine, cimetidine, ketoconazole.

PRESCRIPTION:
Yes.

PBS:
Yes (restricted to some patients with prostate cancer).

Medications

PERMITTED IN SPORT:
Yes.

OVERDOSE:
Serious. Seek urgent medical attention.

OTHER INFORMATION:
Introduced in 1997 to treat cases of prostate cancer that are not responding to other treatment.

Bicarbonates

See ANTACIDS.

Bifonazole

TRADE NAMES:
Canesten Once Daily Bifonazole, Mycospor.

DRUG CLASS:
Antifungal.

USES:
Fungal infections of skin (eg. tinea, ringworm).

DOSAGE:

Apply once a day at bedtime for two to four weeks.

FORMS:
Cream.

PRECAUTIONS:
Use with caution in pregnancy (B3) and breast feeding. Safe to use in children. Avoid using in eye, nostrils, mouth, vagina and anus.

SIDE EFFECTS:
Common: Redness, burning, itch.
Unusual: Irritation, scaling.

INTERACTIONS:
None significant.

PRESCRIPTION:
No.

PBS:
No.

PERMITTED IN SPORT:
Yes.

Bimatoprost

TRADE NAME:
Lumigan.

DRUG CLASS:
Beta blocker.

USES:
Glaucoma.

DOSAGE:

One drop in affected eye once a day. Apply pressure to inner corner of eye (tear duct) immediately after use. Wait five minutes before using in other eye if necessary.

FORMS:
Eye drops.

PRECAUTIONS:
Use with caution in pregnancy (B3).
Not for use in children.
Use with caution in severe lung, liver and kidney disease.
Do not use with contact lenses.
Do not take if:
 breast feeding.
• under other circumstances.

SIDE EFFECTS:
Common: Eyelid darkening, increased eyelash growth, pigment formation in iris (coloured part of eye).
Unusual: Red eye, itchy eye, tiredness, headache.

Severe but rare (stop medication, consult doctor): Slow heart rate, asthma attack.

INTERACTIONS:
None.

PRESCRIPTION:
Yes.

PBS:
No.

PERMITTED IN SPORT:
Yes.

OVERDOSE:
Unlikely to be serious effects if eye drops swallowed.

OTHER INFORMATION:
Introduced in 2002 as an advance in the treatment of glaucoma.
See also Betaxolol, Brimonidine tartrate, Brinzolamide, Pilocarpine, Timolol.

Bioallethrin

TRADE NAME:
Only available in Australia in combination with Piperonyl butoxide.
Paralice (with piperonyl butoxide).

DRUG CLASS:
Antiparasitic

USES:
Head lice.

OTHER INFORMATION:
See Piperonyl butoxide entry for further information.

Biotin
(Vitamin H)

TRADE NAMES:
A large number of preparations include biotin (vitamin H) alone or in combination with other vitamins and minerals.

DRUG CLASS:
Vitamin.

USES:
No specific medical use.

DOSAGE:

Recommended daily allowance: 100 to 200µg per day.

FORMS:
Tablets, capsules, mixture.

PRECAUTIONS:
Safe in pregnancy, breast feeding and children.
Do not take in high doses or for prolonged periods of time.

SIDE EFFECTS:
Minimal.

INTERACTIONS:
None significant.

PRESCRIPTION:
No.

PBS:
No.

PERMITTED IN SPORT:
Yes.

OVERDOSE:
Unlikely to have serious adverse effects.

OTHER INFORMATION:
Remember, vitamins are merely chemicals that are essential for the functioning of the body, and if taken to excess, act as a drug.

Biperiden

TRADE NAME:
Akineton.

DRUG CLASS:
Antiparkinsonian.

USES:
Parkinson's disease, night time leg cramps, head injuries, trigeminal neuralgia, some movement disorders.

DOSAGE:

Night time leg cramps: One or two tablets at night.
Other conditions: Half to two tablets three or four times a day.

FORMS:
Tablets of 2mg (white).

PRECAUTIONS:
Use with caution in pregnancy (B2) and breast feeding.
Use with caution in prostate gland disease, rapid heart rate, epilepsy.
Do not take if:
 suffering from glaucoma, megacolon, intestinal obstruction.

SIDE EFFECTS:
Common: Dry mouth, drowsiness, blurred vision, dizziness.
Unusual: Rapid heart rate, confusion, constipation, rash, uncoordinated movements, difficulty in passing urine, insomnia.
Severe but rare (stop medication, consult doctor): Severe constipation, glaucoma.

INTERACTIONS:
Other drugs:
- Other antiparkinsonian drugs, quinidine, tricyclic antidepressants, tetracyclic antidepressants, metoclopramide.

Other substances:
- Reacts with alcohol to cause sedation.

PRESCRIPTION:
Yes.

PBS:
Yes.

PERMITTED IN SPORT:
Yes.

OVERDOSE:
May be serious. Induce vomiting if taken recently. Seek urgent medical attention.

Biphasic Insulin

See INSULINS

Bisacodyl

TRADE NAMES:
Bisacodyl, Bisalax, Durolax, Fleet. Coloxyl Suppositories (with docusate sodium).
Go Kit (with other ingredients).

DRUG CLASS:
Laxative.

USES:
Constipation, preparing bowel for surgery or x-rays.

DOSAGE:

Tablets: Two to four tablets at night.
Suppository: One or two at night.

FORMS:
Tablets, suppository.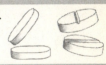

PRECAUTIONS:
Safe in pregnancy (A), breast feeding and children.
Designed for short term use only.
Do not take if:
 suffering from belly pains or bowel obstruction

SIDE EFFECTS:

Common: Minimal.
Unusual: Diarrhoea, belly discomfort.
Severe but rare (stop medication, consult doctor): Severe belly pain.

INTERACTIONS:

Other drugs:
- Do not take antacids within 30 minutes of bisacodyl.

PRESCRIPTION:
No.

PBS:
Suppository: Yes.
Tablets: No.

PERMITTED IN SPORT:
Yes.

OVERDOSE:
Diarrhoea and belly pain only effects likely.

OTHER INFORMATION:
Widely used and very safe.

See also Docusate sodium, Fibre, Frangula, Glycerol, Lactulose, Paraffin, Poloxamer, Psyllium, Senna, Sodium phosphate, Sodium picosulfate, Sorbitol, Sterculia.

Bisoprolol

TRADE NAME:
Bicor.

DRUG CLASS:
Beta blocker.

USES:
Stable chronic heart failure.

DOSAGE:

Slowly increase from 1.25mg a day to necessary dose. Maximum 10mg a day.
Usually prescribed with an ACE inhibitor.

FORMS:
Tablets of 1.25mg (white), 2.5mg (white), 5mg (yellow), 10mg (orange).

PRECAUTIONS:
Not to be used in pregnancy (C), breast feeding and children.
Use with caution in diabetes, liver and kidney disease, congenital heart disease, cardiomyopathy, recent heart attack, Prinzmetal angina, asthma, thyrotoxicosis, psoriasis.
Use with care in the elderly.

Do not take if:
suffering from acute heart failure, low blood pressure, sick heart sinus syndrome, slow heart rate, severe asthma, emphysema, poor circulation, Raynaud syndrome, phaeochromocytoma.

SIDE EFFECTS:
Common: Cold numb feeling in hands and feet, tiredness, dizziness, headache, diarrhoea.

INTERACTIONS:
Other drugs:
- Calcium antagonists, clonidine, Monoamine oxidase inhibitors, insulin, drugs used to control heart rhythm, hypoglycaemics, digoxin, ergotamine,

tricyclic antidepressants, barbiturates, phenothiazines, other beta blockers, rifampicin, mefloquine.

PRESCRIPTION:
Yes.

PBS:
Yes (authority required – limited to patients with heart failure not stabilised on other medication).

PERMITTED IN SPORT:
Yes.

OVERDOSE:
Likely to be serious. Slow heart rate, low blood pressure, asthma and heart failure may result. Administer activated charcoal or induce vomiting if tablets taken recently. Use Salbutamol or other asthma sprays for difficulty in breathing. Seek medical assistance.

OTHER INFORMATION:
Introduced in 2001 for the management of patients whose heart failure could not be controlled by other medications.

BISPHOSPHONATES

DISCUSSION:
Medications that prevent the loss of bone density in osteoporosis.

See Alendronate, Disodium etidronate, Disodium pamidronate, Sodium clodronate, Tiludronate disodium.

Bleomycin sulfate

TRADE NAMES:
Blenamax, Blenoxane, Bleomycin Injection.

DRUG CLASS:
Cytotoxic.

USES:
Some types of spreading skin cancer, head and neck cancer, cancer of the oesophagus (gullet) and larynx (voice box), cancer of the penis and testes, cancer of the uterus, lymphomas, other rare types of cancer.

DOSAGE:

Complex. Must be determined individually for each patient by the doctor.

FORMS:
Injection.

PRECAUTIONS:
Must not be used in pregnancy (D) or breast feeding.
Must be used with caution in patients with lung disease. lung function must be checked regularly in all patients.

SIDE EFFECTS:
Common: Lung damage, mouth ulcers, rashes, fever, headache, diarrhoea, nausea, loss of appetite, tiredness.
Unusual: Kidney and liver damage.

INTERACTIONS:
Other drugs:
- Drugs that may stress the kidneys.

PRESCRIPTION:
Yes.

PBS:
Yes.

PERMITTED IN SPORT:
Yes.

OVERDOSE:
Serious damage to many organs may result. Given only under close medical supervision.

OTHER INFORMATION:
Used to relieve cancer pain in inoperable cases, or as an addition to surgery and/or radiation.

Bosentan

TRADE NAME:
Tracleer.

USES:
High blood pressure in lungs.

DOSAGE:

62.5mg to 125mg twice a day.

FORMS:
Tablets of 62.5mg and 125mg (orange/white).

PRECAUTIONS:
Must never be used in pregnancy (X) as serious damage to the baby will occur.
Use with care in breast feeding and children.
Adequate contraception essential in non-menopausal women.
Use with caution if suffering from low blood pressure and anaemia.
Regular blood tests to check blood cells and liver function recommended.

Do not take if:
 suffering from liver disease.

SIDE EFFECTS:
Common: Headache, flushing.
Unusual: Leg swelling.
Severe but rare (stop medication, consult doctor): Liver damage (jaundice), blood cell damage.

INTERACTIONS:
Other drugs:
- Severe interaction with cyclosporin A, glibenclamide.
- Ketoconazole, warfarin, digoxin, simvastatin.

PRESCRIPTION:
Yes.

PBS:
No.

PERMITTED IN SPORT:
Yes.

OVERDOSE:
Severe liver damage possible. Induce vomiting or give activated charcoal if taken recently. Seek urgent medical attention.

OTHER INFORMATION:
Introduced in 2003 as the first effective treatment for the very complex condition of isolated high blood pressure in the lungs which may be due to scleroderma.

Botulinum toxin

TRADE NAMES:
Botox, Dysport.

USES:
Spasms of eyelids, facial nerve disorders, facial muscle spasms, foot spasticity and deformity in children with cerebral palsy, arm spasms after a stroke.

DOSAGE:

Complex. As determined by doctor for each individual patient.

FORMS:
Injection.

PRECAUTIONS:
Use with caution in pregnancy (B3), breast feeding and children.
Use with caution in myasthenia gravis, Eaton-Lambert syndrome, amyotrophic lateral sclerosis, other nerve-muscle diseases.
Avoid areas of local inflammation when injecting.

SIDE EFFECTS:
General: Nerve damage, muscle weakness and pain, rash, irregular heart rhythm.
Eyelid injections: Eye irritation, drooping eyelid, dry eye surface and ulceration.
Facial spasm: Blurred vision, facial muscle weakness.
Severe but rare (stop medication, consult doctor): Heart attack.

INTERACTIONS:
Other drugs:
- Aminoglycosides, drugs acting on nerves and muscles.

PRESCRIPTION:
Yes.

PBS:
Yes (very restricted to nominated patients only).

PERMITTED IN SPORT:
Yes.

OVERDOSE:
Potentially fatal.

OTHER INFORMATION:
Derived from the bacteria that causes botulism, one of the most severe forms of food poisoning.

Brimonidine tartrate

TRADE NAMES:
Alphagan, Enidin.

USES:
Glaucoma.

DOSAGE:
One drop in affected eye twice a day.

FORMS:
Eye drops (keep refrigerated).

PRECAUTIONS:
Use with caution in pregnancy (B1), breast feeding and children.
Use with caution in severe heart disease, poor liver and kidney function, poor blood supply to heart or brain, low blood pressure.
May aggravate Raynaud's phenomenon. Eye drops are absorbed into the bloodstream and may cause effects in other parts of the body.

Do not take if:
 using soft contact lenses.

SIDE EFFECTS:
Common: Dry mouth, red eyes, irritated eyes, eye stinging, eye itching, headache, tiredness.
Unusual: Eye irritation, eye ulceration, light sensitivity of eye, swelling of eyelid, inflamed eye, intestinal upset.

INTERACTIONS:
Other drugs:
- Must not be used with MAOI (see separate entry).

PRESCRIPTION:
Yes.

PBS:
Yes.

PERMITTED IN SPORT:
Yes.

OVERDOSE:
Unlikely to be serious if swallowed.

OTHER INFORMATION:
Introduced in 1998 for forms of glaucoma that cannot be controlled by other medications.

See also Betaxolol, Bimatroprost, Brinzolamide, Levobunolol, Pilocarpine.

Brinzolamide

TRADE NAME:
Azopt.

USES:
Glaucoma.

DOSAGE:
 One drop in affected eye twice a day. Apply pressure to inner corner of eye (tear duct) for two minutes after use.

FORMS:
Eye drops.

PRECAUTIONS:
Use with caution in pregnancy (B3), breast feeding and children.
Use with care in liver and kidney disease, and with soft contact lenses.
Do not take if:
 suffering from severe kidney disease.
• allergic to sulphas.

SIDE EFFECTS:
Common: Blurred vision, eye discomfort, red eye.
Unusual: Eye pain, dry eye, eye discharge, headache, taste disturbance.

INTERACTIONS:
Other drugs:
• Tablets used to treat glaucoma.

PRESCRIPTION:
Yes.

PBS:
Yes.

PERMITTED IN SPORT:
Yes.

OVERDOSE:
Unlikely to be serious if swallowed.

See also Betaxolol, Bimatroprost, Brimonidine, Levobunolol, Pilocarpine.

Bromazepam

TRADE NAME:
Lexotan.

DRUG CLASS:
Benzodiazepine (Anxiolytic).

USES:
Tension, anxiety and agitation.

DOSAGE:
 3mg to 6mg two or three times a day.

FORMS:
Tables of
3mg (pink) and
6mg (grey-green).

PRECAUTIONS:
Should be used with caution in pregnancy (C), but not at all if delivery of infant imminent as it may decrease desire to breathe in newborn infant. Should be used with caution in breast feeding. Not for use in children.
Lower dose required in elderly.
Should be used intermittently and not constantly as dependency may develop.
Use with caution in glaucoma, myasthenia gravis, heart disease, kidney or liver disease, psychiatric conditions, schizophrenia, depression and epilepsy.
Do not take if:
 suffering from severe lung disease, confusion.
• tendency to addiction or dependence.
• operating machinery, driving a vehicle or undertaking tasks that require concentration and alertness.

SIDE EFFECTS:

Common: Reduced alertness, dependence.
Unusual: Incoordination, tremor, confusion, increased risk of falls in elderly, rash, low blood pressure, nausea, muscle weakness,
Severe but rare (stop medication, consult doctor): Jaundice (yellow skin).

INTERACTIONS:

Other drugs:
- Sedatives, other anxiolytics, disulfiram, cimetidine, anticonvulsants, anticholinergics.

Herbs:
- Guarana, kava kava, passionflower, St John's wort, valerian.

Other substances:
- Reacts with alcohol to cause sedation and confusion.

PRESCRIPTION:
Yes.

PBS:
Yes (authority required)

PERMITTED IN SPORT:
Yes.

OVERDOSE:
Seldom life threatening. May cause drowsiness, confusion and coma. Induce vomiting if tablets taken recently. Seek medical assistance.

OTHER INFORMATION:
Dependency may be a problem, particularly in elderly, due to overuse.
See also Alprazolam, Buspirone, Clobazam, Diazepam, Lorazepam, Oxazepam.

Bromhexine

TRADE NAMES:

Bisolvon Chesty, Duro-Tuss Mucolytic. Chemists' Own Chesty Cough (with pseudoephedrine and guaiphenesin).
Chemists' Own Chesty Mucus Cough, Logicin Expectorant, Robitussin ME, Tussinol Expectorant (with guaiphenesin).
Bisolvon Sinus, Dur-Elix Plus (with pseudoephedrine).
Duro-Tuss Expectorant (with pholcodine).

DRUG CLASS:
Expectorant, mucolytic (liquefies mucus).

USES:
Bronchitis, emphysema, productive cough, thick phlegm.

DOSAGE:

 5 to 10mLs or one to two tablets three times a day.

FORMS:
Tablets of 8mg (white), mixture.

PRECAUTIONS
Safe to use in pregnancy (A), breast feeding and children.
Use only with appropriate antibiotics when suffering from lung infection or tuberculosis.
Use with caution in stomach ulcers.

SIDE EFFECTS:
Common: Minimal
Unusual: Nausea, belly fullness, diarrhoea, indigestion, headache, dizziness, rash.

INTERACTIONS:
None significant.

PRESCRIPTION:
No.

PBS:
No.

PERMITTED IN SPORT:
Yes.

OVERDOSE:
Exacerbation of side effects likely.

OTHER INFORMATION:
A very useful but often overlooked additional treatment in any condition with excessive amounts of thick phlegm. Widely used in Europe.

Bromocriptine

TRADE NAMES:
Bromohexal, Bromolactin, Kripton, Parlodel.

DRUG CLASS:
Antiparkinsonian.

USES:
Parkinson's disease, acromegaly, abnormal production of breast milk, stopping production of breast milk after childbirth.

DOSAGE:
 Depends on purpose. Usually start low, and increase slowly until desired result obtained. Taken three or four times a day.

FORMS:
Tablets, capsules.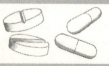

PRECAUTIONS:
Safe in pregnancy (A). Not to be used during breast feeding.
Use with caution in psychiatric conditions, high or low blood pressure, heart disease, diabetes, peptic ulcer, eye disease and liver disease.
Use with caution in women who wish to fall pregnant, as Bromocriptine may reduce fertility.

Do not take if:
suffering from high blood pressure in or immediately after pregnancy, after pregnancy if breast feeding desired, toxaemia of pregnancy, significant heart disease.

SIDE EFFECTS:
Common: Nausea very common. Dizziness, headache, nasal congestion, vomiting, tiredness, reduced blood pressure (fainting).
Unusual: Hallucinations, confusion, behavioural disturbances, unwanted muscle movements, psychiatric disturbances, peptic ulcer.
Severe but rare (stop medication, consult doctor): Vomiting blood, severe psychiatric disturbances.

INTERACTIONS:
Other drugs:
- Medications that lower blood pressure, erythromycin.

Other substances:
- Reacts adversely with alcohol.

PRESCRIPTION:
Yes.

PBS:
Yes (restricted to Parkinson's disease, acromegaly and pituitary tumours causing breast milk production).

PERMITTED IN SPORT:
Yes.

OVERDOSE:
May cause vomiting, tiredness, low blood pressure and hallucinations. Not likely to be life threatening. Administer activated charcoal or induce vomiting if taken recently. Seek medical assistance.

OTHER INFORMATION:
A very useful drug with an extraordinary range of activities. Tumours of the pituitary gland in the brain cause both acromegaly (excess bone growth) and abnormal breast milk production (in both sexes).

Brompheniramine

See ANTIHISTAMINES, SEDATING.

BRONCHODILATORS

DISCUSSION:
Wide range of inhaled and oral medications that open the airways (bronchi) in the lungs to treat conditions such as asthma, chronic bronchitis and emphysema.

See BETA-2 AGONISTS, Eformoterol, Ephedrine, Fenoterol, Ipratropium bromide, Orciprenaline, Salbutamol, Salmeterol, Terbutaline, THEOPHYLLINES.

Budesonide

TRADE NAMES:
Budamax, Entocort, Pulmicort, Rhinocort.
Symbicort (with eformoterol).

DRUG CLASS:
Corticosteroid.

USES:
Prevention of asthma, prevention of hay fever and chronic nasal drip, Crohn's disease.

DOSAGE:
 Asthma spray (Pulmicort, Symbicort): One or two inhalations, once a day.
Nasal sprays (Budamax, Rhinocort): One spray, once a day in each nostril.
Capsules (Entocort): Three capsules in morning with water before breakfast.

FORMS:
Inhaler, nasal spray, nebuliser solution, capsules of 3mg.

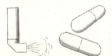

PRECAUTIONS:
Use with caution in pregnancy (B3), breast feeding and children.
Use with caution in lung or throat infection and tuberculosis.
Use capsules with caution in osteoporosis, peptic ulcer, liver disease, glaucoma, diabetes and cataracts.
Lung function should be checked regularly to ensure adequate dose is received.

SIDE EFFECTS:
Common: Capsules: Nausea, diarrhoea, headache, dizziness, palpitations.
Other forms: Fungal (thrush) infections of mouth, sore throat and mouth, dry mouth.
Unusual: Capsules: Bronchitis, rash, Cushing syndrome, back pain, blurred vision.
Other forms: Hoarseness, unusual bleeding and bruising, slowed growth.

INTERACTIONS:
Other drugs:
• Capsules interact with ketoconazole.
Herbs:
• Liquorice.

PRESCRIPTION:
Yes.

PBS:
Asthma inhaler and nebuliser solution: Yes.
Nasal sprays and capsules: No.

PERMITTED IN SPORT:
Most forms: Yes.
Capsules: No.

OVERDOSE:
Inhalers and sprays unlikely to have any serious effects. Capsules may have serious effects. Seek medical attention.

OTHER INFORMATION:
The introduction of the turbuhaler for the inhalation of Budesonide was a significant advance in asthma prevention as it is far easier to use than pressurised sprays. Budesonide is very effective in preventing hay fever and other forms of constantly

dripping nose. Designed for long term use. Does not cause dependence or addiction.

See also Beclomethasone dipropionate, Fluticasone.

Bufexamac

TRADE NAMES:
Paraderm
Fungo Soothing Balm (with miconazole, dimethicone and other ingredients).
Paraderm Plus (with chlorhexidine, lignocaine).

DRUG CLASS:
NSAID (Nonsteroidal anti-inflammatory drug).

USES:
Dermatitis, hives, rashes, insect bites, stings, abrasions.

DOSAGE:

Rub into affected area three or four times a day for up to two weeks.

FORMS:
Cream.

PRECAUTIONS:
May be used in pregnancy (A), breast feeding and children.

SIDE EFFECTS:
Common: Skin irritation.
Unusual: Secondary infection, eczema.

INTERACTIONS:
None significant.

PRESCRIPTION:
No.

PBS:
No.

PERMITTED IN SPORT:
Yes.

See also Aspirin, Celecoxib, Diclofenac, Diflunisal, Flurbiprofen, Ibuprofen, Indomethacin, Ketoprofen, Ketorolac trometanol, Mefenamic Acid, Naproxen, Piroxicam, Rofecoxib, Salicylic acid, Sulindac, Tenoxicam, Tiaprofenic Acid.

Bumetanide

TRADE NAME:
Burinex.

DRUG CLASS:
Diuretic.

USES:
Excess fluid in body.

DOSAGE:

One or more tablets in morning to maximum of 10mg.

FORMS:
Tablet of 1mg (white).

PRECAUTIONS:
Should not be used in pregnancy (C) unless medically essential. Should not be used in breast feeding or children.
Use with caution in elderly, diabetes, gout and heart failure.
May require regular blood tests to check on level of salts (electrolytes) in blood.

Do not take if:

suffering from severe kidney or liver disease.

SIDE EFFECTS:
Common: Muscle cramps, dizziness, headache, nausea.
Unusual: Deafness, rash, itch, weakness, arthritis, belly pains, vomiting.
Severe but rare (stop medication, consult doctor): Fainting.

INTERACTIONS:

Other drugs:
- Digoxin, lithium, probenecid, anticoagulants, indomethacin.
- Medications that lower blood pressure.

Herbs:
- Celery, dandelion, uva ursi.

PRESCRIPTION:
Yes.

PBS:
Yes.

PERMITTED IN SPORT:
No (acts as masking agent for other illegal drugs).

OVERDOSE:
May lead to severe dehydration and blood clots. Symptoms include weakness, dizziness, confusion, cramps and vomiting. Induce vomiting if tablets taken recently. Give extra fluids. Seek medical assistance.

OTHER INFORMATION:
Introduced in 1980's. Similar to frusemide, but faster and shorter acting.
See also Amiloride, Ethacrynic Acid, Frusemide, Indapamide, Spironolactone, THIAZIDE DIURETICS.

Bupivacaine
See ANAESTHETICS, LOCAL.

Buprenorphine

TRADE NAME:
Subutex, Temgesic.

DRUG CLASS:
Narcotic, analgesic.

USES:
Moderate to severe pain, treatment of narcotic addiction.

DOSAGE:

One or two tablets under tongue every six to eight hours as required.

FORMS:
Tablets for use under tongue, injection.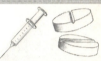

PRECAUTIONS:
Should not be used in pregnancy (C) unless medically essential. Not for use in breast feeding or children.
Use with caution in head injury, liver disease and severe lung disease.
Do not take if:
 operating machinery or driving a vehicle.

SIDE EFFECTS:
Common: Drowsiness, nausea.
Unusual: Headache, vomiting, dry mouth, constipation, dizziness, difficulty in passing urine.
Severe but rare (stop medication, consult doctor): Difficulty in breathing.

INTERACTIONS:
Other drugs:
- MAOI, benzodiazepines, sedatives, other narcotics, some antifungals, erythromycin, calcium channel antagonists.

Other substances:
- Alcohol should be avoided.

PRESCRIPTION:
Yes (very restricted).

PBS:
Yes (authority required – very limited indications).

PERMITTED IN SPORT:
No.

OVERDOSE:
Symptoms may include drowsiness, confusion, difficulty in breathing and coma. Induce vomiting if medication taken recently and patient alert. Seek urgent medical attention.

OTHER INFORMATION:
May cause addiction or dependence if used inappropriately. Introduced in the late 1980s for use in more intractable pain conditions, and now used to treat drug addiction.

See also Alfentanil, Codeine phosphate, Dextromoramide, Dextropropoxyphene, Fentanyl, Heroin, Hydromorphone, Methadone, Morphine, Oxycodone, Pentazocine, Pethidine.

Bupropion
(Amfebutamone)

TRADE NAME:
Zyban.

USES:
Aids cessation of smoking and counteracts nicotine addiction.

DOSAGE:

One tablet a day for three days, increasing to one tablet twice a day.

FORMS:
Tablet of 150mg (white).

PRECAUTIONS:
Not to be used in pregnancy, breast feeding and children.
Use with caution in any liver or kidney disease, head injury, brain tumour, alcoholism and diabetes.
Blood pressure should be checked regularly.

Do not take if:
suffering from epilepsy or other condition causing seizures, bipolar disorder, eating disorder, severe liver disease (eg. cirrhosis).

SIDE EFFECTS:
Common: Sleeplessness, headache, fever, dry mouth, nausea, flushing, rapid heart rate.
Unusual: Diarrhoea or constipation, brain irritation, skin reaction, taste disorders, poor concentration, loss of appetite.
Severe but rare (stop medication, consult doctor): Convulsion, high blood pressure.

INTERACTIONS:
Other drugs:
- MAOI, antipsychotics, antidepressants, theophylline, steroid tablets, benzodiazepines, medications used to treat epilepsy and convulsions, levodopa, beta blockers.

Other substances:
- Alcohol, stimulants.

PRESCRIPTION:
Yes.

PBS:
Yes (authority required).

PERMITTED IN SPORT:
No.

OVERDOSE:
May be serious. Drowsiness, hallucinations, seizures, coma and rarely death may occur. Seek urgent medical attention. Administer activated charcoal or induce vomiting if tablets taken recently and patient alert.

OTHER INFORMATION:
Introduced in late 2000 as an additional aid in the fight against smoking.
See also Nicotine.

Buspirone

TRADE NAME:
Buspar.

DRUG CLASS:
Anxiolytic.

USES:
Relief of anxiety.

DOSAGE:

 5mg to 20mg (one to three tablets), three times a day.

FORMS:
Tablets (white) of 5mg and 10mg.

PRECAUTIONS:
Should only be used in pregnancy if medically essential. Breast feeding should be ceased before Buspirone taken. Not for use in children.
Should be used with caution in epilepsy, liver and kidney disease.
Lower doses required in elderly.

Do not take if:

 suffering from severe liver disease.

- operating machinery, driving a vehicle, or undertaking tasks that require concentration, alertness and coordination.

SIDE EFFECTS:
Common: Dizziness, sleeplessness, drowsiness, light headedness, nausea, headache, nasal congestion.
Unusual: Excitement, chest pain, nightmares, rapid heart rate, palpitations, blurred vision, muscle pains, pins and needles sensation, tremor.

INTERACTIONS:
Other drugs:
- Benzodiazepines and other anxiolytics.
- MAOI.

Other substances:
- No reaction with alcohol.
- Food increases absorption of Buspirone.

PRESCRIPTION:
Yes.

PBS:
No. Available to some Veteran Affairs pensioners under strict guidelines.

PERMITTED IN SPORT:
No.

OVERDOSE:
May cause vomiting, drowsiness and stomach pains. Not believed to be serious. Administer activated charcoal or induce vomiting if tablets taken recently and patient alert. Seek medical attention.

OTHER INFORMATION:
Introduced in early 1990s as an non-addictive alternative to benzodiazepines. Does not cause dependence. Very safe, but not as rapid in its effect as other anxiolytics.
See also Alprazolam, Bromazepam, Clobazam, Diazepam, Lorazepam, Oxazepam.

Busulfan

TRADE NAME:
Myleran.

DRUG CLASS;
Alkylater.

USES:
Leukaemia, polycythaemia rubra vera, myelofibrosis, thrombocythaemia.

DOSAGE:

 Must be individualised by doctor for each patient depending on disease, severity, age and weight of patient.

FORMS:
Tablets (white) of 2mg.

PRECAUTIONS:
Must not be used in pregnancy (D) unless mother's life is at risk as damage to the foetus may occur. Breast feeding must be ceased before use. May be used in children if medically essential.
Regular blood tests to monitor blood cells and liver function essential.
Adequate contraception must be used by women while medication taken.
Must be used with caution in all patients.

SIDE EFFECTS:
Common: Damage to bone marrow, skin pigmentation.
Unusual: Nausea, vomiting, diarrhoea, lung damage (cough), eye damage, liver damage, hair loss, rash, itch.

INTERACTIONS:
Other drugs:
- Phenytoin, itraconazole, thioguanine.

PRESCRIPTION:
Yes.

PBS:
Yes.

PERMITTED IN SPORT:
Yes.

OVERDOSE:
Very serious. Permanent damage to bone marrow with subsequent death likely. Administer activated charcoal or induce vomiting if medication taken recently. Seek urgent medical assistance.

OTHER INFORMATION:
Although busulfan has serious side effects, it may be life saving in patients with some types of malignancy or blood disorders.
See also Amsacrine, **VINCA ALKALOIDS.**

Butyl aminobenzoate pictrate

TRADE NAME:
Butesin Pictrate With Metaphen (with nitromersol).

USES:
Scalds and minor burns.

DOSAGE:
 Apply twice a day.

FORMS:
Ointment.

PRECAUTIONS:
Safe to use in pregnancy, breast feeding and children.
May cause staining of clothing.

SIDE EFFECTS:
Common: Minimal.
Severe but rare (stop medication, consult doctor): Dermatitis.

INTERACTIONS:
None.

PRESCRIPTION:
No.

PBS:
No.

PERMITTED IN SPORT:
Yes.

OTHER INFORMATION:
Old-fashioned but effective and useful home treatment for minor burns.

Medications

Cabergoline

TRADE NAMES:
Cabaser, Dostinex.

USES:
Parkinson's disease, stopping breast milk production, excess production of the hormone prolactin.

DOSAGE:
 Stopping breast feeding: Two tablets taken once.
Excess prolactin production: Half to four tablets, once a week.
Parkinson's disease: Increase dose slowly from 0.5mg a day to maximum of 4mg a day.

FORMS:
Tablets (white) of 0.5 and 1mg.

PRECAUTIONS:
Use with caution in pregnancy (B1), breast feeding and children.
Use with caution in heart disease, kidney disease, liver disease, peptic ulcer disease.
May aggravate some psychiatric conditions.
High blood pressure after childbirth may be made worse.

SIDE EFFECTS:
Common: Low blood pressure, fainting, dizziness, headache, tiredness.
Unusual: Fatigue, depression, stomach upsets, breast pain, hot flushes.
Severe but rare (stop medication, consult doctor): Pleural effusion (collection of fluid around lungs – chest pain and shortness of breath).

INTERACTIONS:
Other drugs:
- Ergot alkaloids, methylergotamine, dopamine agonists, drugs that inhibit liver function, metoclopramide.

PRESCRIPTION:
Yes.

PBS:
Yes (restricted to specific purposes).

PERMITTED IN SPORT:
Yes.

Cadexomer Iodine

TRADE NAMES:
Iodoflex, Iodosorb

USES:
Chronic skin ulcers.

DOSAGE:
 Apply dressing, powder or ointment every one to three days.

FORMS:
Ointment, powder, impregnated dressing.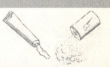

PRECAUTIONS:
Use with caution in in pregnancy (C) and breast feeding.
Not for use in children under 12 years.
Use with caution on large ulcers.
Do not use for more than three months.
Do not take if:
 suffering from kidney failure, Hashimoto thyroiditis, goitre.
- sensitive to iodine.

Home Guide to Medication

Medications

SIDE EFFECTS:
Common: Skin irritation.
Unusual: Swelling of tissue.
Severe but rare (stop medication, consult doctor): Thyroid gland abnormalities (eg. goitre).

INTERACTIONS:
Other drugs:
- Lithium, mercury-based antiseptics (eg. Mercurochrome).

PRESCRIPTION:
No.

PBS:
No. Available to some Veteran Affairs pensioners.

PERMITTED IN SPORT:
Yes.

OTHER INFORMATION:
Introduced in 2001 as a new form of treatment for persistent skin and leg ulcers.

Caffeine

TRADE NAMES:
NoDoz.
Cafergot (with ergotamine).
Dynamo (with glucose, nicotinic acid).
Ergodryl (with ergotamine, diphenhydramine).
NoDoz Plus (with glucose, thiamine, nicotinic acid).
Travacalm (with hyoscine, dimenhydrinate).
Caffeine is also found in a wide range of foods and beverages.

DRUG CLASS:
Stimulant.

USES:
Fatigue, additive to assist motion sickness and migraines.

DOSAGE:

One tablet every three hours or as directed by doctor.
One suppository up to three times a day.

FORMS:
Tablets, suppository.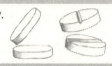

PRECAUTIONS:
Safe in pregnancy and breast feeding. Use with caution in children.
Do not take if:
 suffering from peptic ulcer, heartburn.

SIDE EFFECTS:
Common: Anxiety, nervousness, sleeplessness, passing increased amount of urine.

INTERACTIONS:
Other substances:
- Reacts with coffee, tea and cola drinks containing caffeine.

PRESCRIPTION:
Cafergot, Ergodryl: Yes.
Other forms: No.

PBS:
Most forms: No.
Cafergot suppositories: Yes

PERMITTED IN SPORT:
No.

OVERDOSE:
Anxiety, restlessness, irritability and sleeplessness are likely.

OTHER INFORMATION:
Used for centuries in tea and coffee as a mild stimulant. Also found in cola drinks and chocolate.
100mL of brewed coffee contains 60 to 130mg of caffeine.
100mL of instant coffee contains 40 to 100mg caffeine.
100mL of tea contains 40 to 60mg caffeine.

100mL of cola drink contains 10mg of caffeine.
100g of chocolate contains 20 to 30mg of caffeine.

Calamine

TRADE NAMES:
Found in numerous soothing preparations.

USES:
Minor skin irritations, insect bites, sunburn, leg ulcers.

DOSAGE:
 Apply several times a day as required.

FORMS:
Cream, lotion, bandages.

PRECAUTIONS:
Safe to use in pregnancy, breast feeding and children.
Avoid eyes, mouth and nostrils.
Do not take if:
 suffering from blistered, raw or oozing skin.

SIDE EFFECTS:
Minimal.

INTERACTIONS:
None.

PRESCRIPTION:
No.

PBS:
No.

PERMITTED IN SPORT:
Yes.

OTHER INFORMATION:
Widely used, effective old-fashioned treatment for everything from bites to chickenpox.

Calciferol

See Calcitriol, Cholecalciferol and Ergocalciferol (Vitamin D).

Calcipotriol

TRADE NAME:
Daivonex.

USES:
Psoriasis.

DOSAGE:
 Apply twice a day. Reduce frequency if possible.

FORMS:
Ointment, cream, scalp lotion.

PRECAUTIONS:
Use with caution in pregnancy (B1), breast feeding and children.
Avoid contact with eyes!
Use with caution on face, scalp and in skin flexures.
Use with care long term.
Avoid sun exposure during use.
Do not take if:
 suffering from disorders of calcium metabolism.
• suffering from severe or pustular psoriasis.

SIDE EFFECTS:
Common: Skin irritation, sun sensitivity.
Unusual: Skin pigmentation, excess calcium levels in blood with excess use.

INTERACTIONS:
Other drugs:
• Calcium, vitamin D supplements.

PRESCRIPTION:
Yes.

Medications

PBS:
Cream, lotion: No.
Ointment: Yes

PERMITTED IN SPORT:
Yes

OVERDOSE:
Skin damage possible if overused.

Calcitonin
See Salcatonin.

Calcitriol

TRADE NAMES:
Calcijex, Citrihexal, Kosteo, Rocaltrol, Sitriol.

DRUG CLASS:
A form of vitamin D.

USES:
Osteoporosis prevention and treatment, rickets, hypoparathyroidism, some types of hypocalcaemia.

DOSAGE:
 One or two tablets twice a day.

FORMS:
Capsules of 0.25µg.

PRECAUTIONS:
Use with caution in pregnancy (B3), breast feeding and children. Use with caution in infants.
Use with caution in kidney disease.
Regular blood tests necessary.
Ensure adequate fluid intake.

Do not take if:
 suffering from hypercalcaemia, vitamin D sensitivity.

SIDE EFFECTS:
Common: Drowsiness, nausea, weakness, constipation or diarrhoea, itchy skin.
Unusual: Calcium deposits in tissue, dehydration, kidney damage.

INTERACTIONS:
Other drugs: Cholestyramine, thiazide diuretics, digoxin, magnesium, corticosteroids.

PRESCRIPTION:
Yes.

PBS:
Yes (restricted).

PERMITTED IN SPORT:
Yes.

OVERDOSE:
Serious. Symptoms include loss of appetite, tiredness, vomiting, diarrhoea, sweating, excess urine production, extreme thirst and headache. This may progress to high blood pressure and kidney failure. Administer activated charcoal or induce vomiting if taken recently. Seek medical assistance.

See also Cholecalciferol, Ergocalciferol.

Calcium

TRADE and GENERIC NAMES:
Calcium in various forms is found in numerous nutritional supplements and antacids, some of which are listed below.
Algicon, Andrews Antacids, Degas Extra Chewable, De Witt's Antacid, Gaviscon, Mylanta Heartburn Relief, Titralac (Calcium carbonate with antacids).
Andrews TUMS, Cal-Sup, Caltrate (Calcium carbonate).
Bioglan B Complex, Bioglan Synergy B, Cenovis B Complex, Macro Mega B (Calcium pantothenate with vitamins and other ingredients).
Bioglan Junior (Calcium ascorbate with vitamins and other ingredients).

Medications

Blackmores Bio Calcium (Calcium phosphate with vitamin D and calcium hydrogen phosphate).
Blackmores Bio Magnesium (Calcium ascorbate with magnesium, vitamin B6).
Blackmores for Women Total Calcium (Calcium phosphate and calcium citrate with vitamins).
Caltrate + D (Calcium carbonate with vitamin D).
Caltrate Plus (Calcium carbonate with vitamins and other ingredients).
Citracal (Calcium citrate).
Citracal Plus (Calcium citrate with other vitamins and minerals).
Citracal + D (Calcium citrate with vitamin D).
Didrocal (Calcium carbonate with disodium etidronate).
FAB Trical (Calcium gluconate with vitamins and minerals).
Mylanta Rolltabs, Rennie (Calcium carbonate with magnesium carbonate).
Sandocal 1000 (Calcium carbonate, calcium lactate gluconate).

DRUG CLASS:
Mineral.

USES:
Antacid, improves circulation, poor nutrition, osteomalacia, osteoporosis, excess phosphate in body.

DOSAGE:
 Recommended daily intake 800mg per day.

FORMS:
Tablets, capsules, mixtures, injections.

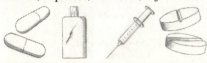

PRECAUTIONS:
Safe in pregnancy, breast feeding and children.
Use with caution in kidney stones, kidney disease and diabetes.

Do not take if:
 suffering from severe kidney disease, high blood calcium.

SIDE EFFECTS:
Common: Constipation, hot flushes, sweating.
Unusual: Low blood pressure.
Severe but rare (stop medication, consult doctor): Kidney stones (severe loin pain).

INTERACTIONS:
Other drugs:
- Iron, digoxin, tetracycline, fluoride, calcium channel blockers, vitamin D.

PRESCRIPTION:
Most forms: No.
Didrocal: Yes.

PBS:
Cal-Sup, Caltrate: Yes.
Didrocal: Yes (authority required).
Other forms: No.

PERMITTED IN SPORT:
Yes.

OVERDOSE:
Exacerbation of side effects likely.

OTHER INFORMATION:
Essential mineral found mainly in dairy products (eg. cheese, milk, yoghurt), bony fish (eg. sardines, salmon); and to a lesser extent in peas, beans, broccoli, almonds and whole grain cereals.

See also ANTACIDS.

Calcium alginate

TRADE NAMES:
Kaltostat, Sorbsan.

USES:
Discharging, purulent, contaminated wounds and ulcers.

DOSAGE:

Dressing applied directly to wound. Changed every 12 to 72 hours depending on nature of wound.

FORMS:
Dressing.

PRECAUTIONS:
Inert agent. Safe to use on all patients. Not for use on dry wounds or if significant infection present.
Infected wounds may need antibiotics to reduce infection.

SIDE EFFECTS:
None.

INTERACTIONS:
None.

PRESCRIPTION:
No.

PBS:
No.

PERMITTED IN SPORT:
Yes.

OTHER INFORMATION:
Derived from seaweed. Soaks up exudate from weeping wounds to keep them dry and aid healing. Forms a protective thick gel over healing tissue.

Calcium carbonate

See ANTACIDS, Calcium.

CALCIUM CHANNEL BLOCKERS (CALCIUM ANTAGONISTS)

DISCUSSION:
Calcium is essential for the contraction of the tiny muscles around the arteries. When these muscles contract, the artery becomes smaller and narrower. Calcium channel blockers prevent the calcium from entering the muscle cells through tiny channels in the membrane surrounding the cell. These muscle cells cannot then contract easily, remain relaxed, and do not narrow the artery. The wider an artery, the less resistance is placed on the blood flowing through it, and the lower the blood pressure. Because they prevent the contraction of all arteries, they reduce the strain on the heart, and some of these drugs can therefore be used to treat angina (a lack of blood to the heart muscle). Calcium channel blockers are quite safe and are normally used in tablet form, although some can be given as injections.

See **Amlodipine**, **Diltiazem**, **Felodipine**, **Lercanidipine**, **Nifedipine**, **Nimodipine**, **Verapamil**.

Calcium folinate

TRADE NAME:
Leucovorin.

USES:
Deficiencies in the body's folic acid level caused by cancer treatment, inadequate intake or anaemia.

DOSAGE:

Depends on disease, and severity of folic acid deficiency.

FORMS:
Tablets (off-white) of 15mg, injection.

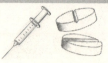

PRECAUTIONS:
May be used safely in pregnancy (A) and children. Use with caution in breast feeding.
Do not take if:
 suffering from pernicious anaemia.

SIDE EFFECTS:
Common: Minimal.
Unusual: Fever, seizures, fainting, diarrhoea, allergy reaction.

INTERACTIONS:
Other drugs:
- Methotrexate, droperidol, fluorouracil, phenobarbitone, phenytoin, primidone.

PRESCRIPTION:
Yes.

PBS:
Tablets: Yes.
Injection: No.

PERMITTED IN SPORT:
Yes.

OVERDOSE:
No adverse effects expected.

OTHER INFORMATION:
Folic acid is essential for formation of red blood cells, but the bacteria that produce it in the gut are destroyed by many anticancer drugs.

Calcium Salts
See ANTACIDS.

Camphor

TRADE NAMES:
Widely used in many cough mixtures, ointments, creams, liniments, lotions and inhalations.

DRUG CLASS:
Expectorant, Liniment.

USES:
Soothes muscle and joint pains, and burns.
Eases productive coughs.
Eases nasal congestion.

DOSAGE:
 Take every four to six hours. Apply to affected areas or inhale as required.

FORMS:
Mixture, ointment, cream, liniment, lotion, inhalation.

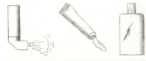

PRECAUTIONS:
Safe to use in pregnancy, breast feeding and children.
Not to be swallowed.

SIDE EFFECTS:
Minimal.

INTERACTIONS:
None significant.

PRESCRIPTION:
No.

PBS:
No.

PERMITTED IN SPORT:
Yes.

OVERDOSE:
Unlikely to cause any significant adverse effects.

CANCER-TREATING DRUGS
(Alkylaters, Antimetabolites, Antineoplastics, Cytotoxics)

DISCUSSION:
The cytotoxics and antineoplastics form a large, diverse group of drugs that are used to destroy cancer cells within the body in a process known as chemotherapy. 'Cyto' means cell, so 'cytotoxic' means toxic (harmful) to cells, while antineoplastic means 'against cancer'. These drugs can be given by tablet or injection, and different drugs are used to attack different types of cancer. Unfortunately they are not all as specific in attacking cancer cells as we would wish, and normal cells may also be attacked and destroyed. The balance between giving enough of the drug to kill the cancer cells and not enough to kill too many normal cells is a very fine one.

The effectiveness of cytotoxic drugs varies dramatically from one patient to another and one disease to another. Some forms of cancer are very susceptible to cytotoxic drugs (eg. acute leukaemias), while others are resistant. Side effects are very common, and again variable. Nausea, vomiting, diarrhoea, muscle pain, loss of hair, weight loss, fatigue and headaches are just a few of the many complications possible. Patients taking this type of medication will be closely monitored by their doctors through regular blood tests and clinic visits. Long-term treatment for many months is usually required, and other medications may be added to control the side effects.

See Altretamine, Aminoglutethamide, Anagrelide, Anastrozole, Bicalutamide, Bleomycin sulfate, Busulfan, Capecitabine, Carboplatin, Carmustine, Chlorambucil, Cisplatin, Cyclophosphamide, Cytarabine, Dactinomycin, Daunorubicin, Etoposide, Exemestane, Fluorouracil, Flutamide, Fosfestrol, Goserelin acetate, Hydroxyurea, Idarubicin, Imatinib, Letrozole, Leuprorelin, Lomustine, Medroxyprogesterone acetate, Megestrol, Melphalan, Mercaptopurine, Methotrexate, Nilutamide, Paclitaxel, Procarbazine, Tamoxifen, Temozolomide, Toremifene, VINCA ALKALOIDS.

Candesartan
See ANGIOTENSIN II RECEPTOR ANTAGONISTS.

Cannabis
See Marijuana.

Capecitabine

TRADE NAME:
Xeloda.

DRUG CLASS:
Antimetabolite.

USES:
Advanced breast cancer not responding to other treatments.

DOSAGE:

As determined by doctor for each individual patient.

FORMS:
Tablets (peach) of 150 and 500mg.

PRECAUTIONS:
Not for use in pregnancy (D) or breast feeding.
Use with caution in heart disease, liver disease, children and the elderly.

Do not take if:
 suffering from severe kidney disease.

SIDE EFFECTS:
Common: Numerous, including diarrhoea, nausea, vomiting, hand and foot discomfort, mouth ulcers and soreness, loss of appetite, rashes, tiredness.
Unusual: Abdominal pain, insomnia, dizziness, taste changes, excessive skin

sensitivity, pins and needles sensation, swelling of tissue.
Severe but rare (stop medication, consult doctor): Damage to blood cells (regular blood tests necessary), liver damage.

INTERACTIONS:
Other drugs:
- Warfarin, phenytoin.

PRESCRIPTION:
Yes.

PBS:
Yes (authority required).

PERMITTED IN SPORT:
Yes.

OVERDOSE:
Very serious. Seek urgent medical attention. Induce vomiting or give activated charcoal if swallowed recently.

OTHER INFORMATION:
Introduced in 2002 as a treatment of last resort for breast cancer.

Capsaicin

TRADE NAME:
Zostrix.

DRUG CLASS:
Rubefacient, analgesic.

USES:
Nerve pain in skin after shingles or with diabetes, arthritis.

DOSAGE:

Apply to affected area three or four times a day.

FORMS:
Cream.

PRECAUTIONS:
Safe in pregnancy, breast feeding and children over 2 years.
Avoid eyes, mouth, nose, anus and vagina.
Avoid broken or infected skin.

Do not use if:
 suffering from active shingles or chickenpox.

SIDE EFFECTS:
Common: Minimal.
Unusual: Burning, skin irritation.

INTERACTIONS:
None significant.

PRESCRIPTION:
No.

PBS:
No.

PERMITTED IN SPORT:
Yes.

OTHER INFORMATION:
Becoming less relevant as more effective treatments for acute shingles (eg. Valaciclovir) to prevent nerve pain have become available.

Captopril

See ACE INHIBITORS.

Carbachol

TRADE NAMES:
Isopto Carbachol, Miostat.

DRUG CLASS:
Miotic.

USES:
Glaucoma, eye surgery.

DOSAGE:

Two drops three times a day.

FORMS:
Eye drops.

PRECAUTIONS:
May be used in pregnancy, breast feeding and children.
Avoid exceeding recommended dose.
Use with caution in heart failure, asthma, stomach ulcer, over-active thyroid gland, Parkinson's disease, gut spasm, difficulty in passing urine.
Do not use if:

Eye injured or grazed.

SIDE EFFECTS:
Common: Blurred vision, constriction of pupil, headache.
Uncommon: Heart disturbances, gut disturbances.
Severe but rare (stop medication, consult doctor): Miostat – Retinal detachment (sudden partial or complete blindness).

INTERACTIONS:
None significant.

PRESCRIPTION:
Yes.

PBS:
Isopto Carbachol: Yes.
Miostat: No.

PERMITTED IN SPORT:
Yes.

OVERDOSE:
Seek medical attention if swallowed. Antidote available.

See also Acetazolamide, Acetylcholine chloride, Apraclonidine, Betaxolol, Bimatoprost, Brimonidine, Brinzolamide, Dipivefrine, Dorzolamide, Latanoprost, Levobunolol, Phenylephrine, Pilocarpine, Timolol, Travoprost.

Carbamazepine

TRADE NAMES:
Tegretol, Teril.

DRUG CLASS:
Anticonvulsant.

USES:
Epilepsy, manic states, mood stabilisation, trigeminal neuralgia (tic doloureux), other forms of neuralgia (nerve pain).

DOSAGE:

Dosage increased slowly under medical supervision until desired effect obtained. Maximum 1200mg a day.
Blood tests may help check on dose required.

FORMS:
Tablet, controlled release tablets, suspension.

PRECAUTIONS:
Not to be used in pregnancy (D) unless medically essential as risk of foetal abnormality is increased by 300%. Breast feeding should be ceased before use. May be used in children over 5 years.
Use with caution in heart disease, glaucoma, psychiatric conditions, prostate disease, kidney and liver disease.
Use with caution in elderly.
Regular blood tests to check liver and

kidney function and blood cells recommended.
Do not stop suddenly, but reduce dose slowly.

Do not take if:

☠ suffering from heart block, lupus erythematosus, liver failure, porphyria, bone marrow suppression.
- sensitive to Tricyclic antidepressants.
- drinking alcohol.

SIDE EFFECTS:

Common: Some side effects are very common for the first few days then lessen. Drowsiness, incoordination, reduced alertness, dizziness, double vision, headache, nausea, skin reactions.
Unusual: Vomiting, hallucinations, depression, dry mouth, fluid retention.
Severe but rare (stop medication, consult doctor): Unusual bleeding or bruising.

INTERACTIONS:

Other drugs:
- Other anticonvulsants, oral contraceptives, MAOI within 14 days, warfarin

Herbs:
- Evening primrose (linoleic acid), Gingko biloba, St John's wort.

Other substances:
- Reacts adversely with alcohol.
- Borage.

PRESCRIPTION:
Yes.

PBS:
Yes.

PERMITTED IN SPORT:
Yes.

OVERDOSE:
Serious. Symptoms very varied but may include vomiting, low blood pressure, rapid heart rate, agitation, hallucinations, blurred vision, coma and death. Administer activated charcoal or induce vomiting if medication recently taken and patient alert. Seek urgent medical assistance.

OTHER INFORMATION:
Used for many decades to control epilepsy and neuralgia. Not addictive or dependence forming. Does not cause dependence or addiction.

See also **BARBITURATES, BENZODIAZEPINES, Clonazepam, Ethosuximide, Gabapentin, Lamotrigine, Levetiracetam, Oxcarbazepine, Phenytoin, Primidone, Sodium valproate, Sulthiame, Tiagabine, Topiramate, Vigabatrin.**

Carbidopa

See **LEVODOPA COMPOUNDS.**

Carbimazole

TRADE NAME:
Neo-Mercazole.

DRUG CLASS:
Antithyroid.

USES:
Over-active thyroid gland.

DOSAGE:

Two to 12 tablets a day, strictly as directed by doctor.

FORMS:
Tablets (pink) of 5mg.

PRECAUTIONS:
Not to be used in pregnancy (C) or breast feeding. Use in children only if medically essential.

SIDE EFFECTS:
Common: Dose related.
Unusual: Nausea, diarrhoea, headache, rash, muscle pains, joint pains, itchy skin, hair loss.
Severe but rare (stop medication, consult doctor): Bone marrow damage, liver damage (detected by regular blood tests).

Medications

INTERACTIONS:
Other drugs:
- Radioactive iodine.

PRESCRIPTION:
Yes.

PBS:
Yes.

PERMITTED IN SPORT:
Yes.

OVERDOSE:
Rash likely. Damage to bone marrow possible.

OTHER INFORMATION:
Often used to control overactive thyroid gland before surgery to remove gland, or irradiation to destroy gland.

Carbomer 940
See EYE LUBRICANTS.

Carbomer 974
See EYE LUBRICANTS.

Carbomer 980
See EYE LUBRICANTS.

Carboplatin

TRADE NAME:
Carboplatin.

DRUG CLASS:
Antineoplastic.

USES:
Some forms of advanced cancer of the ovary.

DOSAGE:
 As determined by doctor for each patient.

FORMS:
Injection.

PRECAUTIONS:
Not to be used in pregnancy (D), breast feeding and children.
Use with caution in debilitated and elderly patients.
Regular blood tests essential.
Hearing and brain function need to be checked regularly.

Do not take if:
 suffering from severe kidney disease.

SIDE EFFECTS:
Common: Blood cell damage, kidney and liver damage, ear damage, nausea, diarrhoea, muscle pains.
Unusual: Vomiting, local skin reactions.
Severe but rare (stop medication, consult doctor): Liver or kidney failure.

INTERACTIONS:
Other drugs:
- Other drugs used to treat cancer, aminoglycosides.

PRESCRIPTION:
Yes.

PBS:
Yes.

PERMITTED IN SPORT:
Yes.

OTHER INFORMATION:
Used only when no other medication will assist patient.

CARDIAC GLYCOSIDE

DISCUSSION:
The cardiac glycosides are an ancient group of medications that regulate heart rate. They are derived from the foxglove flower. Only one is used in modern medicine.
See Digoxin.

Carmellose sodium
See EYE LUBRICANTS.

Carmustine

TRADE NAMES:
Bicnu, Gliadel.

DRUG CLASS:
Antineoplastic.

USES:
Hodgkin's disease, multiple myeloma, lymphomas, some types of brain cancer, palliation of other cancers.

DOSAGE:
 As determined by doctor for each patient.

FORMS:
Injection, implant.

PRECAUTIONS:
Must not be used in pregnancy (D) or breast feeding. Adequate contraception essential.
Blood tests must be performed regularly to monitor liver function and blood cells. Use with caution in lung disease.
Do not take if:
 suffering from bleeding disorders due to low platelet count.

SIDE EFFECTS:
Common: Liver and kidney damage, lung damage, seizures, headache, poor healing, meningitis.
Unusual: Numerous possibilities that should be discussed with your doctor.

INTERACTIONS:
None significant.

PRESCRIPTION:
Yes.

PBS:
No (expensive).

PERMITTED IN SPORT:
Yes.

OVERDOSE:
Serious organ damage likely. Only given under strict medical supervision.

OTHER INFORMATION:
Implants introduced in 2001 to avoid the need for regular injections, but course costs many thousands of dollars.

Carvedilol

TRADE NAMES:
Dilatrend, Kredex.

DRUG CLASS:
Beta blocker.

USES:
Heart failure, high blood pressure.

DOSAGE:
 Start with 3.125mg twice a day with food. Increase dose slowly to maximum of 25mg twice a day (may be higher for very heavy patients).

FORMS:
Tablets of 3.125mg, 6.25mg, 12.5mg and 25mg.

Medications

PRECAUTIONS:
Should not be used in pregnancy (C) unless essential for the mother's health. Use with considerable caution in breast feeding and children.
Use with caution in poor circulation to hands and feet, kidney disease, diabetes, over-active thyroid gland.
Do not stop medication suddenly, but reduce dose slowly.

Do not take if:
 suffering from asthma, slow heart rate, low blood pressure, heart block, poor liver function.

SIDE EFFECTS:
Common: Tissue swelling, slow heart rate, low blood pressure, dizziness, diarrhoea, nausea.
Unusual: Vomiting, ankle swelling, joint pain, muscle pain, blurred vision, fainting, chest pain.
Severe but rare (stop medication, consult doctor): Unusual bleeding, wheezing, shortness of breath.

INTERACTIONS:
Other drugs:
- Rifampicin, cimetidine, clonidine, calcium channel blockers, hypoglycaemics, insulin, quinidine, paroxetine, fluoxetine, digoxin, MAOI, reserpine, other beta blockers.

Other substances:
- Grapefruit eaten at same time as tablets taken.

PRESCRIPTION:
Yes.

PBS:
Yes (authority required).

PERMITTED IN SPORT:
No.

OVERDOSE:
Low blood pressure, fainting, slow heart rate, seizures, reduced breathing, collapse, heart failure and death may occur. Lie patient flat on side in coma position. Induce vomiting or administer activated charcoal if swallowed recently. Seek urgent medical attention.

OTHER INFORMATION:
Introduced in 1998 to treat more difficult cases of heart failure,

See also Esmolol, Labetalol, Metoprolol, Oxprenolol, Pindolol, Propranolol, Sotalol.

Cefaclor, Cefepime, Cefotaxime, Cefotetan, Cefoxitin, Cefpiromine, Ceftazidime, Ceftriaxone, Cefuroxime.

See CEPHALOSPORINS.

Celecoxib

TRADE NAME:
Celebrex.

DRUG CLASS:
COX-2 Inhibitor.

USES:
Rheumatoid arthritis and osteoarthritis.

DOSAGE:
 100 to 400mg a day.

FORMS:
Capsules (white) of 100 and 200mg.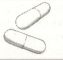

PRECAUTIONS:
Use with considerable caution in pregnancy (B3).
Use with caution in breast feeding and children.
Use with caution with previous peptic ulcer, high blood pressure, fluid retention,

heart failure, asthma, dehydration, liver or kidney disease, sulpha allergy.
Lower doses may be necessary in the elderly and with long term use.

Do not take if:

 asthma occurs with NSAID medications or aspirin.

SIDE EFFECTS:

Common: Fluid retention (swollen feet).
Unusual: Gut irritation, indigestion.
Severe but rare (stop medication, consult doctor): Liver and kidney damage.

INTERACTIONS:

Other drugs:
- Nonsteroidal anti-inflammatory drugs (NSAID), steroids, anticoagulants (eg. warfarin), diuretics, ACE inhibitors, lithium, antacids, fluconazole.

PRESCRIPTION:
Yes.

PBS:
Yes.

PERMITTED IN SPORT:
Yes.

OVERDOSE:
Lethargy, drowsiness, nausea, vomiting and indigestion may occur. Give activated charcoal. Seek medical attention.

OTHER INFORMATION:
Revolutionary new class of medications first released in 1999 to treat all forms of arthritis and inflammation with much reduced side effects.
See also Aspirin, Diclofenac, Diflunisal, Flurbiprofen, Ibuprofen, Indomethacin, Ketoprofen, Mefenamic Acid, Naproxen, Piroxicam, Rofecoxib, Sulindac, Tenoxicam, Tiaprofenic Acid.

Cephalexin
See CEPHALOSPORINS.

CEPHALOSPORINS

TRADE and GENERIC NAMES:
Apatef (Cefotetan).
Ceclor, Cefaclor, Cefkor, GenRx Cefaclor, Keflor (Cefaclor).
Cefazolin, Kefzol (Cephazolin).
Cefrom (Cefpiromine). Injection only.
Cefalexin-BC, Cilex, GenRx Cephalexin, Ibilex, Keflex, Sporahexal (Cephalexin).
Cefotaxime-BC, Claforan (Cefotaxime).
Fortum (Ceftazidime).
Keflin (Cephalothin).
Mandol (Cephamandole).
Maxipime (Cefepime). Injection only.
Mefoxin (Cefoxitin).
Rocephin (Ceftriaxone).
Zinnat (Cefuroxime).

DRUG CLASS:
Antibiotic, broad spectrum.

USES:
Treats infections caused by susceptible bacteria.

DOSAGE:
 One or two capsules two to four times a day.

FORMS:
Capsules, tablets, suspension, injection.

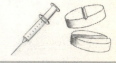

PRECAUTIONS:
Safe to use in pregnancy (cephalexin – A, other forms – B1), breast feeding and children.
Use with caution in severe kidney disease and colitis (inflammation of large bowel). Use short term if possible.

SIDE EFFECTS:
Common: Diarrhoea,
Unusual: Nausea, vomiting, belly pain, rash.

Severe but rare (stop medication, consult doctor): Bloody diarrhoea, severe itchy rash, yellow skin (jaundice).

INTERACTIONS:

Other drugs:
- Diuretics, other cephalosporins.

Other substances:
- May cause false positive test for sugar in urine.

PRESCRIPTION:
Yes.

PBS:
Yes (some forms are excluded).

PERMITTED IN SPORT:
Yes.

OVERDOSE:
Exacerbation of side effects only likely effect.

OTHER INFORMATION:
Cephalosporins are a group of relatively strong antibiotics. They are divided by doctors into first, second and third generation cephalosporins. In general terms, they increase in strength and the number of types of bacteria they are active against decreases as you go from first to third generation drugs.

First generation cephalosporins (cefaclor, cephalexin, cefuroxime) are commonly used by general practitioners. They are active against a very wide range of bacteria, and are particularly useful in chest, urinary, skin and joint infections. Side effects are uncommon with the first generation capsules and mixtures, but more likely with the third generation cephalosporins which are given by injection. They do not cause dependence or addiction.

Cephalothin, Cephamandole, Cephazolin

See CEPHALOSPORINS.

Cetalkonium chloride

TRADE NAMES:
Only available in Australia in combination with other medications.
Applicaine Drops (with benzocaine, cetylpyridinium and other ingredients).
Applicaine Gel (with cetylpyridinium and other ingredients).
Bonjela, Seda-Gel Gel (with choline salicylate).

DRUG CLASS:
Antiseptic.

USES:
Mouth and gum irritation, teething.

DOSAGE:
 Apply every three hours.

FORMS:
Drops, gel, lotion.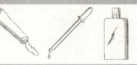

PRECAUTIONS:
Safe in pregnancy, breast feeding, children and infants over four months.

SIDE EFFECTS:
Minimal.

INTERACTIONS:
Most forms: None significant.
Bonjela: Do not take Aspirin.

PRESCRIPTION:
No.

PBS:
No.

PERMITTED IN SPORT:
Yes.

OTHER INFORMATION:
Widely and safely used for infant teething.

Cetirizine

See ANTIHISTAMINES, SEDATING.

Cetomacrogol

TRADE NAMES:
Hydraderm, Sorbolene.

DRUG CLASS:
Moisturiser.

USES:
Dry skin, cracked skin, soap substitute.

DOSAGE:
 Apply as required.

FORMS:
Cream.

PRECAUTIONS:
Safe to use in pregnancy, breast feeding and children.

SIDE EFFECTS:
None.

INTERACTIONS:
None.

PRESCRIPTION:
No.

PBS:
No.

PERMITTED IN SPORT:
Yes.

OTHER INFORMATION:
One of the original moisturising creams that has been available for over a century. Cheap and effective.

Cetrimide

TRADE NAMES:
Available in Australia only in combination with other medications as an antiseptic.
Acnederm, Curacleanse Antiseptic Gel, Savlon Antiseptic (with chlorhexidine).
Pine Tar Lotion with Menthol (with menthol, dimethicone, pine tar).
SOOV (with other ingredients).

DRUG CLASS:
Antiseptic.

USES:
Disinfection of skin and medical equipment, acne, minor burns, grazes.

DOSAGE:
 Apply or use as required.

FORMS:
Cream, wash, lotion, liquid.

PRECAUTIONS:
Safe to use in pregnancy, breast feeding and children.
Avoid eye contact.

SIDE EFFECTS:
Minimal.

INTERACTIONS:
None significant.

PRESCRIPTION:
No.

PBS:
No.

PERMITTED IN SPORT:
Yes.

OVERDOSE:
If swallowed may cause nausea, vomiting, diarrhoea and stomach cramps.

Medications

Cetylpyridinium

TRADE NAMES:
Lemsip Lozenges.
Applicaine Drops (with benzocaine and other ingredients).
Applicaine Gel, Gentlees (with other ingredients).
Cepacaine (with benzocaine).
Cepacol Cough (with dextromethorphan, benzocaine, menthol).
Difflam Lozenges (with benzydamine).
Difflam Anti-inflammatory Cough Lozenges (with pholcodine, benzydamine and other ingredients).
Duro-Tuss Lozenges (with pholcodine).
Seda-Gel Lotion (with lignocaine and chlorhexidine).
Numerous other locally produced preparations.

DRUG CLASS:
Antiseptic.

USES:
Prevention of infection, treatment of minor infections.

DOSAGE:

Depends on form and condition being treated.
Follow instruction on packaging or from doctor.

FORMS:
Lozenges, gargle, spray, gel, lotion, wipes, drops.

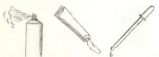

PRECAUTIONS:
Safe to use in pregnancy (A), breast feeding and children.
Use with caution in children under 3 years.

SIDE EFFECTS:
None significant.

INTERACTIONS:
None significant.

PRESCRIPTION:
No.

PBS:
No.

PERMITTED IN SPORT:
Yes.

OVERDOSE:
Swallowing gargle or lozenges may cause belly discomfort, nausea and diarrhoea.

Charcoal

TRADE NAMES:
Ad-Sorb, Charcocaps.
Carbosorb (Activated charcoal).
Carbosorb S (Activated charcoal with sorbitol).
No Gas (with simethicone).

USES:
Excessive amounts of burping, excessive passing of wind, gassy discomfort of stomach, may absorb some forms of poison, drug overdosage.

DOSAGE:

One to four tablets or capsules (200 to 1200mg) up to four times a day.

FORMS:
Capsules, tablets (store capsules away from heat and moisture).
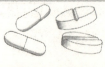

PRECAUTIONS:
Safe in pregnancy and breast feeding. Not for use under 3 years of age.
Do not take from one hour before to two hours after a meal.

Do not take if:
 taking other medications as charcoal may interfere with absorption of many types of medication.
- suffering from diarrhoea.

SIDE EFFECTS:
Common: May alter bowel habits.

INTERACTIONS:
Other drugs:
- Reduces absorption of many other medications.

Other substances:
- Reduces absorption of some foods.

PRESCRIPTION:
No.

PBS:
No.

PERMITTED IN SPORT:
Yes.

OVERDOSE:
Diarrhoea only likely result. No specific treatment necessary.

OTHER INFORMATION:
One of the oldest medications known to mankind, and probably used since prehistoric times for stomach wind and discomfort. Very effective in reducing amount of toxic material absorbed in overdosage of medication or in poisoning. See section on First Aid at front of book.

Chickenpox vaccine
(Varicella zoster vaccine)

TRADE NAMES:
Varilix, Varivax II.

DRUG CLASS:
Vaccine.

USES:
Prevention of chickenpox.

DOSAGE:
 Children from 9 months to 12 years: One injection
Over 12 years: Two injections six weeks apart.

FORMS:
Injection.

PRECAUTIONS:
Not for use in pregnancy.
Use with caution in breast feeding.
Use with caution in HIV (AIDS).

Do not take if:
 sensitive to neomycin.

- blood transfusion received recently.
- suffering from a high fever.
- under nine months of age.

SIDE EFFECTS:
Common: Local soreness at injection site.
Unusual: Rash. Vaccinated person may rarely pass virus onto an unvaccinated person to cause chickenpox.
Severe but rare (stop medication, consult doctor): Allergic reaction.

INTERACTIONS:
Other drugs:
- Other viral vaccines (eg. measles), salicylates.

Other substances:
- Interferes with TB skin tests.

PRESCRIPTION:
Yes.

PBS:
No.

PERMITTED IN SPORT:
Yes.

OTHER INFORMATION:
Introduced in 2000 as the first vaccine against chickenpox. An attenuated live virus vaccine.

Chlorambucil

TRADE NAME:
Leukeran.

DRUG CLASS:
Alkyllater.

USES:
Leukaemia, breast and ovary cancer, Hodgkin's disease, lymphoma, other malignant conditions.

DOSAGE:

Complex. Must be individualised by doctor for each patient.

FORMS:
Tablets (yellow) of 2mg.

PRECAUTIONS:
Must not be used in pregnancy (D) unless the life of the mother is at risk as serious damage to the foetus is likely. Breast feeding must be ceased before use. Use in children only when medically essential. Regular blood tests to monitor blood cells and liver function essential.
Adequate contraception must be used during treatment.
Must be used with extreme caution in all patients.

SIDE EFFECTS:
Common: Bone marrow damage.
Unusual: Nausea, vomiting, diarrhoea, mouth ulcers, lung damage, convulsions in children.
Severe but rare (stop medication, consult doctor): Yellow skin (jaundice).

INTERACTIONS:
Other drugs:
- Phenylbutazone, other cancer treatments.

PRESCRIPTION:
Yes.

PBS:
Yes.

PERMITTED IN SPORT:
Yes.

OVERDOSE:
May cause damage to blood and bone marrow cells, convulsions, incoordination and irrational behaviour. Administer activated charcoal or induce vomiting if medication taken recently. Seek medical assistance.

OTHER INFORMATION:
Although serious side effects are possible, chlorambucil may be life saving in some patients.
See also Amsacrine, **VINCA ALKALOIDS**.

Chloramphenicol

TRADE NAMES:
Chloromycetin, Chlorsig, Minims Chloramphenicol.

DRUG CLASS:
Antibiotic.

USES:
Very severe generalised infections, common eye and ear infections.

DOSAGE:

Capsules: One or two capsules four times a day.
Eye drops: Two drops every three hours.
Eye ointment: Insert three times a day.
Ear drops: Two drops four times a day.

FORMS:
Capsules (white/grey) of 250mg, injection, solution, ear drops, eye drops, eye ointment.

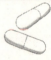
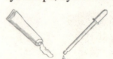

Medications

PRECAUTIONS:
Ear drops, eye drops and ointment may be used in pregnancy, breast feeding and children.
Capsules and solution should not be used in any patient unless no other antibiotic can be successfully used for a severe infection. There are further risks of using capsules and solution in pregnancy (C), breast feeding and children. Capsules and solution never to be used in infants.
Never to be used long term.
Use with additional caution in liver and kidney disease.

SIDE EFFECTS:
Common: Eye preparations – Irritation. Capsules – Nausea.
Unusual: Capsules – Vomiting, sore mouth, diarrhoea, headache.
Severe but rare: Chloramphenicol can cause (sometimes months after the medication is taken) a severe and usually fatal blood disorder with an incidence between 1:25,000 and 1:100,000 patients using the drug. In children under three months, the 'Grey syndrome' may occur as a result of the undeveloped liver's inability to deal adequately with the drug.

INTERACTIONS:
Other drugs:
- Anticonvulsants, anticoagulants.

PRESCRIPTION:
Yes.

PBS:
Yes.

PERMITTED IN SPORT:
Yes.

OVERDOSE:
Exacerbation of side effects and increased risk of serious reactions possible.

OTHER INFORMATION:
Chloramphenicol is a very effective and well tolerated antibiotic, but because if taken by mouth or injection it can rarely cause death by destroying the red blood cells, it is only used when no other antibiotic can control a severe infection. It is widely used in eye and ear preparations quite safely, as the drug is not absorbed in any significant concentration into the blood stream. The use of chloramphenicol is usually restricted to topical creams and eye preparations. It is used by mouth or injection in certain serious life threatening situations, such as meningitis, when it worth the risk of the rare side effects.

Chlorhexidine

TRADE NAMES:
Bactigras, Chlorhexidine Preparations, Hexol, Microshield Preparations, Plaqacide, Savacol.
Acnederm Foaming Wash, Curacleanse Gel, Microshield Antiseptic Concentrate, Pharmacia Chlorhexidine and Cetrimide, Savlon (with cetrimide).
Difflam C Anti-inflammatory Antiseptic (with benzydamine).
Hamilton Cleansing Lotion (with glycerol, paraffin and other ingredients).
Hemocane (with lignocaine and other ingredients).
Lignocaine Gel with Chlorhexidine (with lignocaine).
Medi Creme (with lignocaine, cetrimide and other ingredients).
Medi Pulv (with hexamidine).
Mycil Healthy Feet (with tolnaftate).
Nasalate (with phenylephrine).
Paraderm Plus (with lignocaine and bufexamac).
Seda-Gel Lotion (with lignocaine and cetylpyridinium).
Silvazine (with silver sulfadiazine).
SOOV (with other ingredients).

DRUG CLASS:
Antiseptic.

USES:
Prevention of infection, skin cleaning, minor infections of skin and mouth.

Medications

DOSAGE:
 Depends on form. Normally use several times a day.

FORMS:
Cream, solution, wash, oil, powder, tincture, gel, mouth wash, tulle (netting), suppository.

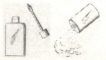

PRECAUTIONS:
Safe to use in pregnancy (A), breast feeding and children.
Avoid eye contact.
Use with caution on open wounds and in nose, mouth and ears.

SIDE EFFECTS:
Uncommon: Skin sensitivity.

INTERACTIONS:
Other drugs:
- None significant.

Other substances:
- Detergents.

PRESCRIPTION:
No.
A prescription is required for some medication combinations.

PBS:
No.

PERMITTED IN SPORT:
Yes.

OVERDOSE:
Diarrhoea, belly discomfort and vomiting only likely effects if swallowed. Seek medical advice, particularly in children.

OTHER INFORMATION:
Widely used antiseptic cleansing agent in hospitals, general practice and operating theatres. Very safe and effective.

Chlormethiazole

TRADE NAME:
Hemineurin M.

DRUG CLASS:
Hypnotic, sedative.

USES:
Control of alcohol withdrawal and delirium tremens, short term control of extreme agitation and confusion.

DOSAGE:
 Two to four capsules at once, then two capsules hourly until symptoms controlled, then reduce dosage slowly, ceasing within 10 days. Only prescribed in circumstances of strict medical supervision.

FORMS:
Capsules of 192mg (brown).

PRECAUTIONS:
Safe in pregnancy (A). Breast feeding should be ceased if medication necessary.
Not for use in children.
Lower doses required in elderly.
Caution needed in patients with heart disease, and severe liver disease.

Do not take if:

 suffering from severe lung disease.
- operating machinery, driving vehicles, or undertaking tasks requiring coordination, concentration and alertness.

SIDE EFFECTS:
Common: Drowsiness, nasal irritation, eye irritation, facial burning.
Unusual: Rash, red skin, itch, excessive phlegm in throat.
Severe but rare (stop medication, consult doctor): Jaundice (liver damage).

Medications

INTERACTIONS:
Other drugs:
- Propranolol, cimetidine, diazoxide, sedatives.

Herbs:
- Celery, camomile, goldenseal, valerian.

Other substances:
- Reacts adversely with alcohol.

PRESCRIPTION:
Yes.

PBS:
No.

PERMITTED IN SPORT:
Yes.

OVERDOSE:
Low blood pressure, low body temperature, slow heart rate and coma may occur. Symptoms worse if taken with alcohol. Rarely fatal. Administer activated charcoal or induce vomiting if patient alert and tablets taken recently. Seek urgent medical attention.

OTHER INFORMATION:
Rarely used outside hospital. Very useful in very disturbed patients or alcohol withdrawal. Addictive.

See also BARBITURATES, Flunitrazepam, Midazolam, Nitrazepam, Temazepam, Triazolam, Zolpidem, Zopiclone.

Chloroquine

TRADE NAME:
Chlorquin.

DRUG CLASS:
Antimalarial.

USES:
Prevention and treatment of malaria, treatment of rheumatoid arthritis, amoebic hepatitis, systemic lupus erythematosus (SLE), other collagen affecting diseases.

DOSAGE:
 Malaria prevention: Two tablets on same day once a week for two weeks before and four weeks after entering malarious area.
Treatment: Start with high daily dose and slowly decrease as directed by doctor.

FORMS:
Tablets of 155mg (white).

PRECAUTIONS:
Not to be used in pregnancy (D) unless mother's life threatened by severe malaria. May be used in breast feeding and children over 1 year.
Use with caution in liver and kidney disease, psoriasis and porphyria.
Regular eye checks required if used daily long term.

Do not take if:
 suffering from alcoholism.

- trying to become pregnant.

SIDE EFFECTS:
Common: Minimal.
Unusual: Nausea, vomiting, diarrhoea, skin pigmentation, hair loss, rash.
Severe but rare (stop medication, consult doctor): Deteriorating vision.

Home Guide to Medication 133

INTERACTIONS:
Other drugs:
- Antacids, kaolin, cimetidine, metronidazole, ampicillin, other antimalarial drugs.

Other substances:
- Reacts with alcohol.

PRESCRIPTION:
Yes.

PBS:
No.

PERMITTED IN SPORT:
Yes.

OVERDOSE:
Very serious. Depresses the function of the heart and lungs, and may cause fatal liver damage. Administer activated charcoal or induce vomiting if taken recently. Seek urgent medical assistance.

OTHER INFORMATION:
Chloroquine is the traditional mainstay for the prevention of malaria, but malaria in many areas (including most of southeast Asia and New Guinea) is now resistant to Chloroquine. Found serendipitously to assist in the treatment of rheumatoid and other autoimmune diseases. Very dangerous to the foetus in pregnancy, and in overdose.

See also Atovaquone, Artemether and Lumefantrine, Doxycycline, Hydroxychloroquine, Mefloquine, Primaquine, Proguanil, Pyrimethamine, Quinine bisulphate, Sulfadoxine.

Chloroxylenol

TRADE NAMES:
Dettol Liquid.
Dettol Cream (with triclosan).
Solyptol, Zeasorb (with other ingredients).

DRUG CLASS:
Antiseptic.

USES:
Minor skin cuts and grazes, minor skin infections.

DOSAGE:
 Apply as required. Dilute liquid before use.

FORMS:
Cream, powder, liquid.

PRECAUTIONS:
Safe in pregnancy, breast feeding and children.
Do not use for prolonged period.
Avoid eye contact.

SIDE EFFECTS:
Minimal.

INTERACTIONS:
None significant.

PRESCRIPTION:
No.

PBS:
No.

PERMITTED IN SPORT:
Yes.

Chlorphenesin

TRADE NAME:
ZSC Powder (with zinc oxide).

DRUG CLASS:
Antifungal.

USES:
Minor fungal infections of skin, prickly heat, nappy rash.

DOSAGE:
 Apply two or three times a day.

FORMS:
Ointment, powder.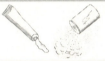

PRECAUTIONS:
Safe to use in pregnancy, breast feeding and children.

SIDE EFFECTS:
Minimal.

INTERACTIONS:
None.

PRESCRIPTION:
No.

PBS:
No.

PERMITTED IN SPORT:
Yes.

OTHER INFORMATION:
Widely used and effective, particularly in preventing recurrent fungal infections.

Chlorpheniramine

See ANTIHISTAMINES, SEDATING.

Chlorpromazine

See PHENOTHIAZINES.

Chlorthalidone

See THIAZIDE DIURETICS.

Cholecalciferol
(Vitamin D)

TRADE NAMES:
Vitamin D consists of a number of chemicals including Cholecalciferol, Calcitriol and Ergocalciferol. It is found in many non-prescription mineral and vitamin supplements.

DRUG CLASS:
Fat soluble essential vitamin.

USES:
Nutritional deficiency, osteomalacia, rickets, hypoparathyroidism, osteoporosis.

DOSAGE:
 Daily requirement is 5μg. Much higher doses used to treat diseases listed above.

FORMS:
Tablets, capsules.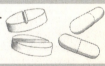

PRECAUTIONS:
Safe for use in pregnancy, breast feeding and children. Use with caution in infants. Use with caution in kidney disease.

SIDE EFFECTS:
Common: Drowsiness, constipation.
Unusual: Calcium deposits in tissue, dehydration.

INTERACTIONS:
Other drugs:
- Cholestyramine, thiazide diuretics, digoxin, magnesium.

Medications

PRESCRIPTION:
No.

PBS:
No.

PERMITTED IN SPORT:
Yes.

OVERDOSE:
Serious. Symptoms include loss of appetite, tiredness, vomiting, diarrhoea, sweating, excess urine production, extreme thirst and headache. This may progress to high blood pressure and kidney failure. Administer activated charcoal or induce vomiting if taken recently. Seek medical assistance.

OTHER INFORMATION:
Remember, vitamins are merely chemicals that are essential in minute doses for the functioning of the body, and if taken to excess, act as a drug. Vitamin D can be found naturally in fatty fish (sardines, tuna, salmon, herrings etc.), margarine and egg yolk. It is also produced in the body by the action of sunlight on the skin.
See also Calcitriol, Ergocalciferol.

Cholera vaccine
(Vibrio cholera vaccine)

TRADE NAME:
Orochol.

DRUG CLASS:
Vaccine.

USES:
Prevention of cholera.

DOSAGE:

Mix contents of one double chambered sachet with 100mL water and drink once. Repeat every six months if necessary.

FORMS:
Powder.

PRECAUTIONS:
May be used with caution in pregnancy (B2). May be used in breast feeding and children over 2 years of age.
Do not take if:
 suffering from significant infection, diarrhoea, vomiting or reduced immunity.

SIDE EFFECTS:
Common: Nausea, diarrhoea, headache.
Unusual: Fever, swelling of tissues.

INTERACTIONS:
Other drugs:
- Sulfonamides, antibiotics, chloroquine, oral typhoid vaccine.

PRESCRIPTION:
Yes.

PBS:
No.

PERMITTED IN SPORT:
Yes.

OVERDOSE:
An unintentional additional dose is unlikely to have any serious effect.

OTHER INFORMATION:
Not effective against all forms of cholera, and additional care in selection of food and drink and in personal hygiene also essential. Introduced in 2000 as a replacement for a far less effective injected cholera vaccine. Used only in travellers to affected areas of Asia, Africa and tropical America who may be living in primitive conditions. Cholera causes a massive diarrhoea which is often fatal, but which can be successfully treated with oral fluids or fluids given by a drip into a vein.

CHOLESTEROL LOWERING DRUGS
(HYPOLIPIDAEMICS)

See Atorvastatin, Cholestyramine, Colestipol, Fluvastatin, Gemfibrizol, Nicotinic acid, Pravastatin, Probucol, Simvastatin.

Cholestyramine

TRADE NAME:
Questran Lite.

DRUG CLASS:
Hypolipidaemic.

USES:
High blood cholesterol level, relief of itch caused by liver failure, relief of diarrhoea caused by small intestine disease.

DOSAGE:

12g to 16g of powder per day with copious fluids in divided doses through the day.

FORMS:
Powder.

PRECAUTIONS:
Should be used with caution in pregnancy (B2). Not to be used in breast feeding. Use with caution in children.
May interfere with vitamin absorption. Lower doses required in elderly.

Do not take if:

suffering from gall bladder obstruction, phenylketonuria.

SIDE EFFECTS:
Common: Constipation.
Unusual: Belly discomfort, excess wind, vomiting, heartburn, loss of appetite, rash, osteoporosis.
Severe but rare (stop medication, consult doctor): Unusual bleeding.

INTERACTIONS:
Other drugs:
- Other medications should be taken 30 minutes before cholestyramine or four to six hours after cholestyramine.
- Warfarin, digoxin, phenylbutazone, chlorthiazide, tetracyclines, phenobarbitone, thyroxine, oestrogen.

Herbs:
- Alfalfa, fenugreek, garlic, ginger.

PRESCRIPTION:
Yes.

PBS:
Yes.

PERMITTED IN SPORT:
Yes.

OVERDOSE:
No significant problems. Severe constipation probable.

OTHER INFORMATION:
One of the earlier forms of treatment for excess blood cholesterol. Effective, but patient compliance often poor due to taste and method of taking.

See also Atorvastatin, Colestipol, Fluvastatin, Gemfibrizol, Nicotinic acid, Pravastatin, Probucol, Simvastatin.

Choline salicylate

TRADE and GENERIC NAMES:
Herron Baby Teething Gel
Applicaine (with cetalkonium chloride, cetylpyridinium chloride).
Bonjela, Seda-Gel (with cetalkonium chloride).
Ora-Sed Jel (with benzalkonium chloride).
Numerous other ointments, creams and liniments contain various salicylates.

DRUG CLASS:
Salicylate.

USES:
Temporary relief of gum pain.

DOSAGE:
 Apply gels every three hours.

FORMS:
Gel, drops.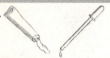

PRECAUTIONS:
Safe in pregnancy and breast feeding and children over four months.

SIDE EFFECTS:
Minimal.

INTERACTIONS:
Other drugs:
• Aspirin interacts with mouth gels.

PRESCRIPTION:
No.

PBS:
No.

PERMITTED IN SPORT:
Yes.

OTHER INFORMATION:
Widely used and very safe.

Choline theophyllinate

See THEOPHYLLINES.

Chorionic gonadotrophin, human
(HCG)

TRADE NAMES:
Pregnyl, Profasi.

DRUG CLASS:
Sex hormone, Trophic hormone.

USES:
Infertility in women, delayed puberty in girls, failure of testicular development, failure of sperm production.

DOSAGE:
 As determined for each patient by doctor.

FORMS:
Injection.

PRECAUTIONS:
Do not use before puberty.
May cause multiple foetus pregnancy.
Use with caution in fluid retention.
Not normally used for more than six months.
Do not take if:
☠ suffering from some types of cancer affecting sex organs.

SIDE EFFECTS:
Common: Minimal.
Unusual: Multiple foetus pregnancy, fluid retention, rash.

INTERACTIONS:
None significant.

PRESCRIPTION:
Yes.

Medications

PBS:
Yes (authority required).

PERMITTED IN SPORT:
No.

OVERDOSE:
Not likely to be serious. Given under strict medical supervision.

Cilastatin and Imipenem

TRADE NAME:
Primaxin (only available as combination of the two medications).

DRUG CLASS:
Antibiotic.

USES:
Serious bacterial infections of the lungs, belly, pelvis, bones, joints, heart and blood stream.

DOSAGE:
 Administered by a slow infusion through a drip into a vein. Dosage determined by doctor.

FORMS:
Injection.

PRECAUTIONS:
Use with caution in pregnancy (B3), breast feeding and infants.
Safe to use in children.
Use with caution in kidney disease, colitis, meningitis, brain abscess and other brain diseases.
Not for long term use.
Regular blood tests necessary during use to monitor blood and liver.

SIDE EFFECTS:
Common: Rash, itch, other infections, fever, abnormal taste.
Unusual: Seizures, confusion, dizziness, tiredness, nausea, diarrhoea.
Severe but rare (stop medication, consult doctor): Vein inflammation, low blood pressure, pseudomembranous colitis (bowel inflammation), abnormal blood cells, abnormal liver function.

INTERACTIONS:
Other drugs:
- Other antibiotics, ganciclovir, probenecid.

PRESCRIPTION:
Yes.

PBS:
No.

PERMITTED IN SPORT:
Yes.

OTHER INFORMATION:
Introduced in 1999 for the treatment of serious infections that do not respond to other antibiotics.

Cimetidine

TRADE NAMES:
Cimehexal, GenRx Cimetidine, Magicul, Sigmetadine, Tagamet.

DRUG CLASS:
Antiulcerant, H2 receptor antagonist.

USES:
Prevention and treatment of ulcers of the stomach, oesophagus (gullet) and duodenum (upper small intestine). Prevention of acid reflux into the oesophagus (heartburn).
Unapproved use: Treatment of widespread warts.

DOSAGE:
 Up to 1600mg a day in one, two or three doses.

FORMS:

Tablets,
soluble tablets,
injection.

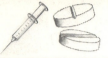

PRECAUTIONS:

Care should be taken with use in pregnancy (B1) and breast feeding. Children under 12 may be treated at the discretion of the doctor.
Use with caution in kidney and liver disease.

Do not take if:

 suffering from severe kidney disease or phenylketonuria.

SIDE EFFECTS:

Common: Headache, diarrhoea, tiredness, dizziness, drowsiness, rash.
Unusual: Constipation, breast enlargement and tenderness (both sexes), confusion in elderly.
Severe but rare (stop medication, consult doctor): Hepatitis (jaundice – yellow skin), pancreatitis (severe stomach pain), rapid or irregular heartbeat.

INTERACTIONS:

Other drugs:
- Toxicity may result with warfarin, phenytoin, lignocaine, theophylline, quinidine, procainamide, flecainide, nifedipine, antacids.
- Effectiveness of many medications affecting the heart, blood pressure and diabetes may be altered.

Herbs:
- Alfalfa, capsicum, eucalyptus, senega.

PRESCRIPTION:
Yes.

PBS:
Yes.

PERMITTED IN SPORT:
Yes.

OVERDOSE:
No serious effects reported.

OTHER INFORMATION:

Introduced in 1978, cimetidine was the first of a group of drugs (H2 antagonists) that radically improved the treatment of peptic ulcers. It is very safe, and available without prescription in some countries, but interacts with many other medications, and as a result has fallen out of favour.

Cinchocaine

see ANAESTHETICS, LOCAL

Ciprofloxacin

TRADE NAMES:

C-Flox, CiloQuin, Ciloxan, Cipro, Ciproxin, Proquin.
Ciproxin HC (with hydrocortisone).

DRUG CLASS:

Quinolone antibiotic.

USES:

Serious bacterial infections.

DOSAGE:

 Tablets: One to three tablets twice a day.
Eye drops: Two drops every 15 to 60 minutes.
Ear drops: Three drops twice a day.

FORMS:

Tablets (white) of 250mg and 500mg, eye drops, ear drops, infusion.

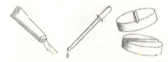

PRECAUTIONS:

Use tablets in pregnancy (B3) and breast feeding only if medically essential.
Tablets not for use in children.
Eye and ear drops may be used with caution in pregnancy and children.
Use with caution in cystic fibrosis and kidney disease.
Designed for short term use.

SIDE EFFECTS:
Common: Nausea.
Unusual: Diarrhoea, vomiting, rash, restlessness, tremor, headache, dizziness, itch.

INTERACTIONS:
Other drugs:
- Antacids, theophylline, probenecid, warfarin, cyclosporin, metoclopramide, glibenclamide, NSAIDs, iron, sucralfate.

Other substances:
- Caffeine (coffee, stimulant drinks and tablets)

PRESCRIPTION:
Yes.

PBS:
Yes (restricted to more severe infections).

PERMITTED IN SPORT:
Yes.

OVERDOSE:
Exacerbation of side effects most likely. Administer activated charcoal or induce vomiting if medication taken recently.

OTHER INFORMATION:
Very effective and useful medication in dealing with severe bacterial infections that are not controlled by other antibiotics. Introduced in the late 1980s.

See also Norfloxacin

Cisapride

TRADE NAME:
Prepulsid.

DRUG CLASS:
Prokinetic agent. Increases emptying rate of stomach.

USES:
Reflux oesophagitis (heartburn), delayed emptying of food from stomach (gastroparesis).

DOSAGE:

5 to 20mg three times a day 15 minutes before food, and last thing at night.

FORMS:
Tablets of 5mg and 10mg, suspension.

PRECAUTIONS:
Caution required with use in pregnancy (B1) and breast feeding.
Safe in children.
Lower doses may be necessary in elderly.
Reassess necessity for treatment every three months.

Do not take if:
Suffering from significant liver or kidney disease, intestinal bleeding or obstruction, irregular heart rhythm, specific heart abnormalities (prolonged QT interval), very slow heart rate, heart failure.
- Premature infant.

SIDE EFFECTS:
Common: Belly cramps and noises, diarrhoea.
Unusual: Blurred vision, increased cholesterol levels.
Severe but rare (stop medication, consult doctor): Jaundice (yellow skin), convulsions, urinary frequency, severe belly pain, irregular heart rhythm.

Medications

INTERACTIONS:
Other drugs:
- Serious interactions with ketoconazole, itraconazole, miconazole, fluconazole, erythromycin, clarithromycin, nefazodone, ritonavir. Digoxin absorption reduced. Many other drugs have their absorption slightly altered due to increased emptying rate of stomach.

Other substances:
- Reacts with alcohol to increase its effect.

PRESCRIPTION:
Yes.

PBS:
Yes (very restricted).

PERMITTED IN SPORT:
Yes.

OVERDOSE:
Abdominal cramps and diarrhoea only problems. Reversed by giving activated charcoal.

OTHER INFORMATION:
Initially widely used in combination with other medications to treat stomach and oesophageal (gullet) ulcers. Still very effective for these indications, but has been found with wide use to very rarely cause a serious irregularity of heart rhythm, and so has now been restricted, and is only used when no other medication is effective.

Cisplatin

TRADE NAMES:
Cisplatin.

USES:
Cancer of the ovary, testes, bladder, skin (squamous cell carcinomas) involving the head and neck.

DOSAGE:
 Injections or by drip infusion as directed by doctor.

FORMS:
Injection, infusion.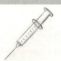

PRECAUTIONS:
Not to be used in pregnancy (D) unless mother's life in danger, as damage to foetus possible. Breast feeding must be ceased before use. Use in children only if medically essential.
Regular blood tests to check blood cells and kidney function essential.
Regular hearing tests recommended.
Ensure adequate fluid intake.
Use with caution in kidney disease.

Do not take if:
 suffering from hearing disorders, kidney failure or bone marrow disease.

SIDE EFFECTS:
Common: Ringing in ears, pins and needles, nausea, vomiting.
Unusual: Tremor, muscle spasms, wheeze, unusual bleeding and bruising.
Severe but rare (stop medication, consult doctor): Abnormal blood test results.

INTERACTIONS:
Other drugs:
- Aminoglycosides, frusemide.

Other substances:
- Aluminium medical instruments.

Medications

PRESCRIPTION:
Yes.

PBS:
Yes.

PERMITTED IN SPORT:
Yes.

OVERDOSE:
Exacerbation of side effects likely.

OTHER INFORMATION:
Despite its significant side effects, cisplatin may be life saving in some patients with cancer.

Citalopram

TRADE NAMES:
Celapram, Cipramil, Talohexal.

DRUG CLASS:
SSRI antidepressant.

USES:
Depression.

DOSAGE:
 20mg to 60mg once a day.

FORMS:
Tablets of 20mg (white).

PRECAUTIONS:
Use with caution in pregnancy (B3), breast feeding and children.
Use with caution in heart disease, slow heart rate, diabetes, fitting tendency, mania and liver disease.
Reduce dose slowly, do not stop suddenly. Use lower doses in elderly.
Do not take if:
 taking other SSRI antidepressants.

SIDE EFFECTS:
Common: Nausea, diarrhoea, tiredness, dry mouth, impotence.
Unusual: Sweating, loss of appetite, tremor, agitation, watery nose, low libido.
Severe but rare (stop medication, consult doctor): Excessive bruising, bleeding or nose bleeds.

INTERACTIONS:
Other drugs:
- Other SSRI and tricyclic antidepressants, MAOI, cimetidine, lithium, moclobemide, tryptophan, tramadol, sumatriptan, ketoconazole, itraconazole, macrolide antibiotics, omeprazole, metoprolol, cimetidine.

Herbs:
- St John's wort, ma huang.

Other substances:
- Alcohol.

PRESCRIPTION:
Yes.

PBS:
Yes.

PERMITTED IN SPORT:
Yes.

OVERDOSE:
Tiredness, vomiting, rapid heart rate, tremor, sweating, poor circulation (blue tinged colour to skin), coma, convulsions and death can occur. Induce vomiting or administer activated charcoal if tablets taken recently. Seek urgent medical attention.

OTHER INFORMATION:
Introduced in 1998 as a further advance within an excellent class of drugs that are very effective and safe in treating depression. Claimed to have a faster effect and fewer side effects than other SSRI antidepressants.

See also Fluoxetine, Fluvoxamine, Paroxetine, Sertraline, Venlafaxine.

Citric acid

See URINARY ALKALINISERS.

Clarithromycin

TRADE NAMES:
Klacid.
Klacid HP7, Losec HP7 (with omeprazole, amoxycillin).
Pylorid KA (with ranitidine, amoxycillin).

DRUG CLASS:
Macrolide antibiotic.

USES:
Treatment of infections caused by susceptible bacteria (eg. Streptococcal throat infection, skin infection, bronchitis), in combination with other drugs to eradicate *Helicobacter pylori*, which may cause peptic ulcers.

DOSAGE:
 250 to 500mg twice a day.

FORMS:
Tablets (yellow) of 250mg and 500mg, suspension.

PRECAUTIONS:
Use with caution in pregnancy (B3), breast feeding and children.
Not designed for prolonged or repeated use.
Use with caution in kidney disease.
Do not take if:
 suffering from severe liver disease, jaundice (yellow skin).

SIDE EFFECTS:
Common: Nausea, vomiting, diarrhoea, rash, headache.
Unusual: Belly pain, loss of appetite, excess wind, dizziness, ear noises, temporary deafness.

Severe but rare (stop medication, consult doctor): Yellow skin (jaundice), irregular heartbeat.

INTERACTIONS:
Other drugs:
- Serious interactions with cisapride and pimozide.
- Alprazolam, carbamazepine, cilastazol, cyclosporin, digoxin, lovastatin, methylprednisolone, midazolam, oral contraceptives, phenytoin, quinidine, sildenafil, simvastatin, theophylline, triazolam, valproate, vinblastine, warfarin, zidovudine,

PRESCRIPTION:
Yes.

PBS:
Tablets: Yes
Suspension: No.

PERMITTED IN SPORT:
Yes.

OVERDOSE:
Severe diarrhoea, stomach pains and deafness may occur.

OTHER INFORMATION:
Very effective and generally safe antibiotic introduced in 1998. Becoming used as a first line antibiotic in many situations.

Clavulanic acid

See Potassium clavulanate.

Clindamycin

TRADE NAMES:
Cleocin, Clindatech, Dalacin C, Dalacin T, Dalacin V.

DRUG CLASS:
Antibiotic.

USES:
Solution: Acne.
Cream: Vaginal infections.
Capsules and injection: Serious bacterial infections (eg. lung, belly and skin abscesses).

DOSAGE:

Solution, lotion: Apply to acne twice a day.
Capsules: One or two capsules, three or four times a day.
Vaginal cream: Insert once a day at bedtime.

FORMS:
Capsules of 150mg, injection, solution, vaginal cream, syrup, lotion.

 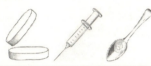

PRECAUTIONS:
Safe to use in pregnancy (A). May be used with caution in breast feeding and infants.
Safe in children.
Capsules and syrup not to be used long term.
Capsules and syrup to be used with caution in kidney and liver disease.
Cream not to be used on skin or in eyes.

SIDE EFFECTS:
Common: Solution, lotion – dry skin.
Capsules and syrup – nausea, rash.
Unusual: Capsules and syrup – vomiting, diarrhoea, belly pains, itch.
Severe but rare (stop medication, consult doctor): Severe or bloody diarrhoea, severe belly pain, yellow skin (jaundice).

INTERACTIONS:
Other drugs:
- Erythromycin.
Other substances:
- Capsules and syrup react with alcohol.

PRESCRIPTION:
Yes.

PBS:
Capsules and syrup: Yes.
Other forms: No.

PERMITTED IN SPORT:
Yes.

OVERDOSE:
Exacerbation of side effects likely.

OTHER INFORMATION:
Effective medication that is reserved for more severe internal infections, but commonly used as a topical preparation to control acne.

Clioquinol

TRADE NAMES:
Hydroform (with hydrocortisone).
Locacorten Vioform (with flumethasone).

DRUG CLASS:
Antiseptic.

USES:
Minor infections of skin, ear canal infections.

DOSAGE:
 Apply four times a day.

FORMS:
Cream, ear drops.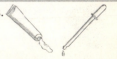

PRECAUTIONS:
Safe to use in pregnancy, breast feeding (avoid application to breasts) and children over two years.
Avoid eye contact.
Not designed for long term use.
May interfere with blood tests for thyroid function.

SIDE EFFECTS:
Common: Staining, skin irritation.
Unusual: Pimples on skin.
Severe but rare (stop medication, consult doctor): Brain irritation in children.

INTERACTIONS:
Other:
- Affects thyroid function tests.

PRESCRIPTION:
Yes.

PBS:
No.

PERMITTED IN SPORT:
Yes.

OTHER INFORMATION:
Dangerous brain inflammation may rarely occur if used in children under 2 years.

Clobazam

TRADE NAME:
Frisium.

DRUG CLASS:
Benzodiazepine (Anxiolytic).

USES:
Short term relief of anxiety and sleep disturbances.

DOSAGE:
 10 to 30mg a day

FORMS:
Tablets of 10mg (white).

PRECAUTIONS:
Should be used with caution in pregnancy (C), but not at all if delivery of infant imminent as it may decrease desire to breathe in newborn infant. Should be used with caution in breast feeding. Not for use in children.
Lower dose required in elderly.
Should be used intermittently and not constantly as dependency may develop.
Use with caution in glaucoma, heart disease, kidney or liver disease, psychiatric conditions, schizophrenia, depression and epilepsy.

Do not take if:
 suffering from severe lung or liver disease, confusion, myasthenia gravis, sleep apnoea.
- tendency to addiction or dependence.
- operating machinery, driving a vehicle or undertaking tasks that require concentration and alertness.

SIDE EFFECTS:
Common: Reduced alertness, dependence, dry mouth, depression.
Unusual: Incoordination, tremor, confusion, increased risk of falls in elderly, rash, low blood pressure, nausea, muscle weakness,
Severe but rare (stop medication, consult doctor): Jaundice (yellow skin).

INTERACTIONS:
Other drugs:
- Sedatives, other anxiolytics, disulfiram, cimetidine, anticonvulsants, narcotics, anticholinergics, lithium.

Herbs:
- Guarana, kava kava, passionflower, St John's wort, valerian.

Other substances:
- Reacts with alcohol to cause sedation and confusion.

Medications

PRESCRIPTION:
Yes.

PBS:
No.

PERMITTED IN SPORT:
Yes.

OVERDOSE:
Seldom life threatening. May cause drowsiness, confusion and coma. Induce vomiting if tablets taken recently. Seek medical assistance.

OTHER INFORMATION:
Very safe if used correctly. Dependency may be a problem, particularly in elderly, due to overuse.

See also Alprazolam, Bromazepam, Buspirone, Diazepam, Lorazepam, Oxazepam.

Clofazime

TRADE NAME:
Lamprene.

USES:
Leprosy in combination with other drugs.

DOSAGE:
 Complex. As directed by doctor.

FORMS:
Capsules (brown) of 50mg.

PRECAUTIONS:
Not to be used in pregnancy (C) or breast feeding.
May be used in children.
Use with caution in liver or kidney disease, history of abdominal pain or diarrhoea.
Use for more than three months should be carefully monitored.

SIDE EFFECTS:
Common: Reversible discolouration of skin and hair, nausea, dry skin and eyes, diarrhoea.
Unusual: Itch, light sensitive skin, acne, vomiting, belly pain, weight loss, impaired vision.
Severe but rare (stop medication, consult doctor): Blood in faeces or urine, severe belly pain.

INTERACTIONS:
Nil significant.

PRESCRIPTION:
Yes.

PBS:
No.

PERMITTED IN SPORT:
Yes.

OVERDOSE:
Serious exacerbation of side effects possible. Seek medical assistance.

Clomiphene

TRADE NAMES:
Clomhexal, Clomid, GenRx Clomiphene, Serophene.

USES:
Female infertility.

DOSAGE:
 One tablet a day for five days. Repeat monthly for a maximum of six cycles.

FORMS:
Tablets (white) of 50mg.

PRECAUTIONS:
Not to be used in pregnancy (B3), breast feeding or children.
Use with caution with ovarian cysts

and fibroids.
Multiple pregnancies (ie: twins, triplets, quads etc.) possible.
Must only be used in carefully selected patients.

Do not take if:

 suffering from liver disease, hormonal tumours, abnormal bleeding from uterus.

SIDE EFFECTS:

Common: Hot flushes, belly discomfort and bloating.
Unusual: Enlarged ovaries. One in 200 chance of birth defect (similar to normal risk).
Severe but rare (stop medication, consult doctor): Blurred vision, yellow skin (jaundice).

INTERACTIONS:

None significant.

PRESCRIPTION:

Yes (restricted to specific doctors in some states).

PBS:

Yes (restricted).

PERMITTED IN SPORT:

Yes.

OVERDOSE:

May increase risk of foetal abnormality if taken during pregnancy. Otherwise no serious effects likely.

OTHER INFORMATION:

Stimulates ovulation in infertile women, but several eggs may be released, resulting in multiple pregnancies. Has revolutionised the lives of many infertile couples since first introduced in the 1970s.

See also Follicle Stimulating Hormone.

Clomipramine

See TRICYCLIC ANTIDEPRESSANTS.

Clonazepam

TRADE NAMES:
Paxam, Rivotril.

DRUG CLASS:
Anticonvulsant, Benzodiazepine.

USES:
Epilepsy.

DOSAGE:
 Given twice a day in individually determined dosage. Follow doctors instructions carefully.

FORMS:
Tablets, drops, injection.

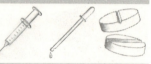

PRECAUTIONS:

Not to be used in pregnancy (D) unless medically essential. Use with caution in breast feeding and infants. Safe for use in children.
Use with caution in glaucoma, myasthenia gravis, low blood pressure, heart disease, kidney and liver disease, depression and psychiatric conditions (eg. schizophrenia).
Use with caution if operating machinery or driving a vehicle.
Do not stop taking medication suddenly, but reduce dose slowly.
Use with caution for long periods of time.

Do not take if:

 suffering from severe lung or liver disease, alcoholism.

SIDE EFFECTS:

Common: Drowsiness (worse in first few days), incoordination, behaviour changes, tiredness, fatigue, muscle weakness, excess salivation, dizziness.

Unusual: Low blood pressure, itch, skin pigmentation, changes in hair distribution, nausea, loss of appetite, weight changes, impotence, low libido, confusion, aggression, depression, irritability, cough.
Severe but rare (stop medication, consult doctor): Unusual bruising or bleeding.

INTERACTIONS:
Other drugs:
- Sedatives, stimulants, phenytoin, carbamazepine, valproate, other anticonvulsants, disulfiram, cimetidine.

Herbs:
- Guarana, borage, kava kava, passionflower, St John's wort, valerian, evening primrose (linoleic acid), Gingko biloba.

Other substances:
- Reacts adversely with alcohol.

PRESCRIPTION:
Yes.

PBS:
Yes (authority required).

PERMITTED IN SPORT:
Depends on sport. Check with governing body.

OVERDOSE:
May cause drowsiness, confusion, incoordination, slow breathing, coma and rarely death. Administer activated charcoal or induce vomiting if taken recently and patient alert. Seek urgent medical attention.

OTHER INFORMATION:
May cause dependence and addiction if used inappropriately.

See also **BARBITURATES, BENZODIAZEPINES, Carbamazepine, Ethosuximide, Gabapentin, Lamotrigine, Levetiracetam, Oxcarbazepine, Phenytoin, Primidone, Sodium valproate, Sulthiame, Tiagabine, Topiramate, Vigabatrin.**

Clonidine

TRADE NAME:
Catapres.

DRUG CLASS:
Antihypertensive, antimigraine.

USES:
High blood pressure, prevention of migraine and vascular headaches, treatment of menopausal flushing.

DOSAGE:

One or two tablets, three times a day to a maximum of 900µg per day.

FORMS:
Tablets (white) of 100µg and 150µg, injection.
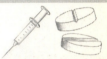

PRECAUTIONS:
Use with significant caution in pregnancy (B3) and breast feeding.
Use with caution in children under 12 years.
Use with caution in depression, poor blood supply to brain, irregular heartbeat, constipation and phaeochromocytoma.
Medication must not be stopped suddenly, but dosage must be slowly decreased over several days or weeks.

Do not take if:

suffering from liver or kidney failure, severe heart disease, diabetes or very slow heart rate.

SIDE EFFECTS:
Common: Drowsiness, dry mouth, stomach upsets.
Unusual: Hair thinning, blurred vision, constipation, delusions, depression, impotence, irritability, low blood pressure on standing.

INTERACTIONS:
Other drugs:
- Sedatives, hypnotics, other medications

for treatment of high blood pressure, antidepressants.

Other substances:
- Reacts with alcohol.

PRESCRIPTION:
Yes.

PBS:
Yes.

PERMITTED IN SPORT:
Yes.

OVERDOSE:
Slow heart rate, low blood pressure and coma result. First aid involves administering activated charcoal or inducing vomiting if awake and alert, and seeking very urgent medical assistance.

OTHER INFORMATION:
Old-fashioned, but often effective treatment for migraines. Only used for most severe forms of high blood pressure. Occasionally used to stop symptoms of narcotic withdrawal.

Clopidogrel

TRADE NAMES:
Iscover, Plavix

DRUG CLASS:
Anticoagulant.

USES:
Prevention of blood clots (eg. strokes, heart attack).

DOSAGE:
 One tablet a day.

FORMS:
Tablets of 75mg (pink).

PRECAUTIONS:
Not for use in pregnancy (B1). Use with caution in breast feeding and children. Use with caution in peptic ulcers, other intestinal ulcers, recent heart attack or stroke, glaucoma.
Cease before any elective surgery.

Do not take if:

 suffering from liver disease or bleeding disorders.

SIDE EFFECTS:
Common: Abnormal bleeding, diarrhoea, rash, agitation.
Unusual: Low level of white blood cells.
Severe but rare (stop medication, consult doctor): Jaundice, heavy bleeding.

INTERACTIONS:
Other drugs: NSAID, aspirin (but may be used with aspirin in low doses), fluvastatin, anticoagulants (eg. warfarin, heparin), phenytoin, tamoxifen, tolbutamide.

PRESCRIPTION:
Yes.

PBS:
Yes (restricted to certain circumstances – authority required).

PERMITTED IN SPORT:
Yes.

OVERDOSE:
May be very serious with excessive internal and external bleeding. Administer activated charcoal or inducing vomiting if awake and alert, and seek urgent medical assistance.

OTHER INFORMATION:
Very useful medication introduced 1999 as an additional treatment for patients who have recurrent episodes of abnormal blood clotting.

See also ANTICOAGULANTS.

Clotrimazole

TRADE NAMES:

Canesten, Clofeme, Clonea, Clotreme, Clozole, Gyne-Lotremin, Tinaderm Extra.
Hydrozole (with hydrocortisone).
Numerous locally produced creams.

USES:

Treatment of fungal infections of skin (tinea, athlete's foot, pityriasis versicolor) and vagina (thrush).

DOSAGE:

Skin: Apply two or three times a day.
Vagina: Insert once a day at night.

FORMS:

Cream, vaginal cream, vaginal pessary, gel, lotion, solution.

PRECAUTIONS:

Safe to use in pregnancy (A), breast feeding and children.
Should not be swallowed or used in eyes.
Use with care on open wounds.

SIDE EFFECTS:

Common: Nil.
Unusual: Skin irritation, rash.

INTERACTIONS:

None significant.

PRESCRIPTION:

No.

PBS:

No. Available to some Veterans Affairs pensioners.

PERMITTED IN SPORT:

Yes.

OTHER INFORMATION:

This class of medication dramatically improved the treatment of fungal infections when introduced in the early 1970s. Very safe and effective.

See Econazole, Fluconazole, Itraconazole, Ketoconazole, Miconazole.

Clozapine

See PHENOTHIAZINES.

Coal tar

See TARS.

Cocaine

OTHER NAMES:

Crack, coke.

DRUG CLASS:

Local anaesthetic, stimulant.

USES:

No recognised medical uses.
Used illegally as a psychoactive drug to cause euphoria (artificial happiness).

FORMS:

Used illegally in many forms including smoked, injected and sniffed.

PRECAUTIONS:

Should never be used in pregnancy (increased risk of malformation and heart disease), breast feeding or children.

Do not use if:

 suffering from psychiatric disturbances.
- driving a car, operating machinery, swimming or undertaking any activity that requires concentration.

SIDE EFFECTS:

Common: Damage to nostrils, fever, headache, irregular heart rate, dilation of pupils, loss of libido, infertility, impotence, breast enlargement and

Medications

tenderness in both sexes, menstrual period irregularities, psychiatric disturbances, abnormal breast milk production, may lead to desire for more frequent use or stronger drugs of addiction.
Unusual: High blood pressure, perforation of nasal septum, difficulty in breathing, convulsions, stroke, dementia, heart attack, death.

INTERACTIONS:
Other drugs:
- Stimulants, MAOI, tricyclic antidepressants, sedatives, other medications acting on the brain.

Other substances:
- Reacts with alcohol, heroin and marijuana.

PRESCRIPTION:
Illegal except in hospitals under specific circumstances.

PBS:
No.

PERMITTED IN SPORT:
No.

OVERDOSE:
Convulsions, difficulty in breathing, irregular heart rate, coma and death may occur. Seek urgent medical assistance.

OTHER INFORMATION:
The more refined version of cocaine known as "crack" is the only form that can be smoked, and is ten times more potent than cocaine base, and is therefore more dangerous. Highly addictive. When smoked, sniffed or injected, cocaine works within seconds to cause euphoria (artificial happiness) and stimulates the brain to increase all sensations. After use many people feel worse than before, hence they want to repeat the artificial high. The more frequently it is used, the higher the dose necessary to achieve the same sensations, and the greater the risk of serious side effects.

Codeine Phosphate

TRADE NAMES:
Actacode.
Aspalgin, Codiphen, Codis, Codral Forte, Disprin Forte, Veganin (with aspirin).
Codalgin, Codalgin Forte, Codapane, Codral Pain Relief, Dolased Day Relief, Dymadon Co, Dymadon Forte, Liquigesic-Co, Mersyndol Day, Panadeine, Panadeine Forte, Panamax Co, Prodeine-15 (with paracetamol).
Biotech Cold & Flu Non-Drowsy, Codral Cold & Flu, Codral Daytime, Nyal Plus Cold & Flu (with paracetamol, pseudoephedrine).
Biotech Cold & Flu, Codral 4 Flu (with paracetamol, chlorpheniramine and pseudoephedrine).
Bis-Pectin (with kaolin, aluminium hydroxide, pectin and other ingredients).
Codral Dry Cough, Nucosef (with pseudoephedrine).
Codalgin Plus, Dolased Analgesic Relaxant, Dolased Night Relief, Fiorinal, Mersyndol, Mersyndol Forte, Panalgesic (with paracetamol, doxylamine succinate).
Nurofen Plus (with ibuprofen).
Painstop (with paracetamol and promethazine).
Also found in numerous other locally marketed pain relievers and cough medications.

DRUG CLASS:
Narcotic.

USES:
Pain, diarrhoea, coughing.

DOSAGE:
 5mg to 60mg every four to six hours.

FORMS:
Tablets as codeine phosphate alone. Tablets and mixtures in combination with other medications.

PRECAUTIONS:

Safe in pregnancy (A). Should be used with caution in breast feeding and children.
Should be used with caution in people with an underactive thyroid gland, liver disease, an enlarged prostate gland or lung disease.
Not for long term use.
Elderly patients should take a reduced dose.

Do not take if:

 addicted to narcotics.

- operating machinery, driving a vehicle or undertaking other activity requiring concentration.

SIDE EFFECTS:

Common: Constipation, nausea, drowsiness.
Unusual: Dizziness, vomiting.

INTERACTIONS:

Other drugs:
- Increases the effects of sedatives and hypnotics.

Herbs:
- Kava kava.

Other substances:
- Do not drink alcohol while taking codeine

PRESCRIPTION:

Tablets with no more than 8mg codeine: No prescription needed.
Tablets with more than 8mg codeine: Prescription required.
Mixtures: No prescription.

PBS:

Panadeine Forte, Dymadon Forte: Yes
Others: No

PERMITTED IN SPORT:

Yes.

OVERDOSE:

Moderately serious. May cause initial stimulation, followed by vomiting, drowsiness, convulsions, reduced breathing, coma and very rarely death. Seek urgent medical attention.

OTHER INFORMATION:

May cause dependency or addiction if used unnecessarily for long periods.
The mildest of the narcotic drugs.
Very effective and, except for risk of dependency, very safe.
Widely used in many cough and cold mixtures, pain relievers and preparations for diarrhoea. Minimal problems if used short term.

See also Alfentanil, Buprenorphine, Dextromoramide, Dextropropoxyphene, Fentanyl, Heroin, Hydromorphone, Methadone, Morphine, Oxycodone, Pentazocine, Pethidine.

Cod liver oil

TRADE NAMES:

Found in a large range of over the counter and health shop medications.

USES:

Tonic, moisturiser.

DOSAGE:

Apply to skin as required, or take one dose a day.

FORMS:

Cream, capsule, mixture etc.

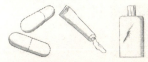

PRECAUTIONS:

Safe in breast feeding and children.
Small amounts safe, but excess may cause birth defects in pregnancy (D).

SIDE EFFECTS:

Common: Foul taste.
Unusual: Nausea, diarrhoea.

INTERACTIONS:

None significant.

PRESCRIPTION:
No.

PBS:
No.

PERMITTED IN SPORT:
Yes.

OVERDOSE:
Vomiting and diarrhoea only likely effects.

OTHER INFORMATION:
Very old form of multivitamin (particularly A and D) and fatty acid supplementation.
See also Retinol.

Colchicine

TRADE NAME:
Colgout.

USES:
Treatment of acute gout, prevention of gout.

DOSAGE:

Two tablets at once, then one tablet every two hours until relief obtained, diarrhoea starts or six tablets taken.

FORMS:
Tablets (white) of 500µg.

PRECAUTIONS:
Not for use in pregnancy (D) and breast feeding, or children under 2 years.
Use with caution in heart disease, kidney disease and bowel disease.
Lower doses necessary in elderly and debilitated.
Do not take if:
 suffering from severe liver, kidney or heart disease.
• suffering from blood cell disorders or diarrhoea.

SIDE EFFECTS:
Common: Diarrhoea.
Unusual: Reduced body temperature, reduced urge to breathe, muscle weakness, cold extremities, high blood pressure, rash.
Severe but rare (stop medication, consult doctor): Abnormal bleeding or bruising, muscle pain, hair loss, changes to vision.

INTERACTIONS:
Other drugs:
• Sedatives, cyclosporin, erythromycin, warfarin.
Other substances:
• Alcohol may aggravate gout.

PRESCRIPTION:
Yes.

PBS:
Yes.

PERMITTED IN SPORT:
Yes.

OVERDOSE:
Very serious. Symptoms may be delayed in onset and may include burning mouth, vomiting, diarrhoea, gut pain and spasms, delirium, convulsions and death. Administer activated charcoal or induce vomiting if medication taken recently. Give copious fluids. Seek urgent medical attention.

OTHER INFORMATION:
Does not cause addiction or dependence. Effective, but diarrhoea limits its usefulness.

Colestipol

TRADE NAME:
Colestid.

DRUG CLASS:
Hypolipidaemic.

USES:
Lowering high levels of cholesterol in blood.

DOSAGE:
 15g to 30g two to four times a day with water.

FORMS:
Granules (sachets of 5g).

PRECAUTIONS:
Should be used with caution in pregnancy (B2). Should not be used in breast feeding. Use only if medically essential in children.
Regular blood tests to check blood fat levels are recommended.

Do not take if:
 suffering from underactive thyroid gland, diabetes, severe kidney or liver disease.

SIDE EFFECTS:
Common: Constipation.
Unusual: Vitamin deficiency.
Severe but rare (stop medication, consult doctor): Chest pain, rapid heart rate.

INTERACTIONS:
Other drugs:
- Numerous other drugs – check with doctor.
- Do not take at same time as any other medication.

Herbs:
- Alfalfa, fenugreek, garlic, ginger.

PRESCRIPTION:
Yes.

PBS:
Yes.

PERMITTED IN SPORT:
Yes.

OVERDOSE:
Constipation only likely problem.

See also Atorvastatin, Cholestyramine, Fluvastatin, Gemfibrizol, Nicotinic acid, Pravastatin, Probucol, Simvastatin

CONTRACEPTIVES

See Etonogestrel, Levonorgestrel, Medroxyprogesterone acetate, ORAL CONTRACEPTIVES, SPERMICIDES.

Copper

TRADE NAMES:
Caltrate Plus, Citracal Plus (with calcium, manganese, zinc, magnesium). Also found in numerous other vitamin and mineral supplements, and soothing creams.

DRUG CLASS:
Mineral.

USES:
Soothing and healing cream and gel, mild antiseptic, mineral supplement.

DOSAGE:
 Tablets: As directed.
Cream and gel: Massage into skin twice a day.

FORMS:
Tablets, liniment, cream.

PRECAUTIONS:
May be used in pregnancy and breast feeding.
Not for use under 2 years of age.

Do not swallow mouthwash tablets.
Use with caution in kidney and liver failure.

Do not use if:

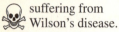 suffering from Wilson's disease.
- under other circumstances

SIDE EFFECTS:
Common: Creams, gels – Dry skin, skin irritation.
Tablets – Minimal.

INTERACTIONS:
None significant.

PRESCRIPTION:
No.

PBS:
No.

PERMITTED IN SPORT:
Yes.

CORTICOSTEROIDS

DISCUSSION:
A diverse group of drugs that act as powerful reducers of inflammation anywhere in the body, depending on the way in which they are administered (eg. creams act only on skin, inhalers act mainly in lungs, tablets are absorbed and work throughout the body). Unfortunately, if inappropriately used, they may have significant side effects.

See Alclometasone, Beclomethasone dipropionate, Betamethasone, Budesonide, Cortisone acetate, Desonide, Dexamethasone, Fludrocortisone, Flumethasone, Fluorometholone, Fluticasone, Hydrocortisone, Medrysone, Methylprednisolone, Mometasone, Prednisolone and Prednisone, STEROIDS, Triamcinolone.

Cortisol
See Hydrocortisone.

Cortisone Acetate

TRADE NAME:
Cortate.

DRUG CLASS:
Corticosteroid.

USES:
Severe asthma, rheumatoid and other forms of severe arthritis, autoimmune diseases (eg. Sjögren syndrome), severe allergy reactions, and other severe and chronic inflammatory diseases.

DOSAGE:
 One to five tablets a day as directed by doctor.

FORMS:
Tablets (white) of 5mg and 25mg.

PRECAUTIONS:
May be used with caution in pregnancy (A), breast feeding and children.
Use with caution if under stress, and in patients with under-active thyroid gland, liver disease, diverticulitis, high blood pressure, myasthenia gravis, or kidney disease.
Use for shortest period of time possible.

Do not use if:

 suffering from an uncontrolled infection, peptic ulcer, or osteoporosis.
- having a vaccination.

SIDE EFFECTS:
Common: May cause bloating, weight gain, rashes and intestinal disturbances.
Unusual: Biochemical disturbances of blood, muscle weakness, bone weakness,

impaired wound healing, skin thinning, tendon weakness, peptic ulcers, gullet ulcers, bruising, increased sweating, loss of fat under skin, premature ageing, excess facial hair growth in women, pigmentation of skin and nails, acne, convulsions, headaches, dizziness, growth suppression in children, aggravation of diabetes, worsening of infections, cataracts, aggravation of glaucoma, blood clots in veins and sleeplessness.

Most significant side effects occur only with prolonged use.

Medication should not be ceased abruptly, but dosage should be slowly reduced.

Severe but rare (stop medication, consult doctor): Any significant side effect should be reported to a doctor immediately.

INTERACTIONS:

Other drugs:
- Oral contraceptives, aspirin, ketoconazole, antacids, barbiturates, diabetes medications, digoxin, diuretics, phenytoin, rifampicin.

PRESCRIPTION:
Yes.

PBS:
Yes.

PERMITTED IN SPORT:
No.

OVERDOSE:
Medical treatment is required. Serious effects and death rare.

OTHER INFORMATION:
Extremely effective and useful medication if used correctly. Must be used with extreme care under strict medical supervision. Lowest dose and shortest possible course should be used. Not addictive.

Co-trimoxazole

See Sulfamethoxazole, Trimethoprim.

COUGH SUPPRESSANTS

DISCUSSION:
Antitussives are the mixtures, lozenges or tablets that stop coughing. They act by directly soothing the inflamed throat, decreasing the sensitivity of the part of the brain that triggers the spasm of coughing, decreasing the amount of phlegm in the throat, anaesthetising the throat, reducing inflammation, reducing pain, and by almost any combination of these methods. There are several different ingredients used in cough mixtures. They differ from the expectorants (see separate entry), which are designed to increase coughing but make the coughing more effective so that phlegm can be cleared from the lungs and throat.

See Ammonium chloride, Codeine Phosphate, Dextromethorphan, Dihydrocodeine, EXPECTORANTS, Pentoxyverine citrate, Pholcodine.

COX -2 INHIBITORS

DISCUSSION:
Anti-inflammatory medication for the treatment of arthritis with minimal effects on the stomach compared to other nonsteroidal anti-inflammatory drugs – NSAIDs.

See Celecoxib, Meloxicam, Rofecoxib.

Coxiella burnetti vaccine
(Q fever vaccine)

TRADE NAME:
Q-Vax.

DRUG CLASS:
Vaccine.

USES:
Prevention of Q fever.

DOSAGE:
 Single injection gives long term immunity.

FORMS:
Injection.

PRECAUTIONS:
Not designed to be used in pregnancy (B2), but inadvertent use in pregnancy is unlikely to be harmful. May be used in breast feeding. Not designed for use in children. Use with caution in immune system diseases.

Do not take if:
 previously vaccinated.
- previously infected by Q fever.
- allergic to poultry or eggs.

SIDE EFFECTS:
Common: Local redness and tenderness at injection site, headache.
Unusual: Muscle pains, fever, sweating.

INTERACTIONS:
None significant.

PRESCRIPTION:
Yes.

PBS:
No.

PERMITTED IN SPORT:
Yes.

OVERDOSE:
An additional inadvertent vaccination may cause significant allergic or other adverse reactions. Seek medical assistance.

OTHER INFORMATION:
Not in general use, but restricted to abattoir workers, veterinarians and laboratory workers who may be exposed to Q fever. Q fever is an infection caught from cattle, sheep and goats.

Cromoglycate, sodium
See Sodium cromoglycate.

Cromolyn sodium
See Sodium cromoglycate.

Crotamiton

TRADE NAME:
Eurax.

DRUG CLASS:
Antiseptic.

USES:
Itchy skin, scabies.

DOSAGE:
 Itch: Apply to affected area two or three times a day.
Scabies: Rub over entire body surface except scalp and face after bathing for three to five consecutive days.

FORMS:
Cream, lotion.

PRECAUTIONS:
Use with caution in first three months of pregnancy (B2) and small children. May be used safely in breast feeding (not on breasts) and older children.
Avoid eye contact.

Medications

Do not use if:

 suffering from weeping or broken skin.

SIDE EFFECTS:

Common: Slight stinging, sensitive skin.

INTERACTIONS:

None significant.

PRESCRIPTION:

No.

PBS:

No.

PERMITTED IN SPORT:

Yes.

Cyanocobalamin
(Vitamin B12)

TRADE NAMES:

Blackmores B12, Cytamen.
A large number of other preparations include various forms of Vitamin B12 alone or in combination with other medications.

DRUG CLASS:

Vitamin.

USES:

Pernicious anaemia, pins and needles sensation of feet.

DOSAGE:

 Injection: Once every three months, or as determined by doctor.
Recommended daily allowance: 2µg a day.

FORMS:

Tablets, capsules, mixture, drops, injection.

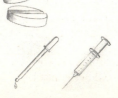

PRECAUTIONS:

Safe in pregnancy, breast feeding and children.
Do not take in high doses or for prolonged periods of time.

Do not take if:

 suffering from megaloblastic anaemia of pregnancy.

SIDE EFFECTS:

Common: Injection site reaction.
Unusual: Diarrhoea, abdominal pain, skin rash, allergy reaction.
Severe but rare (stop medication, consult doctor): Vision changes (Leber's disease).

INTERACTIONS:

Other drugs:
- Chloramphenicol, oral contraceptives, folic acid, colchicine, phenytoin, some antibiotics (aminoglycosides), phenobarbitone, primidone, cimetidine, ranitidine, nizatadine, famotidine.

Other substances:
- Alcohol.

PRESCRIPTION:

No.

PBS:

Injection: Yes
Other forms: No.

PERMITTED IN SPORT:

Yes.

OVERDOSE:

Unlikely to cause any serious effects.

OTHER INFORMATION:

Several chemical variations of vitamin B12 exist including cyanocobalamin and hydroxycobalamin. They are identical in their actions and use. Cyanocobalamin was the original form of vitamin B12 used medically. Vitamin B12 is a water soluble vitamin found in animal products. It is essential for the formation of red blood cells, normal growth, and normal fat and sugar metabolism. In pernicious anaemia, the body loses the ability to absorb vitamin

B12 from the stomach. Remember, vitamins are merely chemicals that are essential for the functioning of the body, and if taken to excess, act as a drug.
See also Hydroxycobalamin.

Cyclopentolate
See MYDRIATICS.

Cyclophosphamide

TRADE NAMES:
Cycloblastin, Endoxan.

DRUG CLASS:
Alkylater.

USES:
Leukaemia, lymphomas, multiple myeloma, Hodgkin's disease, cancer of the ovary and retina (eye).
Prevents rejection of transplanted organs.

DOSAGE:
 Must be individualised by doctor for each patient depending on disease, severity, response, weight and age of patient.

FORMS:
Tablets of 50mg (brown), injection.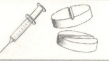

PRECAUTIONS:
Use in pregnancy (D) will cause damage or death to the foetus, and therefore Cyclophosphamide must not be used unless life of mother is threatened. Breast feeding must be ceased before use. Use in children only if child's life at risk.
Regular blood tests to follow course of disease and the effect of medication on blood cells, bone marrow and liver function essential.
Adequate contraception must be used during use of Cyclophosphamide.

Must be used with caution in all patients. Ensure adequate fluid intake.
Do not take if:
 suffering from recent surgery.

SIDE EFFECTS:
Common: Nausea, vomiting, mouth ulcers, hair loss, dermatitis, nail damage, delayed wound healing, infertility.
Unusual: Yellow skin (jaundice), blood in urine, fluid retention, testicle and ovary damage, skin pigmentation, diarrhoea
Severe but rare (stop medication, consult doctor): Lung and kidney damage, further cancer development.

INTERACTIONS:
Other drugs: Barbiturates, imipramine, allopurinol, phenothiazines, indomethacin, insulin, diabetic medications, digoxin, cytotoxics, warfarin.

PRESCRIPTION:
Yes.

PBS:
Yes.

PERMITTED IN SPORT:
Yes.

OVERDOSE:
Extremely serious. May cause severe damage to kidney, bone marrow and blood cells leading to destruction of immune system and subsequent fatal infections. Administer activated charcoal or induce vomiting if medication taken recently. Seek urgent medical assistance.

OTHER INFORMATION:
Although cyclophosphamide has multiple serious side effects, it may be life saving in patients with severe or widespread cancer or leukaemia.
See also VINCA ALKALOIDS.

Cycloserine

TRADE NAME:
Cycloserine.

DRUG CLASS:
Antibiotic.

USES:
Tuberculosis, severe urinary tract infections.

DOSAGE:

250 to 500mg twice a day.

FORMS:
Capsules of 250mg (red/grey).

PRECAUTIONS:
May be used with caution in pregnancy, breast feeding and children.
Regular blood tests essential to check blood cells, liver and kidney function, and drug levels.

Do not take if:
suffering from epilepsy, depression, severe anxiety, psychoses, severe kidney disease or alcoholism.

SIDE EFFECTS:
Common: Allergy, rash, brain irritation.
Unusual: Liver and heart damage.
Severe but rare (stop medication, consult doctor): Jaundice (yellow skin).

INTERACTIONS:
Other drugs:
- Ethionamide, isoniazid.

Other substances:
- Alcohol.

PRESCRIPTION:
Yes.

PBS:
No.

PERMITTED IN SPORT:
Yes.

OVERDOSE:
Likely to be very serious. Seek urgent medical attention.

OTHER INFORMATION:
Only used after other forms of treatment have failed.
See also Ethambutol, Isoniazid, Pyrazinamide, Rifampicin.

Cyclosporin

TRADE NAMES:
Cysporin, Neoral, Sandimmun.

DRUG CLASS:
Immunomodifier.

USES:
Prevents rejection of transplanted organs (eg. kidney, liver, heart), severe rheumatoid arthritis, severe psoriasis, nephrotic syndrome.

DOSAGE:

Taken twice a day with milk or food.

FORMS:
Capsules of 10mg, 25mg, 50mg and 100mg, solution, infusion.

PRECAUTIONS:
Not to be used in pregnancy (C) unless mother's life at risk. Breast feeding must be ceased before use. Must be used with caution in children.
Careful monitoring of all patients by clinical examination and blood tests essential.

Do not take if:
suffering from high blood pressure, significant infection, immune deficiency, poor kidney function.

SIDE EFFECTS:

Common: Excess hair growth, tremor, sore gums, nausea, vomiting, high blood pressure, increased risk of infection.
Unusual: Fluid retention, convulsions, diarrhoea, peptic ulcer formation, acne, rash, itch, muscle cramps, headache, hearing loss, ringing in ears, confusion, tiredness, anaemia, pins and needles, flushing, sinusitis, weight loss.

INTERACTIONS:

Other drugs:
- Reacts with a wide range of medications. Check all with a doctor.

Herbs:
- St John's wort, echinacea.

Other substances:
- Zinc.

PRESCRIPTION:

Yes

PBS:

Infusion: Yes (authority required).
Other forms: No

PERMITTED IN SPORT:

Yes.

OVERDOSE:

Serious. Administer activated charcoal or induce vomiting if medication taken recently. Seek urgent medical assistance.

OTHER INFORMATION:

Potent medication which can be of great benefit if used appropriately and carefully.

Cyproheptadine

See ANTIHISTAMINES, SEDATING.

Cyproterone Acetate

TRADE NAMES:

Androcur, Cyprone, Cyprostat, Procur. Brenda, Diane, Juliet (with ethinyloestradiol – see oral contraceptives).
Climen (with oestradiol valerate).

DRUG CLASS:

Antiandrogen (acts against testosterone).

USES:

Excessive body hair in women, loss of scalp hair in women, severe acne in women.
Reduction of sexual drive in men, premature puberty, cancer of the prostate gland.
Brenda, Diane: Oral contraception.
Climen: Hormone replacement therapy.

DOSAGE:

Androcur, Cyprone, Cyprostat, Procur: Depends on use and response to medication. Usually 100 to 300mg a day. Follow doctor's instructions.
Brenda, Diane, Juliet: Take one daily, including seven days of sugar drug free pills.
Climen: Take one tablet a day for three weeks, then stop for seven days before restarting.

FORMS:

Tablets.

PRECAUTIONS:

Not to be used in pregnancy (D) or breast feeding. Adequate contraception must be used in sexually active women. Not to be used in girls. For use in boys only if medically indicated.
Use Androcur, Cyprone, Cyprostat and Procur with caution if operating machinery or undertaking tasks that require concentration.
Use with caution in diabetes, liver tumours.

Do not take if:

☠ suffering from severe liver disease, blood clots, sickle cell anaemia, severe depression or diabetes.

SIDE EFFECTS:

Common: Male infertility, reduced libido, tiredness, increased weight, nausea, headache, irregular menstrual periods (Androcur and Cyprone only).
Unusual: Breast enlargement in men, depression, breast milk production, sleeplessness, hot flushes.
Severe but rare (stop medication, consult doctor): Calf or chest pain.

INTERACTIONS:
None significant.

PRESCRIPTION:
Yes.

PBS:
Climen: Yes.
Androcur, Cyprone, Cyprostat, Procur: Yes (restricted to certain specific conditions – authority required).
Brenda, Diane, Juliet: No.

PERMITTED IN SPORT:
Yes.

OVERDOSE:
Aggravation of side effects likely.

OTHER INFORMATION:
Does not cause addiction or dependence. Must be used strictly according to doctor's instructions.
See also Danazol, Dydrogesterone, Ethinyloestradiol, Etonogestrel, HORMONE REPLACEMENT THERAPY, Medroxyprogesterone acetate, Oestradiol, Oestriol, Oestrogen, ORAL CONTRACEPTIVES, Oxandrolone, Piperazine oestrone sulfate, Testosterone.

Cysteamine

TRADE NAME:
Cystagon.

DRUG CLASS:
Detoxifying agent.

USES:
Cystinosis affecting the kidneys.

DOSAGE:

Depends on body weight. Gradually increased over six weeks to maintenance dose level.

FORMS:
Capsules (white) of 50mg and 150mg.

PRECAUTIONS:
Use with caution in pregnancy (B2), breast feeding and children.
Use with caution if brain symptoms or rash present due to cystinosis.
Liver function and blood condition must be monitored regularly by blood tests.

Do not take if:
 hypersensitive to penicillamine.

SIDE EFFECTS:
Common: Rash, drowsiness, depression, stomach ulcers, nausea.
Unusual: Bleeding from bowel, vomiting blood, abnormal liver function, fever, low white blood cell count.
Severe but rare (stop medication, consult doctor): Seizures, brain inflammation.

INTERACTIONS:
None significant.

PRESCRIPTION:
Yes.

PBS:
No.

Medications

PERMITTED IN SPORT:
Yes.

OTHER INFORMATION:
Introduced in 1997 for treatment of the rare condition, cystinosis.

Cytarabine

TRADE NAME:
Cytarabine.

DRUG CLASS:
Antimetabolite.

USES:
Treatment of leukaemia and lymphomas.

DOSAGE:

As determined for each patient by doctor.

FORMS:
Injection.

PRECAUTIONS:
Never to be used in pregnancy (D). Use with caution in breast feeding. Regular blood tests necessary to monitor function of kidney, liver and blood cells.

SIDE EFFECTS:
Common: Ulcers of mouth and anus, nausea, vomiting, fever, muscle pain, bone pain, chest pain, rash, tiredness, red irritated eyes, diarrhoea, loss of appetite.
Unusual: Liver dysfunction, infections, skin ulcers, nerve inflammation, sore throat, pain on swallowing, retention of urine, dizziness, hair loss, itchy skin, headache.
Severe but rare (stop medication, consult doctor): Pneumonia, blood clots, severe belly pain.

INTERACTIONS:
Other drugs:
- Methotrexate, digoxin, gentamicin, fluorocytosine.

PRESCRIPTION:
Yes.

PBS:
Yes.

PERMITTED IN SPORT:
Yes.

OVERDOSE:
Very serious. Only given under strict medical supervision.

See also Amsacrine, Chlorambucil, VINCA ALKALOIDS.

CYTOTOXICS

See CANCER-TREATING DRUGS.

Dactinomycin

TRADE NAME:
Cosmegen.

DRUG CLASS:
Cytotoxic.

USES:
Cancer of the kidney (Wilm's tumour), brain, testes, uterus, muscle (rhabdomyosarcoma) and bone.

DOSAGE:
 By drip into vein as determined for each patient by doctor.

FORMS:
Injection.

PRECAUTIONS:
Not to be used in pregnancy (D), breast feeding or infants.
Use with caution in children.
Use with caution if having radiotherapy.
Do not allow solution to touch skin – extremely corrosive. Ensure there is no leakage from drip into tissues outside vein.
Regular blood tests essential to check function of liver, kidney, bone marrow and blood cells.

Do not take if:
 suffering from chickenpox or shingles.

SIDE EFFECTS:
Common: Skin rashes, nausea, vomiting, tiredness, muscle pain, fever, anal pain, belly pain, loss of appetite.
Unusual: Liver damage, anaemia.

INTERACTIONS:
None significant.

PRESCRIPTION:
Yes.

PBS:
No.

PERMITTED IN SPORT:
Yes.

OVERDOSE:
Very serious. Only given under strict medical supervision.

Dalteparin

TRADE NAME:
Fragmin.

DRUG CLASS:
Anticoagulant.

USES:
Prevention and treatment of blood clots.

DOSAGE:
 Injection under skin into fat tissue once a day.

FORMS:
Injection.

PRECAUTIONS:
Use only if essential in pregnancy (C) as damage to foetus may occur. Use with caution in breast feeding and children.
Bleeding times must be checked regularly by blood test.
Liver and kidney function must be checked regularly by blood tests if used for prolonged period.
Use with caution in osteoporosis and elderly.

Do not take if:

☠ suffering from bleeding disorder, active bleeding, severe coagulation disorders, heart infection, uncontrolled high blood pressure.
- having eye, ear, brain or spinal cord surgery.
- using aspirin or NSAIDs (anti-inflammatory drugs used for joint pain).

SIDE EFFECTS:

Common: Abnormal bruising and bleeding.
Severe but rare (stop medication, consult doctor): Excessive bleeding or bruising, loss of blood from anus, vagina or mouth, coughing blood.

INTERACTIONS:

Other drugs:
- Aspirin, NSAIDs, vitamin K antagonists, dipyridamole, dextran, sulfinpyrazone, probenecid, ethacrynic acid, antihistamines, digoxin, tetracycline antibiotics, ascorbic acid.

Other substances:
- Vitamin C.

PRESCRIPTION:
Yes.

PBS:
Yes.

PERMITTED IN SPORT:
Yes.

OVERDOSE:
Very serious. May cause catastrophic excessive bleeding. Seek emergency medical treatment.

OTHER INFORMATION:
Used instead of heparin in some patients as it is less likely to have serious side effects.

See also Danaparoid, Heparin.

Danaparoid

TRADE NAME:
Orgaran.

DRUG CLASS:
Anticoagulant.

USES:
Prevention of blood clots in veins after surgery.

DOSAGE:
 One injection twice a day.

FORMS:
Injection.

PRECAUTIONS:
Not to be used in pregnancy (C).
Use with caution in breast feeding and children.
Use with caution in kidney and liver disease, or stomach ulcers.
Use with caution if having a spinal anaesthetic.
Regular blood tests necessary to monitor effect.

Do not take if:

☠ suffering from bleeding disorder, active bleeding, severe coagulation disorders, heart infection, uncontrolled high blood pressure, diabetic eye damage.
- Using aspirin or NSAIDs (anti-inflammatory drugs used for joint pain).

SIDE EFFECTS:
Common: Local irritation, rash.
Unusual: Abnormal bleeding.
Severe but rare (stop medication, consult doctor): Significant bleeding.

INTERACTIONS:

Other drugs:
- Aspirin, NSAIDs, vitamin K antagonists, dipyridamole, dextran, sulfinpyrazone, probenecid, ethacrynic acid,

antihistamines, digoxin, tetracycline antibiotics, ascorbic acid.
Other substances:
- Vitamin C.

PRESCRIPTION:
Yes.

PBS:
No.

PERMITTED IN SPORT:
Yes.

OVERDOSE:
Very serious. May cause catastrophic excessive bleeding. Seek emergency medical treatment.

See also Dalteparin, Heparin.

Danazol

TRADE NAMES:
Azol, Danocrine.

DRUG CLASS:
Sex hormone.

USES:
Endometriosis, severe intractable period pain, severe breast pain, rare form of severe tissue swelling (angioedema).

DOSAGE:

One capsule two to four times a day for three to nine months.

FORMS:
Capsules of 100mg and 200mg.

PRECAUTIONS:
Not to be used during pregnancy (D) or breast feeding. Adequate non-hormonal contraception must be used by women taking Danazol. Not to be used in children. Regular blood tests to check liver function recommended.

Use with caution in liver disease, high blood pressure, heart disease, diabetes.

Do not take if:
suffering from undiagnosed genital disease, severe liver disease, pelvic infection, cancer of sex organs, heart failure, recent blood clot, porphyria.

SIDE EFFECTS:
Common: Acne, weight gain, fluid retention, excess body hair growth, voice deepening, flushing, sweating, dry vagina, menstrual period irregularities.
Unusual: Oily skin, hoarseness, reduced breast size, enlargement of clitoris, nervousness.
Severe but rare (stop medication, consult doctor): Yellow skin (jaundice), blood clot in vein, chest pain (embolism).

INTERACTIONS:
Other drugs:
- Warfarin, carbamazepine, cyclosporin, oral contraceptives, phenytoin, steroids, diabetes medications.

PRESCRIPTION:
Yes.

PBS:
Yes (authority required – restricted to specific diseases and conditions).

PERMITTED IN SPORT:
No.

OVERDOSE:
May cause vomiting, tissue swelling and indigestion.

OTHER INFORMATION:
Very effective medication, but significant side effects a problem for some patients. Used for six to nine months only. Does not cause addiction or dependence.

See also Cyproterone acetate, Dydrogesterone, Ethinyloestradiol, Etonogestrel, HORMONE REPLACEMENT THERAPY, Medroxyprogesterone acetate, Oestradiol, Oestriol, Oestrogen, ORAL CONTRACEPTIVES, Oxandrolone, Piperazine oestrone sulfate, Testosterone.

Dantrolene

TRADE NAME:
Dantrium.

USES:
Muscle spasm caused by cerebral palsy, stroke, multiple sclerosis or spinal cord injury.

DOSAGE:

25mg once a day initially, then slowly increase as directed by doctor to a maximum of 50mg four times a day.

FORMS:
Capsules (orange/tan) of 25 and 50mg, injection.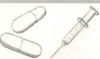

PRECAUTIONS:
Use with caution in pregnancy (B2), breast feeding and children.
Use with caution in liver disease. Regular blood tests to check on liver function recommended.
Do not take if:
 suffering from severe liver disease.
- operating machinery or driving a vehicle.

SIDE EFFECTS:
Common: Drowsiness, weakness, dizziness, diarrhoea.
Unusual: Constipation, bleeding from bowel, slurred speech, headache, rapid heart rate, depression, urinary frequency, skin sensitised to sunlight.
Severe but rare (stop medication, consult doctor): Yellow skin (jaundice).

INTERACTIONS:
Other drugs:
- Tranquillisers, verapamil, oral contraceptives.

Other substances:
- Reacts adversely with alcohol.

PRESCRIPTION:
Yes.

PBS:
Yes.

PERMITTED IN SPORT:
Yes.

OVERDOSE:
May cause drowsiness, irregular heart rate, convulsions and coma. Induce vomiting if medication taken recently and patient alert. Seek urgent medical assistance.

OTHER INFORMATION:
Does not cause addiction or dependence.

Daunorubicin

TRADE NAMES:
Daunorubicin, Daunoxome.

DRUG CLASS:
Cytotoxic.

USES:
Leukaemia, neuroblastoma, other cancers.

DOSAGE:
 As determined by doctor for each patient. Given by drip into vein.

FORMS:
Injection.

PRECAUTIONS:
Must not be used in pregnancy (D). Use with caution in breast feeding.
Second full course must not be used unless clinically essential.
Use with caution in heart, kidney and liver disease.
Regular blood tests to monitor kidney, liver and bone marrow function essential.

Ensure medication does not leak out of drip into surrounding tissues outside vein.

Do not take if:

 suffering from suppressed bone marrow from radiotherapy or chemotherapy.
- under other circumstances.

SIDE EFFECTS:

Common: Nausea, vomiting, hair loss, ulceration of mouth, anus and vagina, inflammation around drip site.
Unusual: Anaemia, diarrhoea, belly pain, fever, chills.
Severe but rare (stop medication, consult doctor): Bone marrow, heart and kidney damage.

INTERACTIONS:

Other drugs:
- Doxorubicin, cyclophosphamide, allopurinol, colchicine, heparin, fluorouracil, dexamethasone.

PRESCRIPTION:
Yes.

PBS:
No.

PERMITTED IN SPORT:
Yes.

OVERDOSE:
Very serious. Given under strict medical supervision.

See also **VINCA ALKALOIDS**.

DECONGESTANTS
(SYMPATHOMIMETICS)

DISCUSSION:
Medications that clear blocked nose and sinuses in patients with a cold, flu or hay fever.

See **Phenylephrine, Pseudoephedrine**.

Delavirdine

TRADE NAME:
Rescriptor.

DRUG CLASS:
Antiviral.

USES:
AIDS, HIV infection.

DOSAGE:
 Four tablets, three times a day, in combination with other AIDS treatments.

FORMS:
Tablets of 100mg (white).

PRECAUTIONS:
Use with considerable caution in pregnancy (B3). Use with caution in breast feeding and children.
Use with caution in kidney and liver disease.
Use with caution in elderly.

Do not take if:

 taking no other treatment for HIV/AIDS.

SIDE EFFECTS:
Common: Nausea, headache, tiredness, inability to sleep, rashes.
Unusual: Low white blood cell count.

INTERACTIONS:
Other drugs:
- Rifampicin, rifabutin, phenytoin, phenobarbitone, carbamazepine, saquinavir, didanosine, clarithromycin, ketoconazole, fluoxetine, cimetidine, famotidine, nizatadine, ranitidine, cisapride, triazolam, alprazolam, midazolam, some calcium channel blockers, amphetamines, simvastatin, sildenafil.
- Antacids must be taken an hour before or after.

Herbs:
- St Johns wort.

Medications

PRESCRIPTION:
Yes.

PBS:
Yes (very restricted to specific patients).

PERMITTED IN SPORT:
Yes.

OVERDOSE:
Very serious. Administer activated charcoal or induce vomiting if tablets taken recently. Seek urgent medical attention.

OTHER INFORMATION:
Introduced in 1997 as additional therapy for AIDS.

See Abacavir, Didanosine, Efavirenz, Indinavir, Lamivudine, Nelfinavir, Nevirapine, Ritonavir, Saquinavir, Stavudine, Tenofovir, Zidovudine.

Demeclocycline

TRADE NAME:
Ledermycin.

DRUG CLASS:
Tetracycline antibiotic.

USES:
Infections caused by susceptible bacteria, low salt levels in blood (hyponatraemia).

DOSAGE:

150mg four times a day, or 300mg twice a day.

FORMS:
Capsules (red/rose) of 150mg.

PRECAUTIONS:
Not to be used in pregnancy (D) or children under eight as it may cause permanent staining of teeth of foetus or child. Use with caution in breast feeding. Use with caution in kidney and liver disease.

Do not take if:
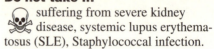 suffering from severe kidney disease, systemic lupus erythematosus (SLE), Staphylococcal infection.

SIDE EFFECTS:
Common: Loss of appetite, nausea, sore mouth, diarrhoea, difficulty in swallowing, inflamed colon.
Unusual: Vomiting, inflamed pancreas, rash, secondary fungal infection (thrush).
Severe but rare (stop medication, consult doctor): Severe belly pain, severe diarrhoea, tooth discolouration.

INTERACTIONS:
Other drugs:
- Anticoagulants, penicillin, antacids, iron, oral contraceptives.

Other substances:
- Milk may reduce absorption from gut.

PRESCRIPTION:
Yes.

PBS:
Yes.

PERMITTED IN SPORT:
Yes.

OVERDOSE:
Exacerbation of side effects only likely effect.

See also Doxycycline, Minocycline, Tetracycline.

Desferrioxamine

TRADE NAME:
Desferal.

DRUG CLASS:
Detoxifying agent.

USES:
Iron poisoning.

DOSAGE:

By drip into vein as determined by doctor for each patient.

FORMS:
Injection.

PRECAUTIONS:
Use with caution in pregnancy (B3), breast feeding and children.
Not for long term use.
Not to be given rapidly.
Test eye and ear function regularly.
Use with caution in kidney disease.

Do not take if:
 iron stores in body are normal.

SIDE EFFECTS:
Common: Reaction at injection site, nausea, vomiting, diarrhoea.
Unusual: Disturbances to lung, heart, blood, kidney and nerve function. Increased risk of infection.
Severe but rare (stop medication, consult doctor): Growth disturbance in children.

INTERACTIONS:
Other drugs:
- Phenothiazines, prochlorperazine, methyldopa, ascorbic acid.

Other substances:
- Vitamin C.

PRESCRIPTION:
Yes.

PBS:
Yes (authority required).

PERMITTED IN SPORT:
Yes.

OVERDOSE:
Excessively low iron levels and organ damage may occur.

Desmopressin acetate

TRADE NAMES:
Minirin, Octostim.

DRUG CLASS:
Antidiuretic.

USES:
Diabetes insipidus, bed wetting, abnormally frequent passing of urine, rare blood disorders.

DOSAGE:

Nasal spray: 10µg to 40µg a day.

FORMS:
Nasal spray, injection.

PRECAUTIONS:
Use with caution in pregnancy (B2), breast feeding and children.
Use nasal spray with caution in nasal infection and hay fever.
Use all forms with caution in heart disease and after operations.
Lower doses necessary in elderly.

Do not take if:
suffering from some types of von Willebrand's disease, frequent passing of urine due to habit or psychological factors, heart failure.

SIDE EFFECTS:
Common: Minimal
Unusual: Fluid retention, rapid heart rate, low blood pressure, headache, nausea, gut cramps, nasal congestion.

INTERACTIONS:
Other drugs:
- Glibenclamide, clofibrate, indomethacin, tricyclic antidepressants, chlorpromazine, carbamazepine, chlorpropamide.

PRESCRIPTION:
Yes.

PBS:
Nasal spray: Yes (authority required – restricted to use with diabetes insipidus). Injection: No.

PERMITTED IN SPORT:
Yes.

OVERDOSE:
No serious effects expected.

OTHER INFORMATION:
One of the few effective treatments for the rare condition of diabetes insipidus which is a totally separate condition to sugar diabetes (diabetes mellitus). Very effective, but expensive, treatment for bed wetting.

Desogestrel
See ORAL CONTRACEPTIVES.

Desonide

TRADE NAME:
Desowen.

DRUG CLASS:
Corticosteroid.

USES:
Dermatitis.

DOSAGE:

Apply two or three times a day for one or two months.

FORMS:
Lotion.

PRECAUTIONS:
Use with caution in pregnancy (B3), breast feeding and children.
Not for long term use.
Use with caution if bacterial or fungal infection present on skin.
Do not take if:
 suffering from viral skin infection (eg. shingles, cold sore), rosacea or tuberculosis.
- child under 2 years.

SIDE EFFECTS:
Common: Skin reaction and dryness.
Unusual: Hair follicle infection, increased hair growth on skin, pimple formation, loss of pigmentation, skin infection.
Severe but rare (stop medication, consult doctor): Thinning of skin.

INTERACTIONS:
None significant.

PRESCRIPTION:
Yes.

PBS:
No.

PERMITTED IN SPORT:
Yes.

OTHER INFORMATION:
Introduced in 2002 as an additional treatment for difficult to treat dermatitis.
See also Betamethasone, Hydrocortisone, Methylprednisolone, Mometasone, Triamcinolone.

Dexamethasone

TRADE NAMES:
Dexmethsone, Maxidex.
Otodex, Sofradex (with framycetin, gramicidin).

DRUG CLASS:
Corticosteroid.

USES:
Severe inflammation of eyes and ears. Severe asthma, rheumatoid and other forms of severe arthritis, autoimmune diseases (eg. Sjögren syndrome), severe allergy reactions, other severe and chronic inflammatory diseases.

DOSAGE:

Eye drops: Insert every two to four hours.
Ear drops: Two drops three times a day.
Tablets: 0.5mg to 4mg a day strictly as directed by doctor.

FORMS:
Injection, tablets, eye drops, ear drops.

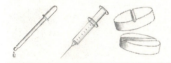

PRECAUTIONS:
May be used in pregnancy (A), breast feeding and children with caution.
Eye and ear preparations safe in pregnancy, breast feeding and children.
Use tablets with caution if under stress, and in patients with under-active thyroid gland, liver disease, diverticulitis, high blood pressure, myasthenia gravis, or kidney disease.
Avoid eyes with all forms except eye drops.
Use for shortest period of time possible.

Do not use if:

- suffering from any form of infection, peptic ulcer, or osteoporosis.
- having a vaccination.

SIDE EFFECTS:
Common: Tablets and injection – May cause bloating, weight gain, rashes and intestinal disturbances.
Eye and ear drops rarely cause adverse reactions.
Unusual: Tablets and injections – Biochemical disturbances of blood, muscle weakness, bone weakness, impaired wound healing, skin thinning, tendon weakness, peptic ulcers, gullet ulcers, bruising, increased sweating, loss of fat under skin, premature ageing, excess facial hair growth in women, pigmentation of skin and nails, acne, convulsions, headaches, dizziness, growth suppression in children, aggravation of diabetes, worsening of infections, cataracts, aggravation of glaucoma, blood clots in veins and sleeplessness.
Most significant side effects occur only with prolonged use of tablets.
Medication should not be ceased abruptly, but dosage should be slowly reduced.
Severe but rare (stop medication, consult doctor): Any significant side effect should be reported to a doctor immediately.

INTERACTIONS:
Other drugs:
- Tablets – Oral contraceptives, barbiturates, phenytoin, rifampicin.

Herbs:
- Echinacea.

PRESCRIPTION:
Yes.

PBS:
Yes.

PERMITTED IN SPORT:
Tablets and injection: No
Ear and eye drops: Yes.

OVERDOSE:
Medical treatment is required. Serious effects and death rare.

OTHER INFORMATION:
Extremely effective and useful medication

if used correctly. Tablets must be used with extreme care under strict medical supervision. Lowest dose and shortest possible course should be used. Not addictive.

Dexamphetamine

TRADE NAME:
Dexamphetamine.

DRUG CLASS:
Stimulant, amphetamine.

USES:
Hyperactivity disorders in children, narcolepsy.

DOSAGE:

2.5mg to 80mg a day in several doses depending upon age, condition and response.

FORMS:
Tablets of 5mg (white).

PRECAUTIONS:
Should be used in pregnancy (B3) and breast feeding only if medically essential. May be used in children over three years only.
Use with caution in kidney disease.
Do not take if:
- suffering from heart disease, high blood pressure, over-active thyroid gland, anxiety, excitability, Tourette syndrome or twitching.
- MAOI taken within two weeks.
- history of drug abuse.

SIDE EFFECTS:
Common: Drug dependence, dry mouth, restlessness, difficulty passing urine, sleeplessness, tremor, loss of appetite, twitching, diarrhoea, nausea, headache.
Unusual: Rapid heart rate, high blood pressure, irregular heartbeat, angina.

INTERACTIONS:
Other drugs:
- Urinary alkalinisers, MAOI, tricyclic antidepressants, antihistamines, medications that lower blood pressure, chlorpromazine, ethosuximide, haloperidol, lithium, pethidine, dextropropoxyphene, phenobarbitone, phenytoin.

Herbs:
- Ma huang.

Other substances:
- Alcohol.

PRESCRIPTION:
Yes (may be restricted to certain doctors in some states).

PBS:
Yes (Authority required from both state and federal governments).

PERMITTED IN SPORT:
No.

OVERDOSE:
Very serious. May cause vomiting, agitation, tremors, twitching, confusion, hallucinations, convulsions, coma and death. Administer activated charcoal or induce vomiting if tablets taken recently. Seek urgent medical attention.

OTHER INFORMATION:
May be addictive if used inappropriately. Very effective in improving the lives of some children with hyperactivity, but there are concerns that it may be used when not necessary or excessively. All forms of behaviour therapy should be tried before this is used as a last resort. Treatment rarely necessary into adult life.

Dexchlorpheniramine
See ANTIHISTAMINES, SEDATING.

Dextran
See EYE LUBRICANTS.

Dextromethorphan

TRADE NAMES:
Benadryl for the Family Dry Forte, Bisolvon Dry, Bisolvon Dry Junior, Dexi-Tuss, Nucosef DM, Robitussin DX, Robitussin Honey Cough, Strepsils Cough Relief, Tussinol for Dry Coughs.
Actifed CC Junior (with triprolidine).
Actifed Dry (with triprolidine and pseudoephedrine).
Benadryl for the Family – Dry (with pseudoephedrine, diphenhydramine).
Cepacol Cough (with benzocaine, menthol, cetylpyridinium and other ingredients).
Chemist's Own Dry Raspy Cough, Tussinol Cough & Cold Infant, Tussinol Night Time Cough & Cold (with chlorpheniramine, pseudoephedrine).
Codral Cough Cold and Flu, Dimetapp Cold & Flu, Logicin Flu, Orthoxicol Cold & Flu, Panadol Cold & Flu, Parke-Davis Cold and Flu, Pharma-Col Junior, Tylenol Cold & Flu Nondrowsy (with paracetamol and pseudoephedrine).
Day & Night Cold & Flu, Dimetapp Cold Cough & Flu Day & Night, Logicin Flu Day & Night, Orthoxicol Day & Night Cold & Flu (with paracetamol and other ingredients).
Dimetapp Cold Cough & Flu (with pseudoephedrine, guaiphenesin, paracetamol).
Dimetapp Cold Cough & Sinus (with pseudoephedrine, guaiphenesin).
Dimetapp DM (with brompheniramine, phenylephrine and other ingredients).
Lemsip Flu, Tylenol Cold & Flu (with paracetamol, pseudoephedrine, chlorpheniramine).
Logicin Cough – Dry, Logicin Junior Children's Cough, Robitussin DM-P, Tussinol Actifed Dry Cough and Nasal Congestion (with pseudoephedrine).
Neo-Diophen (with mepyramine maleate, phenylpropanolamine, atropine).
Orthoxicol Night Cold & Flu (with chlorpheniramine, paracetamol).
Robitussin DM (with guaiphenesin).
Sigma Relief (with guaiphenesin and pseudoephedrine).

Also found in numerous locally marketed cough medications.

DRUG CLASS:
Cough suppressant.

USES:
Control of hard dry cough.

DOSAGE:
 Take recommended amount every six to eight hours.

FORMS:
Mixture, syrup, capsules, lozenges.

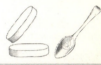

PRECAUTIONS:
Use with care in pregnancy (A) and infants under two years. Not for use in breast feeding. Safe in children.
Not to be used to treat asthma, pneumonia, emphysema or chronic bronchitis.
Not for long term use.
Use with care in liver disease.
Do not take if:
 suffering from clinical depression.

SIDE EFFECTS:
Common: Minimal.
Unusual: Drowsiness, dizziness, nausea, diarrhoea.

INTERACTIONS:
Other drugs:
- MAOI, amiodarone, quinidine, amiodarone, fluoxetine, fluvoxamine, paroxetine.

Other substances:
- Alcohol

PRESCRIPTION:
No.

PBS:
No.

PERMITTED IN SPORT:
Yes, provided it is not combined with pseudoephedrine.

OVERDOSE:
Unlikely to cause any significant serious effects.

See also **Ammonium chloride, Codeine Phosphate, Dihydrocodeine, EXPECTORANTS, Pentoxyverine citrate, Pholcodine.**

Dextromoramide

TRADE NAME:
Palfium.

DRUG CLASS:
Narcotic, Analgesic.

USES:
Severe pain.

DOSAGE:

One to four tablets as required for pain before meals. Patient should lie down for 30 minutes after first dose.

FORMS:
Tablets (white) of 5mg.

PRECAUTIONS:
Should not be used in the last few weeks of pregnancy (C) as medication may cause difficulty in breathing in newborn infant. Use with caution in breast feeding and children.
Not designed for prolonged use except in patients with terminal disease.

Do not take if:
 suffering from severe lung disease, low blood pressure.
- operating machinery, driving a vehicle or undertaking tasks that require concentration.

SIDE EFFECTS:
Common: Lightheadedness, dizziness, drowsiness, fainting, nausea.
Unusual: Vomiting, difficulty in breathing, perspiration.

INTERACTIONS:
Other drugs:
- MAOI, barbiturates, tranquillisers, anaesthetics.

Other substances:
- Do not use alcohol with dextromoramide.

PRESCRIPTION:
Yes (very restricted).

PBS:
No.

PERMITTED IN SPORT:
No.

OVERDOSE:
Serious. Administer activated charcoal or induce vomiting if medication taken recently and patient alert. May cause drowsiness, difficulty in breathing, convulsions, coma and death. Especially dangerous when taken with other sedatives including alcohol. Seek urgent medical assistance. Antidote available.

OTHER INFORMATION:
May cause dependence or addiction if used inappropriately.

See also **Alfentanil, Buprenorphine, Codeine Phosphate, Dextropropoxyphene, Fentanyl, Heroin, Hydromorphone, Methadone, Morphine, Oxycodone, Pentazocine, Pethidine.**

Dextropropoxyphene

TRADE NAMES:
Doloxene.
Capadex, Digesic, Paradex (with paracetamol).

DRUG CLASS:
Narcotic, Analgesic.

USES:
Pain relief.

DOSAGE:

One or two capsules or tablets, three or four times a day.

FORMS:
Tablets, capsules.
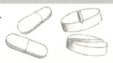

PRECAUTIONS:
Should only be used in pregnancy (C) if medically essential. May cause difficulty in breathing of newborn if used during labour. Use with caution in breast feeding. Not for use in children.
Use with caution in severe lung disease.
Designed for short term use.
Do not exceed recommended dose.

Do not take if:

- suffering from alcoholism.
- prone to suicide.
- suffering from significant kidney or liver disease.
- operating machinery or driving a vehicle.

SIDE EFFECTS:
Common: Sleeplessness, mood changes, rash, dizziness, sedation, nausea.
Unusual: Constipation, belly pains, headache, lightheadedness, weakness, blurred vision.
Severe but rare (stop medication, consult doctor): Yellow skin (jaundice).

INTERACTIONS:
Other drugs:
- Sedatives, anticoagulants, orphenadrine, beta blockers, diazepam, phenytoin, carbamazepine.

Other substances:
- Do not use with alcohol.

PRESCRIPTION:
Yes.

PBS:
No. Available to some Veteran Affairs pensioners.

PERMITTED IN SPORT:
No.

OVERDOSE:
Serious. Induce vomiting if medication taken recently and patient alert. Symptoms include drowsiness, convulsions, reduced breathing, low blood pressure, coma and possibly death. Seek emergency medical assistance.

OTHER INFORMATION:
Widely used for many decades to treat moderate severity pain. May cause dependence if used long term and inappropriately.
See also Alfentanil, Buprenorphine, Codeine, Dextromoramide, Fentanyl, Heroin, Hydromorphone, Methadone, Morphine, Oxycodone, Pentazocine, Pethidine.

DIABETES MEDICATIONS

See HYPOGLYCAEMICS, INSULINS.

Diazepam

TRADE NAMES:
Antenex, Ducene, Valium, Valpam.

DRUG CLASS:
Benzodiazepine (Anxiolytic).

USES:
Short term relief of anxiety, relief of muscle spasm, withdrawal from alcohol dependence, preoperative sedation, uncontrolled epileptic fit (injection).

DOSAGE:

One to four tablets a day in one or more doses. Do not exceed dose directed by doctor.

FORMS:
Tablets of 2mg and 5mg, injection.
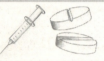

PRECAUTIONS:
Should be used with caution in pregnancy (C), but not at all if delivery of infant imminent as it may decrease desire to breathe in newborn infant.
Should be used with caution in breast feeding.
Not for use in children.
Lower dose required in elderly.
Should be used intermittently and not constantly as dependency may develop.
Use with caution in glaucoma, heart disease, kidney or liver disease, psychiatric conditions, depression and epilepsy.

Do not take if:
suffering from severe lung disease, confusion, myasthenia gravis, sleep apnoea or psychotic illness (eg. schizophrenia).
- tendency to addiction or dependence.
- operating machinery, driving a vehicle or undertaking tasks that require concentration and alertness.

SIDE EFFECTS:
Common: Reduced alertness, dependence.
Unusual: Incoordination, tremor, muscle weakness, confusion, increased risk of falls in elderly, rash, low blood pressure, nausea, muscle weakness, memory loss, nausea, diarrhoea.
Severe but rare (stop medication, consult doctor): Jaundice (yellow skin).

INTERACTIONS:
Other drugs:
- Sedatives, other anxiolytics, disulfiram, cimetidine, anticonvulsants (eg. phenytoin), ketoconazole, fluvoxamine, omeprazole, cisapride, anticholinergics.

Herbs:
- Guarana, kava kava, passionflower, St John's wort, valerian.

Other substances:
- Reacts with alcohol to cause sedation and confusion.

PRESCRIPTION:
Yes.

PBS:
Yes.

PERMITTED IN SPORT:
Yes.

OVERDOSE:
Seldom life threatening. May cause drowsiness, confusion and coma. Induce vomiting if tablets taken recently. Seek medical assistance.

OTHER INFORMATION:
Widely used, and very safe if used correctly. Dependency becoming a significant problem, particularly in elderly, due to overuse. First introduced in 1960s.

See also Alprazolam, Bromazepam, Buspirone, Clobazam, Lorazepam, Oxazepam.

Diazoxide

TRADE NAME:
Diazoxide.

DRUG CLASS:
Vasodilator, Antihypertensive, Thiazide diuretic.

USES:
Severe high blood pressure.

DOSAGE:

Injection into vein every four or more hours as necessary.

FORMS:
Injection.

PRECAUTIONS:
Use only if essential in pregnancy (C).
Use with caution in breast feeding and children.
Use with caution in kidney disease, brain damage, severe heart disease, diabetes and gout.
Patient must be monitored very carefully during use.
Not for prolonged use.

Do not take if:

suffering from arteriovenous shunt, sensitive to thiazides.

SIDE EFFECTS:
Common: High blood sugar, fluid retention, low blood pressure, headache, sensation of warmth, rapid heart rate.
Unusual: High blood salt levels, vomiting, diarrhoea.
Severe but rare (stop medication, consult doctor): Heart attack, stroke, coma.

INTERACTIONS:
Other drugs:
- Thiazide diuretics, anticoagulants, other medications that lower blood pressure.

PRESCRIPTION:
Yes.

PBS:
No.

PERMITTED IN SPORT:
Yes.

OVERDOSE:
Extremely serious. Only given under close medical supervision.

OTHER INFORMATION:
Only used in cases of extremely high, life threatening high blood pressure.
See also Betahistine, Guanethidine, Nicotinic Acid, Phenoxybenzamine.

Dibromopropamidine isethionate

See Propamidine isethionate and Dibromopropamide.

Diclofenac

TRADE NAMES:
Diclohexal, Dinac, Fenac, GenRx Diclofenac, Hexal Diclac, Voltaren Arthrotec (with misoprostol).

DRUG CLASS:
NSAID (Nonsteroidal anti-inflammatories drug).

USES:
All forms of arthritis, inflammatory disorders, gout, back pain, ankylosing spondylitis, bone pain, prevention of miosis (eye contraction) during eye surgery.

DOSAGE:

Tablets: One tablet, two or three times a day with food.
Gels: Rub into affected area three or four times a day for up to two weeks.
Eye drops: As directed by eye doctor.

FORMS:
Tablets, gel, eye drops.
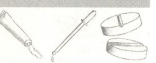

PRECAUTIONS:
Should not be used in pregnancy (C) unless medically essential. Breast feeding should be ceased if necessary to use NSAID. Not for use in children under two. Gel safe in pregnancy.
Use tablets and capsules with caution in psychiatrically disturbed patients, epilepsy, severe infection, heart failure and kidney disease.
Lower doses required in elderly, who may suffer more side effects.

Do not take if:

- suffering from peptic ulcer at present or in recent past.
- due for surgery (including dental surgery).
- suffering from bleeding disorder or anaemia.

SIDE EFFECTS:
Common: Gel – Minimal.
Other forms – Stomach discomfort, diarrhoea, constipation, heartburn, nausea, headache, dizziness.
Unusual: Blurred vision, stomach ulcer, ringing noise in ears, retention of fluid, swelling of tissue, drowsiness, itch, rash, shortness of breath.
Severe but rare (stop medication, consult doctor): Vomiting blood, passing blood in faeces, other unusual bleeding, asthma induced by medication.

INTERACTIONS:
Other drugs:
- Must never be used with anticoagulants (eg. warfarin).
- Probenecid, diuretics, lithium, methotrexate, beta blockers, ACE inhibitors, digoxin, cyclosporin, diabetes medication (hypoglycaemics), steroids.
- Gel has minimal interactions.

Herbs:
- Feverfew.

PRESCRIPTION:
Tablets: Yes.
Gel: No.

PBS:
Tablets: Yes.
Gel: No.

PERMITTED IN SPORT:
Yes.

OVERDOSE:
Causes nausea, vomiting, severe headache, dizziness, confusion and convulsions. Administer activated charcoal or induce vomiting if taken recently. Seek medical assistance.

OTHER INFORMATION:
Extensively used to give excellent relief to a wide variety of inflammatory conditions. Significant side effects (particularly on the stomach) in about 5% of patients limit their use. Special forms

with added misoprostol reduces stomach effects. Minimal side effects gel, but less effective.

See also Aspirin, Bufexamac, Celecoxib, Diflunisal, Flurbiprofen, Ibuprofen, Indomethacin, Ketoprofen, Ketorolac trometanol, Mefenamic Acid, Naproxen, Piroxicam, Rofecoxib, Salicylic acid, Sulindac, Tenoxicam, Tiaprofenic Acid.

Dicloxacillin

TRADE NAMES:
Diclocil, Dicloxsig, Distaph.

DRUG CLASS:
Penicillin antibiotic.

USES:
Serious skin and soft tissue infections, bone infections, pneumonia.

DOSAGE:
 One capsule four times a day more than an hour before food.

FORMS:
Capsules of 250mg and 500mg, injection.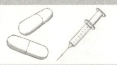

PRECAUTIONS:
May be used with caution in pregnancy (B2), breast feeding and infants. Safe in children.
Use lower doses in elderly.
Not designed for prolonged use.
Do not take if:
 allergic to penicillin.

SIDE EFFECTS:
Common: Nausea, diarrhoea.
Unusual: Blood clots, liver damage.
Severe but rare (stop medication, consult doctor): Bloody diarrhoea, worsening infection, jaundice.

INTERACTIONS:
Other drugs:
- Warfarin, aminoglycoside antibiotics, phenytoin.

PRESCRIPTION:
Yes.

PBS:
Yes.

PERMITTED IN SPORT:
Yes.

OVERDOSE:
Vomiting and diarrhoea only likely effects.

OTHER INFORMATION:
Introduced in 1997. Same effects as Flucloxacillin, but slightly less risk of rare serious side effects. Used for more severe infections. Some bacteria can break down simpler forms of penicillin. Cloxacillin, dicloxacillin and flucloxacillin are not able to be broken down this way and so can be effective when other penicillins fail. Does not cause dependence or addiction.

See also Amoxycillin, Ampicillin, Benzathine penicillin, Benzylpenicillin, Dicloxacillin, Phenoxymethyl penicillin, Piperacillin, Procaine penicillin, Ticarcillin.

Dicyclomine

TRADE NAME:
Merbentyl.

DRUG CLASS:
Anticholinergic, Spasmolytic.

USES:
Spasm of the intestine, irritable bowel syndrome, colic.

DOSAGE:

Tablets: One to four tablets, three or four times a day.
Syrup: 5 to 10mLs three or four times a day.

FORMS:
Tablets, syrup.
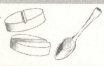

PRECAUTIONS:
Use with caution in pregnancy (B1) and breast feeding.
Should not be used in children under six months of age.
Safe to use in older children.
Use with caution in glaucoma, and enlarged prostate.

Do not take if:
 suffering from difficulty in passing urine
- suffering from ulcerative colitis, intestinal obstruction or intestinal underactivity.
- suffering from myasthenia gravis.

SIDE EFFECTS:
Common: Dry mouth, difficulty in passing urine, blurred vision.
Unusual: Rapid heart rate, loss of taste, headache, nervousness, weakness, dizziness, constipation, sleeplessness, bloating, rashes.
Severe but rare (stop medication, consult doctor): Cessation of breathing in infants.

INTERACTIONS:
None significant.

PRESCRIPTION:
Tablets: Yes.
Mixture: No.

PBS:
No.

PERMITTED IN SPORT:
Yes.

OVERDOSE:
Causes headache, dizziness, vomiting, hot dry skin and difficulty in swallowing.

OTHER INFORMATION:
Commonly used in children (but not infants) for colic. Does not cause dependence.
See also Alverine Citrate, Mebeverine

Didanosine

TRADE NAME:
Videx.

DRUG CLASS:
Antiviral.

USES:
Treatment of advanced AIDS.

DOSAGE:

One to three crushed tablets twice a day on an empty stomach.

FORMS:
Chewable tablets (25mg, 100mg), capsules (125mg, 200mg, 250mg, 400mg), powder for solution.

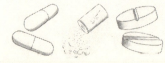

PRECAUTIONS:
Should not be used in pregnancy (B2) and children unless medically essential. Breast feeding should be ceased before use. Use with caution in kidney and liver disease, pancreatitis.

SIDE EFFECTS:
Common: Diarrhoea, nausea, vomiting.
Unusual: Pins and needles, chills, fever, headache, pancreatitis, muscle pain, tiredness, convulsions, confusion, sleeplessness, rash, itch, arthritis.

INTERACTIONS:
Other drugs:
- Ketoconazole, dapsone, pentamidine, tetracycline, phenylalanine, allopurinol, stavudine, hydroxyurea (serious).

PRESCRIPTION:
Yes.

PBS:
Yes (very restricted to specific patients).

PERMITTED IN SPORT:
Yes.

OVERDOSE:
Very serious. Liver damage likely. Seek medical assistance.

OTHER INFORMATION:
Introduced in 1993 to help slow the progress of (but not cure) HIV/AIDS.
See Abacavir, Delavirdine, Efavirenz, Indinavir, Lamivudine, Nelfinavir, Nevirapine, Ritonavir, Saquinavir, Stavudine, Tenofovir, Zalcitabine, Zidovudine.

Diethylamine salicylate

TRADE NAME:
Rubesal (with camphor, menthol and other ingredients).
Numerous other ointments, creams and liniments contain various salicylates.

DRUG CLASS:
Rubefacient.

USES:
Temporary relief of pain (eg. muscular, arthritic, gums).

DOSAGE:
 Massage into clean dry skin two or three times a day.

FORMS:
Cream, spray.

PRECAUTIONS:
Safe in pregnancy and breast feeding.
Use with caution in children under 5 years.
Avoid contact with eyes, mouth, nose, anus and vagina.
Use sparingly on face, skin folds and thin skin.
May stain clothing.
Do not use if:
 suffering from broken or infected skin.

SIDE EFFECTS:
Minimal.

INTERACTIONS:
None significant.

PRESCRIPTION:
No.

PBS:
No.

PERMITTED IN SPORT:
Yes.

OVERDOSE:

May have serious effects in the unlikely event of the liniment being swallowed.

See also Salicylic acid.

Diethylpropion hydrochloride

TRADE NAMES:
Tenuate, Tenuate Dospan (long acting version).

DRUG CLASS:
Anorectic.

USES:
Reduction in appetite in obesity. Must be used in conjunction with an appropriate diet.

DOSAGE:

Tenuate: One tablet an hour before each meal.
Tenuate Dospan: One tablet mid morning.

FORMS:
Tablets of 25mg and 75mg.

PRECAUTIONS:
Not designed for use in pregnancy (B2), breast feeding or children under 12 years. Use with caution in high blood pressure, heart disease, epilepsy, history of drug abuse and psychiatric disturbances.
Not for long term use.
Do not exceed recommended dose.

Do not take if:
 suffering from hardening of arteries, overactive thyroid gland, glaucoma, agitation, significant lung disease, uncontrolled high blood pressure, drug addiction.

SIDE EFFECTS:
Common: Overstimulation, sedation, depression, dry mouth, palpitations, heartbeat irregularities, high blood pressure, bad taste, rash, impotence, diarrhoea, nausea, dependence.
Unusual: Chest pain, nervousness, tremor, excess happiness, headache, vomiting, changes in libido, breast enlargement and tenderness, damage to blood cells and bone marrow.

INTERACTIONS:
Other drugs:
- MAOI, general anaesthetics, drugs used to treat diabetes (hypoglycaemics).

Other substances:
- Reacts with alcohol and caffeine.

PRESCRIPTION:
Yes (highly restricted in some states).

PBS:
No.

PERMITTED IN SPORT:
No.

OVERDOSE:
Serious. May cause restlessness, tremor, rapid breathing, irregular heartbeat, high blood pressure, confusion, hallucinations, violence, panic state, vomiting, diarrhoea, coma, convulsions and death. Administer activated charcoal or induce vomiting if medication taken recently. Seek urgent medical attention.

OTHER INFORMATION:
May cause dependence and addiction.

See also Orlistat, Phentermine, Silbutramine.

Diflunisal

TRADE NAME:
Dolobid.

DRUG CLASS:
NSAID (Nonsteroidal anti-inflammatories drug).

USES:
All forms of arthritis, inflammatory disorders, gout, back pain, bone pain, general pain relief.

DOSAGE:
 One tablet twice a day with food.

FORMS:
Tablets of 250mg (peach) and 500mg (orange).

PRECAUTIONS:
Should not be used in pregnancy (C) unless medically essential. Breast feeding should be ceased if necessary to use. Not for use in children.
Use with caution in Reye syndrome, epilepsy, severe infection, high blood pressure, heart failure and kidney disease. Lower doses required in elderly, who may suffer more side effects.

Do not take if:
 suffering from peptic ulcer at present or in recent past.
- due for surgery (including dental surgery).
- suffering from bleeding disorder or anaemia.
- urticaria.

SIDE EFFECTS:
Common: Stomach discomfort, diarrhoea, constipation, heartburn, nausea, headache, dizziness.
Unusual: Blurred vision, stomach ulcer, ringing noise in ears, retention of fluid, swelling of tissue, drowsiness, itch, rash, shortness of breath.
Severe but rare (stop medication, consult doctor): Vomiting blood, passing blood in faeces, other unusual bleeding, asthma induced by medication.

INTERACTIONS:
Other drugs:
- Must never be used with anticoagulants (eg. warfarin).
- Probenecid, diuretics, lithium, methotrexate, beta blockers, ACE inhibitors.

PRESCRIPTION:
Yes.

PBS:
Yes.

PERMITTED IN SPORT:
Yes.

OVERDOSE:
Causes nausea, vomiting, severe headache, dizziness, confusion and convulsions. Administer activated charcoal or induce vomiting if taken recently. Seek medical assistance.

OTHER INFORMATION:
Used to give relief to a wide variety of inflammatory conditions. Significant side effects (particularly on the stomach) in about 5% of patients limit their use.

See also Aspirin, Bufexamac, Celecoxib, Diclofenac, Flurbiprofen, Ibuprofen, Indomethacin, Ketoprofen, Ketorolac trometanol, Mefenamic Acid, Naproxen, Piroxicam, Rofecoxib, Salicylic acid, Sulindac, Tenoxicam, Tiaprofenic Acid.

Digitalis
See Digoxin.

Digoxin

TRADE NAMES:
Lanoxin, Sigmaxin.

DRUG CLASS:
Cardiac glycoside.

USES:
Heart failure, irregular heartbeat originating in heart atrium (atrial fibrillation).

DOSAGE:

Must be carefully individualised by regular blood tests. Usually one or two tablets once a day.

FORMS:
Tablets of 250µg (white) and 62.5µg (blue), elixir, injection.

 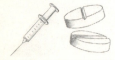

PRECAUTIONS:
Safe in pregnancy (A), breast feeding and children.
Should be used with care in thyroid disease, malabsorption, poor kidney function and elderly.
Regular blood tests recommended to check blood level of medication.

Do not take if:

 suffering from heart block, very rapid heart rate, very slow heart rate.

SIDE EFFECTS:
Common: Usually associated with overdosage. Loss of appetite, nausea.
Unusual: Vomiting, weakness, breast enlargement (both sexes), depression, headache.
Severe but rare (stop medication, consult doctor): Unusual bleeding, slow heart rate.

INTERACTIONS:
Other drugs:
- Blood levels of digoxin increased by diuretics, lithium, steroids, carbenoxolone, amiodarone, captopril, flecainide, prazosin, quinidine, spironolactone, tetracyclines, erythromycin, propantheline and other drugs.
- Blood levels of digoxin decreased by antacids, kaolin, pectin, bulking agents, laxatives, cholestyramine, sulfasalazine, neomycin, rifampicin, phenytoin, metoclopramide, penicillamine and other drugs.
- Variable effects from calcium channel blockers.

Herbs:
- St John's wort, fenugreek, liquorice, guarana, hawthorn, ginseng, golden seal, kyushin, parsley plantain, uzara root.

PRESCRIPTION:
Yes.

PBS:
Yes.

PERMITTED IN SPORT:
Yes.

OVERDOSE:
May result in life threatening heartbeat irregularities. Early symptom of overdosage is a slow heart rate. Administer activated charcoal or induce vomiting if tablets taken recently. Seek urgent medical assistance.

OTHER INFORMATION:
In 1785, William Withering identified the active ingredient of an English folk remedy for dropsy (heart failure) distilled from the purple foxglove as digitalis. This has been further refined into digoxin, which has been a most important medication for the treatment of heart disease for over two centuries.

Dihydrocodeine

TRADE NAMES:
Paracodin, Rikodeine.
Codox (with aspirin).

DRUG CLASS:
Cough suppressant, analgesic.

USES:
Cough, pain.

DOSAGE:

5mLs to 10mLs every four to six hours.
One or two tablets, or one lozenge, every two to three hours.

FORMS:
Mixture, tablets, lozenges.

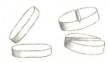

PRECAUTIONS:
Safe to use in pregnancy (A), breast feeding and children over 2 years.

SIDE EFFECTS:
Common: Constipation.

INTERACTIONS:
Other drugs:
• Sedatives.
Other substances:
• Alcohol

PRESCRIPTION:
No.

PBS:
No.

PERMITTED IN SPORT:
Yes.

OVERDOSE:
Sedation and constipation only likely effects.

OTHER INFORMATION:
Safe and effective. Minimal risk of dependence if used long term in high doses.
See also **Ammonium chloride**, **Codeine Phosphate**, **Dextromethorphan**, **EXPECTORANTS**, **Pentoxyverine citrate**, **Pholcodine**.

Dihydroergotamine

TRADE NAME:
Dihydergot.

USES:
Migraine, cluster headaches, vascular headaches, low blood pressure.

DOSAGE:

Tablets: Half to one tablet three times a day.

FORMS:
Tablet (used for low blood pressure).
Injection (used for headaches).

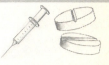

PRECAUTIONS:
Not for use in pregnancy (C), breast feeding or children.
Use with caution in high blood pressure.

Do not take if:
 suffering from kidney or liver disease, heart disease, angina, major infections, poor circulation to legs and arms.

SIDE EFFECTS:
Common: Nausea, vomiting, pins and needles sensation, muscle cramps, chest pain.

INTERACTIONS:
Other drugs:
• Macrolide antibiotics (eg. erythromycin), glyceryl trinitrate, drugs used to treat AIDS.

Medications

PRESCRIPTION:
Yes.

PBS:
Injections: Yes.
Tablets: No.

PERMITTED IN SPORT:
Yes.

OVERDOSE:
Very serious. May cause arterial spasm, cessation of breathing, heart attack and death. Administer activated charcoal or induce vomiting if tablets taken recently. Seek emergency medical assistance.

OTHER INFORMATION:
The ergot alkaloids are naturally occurring substances from a fungus that grows on rye. In the Middle Ages, accidental overdose of ergotamine and similar substances could follow the use of contaminated rye.

Dihydroxyacetone

TRADE NAME:

Vitadye.

USES:
Vitiligo (loss of skin pigmentation).

DOSAGE:

Apply one to three coats to affected area one hour apart. Reapply every one to three days.

FORMS:
Solution.

PRECAUTIONS:
Safe in pregnancy, breast feeding and children.
Avoid contact with eyes, eyelids and broken skin.
May stain clothing.

SIDE EFFECTS:
Common: Minimal.
Unusual: Skin irritation and sensitivity.

INTERACTIONS:
None.

PRESCRIPTION:
No.

PBS:
No.

PERMITTED IN SPORT:
Yes.

OVERDOSE:
Seek urgent medical attention if swallowed.

OTHER INFORMATION:
Dye that stains skin that has lost its pigment and appears excessively white.

Diltiazem

TRADE NAMES:

Auscard, Cardizem, Coras, Diltahexal, Dilzem, GenRx Diltiazem, Vasocardol CD.

DRUG CLASS:
Calcium channel blocker (calcium antagonist).

USES:
High blood pressure, angina.

DOSAGE:

120 to 240mg a day in one or more doses, depending on formulation.

FORMS:
Tablets, capsules, injection.

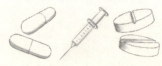

PRECAUTIONS:
Should only be used in pregnancy (C) and breast feeding if medically essential. Not designed for use in children.

Do not take if:

 suffering from severe heart failure, low blood pressure, atrial flutter or fibrillation.

SIDE EFFECTS:
Common: Constipation, tiredness, headache, dizziness, indigestion, swelling of feet and ankles.
Unusual: Flushing, palpitations, slow heart rate, scalp irritation, depression, flushes, nightmares, excess wind.
Severe but rare (stop medication, consult doctor): Fainting.

INTERACTIONS:
Other drugs:
- Beta blockers (eg. propranolol), cyclosporin, digoxin, cimetidine, diazepam, amiodarone, quinidine, rifampicin, phenytoin, cisapride, theophylline, terbutaline, salbutamol, diltiazem.
- Additive effect with other medications for high blood pressure.

Herbs:
- Goldenseal, guarana, hawthorn, Korean ginseng, liquorice.

Other substances:
- Smoking may aggravate conditions that these medications are treating.
- Grapefruit juice.

PRESCRIPTION:
Yes.

PBS:
Yes.

PERMITTED IN SPORT:
Yes.

OVERDOSE:
May continue to be absorbed for up to 48 hours after overdose. Administer activated charcoal or induce vomiting. Purging should be encouraged to eliminate drug from gut. Overdose may cause low blood pressure, irregular heart rhythm, difficulty in breathing, heart attack and death. Obtain urgent medical attention.

OTHER INFORMATION:
Commonly used as a first line medication in high blood pressure and to prevent angina.

See also **Amlodipine, Felodipine, Nifedipine, Nimodipine, Verapamil**

Dimenhydrinate

TRADE NAMES:
Dramamine.
Travacalm (with hyoscine and caffeine).

DRUG CLASS:
Antiemetic, Antihistamine (sedating).

USES:
Nausea, vomiting, dizziness, Ménière's disease.

DOSAGE:
 One tablet every four hours as required.

FORMS:
Tablets, syrup.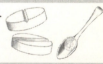

PRECAUTIONS:
Safe in pregnancy (A), breast feeding and children over 2 years.
Use with caution in asthma, epilepsy, heart disease, difficulty in passing urine, enlarged prostate gland, glaucoma, high blood pressure, peptic ulcer and overactive thyroid gland.
Use with caution if operating machinery or driving a vehicle.

Do not take if:

 sensitive to antihistamines.

SIDE EFFECTS:
Common: Drowsiness, thick mucus.

INTERACTIONS:
Other drugs:
- Sedatives, hypnotics, MAOI, tricyclic antidepressants, atropine.

Other substances:
- Reacts with alcohol to increase sedation.

PRESCRIPTION:
No.

PBS:
No.

PERMITTED IN SPORT:
Yes.

OVERDOSE:
Severe, particularly in children. May cause incoordination, flushing, hallucinations, drowsiness, dry mouth, vomiting, stomach pains, fever, shortness of breath, convulsions and death. Administer activated charcoal or induce vomiting if taken recently. Seek urgent medical assistance.

OTHER INFORMATION:
Widely used to prevent motion sickness, and very safe if taken correctly. Does not cause dependence or addiction.

Dimethicone

TRADE NAMES:
Dimethicream, Egozite Protective Baby Lotion, Hamilton Skin Repair, QV Bar, Rosken Skin Repair, Silic 15.
Acnederm Ointment, Egozite Baby Cream, QV Lip Balm, Silcon Cream (with other ingredients).
Eulactol Heel Balm (with urea, lanolin and other ingredients).
Fungo Cream (with miconazole).
Fungo Soothing Balm (with miconazole, bufexamac).
Fungo Vaginal Cream (with miconazole).
Hamilton Eczema Cream (with coal tar, zinc oxide and other ingredients).
Nutra D Cream (with mineral oil).
Also found in numerous other preparations.

USES:
Skin protection.

DOSAGE:
 Apply freely as required.

FORMS:
Cream.

PRECAUTIONS:
Safe to use in pregnancy, breast feeding and children.

SIDE EFFECTS:
Nil.

INTERACTIONS:
None.

PRESCRIPTION:
No.

PBS:
No.

PERMITTED IN SPORT:
Yes.

Dinoprostone

TRADE NAMES:
Prostin E2, Dinoprost F2 Alpha.

USES:
Inducing labour in late pregnancy.

DOSAGE:

Gel inserted into vagina by doctor.
Injection as determined by doctor.

FORMS:
Vaginal gel (Prostin E2), injection (Dinoprost F2 Alpha).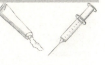

PRECAUTIONS:
Not to be used until late in pregnancy (C).
Use with caution in liver, heart and kidney disease.
Use with caution in asthma, epilepsy and glaucoma.
Contractions of uterus and health of baby must be monitored regularly.

Do not use if:
suffering from ruptured membranes around the baby, head of baby is high, previous pregnancies delivered by Caesarean section, patient has had surgery to uterus, breech or other inappropriate presentation, abnormal vaginal bleeding, more than five previous childbirths.

SIDE EFFECTS:
Common: Excessive contractions of uterus, altered heart rate in baby, nausea, diarrhoea, excess bleeding after delivery.
Unusual: Infection after delivery.
Severe but rare: Lung embolism.

INTERACTIONS:
Other drugs:
- Oxytocin, alcohol.

PRESCRIPTION:
Yes.

PBS:
No.

OVERDOSE:
Excessive contractions of uterus may lead to rupture of the uterus, a condition which is potentially fatal to mother and child.

OTHER INFORMATION:
Normally used when a woman is overdue for delivery and the health of the baby is being affected by a prolonged pregnancy.

Diphemanil methylsulfate

TRADE NAME:
Prantal.

DRUG CLASS:
Anticholinergic.

USES:
Excessive sweating.

DOSAGE:

Apply twice a day.

FORMS:
Powder.

PRECAUTIONS:
Use with caution in pregnancy, breast feeding and children under 12 years.
Apply to limited area only.

SIDE EFFECTS:
Minimal.

INTERACTIONS:
Unlikely with skin use.

PRESCRIPTION:
No.

PBS:
No. Available to some Veteran Affairs pensioners.

PERMITTED IN SPORT:
Yes.

OTHER INFORMATION:
Simple and long used medication for excessive sweating.

Diphenhydramine
See ANTIHISTAMINES, SEDATING.

Diphenoxylate hydrochloride

TRADE NAMES:
Lofenoxal, Lomotil (with atropine sulfate).

DRUG CLASS:
Antidiarrhoeal.

USES:
Diarrhoea.

DOSAGE:
 Two tablets, three or four times a day as required for diarrhoea.

FORMS:
Tablets (white).

PRECAUTIONS:
Should not be used in the last part of pregnancy (C). Should be used with caution in breast feeding.
Should not be used in children under 12 years.

Do not take if:
 suffering from diarrhoea caused by use of antibiotics.
- suffering from jaundice, ulcerative colitis, Crohn's disease, bacterial colitis or amoebic colitis.

SIDE EFFECTS:
Common: Tiredness, dizziness, confusion, rapid heart rate.

Unusual: Restlessness, mood changes, headache, tissue swelling, rash, vomiting, belly discomfort.

INTERACTIONS:
Other drugs:
- Interacts with barbiturates, tranquillisers and monoamine oxidase inhibitors (MAOI).

Other substances:
- Should not be taken with alcohol.

PRESCRIPTION:
Yes.

PBS:
Yes.

PERMITTED IN SPORT:
Yes.

OVERDOSE:
Serious. May cause dry skin and mouth, restlessness, rapid heart rate, coma and reduced breathing. Seek urgent medical attention.

OTHER INFORMATION:
Possibility of addiction with prolonged use. Very effective medication.

See also Atropine, Attapulgite, Codeine Phosphate, Kaolin, Loperamide, Pectin.

Diphtheria vaccine

TRADE NAMES:
Diphtheria Vaccine.
ADT, CDT (with tetanus vaccine).
Boostrix, Infanrix, Triple Antigen (discontinued), **Tripacel** (with tetanus and whooping cough vaccines).
Infanrix HepB (with hepatitis B, tetanus and whooping cough vaccines).

DRUG CLASS:
Vaccine.

USES:
Prevention of diphtheria (life threatening throat infection).

Medications

DOSAGE:

Three doses two months apart at two, four and six months of age; repeat at 18 months, 5 years and then every 10 years.

FORMS:
Injection.

PRECAUTIONS:
May be used safely in pregnancy (A), breast feeding and children.

SIDE EFFECTS:
Common: Local redness, soreness and lump at injection site; fever.
Unusual: Tiredness, irritability.

INTERACTIONS:
None significant.

PRESCRIPTION:
Yes.

PBS:
Yes.

PERMITTED IN SPORT:
Yes.

OVERDOSE:
No serious effect expected if unintentional additional dose given.

OTHER INFORMATION:
Normally given in combination with hepatitis B, tetanus and whooping cough vaccines. Should be given to all infants starting at two months of age. Diphtheria is a very serious infectious disease causing severe and often fatal throat infection. It can be completely prevented by vaccination.

Dipivefrine hydrochloride

TRADE NAMES:
Dipoquin (discontinued)**, Propine.**

USES:
Some types of glaucoma.

DOSAGE:

One drop twice a day.

FORMS:
Eye drops.

PRECAUTIONS:
May be used in pregnancy (B2), breast feeding and children.

Do not take if:
 suffering from narrow angle glaucoma.

SIDE EFFECTS:
Common: Red eyes, eye burning and stinging.
Unusual: Rapid heart rate.

INTERACTIONS:
None significant.

PRESCRIPTION:
Yes.

PBS:
Yes.

PERMITTED IN SPORT:
Yes.

See Acetazolamide, Apraclonidine, Betaxolol, Bimatoprost, Brimonidine tartrate, Brinzolamide, Carbachol, Dorzolamide hydrochloride, Latanoprost, Levobunolol, Phenylephrine, Pilocarpine, Timolol, Travoprost.

Dipyridamole

TRADE NAMES:
Persantin, Persantin SR.
Asasantin SR (with aspirin).

DRUG CLASS:
Anticoagulant.

USES:
Prevention and treatment of blood clots and strokes, particularly in patients with previous strokes, transient ischaemic attacks (mini-strokes), kidney disease and after transplantation of heart valves.

DOSAGE:

Persantin: One tablet four times a day one hour before meals.
Asasantin SR, Persantin SR: One tablet twice a day.

FORMS:
Persantin: Tablet of 100mg (orange), injection.
Persantin SR: Capsule of 200mg (red/orange)
Asasantin SR: Capsule (red/white) (dipyridamole 200mg, aspirin 25mg)

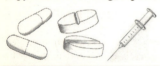

PRECAUTIONS:
Should be used with caution in pregnancy (B1). Not for use in breast feeding. Use with caution in children.
Use with caution in severe heart disease (eg. unstable angina), and aortic stenosis (heart valve disease)

SIDE EFFECTS:
Common: Headache.
Unusual: Diarrhoea, nausea, flushing, low blood pressure, dizziness, rapid heart rate
Severe but rare (stop medication, consult doctor): Abnormal bruising or bleeding.

INTERACTIONS:
Other drugs:
- Xanthinates, adenosine, blood pressure medications (but may be used with most of them).

PRESCRIPTION:
Yes.

PBS:
Yes (SR versions only).

PERMITTED IN SPORT:
Yes.

OVERDOSE:
Unlikely to be serious, but medical assistance should be sought.

OTHER INFORMATION:
Often used in combination with other anticoagulants. Very safe and can be taken long term to prevent heart attacks and strokes.

Disodium cromoglycate

See Sodium cromoglycate.

Disodium etidronate

TRADE NAMES:
Didronel.
Didrocal (with calcium carbonate).

USES:
Paget's disease, osteoporosis.

DOSAGE:

Once a day at bedtime on an empty stomach.

FORMS:
Tablets.

Medications

PRECAUTIONS:
Use in pregnancy only if medically essential. Not for use in breast feeding or children.
Use with caution in peptic ulcer, inflamed bowel, kidney stones.
Diet must contain adequate calcium and vitamin D.

Do not take if:

 suffering from osteomalacia or bone cancer.

SIDE EFFECTS:
Common: Diarrhoea, nausea.
Unusual: Bone pain.
Severe but rare (stop medication, consult doctor): Bleeding from bowel.

INTERACTIONS:
Other drugs:
- Antacids, vitamin and mineral supplements.

Other substances:
- High calcium foods (eg. cheese, sardines).

PRESCRIPTION:
Yes.

PBS:
Yes (Restricted to specific disease states – authority required).

PERMITTED IN SPORT:
Yes.

OVERDOSE:
Unlikely to be serious unless taken long term in excessive doses.

OTHER INFORMATION:
Does not cause dependence or addiction.

Disodium pamidronate

TRADE NAMES:
Aredia, Pamisol.

DRUG CLASS:
Biphosphonate.

USES:
High blood calcium levels, Paget's disease, bone secondary cancer, multiple myeloma.

DOSAGE:
 As determined by doctor.

FORMS:
Intravenous infusion.

PRECAUTIONS:
Use with caution in pregnancy (B3) and breast feeding.
Not for use in children.
Not to be injected into muscle or quickly into vein.
Use with caution in hyperparathyroidism, kidney and heart disease.
Regular blood tests to check calcium, and phosphate levels, and kidney function, are necessary.

SIDE EFFECTS:
Common: Low blood calcium, fever, other biochemical abnormalities, muscle pain, nausea, diarrhoea.
Unusual: Vomiting, headache, drowsiness.
Severe but rare (stop medication, consult doctor): Seizures, damaged blood cells, fluid in lungs, high or low blood pressure, heart failure, kidney failure.

INTERACTIONS:
Other drugs:
- Other biphosphonates, calcium.

Medications

PRESCRIPTION:
Yes.

PBS:
Yes (Authority required)

PERMITTED IN SPORT:
Yes.

Disopyramide

TRADE NAME:
Rythmodan.

DRUG CLASS:
Antiarrhythmic.

USES:
Control of heartbeat irregularities.

DOSAGE:

One or two tablets, three to four times a day.

FORMS:
Capsules of 100mg and 150mg.

PRECAUTIONS:
Should be used with caution in pregnancy (B2) and breast feeding. Not designed for use in children.
Use with caution in low blood pressure, soon after heart attack, low blood potassium, diabetes, glaucoma, prostate disease, kidney and liver failure.
Regular blood tests to check potassium levels necessary.

Do not take if:

suffering from heart failure.

SIDE EFFECTS:
Common: Dose related effects may cause dry mouth, nausea, indigestion, belly pains, bloating, constipation, blurred vision, difficulty in passing urine, dry eyes, dry nose.
Unusual: Dizziness, angina, itch, rash, loss of appetite, bad taste, diarrhoea, frequent urination, burning on urination, impotence, tiredness, pins and needles sensation, headache.
Severe but rare (stop medication, consult doctor): Unable to pass urine, yellow skin.

INTERACTIONS:
Other drugs:
- Other drugs for treatment of irregular heart rhythm.
- Phenothiazines, tricyclic antidepressants, phenytoin, beta blockers, astemizole, cisapride, pentamidine, pimozide, roxithromycin, some laxatives.

PRESCRIPTION:
Yes.

PBS:
Yes.

PERMITTED IN SPORT:
Yes.

OVERDOSE:
Extremely serious. Administer activated charcoal or induce vomiting if conscious. Seek emergency medical assistance. Symptoms include shortness of breath, cessation of breathing, coma and death.

See also Amiodarone, Flecainide, Mexiletine, Procainamide, Quinidine, Sotalol, Verapamil.

Medications

Disulfiram

TRADE NAME:
Antabuse.

USES:
Alcoholism deterrent. Causes violent vomiting if alcohol taken within 24 hours.

DOSAGE:

Half to two tablets once a day.

FORMS:
Tablets (white) of 250mg.

PRECAUTIONS:
Use in pregnancy (B2) and breast feeding only if medically essential.
Not designed for use in children.
Patient and close relatives must be made completely aware of effects of medication before use.
Use with caution in diabetes, thyroid disease, epilepsy, allergic dermatitis, eczema and asthma.
Not designed for prolonged use.

Do not take if:
- suffering from significant heart disease, severe liver or kidney disease, psychiatric disturbances.
- using cough mixtures or other medicines containing alcohol.
- alcohol taken within previous 24 hours.

SIDE EFFECTS:
Common: Numbness, tingling, pain or weakness in hands and feet.
Unusual: Eye pain, blurred vision, psychiatric disturbances, impotence, headache, tiredness, bad taste.

INTERACTIONS:
Other drugs:
- Metronidazole and paraldehyde must not be used.
- Phenytoin, isoniazid, chlordiazepoxide, diazepam, anticoagulants (eg. warfarin).

Other substances:
- Reacts severely with alcohol.

PRESCRIPTION:
Yes.

PBS:
No.

PERMITTED IN SPORT:
Yes

OVERDOSE:
Severe adverse effects unlikely provided alcohol avoided. Induce vomiting if medication taken recently. Seek medical attention.

OTHER INFORMATION:
A very useful incentive in encouraging alcoholics to completely abstain from alcohol.
Must be accompanied by appropriate counselling and support.
In use for many decades. Does not cause addiction or dependence.

See also Acamprosate, Naltrexone.

Dithranol
(Anthralin)

TRADE NAMES:
Dithrasal, Dithrocream, Micanol.

USES:
Psoriasis, fungal skin infections.

DOSAGE:

Apply sparingly twice a day. Wash off if redness occurs.

FORMS:
Cream, ointment.

Home Guide to Medication 197

PRECAUTIONS:
Safe in pregnancy and breast feeding. Use with caution on children.
Avoid eyes, nostrils, mouth, vagina, penis head and anus.
Use with care in skin folds and thin skin. Wash hands after use.

Do not use if:
- suffering from severe or pustular psoriasis.
- suffering from broken skin.

SIDE EFFECTS:
Common: Skin irritation.
Unusual: Fever, skin staining.

INTERACTIONS:
None significant.

PRESCRIPTION:
Yes.

PBS:
No.

PERMITTED IN SPORT:
Yes.

OTHER INFORMATION:
Very effective medication for psoriasis, but must be used carefully, starting with lowest concentration cream then slowly increasing strength depending on response.

DIURETICS

DISCUSSION:
Diuretics are commonly called fluid tablets because they increase the rate at which the kidney produces urine, and therefore the frequency with which the patient has to visit the toilet to pass urine. Common diuretics all come as tablets, and some are available as injections. The most common side effect of diuretics is washing out of the body (with the increased urine production) essential elements that should remain in the body. Potassium is the element most commonly lost, and as a result, many patients are given potassium (K) supplements to take while using diuretics. This side effect may also be overcome by taking the tablets only five days a week, or in some other intermittent pattern. Blood tests are often ordered to assess the levels of potassium (and other elements) in patients on diuretics.

See Amiloride, Bumetanide, Ethacrynic Acid, Frusemide, Indapamide, Spironolactone, THIAZIDE DIURETICS.

Docosahexaenoic acid
See FATTY ACIDS.

Docusate sodium

TRADE NAMES:
Coloxyl Enema, Coloxyl Tablets, Sennesoft, Waxsol.
Coloxyl Suppositories (with bisacodyl).
Coloxyl with Senna (with senna).

DRUG CLASS:
Laxative, softener.

USES:
Constipation, softening faeces, softening ear wax.

DOSAGE:
Tablets: Two tablets, once a day after evening meal.
Suppositories: One a day in evening.
Ear drops: Ten drops nightly for two or three nights.

FORMS:
Tablets, suppository, liquid enema, ear drops.

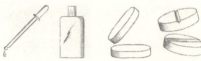

PRECAUTIONS:
Safe in pregnancy (A), breast feeding and after medical advice in children.
Designed for short term use only, unless advised otherwise by a doctor.

Do not take if:
 suffering from undiagnosed belly pains or bowel obstruction.

SIDE EFFECTS:
Common: Ear drops – None.
Other forms – Belly discomfort.
Unusual: Diarrhoea. Blood chemistry imbalances with prolonged use.
Severe but rare (stop medication, consult doctor): Severe belly pains.

INTERACTIONS:
Other drugs:
- Do not use within two hours of any other laxative.

PRESCRIPTION:
No.

PBS:
No. Available in some forms to Veterans Affairs pensioners.

PERMITTED IN SPORT:
Yes.

OVERDOSE:
Diarrhoea and loss of vital body chemicals may occur.

OTHER INFORMATION:
Safe and frequently used medication. Use of ear drops before ear syringing makes wax removal far easier.
See also Bisacodyl, Fibre, Frangula, Glycerol, Lactulose, Paraffin, Poloxamer, Psyllium, Senna, Sodium phosphate, Sodium picosulfate, Sorbitol, Sterculia.

Dolasetron

TRADE NAME:
Anzemet.

USES:
Prevention of nausea and vomiting in patients having chemotherapy for cancer, postoperative nausea and vomiting.

DOSAGE:
 One tablet or injection a day.

FORMS:
Tablets of 50mg (light pink) and 200mg (dark pink), injection.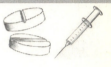

PRECAUTIONS:
May be used with caution in pregnancy (B1), breast feeding and children.
Use with caution in heart and blood vessel disease.

SIDE EFFECTS:
Common: Headache, dizziness, drowsiness, tiredness, sleeplessness, diarrhoea.
Unusual: Altered heart rate, low blood pressure, itch, liver damage.
Severe but rare (stop medication, consult doctor): Heart damage noted on ECG (electrocardiograph).

INTERACTIONS:
Other drugs:
- Some drugs used for irregular heart rhythm.

PRESCRIPTION:
Yes.

PBS:
Yes (restricted to patients suffering nausea from cancer-treating drugs).

PERMITTED IN SPORT:
Yes.

Domperidone

TRADE NAME:
Motilium.

DRUG CLASS:
Antiemetic.

USES:
Nausea, vomiting, delayed stomach emptying.

DOSAGE:

One tablet, three or four times a day, 30 minutes before meals.

FORMS:
Tablets (white) of 10mg.

PRECAUTIONS:
Should be used with caution in pregnancy (B2) and breast feeding and children.
Use with caution in breast cancer, liver and kidney disease.
Do not take if:
 suffering from some forms of pituitary gland tumour.

SIDE EFFECTS:
Common: Minimal.
Unusual: Dry mouth, stomach cramps.

INTERACTIONS:
Other drugs:
- Antacids, anticholinergics, imidazole antifungals, macrolide antibiotics, nefazodone.

PRESCRIPTION:
Yes.

PBS:
Yes.

PERMITTED IN SPORT:
Yes.

OVERDOSE:
No serious effects likely. Seek medical advice.

OTHER INFORMATION:
A remarkably safe and effective medication introduced in the mid 1980s. Marvellous for motion sickness. Does not cause dependence or addiction, but is designed for short term use.
See also Metoclopramide, Prochlorperazine.

Donepezil

TRADE NAME:
Aricept.

DRUG CLASS:
Anticholinesterase.

USES:
Alzheimer's disease.

DOSAGE:
 5 to 10mg a day before bed.

FORMS:
Tablets of 5mg (white) and 10mg (yellow).

PRECAUTIONS:
Not for use in pregnancy (B3), breast feeding or children.
Use with caution in irregular heart rhythm, peptic ulcers, asthma, emphysema, seizures, difficulty in passing urine.
Only prescribed after very careful assessment of the patient's mental state and level of dementia.

SIDE EFFECTS:
Common: Nausea, diarrhoea, tiredness, sleeplessness.
Unusual: Muscle cramps, difficulty in passing urine, seizures, dizziness, headache, loss of appetite.

Medications

Severe but rare (stop medication, consult doctor): Liver damage (jaundice), psychiatric disturbances, irregular heart rhythm, peptic ulcer.

INTERACTIONS:

Other drugs:
- Some anaesthetics, beta blockers, other anticholinergics, NSAID, ketoconazole, phenytoin, quinidine, carbamazepine, dexamethasone, rifampicin, phenobarbitone.

PRESCRIPTION:
Yes.

PBS:
Yes (authority required. Restricted to specialists only).

PERMITTED IN SPORT:
Yes.

OVERDOSE:
Serious. May cause diarrhoea, vomiting, difficulty in breathing, weakness, low blood pressure, slow heart rate and heart attack. Seek urgent medical attention.

OTHER INFORMATION:
Introduced in 1999 as a form of treatment for the otherwise untreatable early stages of Alzheimer's disease. Successful in only a limited number of patients.

See also Galantamine, Neostigmine, Pyridostigmine, Rivastigmine, Tacrine.

Dorzolamide hydrochloride

TRADE NAMES:
Trusopt.
Cosopt (with timolol).

USES:
Glaucoma.

DOSAGE:

One drop two or three times a day in affected eye.

FORMS:
Eye drops.

PRECAUTIONS:
Use with caution in pregnancy (B3), breast feeding and children.
Only suitable for certain types of glaucoma (open angle glaucoma).
Use with caution in severe liver and kidney disease.
Use with caution if eye painful from ulcers on surface or other eye disease present.

Do not use if:

 wearing contact lenses.

- suffering from acute angle closure glaucoma

SIDE EFFECTS:
Common: Eye irritation, bitter taste.
Uncommon: Blurred vision, eye pain, eye redness, eyelid crusting, throat irritation, wheeze.

INTERACTIONS:

Other drugs:
- Oral carbonic anhydrase inhibitors (eg. acetazolamide, dichlorphenamide, methazolamide).

PRESCRIPTION:
Yes.

Home Guide to Medication   201

PBS:
Yes.

PERMITTED IN SPORT:
Yes.

OVERDOSE:
May cause heart and blood pressure irregularities.

OTHER INFORMATION:
Introduced in 1996.

See Acetazolamide, Apraclonidine, Betaxolol, Bimatoprost, Brimonidine tartrate, Brinzolamide, Carbachol, Dipivefrine hydrochloride, Latanoprost, Levobunolol, Phenylephrine, Pilocarpine, Timolol, Travoprost

Dothiepin
See TRICYCLIC ANTIDEPRESSANTS.

Doxepin
See TRICYCLIC ANTIDEPRESSANTS.

Doxycycline

TRADE NAMES:
Doryx, Doxsig, Doxy, Doxyhexal, Doxylin, GenRx Doxycycline, Vibramycin, Vibra-Tabs.

DRUG CLASS:
Tetracycline antibiotic, Antimalarial.

USES:
Treatment or prevention of infections caused by susceptible bacteria. Treatment and prevention of acne. Prevention of malaria.

DOSAGE:
 Treatment of infection: 200mg at once, then 100mg a day.
Acne: 50 to 100mg a day.
Prevention of malaria and acne: 100mg a day.

FORMS:
Capsules and tablets of 50mg and 100mg.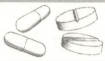

PRECAUTIONS:
Not to be used in pregnancy (D) or children under 12 as it may cause permanent staining of teeth of foetus or child. Use with caution in breast feeding.
Use with caution in kidney and liver disease, and venereal diseases.

Do not take if:
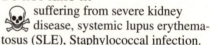 suffering from severe kidney disease, systemic lupus erythematosus (SLE), Staphylococcal infection.
• taking vitamin A or retinoids.

SIDE EFFECTS:
Common: Loss of appetite, nausea, sore mouth, diarrhoea, difficulty in swallowing, inflamed colon.
Unusual: Vomiting, inflamed pancreas, rash, sun-sensitive skin, secondary fungal infection (thrush).
Severe but rare (stop medication, consult doctor): Severe belly pain, severe bloody diarrhoea, tooth discolouration.

INTERACTIONS:
Other drugs:
• Vitamin A, retinoids, anticoagulants (eg. warfarin), penicillin, antacids, iron, oral contraceptives, methoxyflurane, bismuth, barbiturates, anticonvulsants, acetazolamide.

Other substances:
• Milk and food may reduce absorption from gut.

PRESCRIPTION:
Yes.

Medications

PBS:
Yes.

PERMITTED IN SPORT:
Yes.

OVERDOSE:
Exacerbation of side effects only likely effect.

OTHER INFORMATION:
Used to prevent acne and malaria. Used to treat a wide variety of bacterial infections. Does not cause dependence or addiction.
See also ANTIMALARIALS, Demeclocycline, Methacycline, Minocycline, Tetracycline.

Doxylamine

See ANTIHISTAMINES, SEDATING.

Droperidol

TRADE NAME:
Droleptan.

DRUG CLASS:
Antipsychotic.

USES:
Control of acute psychotic agitation, anaesthesia, premedication before surgery.

DOSAGE:

 As determined by doctor as necessary for each patient depending on use.

FORMS:
Injection.

PRECAUTIONS:
Not to be used in pregnancy (C) unless essential. Use with caution in breast feeding and infants.
Use with caution in heart, liver and kidney disease.
Use lower dose in elderly and debilitated.
Do not use if:
- suffering from severe depression, Parkinson's disease, very slow heart rate, heart conduction problems or low potassium or magnesium levels.
- in a coma.

SIDE EFFECTS:
Common: Drowsiness, low blood pressure, incoordination.
Unusual: Irregular heartbeat, tremor, muscle rigidity.

INTERACTIONS:
Other drugs:
- Narcotics, medications which cause brain activity depression, medications that lower blood pressure, medications that put stress on liver function.

Herbs:
- Evening primrose (linoleic acid).

Other substances:
- Marijuana, heroin.

PRESCRIPTION:
Yes.

PBS:
No.

OVERDOSE:
Sedation and low blood pressure leading to coma with muscle rigidity.

OTHER INFORMATION:
Often used during gastroscopy and colonoscopy procedures to relax patient.
See also Amisulpride, Flupenthixol, Haloperidol, Lithium Carbonate, Olanzapine, PHENOTHIAZINES, Pimozide, Quetiapine, Risperidone, Thiothixene, Zuclopenthixol.

Drosperidone

See ORAL CONTRACEPTIVES.

Dydrogesterone

TRADE NAMES:
Duphaston.
Femoston (with oestradiol).

DRUG CLASS:
Sex hormone.

USES:
Abnormal bleeding from uterus, failure of menstrual periods, endometriosis, painful menstrual periods.
Used with oestrogens in postmenopausal hormone replacement.

DOSAGE:

Duphaston: Must be individualised by doctor.
Femoston: One tablet a day.

FORMS:
Duphaston: Tablets (white) of 10mg
Femoston: Tablets (yellow).

PRECAUTIONS:
Not to be used in pregnancy (D), breast feeding or children.
Use with caution in high blood pressure, heart failure, fluid retention, and depression.

Do not take if:
- suffering from blood clots, inflamed veins, stroke, angina, heart attack, breast or genital cancer, liver disease, jaundice, sickle cell anaemia, miscarriage, Dubin-Johnson syndrome, Rotor syndrome.
- suffering undiagnosed vaginal bleeding.

SIDE EFFECTS:
Common: Dizziness, breast pain.
Uncommon: Headache, nausea, abnormal vaginal bleeding, weight gain, fluid retention.
Severe but rare (stop medication, consult doctor): Blood clot, yellow skin (jaundice).

INTERACTIONS:
Other drugs:
- Other sex hormones.

PRESCRIPTION:
Yes.

PBS:
Yes.

PERMITTED IN SPORT:
Yes.

OVERDOSE:
Vomiting and abnormal vaginal bleeding only likely effects.

OTHER INFORMATION:
Does not cause addiction or dependence.

See also Cyproterone acetate, Danazol, Ethinyloestradiol, Etonogestrel, HORMONE REPLACEMENT THERAPY, Medroxyprogesterone acetate, Oestradiol, Oestriol, Oestrogen, ORAL CONTRACEPTIVES, Oxandrolone, Piperazine oestrone sulfate, Testosterone.

Medications

Echinacea

USES:
Cold symptoms, cough, fever, mouth inflammation, minor wounds and burns.

DOSAGE:
 Up to 900mg a day, divided into several doses.

FORMS:
Capsules, liquid, tincture, cream.

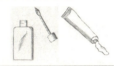

PRECAUTIONS:
Do not use in pregnancy or breast feeding or children. Use with caution in children over 12 years.
Use with caution in diabetes.
Do not take if:
suffering from AIDS, multiple sclerosis, tuberculosis, autoimmune or connective tissue diseases (eg. SLE), allergic tendencies.
- trying to fall pregnant.

SIDE EFFECTS:
Common: Nausea, vomiting, rash.
Unusual: Dizziness, low blood pressure.
Severe but rare (stop medication, consult doctor): Breathing difficulties, swelling of face, infertility.

INTERACTIONS:
Other drugs:
- Cyclosporin, steroids, some cancer-treating drugs

PRESCRIPTION:
No.

PERMITTED IN SPORT:
Yes.

OVERDOSE:
Exacerbation of side effects expected. Seek medical advice.

OTHER INFORMATION:
Not used in orthodox medicine.

Econazole

TRADE NAMES:
Dermazole, Pevaryl.

USES:
Treatment of fungal infections of skin (tinea, athlete's foot, pityriasis versicolor) and vagina (thrush).

DOSAGE:
 Skin: Apply two or three times a day.
Vagina: Insert once a day at night.

FORMS:
Cream, vaginal cream, vaginal pessary, solution.

PRECAUTIONS:
Safe to use in pregnancy (A), breast feeding and children.
Should not be swallowed or used in eyes.
Use with care on open wounds.

SIDE EFFECTS:
Common: Nil.
Unusual: Skin irritation, rash.

INTERACTIONS:
None significant.

PRESCRIPTION:
No.

Home Guide to Medication

PBS:
No. Available to some Veterans Affairs pensioners.

PERMITTED IN SPORT:
Yes.

OTHER INFORMATION:
This class of medication dramatically improved the treatment of fungal infections when introduced in the early 1970s. Very safe and effective.

See Clotrimazole, Fluconazole, Itraconazole, Ketoconazole, Miconazole.

Efavirenz

TRADE NAME:
Stocrin.

DRUG CLASS:
Antiviral.

USES:
Treatment of HIV/AIDS in combination with other medications.

DOSAGE:

Up to 600mg once a day.

FORMS:
Capsules (white/gold) of 50mg, (white) 100 and (gold) 200mg.

PRECAUTIONS:
Never to be used in pregnancy (D). Use with caution in breast feeding and children.
Use with caution in liver and kidney disease, psychiatric disturbances, epilepsy. Use lower doses in elderly.
Monitor blood cholesterol and liver enzyme levels by regular blood tests.

Do not take:
 if suffering from severe liver disease.
- unless using other medications to control HIV/AIDS.

SIDE EFFECTS:
Common: Rash, dizziness, sleeplessness, nausea, diarrhoea, tiredness.
Unusual: Poor concentration, psychotic reactions, headache.
Severe but rare (stop medication, consult doctor): Liver damage.

INTERACTIONS:
Other drugs:
- Astemizole, cisapride, midazolam, triazolam, ergots (all preceding give severe interaction), oral contraceptives, phenobarbitone, phenytoin, carbamazepine, warfarin, rifampicin, sertraline.

Other substances:
- Grapefruit, St John's wort.
- May give false positive test for cannabis use.

PRESCRIPTION:
Yes.

PBS:
Yes (authority required).

PERMITTED IN SPORT:
Yes.

OVERDOSE:
Serious liver and brain damage may occur. Seek urgent medical attention. Induce vomiting or give activated charcoal if alert and medication taken recently.

OTHER INFORMATION:
One of numerous antivirals that are used in combination to control HIV/AIDS.

See Abacavir, Delavirdine, Didanosine, Indinavir, Lamivudine, Nelfinavir, Nevirapine, Ritonavir, Saquinavir, Stavudine, Tenofovir, Zidovudine.

Eformoterol

TRADE NAMES:
Foradile, Oxis.
Symbicort (with budesonide).

DRUG CLASS:
Bronchodilator.

USES:
Long term treatment of asthma.

DOSAGE:

Powder from one or two Foradile capsules inhaled twice daily through purpose made inhaler. Use Oxis Turbuhaler and Symbicort twice a day.

FORMS:
Capsules containing powder for inhalation, inhaler.

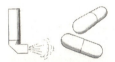

PRECAUTIONS:
Use with caution in pregnancy (B3). Safe in breast feeding and children over 5 years.
Not for use in unstable or deteriorating asthma.
Do not exceed recommended dose.
Do not swallow capsules.
Use with caution in diabetes, liver, heart and thyroid disease.
Lung function should be monitored regularly by use of spirometer.

Do not take if:

lactose sensitive.

SIDE EFFECTS:
Common: Tremor, palpitations, rapid heart rate, headache, throat irritation, dizziness.
Unusual: Lung irritation, nausea, taste disturbance, low blood potassium levels.
Severe but rare (stop medication, consult doctor): Angina (chest pain).

INTERACTIONS:
Other drugs:
- Other bronchodilators used for treatment of asthma (check with doctor).
- Digoxin, beta blockers, xanthinates, diuretics, MAOI, tricyclic antidepressants, quinidine, disopyramide, procainamide, phenothiazines, some antihistamines, oxytocin.

Other substances:
- Alcohol.

PRESCRIPTION:
Yes.

PBS:
Yes.

PERMITTED IN SPORT:
No.

OVERDOSE:
Palpitations, tremor and exacerbation of side effects likely.

OTHER INFORMATION:
Introduced in 1996. Enables patients who would otherwise use large quantities of inhaled bronchodilators (eg. Ventolin) to reduce their usage of these medications dramatically.

See also Salmeterol.

Eicosapentaenoic acid

TRADE NAMES:
Used as an ingredient in many acne skin preparations (eg. **Curacel Acne and Pimple Gel**), eczema creams (eg. **ER Cream**), and nutritional supplements (eg. **Bioglan Maxepa, Himega, Hypol, Fishaphos**).

DRUG CLASS:
Nutritional supplement.

USES:
Fatty acid supplement, acne, eczema, psoriasis.

DOSAGE:

One or two capsules a day.
Apply to skin three times a day.

FORMS:
Capsules, gel, cream.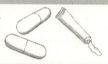

PRECAUTIONS:
Safe in pregnancy (A), breast feeding and children.
Do not exceed recommended dose.

SIDE EFFECTS:
Common: Nausea.

INTERACTIONS:
None significant.

PRESCRIPTION:
No.

PBS:
No.

PERMITTED IN SPORT:
Yes.

OVERDOSE:
Vomiting and diarrhoea only likely effects.

OTHER INFORMATION:
Derived from fish oil.
See also **FATTY ACIDS**.

ELECTROLYTES

TRADE and GENERIC NAMES:
Alka-Seltzer (Sodium bicarbonate with aspirin).
Chlorvescent (Potassium bicarbonate, potassium chloride).
Citravescent (Sodium bicarbonate with citric acid, tartaric acid).
Gastrolyte, Repalyte (Sodium chloride, potassium chloride, sodium acid citrate, glucose).
Gastrolyte-R (Sodium chloride, potassium chloride, sodium acid citrate, glucose, rice).
K-Mag, Magnesium Plus (Potassium aspartate, magnesium aspartate).
KSR, Slow-K, Span-K (Potassium chloride).
Medefizz (Potassium bicarbonate, citric acid). Used only in x-ray centres.
ORS, Pedialyte (Sodium chloride, potassium chloride, glucose and other ingredients).
Salt, Slow Sodium (Sodium chloride – common salt).
Sodibic (Sodium bicarbonate).
Electrolytes are underlined.
Electrolytes are also found in many ANTACIDS (see separate entry).

USES:
Replacement of essential electrolytes lost because of diarrhoea, vomiting, excess passing of urine, heart disease and other diseases.

DOSAGE:

Tablets: One to four tablets a day in one or more doses.
Powder: Dissolve in water and use as often as necessary to prevent dehydration.

FORMS:

Tablets, powder, mixture, injection.

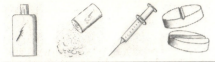

PRECAUTIONS:

Safe in pregnancy, breast feeding and children.
Be careful not to exceed necessary dose. Blood tests to measure severity of electrolyte depletion and response to treatment may be necessary.
Use with caution in kidney and liver disease, stomach ulcers.
Dilute powders with water only, not milk, juice etc.
Use with caution in dehydration as adequate fluid replacement also necessary.

Do not take if:

 suffering from Addison's disease, severe kidney disease, severe injuries or burns.

SIDE EFFECTS:

Common: Minimal.
Unusual: Fluid retention.

INTERACTIONS:

Other drugs: Triamterene, amiloride.

PRESCRIPTION:

No.

PBS:

Chlorvescent, KSR, Slow-K, Span-K: Yes. Other forms: No.

PERMITTED IN SPORT:

Yes.

OVERDOSE:

Most forms: No serious effects expected.
Potassium salts: Serious. May cause low blood pressure, irregular heartbeat, pins and needles sensation, convulsions, paralysis, heart attack, inability to breathe and death. Administer activated charcoal or induce vomiting if medication taken recently. Seek urgent medical assistance.

OTHER INFORMATION:

Electrolytes are elements such as Potassium, Sodium, Chlorine and Magnesium that are essential for the biochemical functioning of the body. Diuretics cause increased loss of potassium and specific replacement and regular checks of blood potassium level are advisable.

Enalapril

See ACE INHIBITORS.

Enoxaparin

TRADE NAME:

Clexane.

DRUG CLASS:

Anticoagulant.

USES:

Prevention and treatment of blood clots in veins. Often used after major surgery, in unstable angina, or in bedridden patients.

DOSAGE:

 As determined by doctor for each patient.

FORMS:

Injection.

PRECAUTIONS:

Not to be used in pregnancy (C) unless essential. Use with caution in breast feeding.
Must not be injected into muscle.
Use with caution in severe kidney and liver disease, artificial heart valves, diabetic eye damage, very thin people, history of peptic ulcer and uncontrolled

high blood pressure.
Not for use in association with a spinal or epidural anaesthetic.
Regular blood tests to measure effect essential.

Do not use if:

☠ suffering from heart infections, bleeding disorders, active peptic ulcer, stroke caused by bleeding in brain.
- taking aspirin, heparin or NSAIDs (anti-inflammatory drugs used for arthritis).

SIDE EFFECTS:

Common: Abnormal bruising and bleeding, bruising at injection site.
Unusual: Liver damage.
Severe but rare (stop medication, consult doctor): Bleeding from anus, coughing blood.

INTERACTIONS:

Other drugs:
- Warfarin, other anticoagulants, NSAIDs, aspirin, dextran, clopidrogel, steroids.

Other substances:
- Celery tablets.

PRESCRIPTION:
Yes.

PBS:
Yes.

PERMITTED IN SPORT:
Yes.

OVERDOSE:
Very serious. Excessive bleeding may occur. Antidote available. Given under strict medical supervision.

OTHER INFORMATION:
Introduced in 1996. Has fewer side effects than Heparin.
See also Heparin.

Entacapone

TRADE NAME:
Comtan.

DRUG CLASS:
Antiparkinsonian.

USES:
Severe Parkinson's disease unmanageable by other medications.

DOSAGE:

One tablet, four to seven times a day.

FORMS:
Tablets of 200mg.

PRECAUTIONS:
Use with caution in pregnancy (B3), breast feeding and children.
Use with caution in low blood pressure.
Avoid taking with fatty meal. Do not cease suddenly, but reduce dose slowly.

Do not take if:

 suffering from phaeochromocytoma, liver disease.

SIDE EFFECTS:

Common: Incoordination, dry mouth, nausea, diarrhoea, belly pains, discoloured urine.
Unusual: Sleep disturbances, psychiatric disturbances, chest pain, confusion, shortness of breath.
Severe but rare (stop medication, consult doctor): Pneumonia, anaemia.

INTERACTIONS:

Other drugs:
- MAOI, Isoprenaline, adrenaline, methyldopa, apomorphine, iron, diazepam, venlafaxine, antidepressants, ibuprofen, benserazide, levodopa, other medications used to treat Parkinson's disease.

Other substances:
- Fatty foods.

Medications

PRESCRIPTION:
Yes.

PBS:
Yes (authority required).

PERMITTED IN SPORT:
Yes.

OVERDOSE:
Likely to be serious. Seek urgent medical attention.

OTHER INFORMATION:
Introduced in 1999 to assist the most severely affected cases of Parkinson's disease.
See also ANTIPARKINSONIANS.

Ephedrine

TRADE NAME:
Ephedrine.

DRUG CLASS:
Sympathomimetic, Bronchodilator.

USES:
Asthma, spasm of bronchi in lungs, severe allergy, bed wetting.

DOSAGE:

One or two tablets, three or four times a day.

FORMS:
Tablets of 30mg, injection.
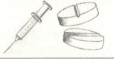

PRECAUTIONS:
May be used in pregnancy (A), breast feeding and children.
Use with caution in heart disease, angina and prostate gland enlargement.
Do not exceed recommended dose.

Do not take if:
suffering from narrowing of heart arteries, heart attack, glaucoma, high blood pressure, overactive thyroid gland, neuroses.

SIDE EFFECTS:
Common: Alertness, sleeplessness, dizziness, headache, nausea, sweating, palpitations.
Unusual: Vomiting, diarrhoea, rapid heart rate, difficulty in passing urine, weakness.

INTERACTIONS:
Other drugs:
- MAOI, digoxin, theophylline, frusemide, cyclopropane, some general anaesthetics.

Other substances:
- Reacts with caffeine.

PRESCRIPTION:
Yes.

PBS:
No. Used in hospitals only.

PERMITTED IN SPORT:
No.

OVERDOSE:
Exacerbation of side effects leading to convulsions and possible heart attack possible. Seek urgent medical assistance.

EPILEPSY TREATMENTS

See ANTICONVULSANTS.

Epoeitin
(Erythropoietin)

TRADE NAME:
Eprex.

USES:
Anaemia associated with kidney failure or some types of cancer, before surgery when significant blood loss expected.

DOSAGE:

Complex. As determined by doctor for each patient. usually one to three injections a week.

FORMS:
Injection.

PRECAUTIONS:
May be used with caution in pregnancy (B3), breast feeding and children.
Use with caution in heart disease, cancer, low and high blood pressure, liver disease, epilepsy, high potassium levels, porphyria and gout.

Do not take if:

suffering uncontrolled high blood pressure, severe heart disease.

SIDE EFFECTS:
Common: Bone pains, muscle aches.
Unusual: High blood pressure, fits, blood clots, rash, allergy reaction.

INTERACTIONS:
Other drugs:
- Cyclosporin, iron.

PRESCRIPTION:
Yes.

PBS:
Yes (very restricted to specific patients for particular conditions).

PERMITTED IN SPORT:
No.

OTHER INFORMATION:
Used illegally by some endurance sports people to enhance performance. Has dramatically improved life expectancy and quality of life for patients on dialysis for kidney failure, but expense limits its use.

Eprosartan
See ANGIOTENSIN II RECEPTOR ANTAGONISTS.

Ergocalciferol

TRADE NAMES:
Ostelin.
May be combined with vitamins and minerals in other preparations.

DRUG CLASS:
Fat soluble essential vitamin. Form of vitamin D.

USES:
Nutritional deficiency of vitamin D, osteomalacia, rickets.

DOSAGE:

One capsule a day.
Daily requirement is 5µg.

FORMS:
Capsules.

PRECAUTIONS:
Use with caution in pregnancy, breast feeding and children.
Use with caution in kidney disease or kidney stones, and heart disease.

Do not take if:

suffering from high blood calcium levels or excess vitamin D.

SIDE EFFECTS:
Common: Constipation, nausea.
Unusual: Calcium deposits in tissue, dehydration, high blood pressure, muscle weakness, headache, irregular heartbeat.

INTERACTIONS:
Other drugs:
- Barbiturates, anticonvulsants.

PRESCRIPTION:
No.

PBS:
No.

PERMITTED IN SPORT:
Yes.

OTHER INFORMATION:
Remember, vitamins are merely chemicals that are essential in minute doses for the functioning of the body, and if taken to excess, act as a drug. Vitamin D can be found naturally in fatty fish (sardines, tuna, salmon, herrings etc.), margarine and egg yolk. It is also produced in the body by the action of sunlight on the skin.

Ergometrine

TRADE NAMES:
Ergometrine.
Syntometrine (with oxytocin).

USES:
Stopping abnormal bleeding after delivery or abortion.

DOSAGE:
 One injection immediately after delivery of baby.

FORMS:
Injection.

PRECAUTIONS:
Safe to use after delivery in pregnancy (A), but should not otherwise be used in pregnancy. Safe for use in breast feeding. Not for use in children.
Use with caution in heart disease, high blood pressure, porphyria.
Usually given as an injection into muscle, not a vein.

Do not take injection if:
 previous Caesarean section, retained placenta.

SIDE EFFECTS:
Common: Rapid heart rate, retention of fluid.
Unusual: Low or high blood pressure, irregular heart rhythm, nausea, diarrhoea, dizziness, hallucinations, sweating.

INTERACTIONS:
Other drugs:
- Glyceryl trinitrate, beta blockers, bromocriptine, dopamine, doxycycline, sumatriptan, erythromycin, tetracycline, general anaesthetics, methysergide, nicotine.

PRESCRIPTION:
Yes.

PBS:
No.

PERMITTED IN SPORT:
Yes.

OVERDOSE:
Unlikely to have serious effects.

OTHER INFORMATION:
Injection commonly used to increase intensity of labour and immediately after delivery to reduce bleeding.

Ergotamine

TRADE NAMES:
Ergodryl Mono.
Ergodryl (with caffeine, diphenhydramine).
Cafergot (with caffeine).

DRUG CLASS:
Antimigraine.

USES:
Migraine, vascular headaches.

DOSAGE:
Tablets and capsules: One or two tablets or capsules immediately symptoms detected. Repeat every half hour. Maximum six a day.
Suppository: One immediately symptoms detected. Maximum three a day.

FORMS:
Tablets, capsules, suppositories.

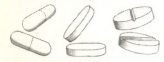

PRECAUTIONS:
Should not be used in pregnancy (C) as it may cause premature labour. Not for use in breast feeding or children.
Should not be used for prolonged period. Not designed for prevention of migraine.
Do not take if:
suffering from poor circulation to arms or legs, angina, high blood pressure, hardening of arteries, severe infection, severe liver or kidney disease.

SIDE EFFECTS:
Common: Nausea, vomiting, diarrhoea, leg weakness, pins and needles sensation, chest pain.
Unusual: Swelling of feet, itch, slow or rapid heart rate.
Severe but rare (stop medication, consult doctor): Severe chest pain, irregular heartbeat.

INTERACTIONS:
Other drugs:
- Vasoconstrictors, macrolide antibiotics (eg. erythromycin).

Other substances:
- Alcohol, caffeine, smoking and exercise may be migraine triggers.

PRESCRIPTION:
Yes.

PBS:
No.

PERMITTED IN SPORT:
Yes

OVERDOSE:
May be serious. Symptoms include vomiting, diarrhoea, thirst, tingling, itching, cold skin, rapid weak pulse, confusion and coma. If tablets or capsules taken recently, induce vomiting. Seek urgent medical assistance.

OTHER INFORMATION:
May become ineffective if used too frequently.

See also Dihydroergotamine, Naratriptan, Sumatriptan, Zolmitriptan.

Erythromycin

TRADE NAMES:
EES, E-Mycin, Eryacne, Eryc, Erythrocin.

DRUG CLASS:
Macrolide antibiotic.

USES:
Treatment of infections of lung (eg. pneumonia, bronchitis), throat, heart, skin (eg. acne, cellulitis), eye (eg. trachoma), teeth and urethra (eg. NSU, syphilis, gonorrhoea).

DOSAGE:
 Orally: One tablet or capsule, two to four times a day.
Gel: Apply twice a day.

FORMS:
Tablets, capsules, filmtabs, injection, syrup, suspension, gel.

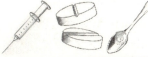

PRECAUTIONS:
Safe to use in pregnancy (A), breast feeding and children.
Not designed for prolonged or repeated use.
Use with caution in liver disease.

Do not take if:
 suffering from severe liver disease, jaundice (yellow skin).

SIDE EFFECTS:
Common: Nausea, vomiting, diarrhoea, rash, headache.
Unusual: Belly pain, loss of appetite, excess wind, dizziness, ear noises, temporary deafness.
Severe but rare (stop medication, consult doctor): Yellow skin (jaundice), irregular heartbeat, worsening infection, seizures, pancreatitis (severe belly pain).

INTERACTIONS:
Other drugs:
- Theophylline, cisapride, pimozide, carbamazepine, warfarin, cyclosporin, triazolam, phenytoin, digoxin, oral contraceptives, dihydroergotamine, disopyramide, bromocriptine, valproate, quinidine, methylprednisolone, sildenafil, triazolam, dihydroergotamine, lovastatin, simvastatin, zopiclone.

PRESCRIPTION:
Yes.

PBS:
Most forms: Yes.
Gel: No.

PERMITTED IN SPORT:
Yes.

OVERDOSE:
Severe diarrhoea, stomach pains and deafness may occur.

OTHER INFORMATION:
Used for a wide range of infections in general practice. Does not cause addiction or dependence. Some forms may cause fewer side effects than others.

Erythropoietin
See Epoetin.

Esmolol

TRADE NAME:
Brevibloc.

DRUG CLASS:
Beta blocker.

USES:
Rapid or irregular heartbeat, paroxysmal atrial tachycardia.

DOSAGE:
 Slow infusion. Rate determined by doctor.

FORMS:
Injection.

PRECAUTIONS:
Should be used in pregnancy (C) only if medically essential.
Safe to use in breast feeding.
May be used with caution in children.
Use with care if suffering from alcoholism, liver or kidney failure or about to have surgery.

Do not take if:
 suffering from diabetes, asthma, or allergic conditions.
- suffering from heart failure, shock, slow heart rate, or enlarged right heart.
- undertaking prolonged fast.

SIDE EFFECTS:
Common: Low blood pressure, slow heart rate, cold hands and feet, asthma.
Unusual: Loss of appetite, nausea, diarrhoea, impotence, tiredness, sleeplessness, nightmares, rash, loss of libido, hair loss, noises in ears.
Severe but rare (stop medication, consult doctor): Severe asthma.

INTERACTIONS:
Other drugs:
- Calcium channel blockers, disopyramide, clonidine, adrenaline, other medications for irregular heartbeat, lignocaine, ergotamine, indomethacin, chlorpromazine.

PRESCRIPTION:
Yes.

PBS:
No.

PERMITTED IN SPORT:
Yes.

OVERDOSE:
Slow heart rate, low blood pressure, asthma and heart failure may result.
See also Atenolol, Carvedilol, Labetalol, Metoprolol, Oxprenolol, Pindolol, Propranolol, Sotalol.

Estradiol
See Oestradiol.

Esomeprazole
See PROTON PUMP INHIBITORS.

Ethacrynic Acid

TRADE NAME:
Edecril.

DRUG CLASS:
Diuretic.

USES:
Excess fluid in body, heart failure resulting in excess fluid in lungs, liver failure with fluid retention, nephrotic syndrome.

DOSAGE:
 One or more tablets after breakfast in morning to a maximum of 400mg a day.

FORMS:
Tablet of 50mg (white).

PRECAUTIONS:
Should be used in pregnancy (C) only if medically essential. Should not be used in breast feeding. Safe in children over 2 years.
Regular blood tests to measure level of chemicals (electrolytes) in blood are recommended.
Should be used intermittently rather than constantly if possible.
Potassium supplements may be required. Use with caution in severe liver disease, angina and heart disease.

Do not take if:
 suffering from severe kidney failure.

SIDE EFFECTS:
Common: Minimal.
Unusual: Loss of appetite, tiredness, belly discomfort, nausea, vomiting, diarrhoea, gout.
Severe but rare (stop medication, consult doctor): Bloody diarrhoea, other unusual bleeding, fainting, fits.

INTERACTIONS:
Other drugs:
- Digoxin, aminoglycosides, warfarin, lithium, steroids.
- Medications that reduce blood pressure.

Herbs:
- Celery, dandelion, uva ursi.

PRESCRIPTION:
Yes.

PBS:
Yes.

PERMITTED IN SPORT:
No, acts as masking agent for other illegal drugs.

OVERDOSE:
Severe dehydration may result.

See also Amiloride, Bumetanide, Frusemide, Indapamide, Spironolactone, THIAZIDE DIURETICS.

Ethambutol

TRADE NAME:
Myambutol.

USES:
Tuberculosis (TB).

DOSAGE:
 In combination with other medications for tuberculosis as directed by doctor.

FORMS:
Tablets of 100mg (yellow) and 400mg (grey).

PRECAUTIONS:
May be used safely in pregnancy (A), breast feeding and children.
Use with caution in kidney and eye disease.
Not designed for prolonged use.

Do not take if:
 suffering from optic neuritis.

SIDE EFFECTS:
Common: Minimal.
Unusual: Blurred vision, nausea, vomiting, diarrhoea, rash, joint pain.
Severe but rare (stop medication, consult doctor): Significant deterioration of vision.

INTERACTIONS:
None significant.

PRESCRIPTION:
Yes.

PBS:
No.

PERMITTED IN SPORT:
Yes.

OVERDOSE:
May cause eye damage.

See also Cycloserine, Isoniazid, Pyrazinamide, Rifampicin.

Ethanol

TRADE NAMES:

Ethanol is common alcohol (ethyl alcohol), and is used in a large number of medications, particularly as a solvent in mixtures, gels and lotions. Ethanol is the alcohol that is present in all alcoholic drinks (beer, wine, spirits etc.).

DRUG CLASS:

Alcohol.

USES:

In medication: Dissolves other medications, acts as a preservative, mild sedative, mild cough suppressant.
In drinks: Relaxes, reduces inhibitions.

DOSAGE:

 As directed or desired.

FORMS:

Mixture, liquid, gel, lotion.

PRECAUTIONS:

Use in pregnancy should be avoided. May be used in small quantities in breast feeding. Not to be given to children except when used in approved medications.

Do not take if:

☠ suffering from liver damage, alcoholism, depression, other psychiatric conditions, pancreatitis, any abnormal bleeding.
- operating machinery, driving a vehicle or undertaking tasks that require concentration.

SIDE EFFECTS:

Common: Drowsiness, flush, rapid heart rate.
Unusual: Nausea, vomiting, headache.

INTERACTIONS:

Other drugs:
- Interacts with a wide range of medications. Should not be taken while using any other medication without consulting a pharmacist or doctor.

Herbs;
- Valerian.

Other substances:
- Reacts adversely with exercise, cocaine, marijuana and narcotics.

PRESCRIPTION:

No.

PBS:

No.

PERMITTED IN SPORT:

Yes. Impairs sport performance.

OVERDOSE:

Vomiting, poor coordination, loss of inhibitions, headache, blurred vision, loss of control of bodily functions, convulsions, coma and rarely death may occur. Seek medical assistance if massive rapid overdose consumed.

OTHER INFORMATION:

Ethanol has been produced by fermenting various fruits, vegetables and cereals for thousands of years and is mankind's most widely used drug. May cause dependence and addiction. Long term use at moderate to high dosage can cause damage to liver, brain and other organs.

Ethinyloestradiol

See ORAL CONTRACEPTIVES.

Ethosuximide

TRADE NAME:
Zarontin.

DRUG CLASS:
Anticonvulsant.

USES:
Petit mal epilepsy (absences).

DOSAGE:
 One to four capsules twice a day.

FORMS:
Capsule (clear/brown) of 250mg, syrup.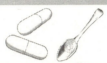

PRECAUTIONS:
Not to be used in pregnancy (D) unless medically essential. Breast feeding should be ceased before use. May be used in children.
Regular blood tests to check on liver function and blood cells recommended.
 Do not stop medication suddenly, but reduce dosage slowly.
Use with caution if operating machinery or driving a vehicle.

SIDE EFFECTS:
Common: Loss of appetite, nausea, belly cramps, drowsiness, headache.
Unusual: Belly pain, weight loss, diarrhoea, hiccups, irritability, rash, abnormal liver function, incoordination, hyperactive.
Severe but rare (stop medication, consult doctor): Blood cell damage (detected by blood tests).

INTERACTIONS:
Other drugs:
- Other medications used to treat epilepsy.

Herbs:
- Evening primrose (linoleic acid), Gingko biloba.

Other substances:
- Reacts adversely with alcohol.
- Borage.

PRESCRIPTION:
Yes.

PBS:
Yes.

PERMITTED IN SPORT:
Yes.

OVERDOSE:
Administer activated charcoal or induce vomiting if medication taken recently and patient alert. Seek medical attention.

OTHER INFORMATION:
Widely and successfully used in treatment of petit mal absences. Does not cause dependence or addiction.

See also BARBITURATES, BENZODIAZEPINES, Carbamazepine, Clonazepam, Gabapentin, Lamotrigine, Levetiracetam, Oxcarbazepine, Phenytoin, Primidone, Sodium valproate, Sulthiame, Tiagabine, Topiramate, Vigabatrin.

Etonogestrel

TRADE NAME:
Implanon.

DRUG CLASS:
Sex hormone.

USES:
Long term contraception. One implant gives three years' protection.

DOSAGE:
 One implant inserted under skin at inside of upper arm every three years. Implant initially during a menstrual period.

FORMS:
Implant.

PRECAUTIONS:
Not for use in pregnancy (B3), breast feeding or children.
Implantation must be preceded by a thorough medical history and examination.
Use with caution in diabetes and liver disease.
Must be removed three years after insertion or complications may occur.

Do not take if:

☠ suffering from blood clots (thromboses), liver disease or tumours, breast cancer.
- cause of any abnormal vaginal bleeding has not been diagnosed.

SIDE EFFECTS:
Common: Breast discomfort, heavy periods, acne, headaches, belly pain, emotional upsets, weight increase, pain at implant site.
Unusual: Chloasma (skin pigmentation), hair loss, dizziness, nausea, depression, increased libido.
Severe but rare (stop medication, consult doctor): Blood clot in vein or artery, lumps in breast, constant vaginal bleeding, jaundice (yellow skin).

INTERACTIONS:
Other drugs:
- Barbiturates, primidone, carbamazepine, oxcarbazepine, griseofulvin, rifampicin, rifabutin, other sex hormones.

PRESCRIPTION:
Yes.

PBS:
Yes.

PERMITTED IN SPORT:
Yes.

OTHER INFORMATION:
Introduced in 2000 as an improved long term contraceptive that requires no regular dosing schedule or planning. Must be carefully implanted in the correct position.
See Medroxyprogesterone acetate, Oestradiol, Oestriol, Oestrogen, ORAL CONTRACEPTIVES.

Etoposide

TRADE NAMES:
Vepesid.
Etopophos (Etoposide phosphate).

USES:
Leukaemia, lung cancer, Hodgkin's disease, lymphoma.

DOSAGE:

Complex. Must be determined individually for each patient by doctor depending on diseases, severity, response and size of patient.

FORMS:
Capsules (pink) of 50mg and 100mg, drip infusion.

PRECAUTIONS:
Not to be used in pregnancy (D) unless mother's life is threatened. Breast feeding must be ceased before use. Use in children only if medically essential.
Adequate contraception must be used by women while taking etoposide.
Regular blood tests to check blood cells, kidney and liver function essential.
Use with caution in infections.
Do not allow infusion to come in contact with skin.

Do not take if:

 suffering from severe liver or bone marrow disease.

SIDE EFFECTS:
Common: Reduced blood white cells and increased risk of infection, unusual bleeding and bruising, total hair loss, nausea, vomiting, loss of appetite, sore mouth, diarrhoea.
Unusual: Low blood pressure, fever, rapid heart rate, shortness of breath, pins and needles.

INTERACTIONS:
Other drugs:
- Other medications used to treat cancer, cyclosporin.

Medications

PRESCRIPTION:
Yes.

PBS:
Yes.

PERMITTED IN SPORT:
Yes.

OVERDOSE:
Worsening of side effects likely. Seek medical attention.

OTHER INFORMATION:
Despite serious side effects, etoposide may be life saving for patients with some severe forms of cancer.

Evening primrose oil
(Linoleic acid)
See FATTY ACIDS.

Exemestane

TRADE NAME:
Aromasin.

DRUG CLASS:
Antineoplastic.

USES:
Treatment of advanced breast cancer.

DOSAGE:
 One tablet a day after a meal.

FORMS:
Tablets of 25mg.

PRECAUTIONS:
Not to be used in pregnancy (C), breast feeding and children.
Only to be used in postmenopausal women.
Regular blood tests to check liver and blood cell function advisable.

SIDE EFFECTS:
Common: Hot flushes, liver damage, tiredness, pain, nausea, diarrhoea, sweating, dizziness, sleeplessness, tissue swelling, fluid retention.
Unusual: Headache, depression, rash, hair loss, white blood cell damage.

INTERACTIONS:
Other drugs:
• Oestrogen.

PRESCRIPTION:
Yes.

PBS:
Yes.

PERMITTED IN SPORT:
Yes for women, no for men.

OVERDOSE:
Unlikely to be serious.

OTHER INFORMATION:
Released in 2001 to treat only the most serious forms of breast cancer.

EXPECTORANTS

DISCUSSION:

Expectorants aid the removal of phlegm and mucus from the respiratory passages of the lung and throat by coughing. They act by liquefying tenacious, sticky mucus so that it does not adhere firmly to the walls of the air passages, and can be shifted up and out by the microscopic hairs that line these passages and by the forced expiration of air in coughing. They are usually combined in a mixture with other medications such as mucolytics, decongestants, antihistamines, bronchodilators or antitussives. The traditional expectorants include senega, ammonium chloride, and potassium iodide, all of which taste absolutely foul. Bromhexine is a more recently developed expectorant that has a slightly better taste. The side effects of expectorants are minimal.

Many different brands are available from chemists without a prescription.

See Ammonium bicarbonate, Bromhexine, Camphor, COUGH SUPPRESSANTS, Guaiphenesin, Senega.

EYE LUBRICANTS

TRADE and GENERIC NAMES:

Aquae (Carmellose sodium, sorbitol).
Bion Tears, Poly-Tears, Tears Naturale (Hypromellose, dextran).
Cellufresh, Celluvisc, Refresh Liquigel, Refresh Tears Plus (Carmellose sodium).
Clerz, In a Wink Moisturising Drops, Rhoto Zi Fresh Eye Drops (Povidone)
Duratears, Lacri Lube (Paraffin).
Gel Tears (Carbomer 940).
Genteal Eye Drops, Isopto Tears, Methopt (Hypromellose).
Genteal Moisturising Eye Gel (Carbomer 980, hypromellose).
Lacrisert (Hydroxypropylcellulose).
Liquifilm, PVA Forte, PVA Tears (Polyvinyl alcohol).
Minims Artificial Tears, Rhoto Zi Contact Eye Drops (Hydroxyethylcellulose).
Murine Contact (Hypromellose, Glycerol).
Murine Revital, Murine Tears, Refresh, Teardrops (Polyvinyl alcohol, povidone).
Poly Gel Lubricant (Carbomer 974).
Poly Visc (Paraffin, wool fat).
Tears Plus (Polyvinyl alcohol and povidone with chlorbutol).
Viscotears (Carbomer 980).
Visine Advanced Relief (Povidone, macrogol 400, tetrahydrozoline, dextran).
Visine True Tears (Hypromellose, macrogol, glycerol).
NB: Eye lubricants are underlined.

USES:
Dry, itchy, irritated eyes.

DOSAGE:

Use drops as required several times a day.

FORMS:
Eye drops, eye ointment, eye inserts, skin gel.

PRECAUTIONS:
May be used safely in pregnancy (use Carbomer 940 with caution), breast feeding and children.
Use with caution if wearing contact lenses.

SIDE EFFECTS:
Common: Mild stinging, blurred vision.

INTERACTIONS:
None significant.

PRESCRIPTION:
No.

PBS:
Cellufresh, Duratears, Minims Artificial Tears, Refresh, Tear Drops,
Viscotears: No.
Other forms: Yes.

PERMITTED IN SPORT:
Yes.

OVERDOSE:
No adverse effects likely if swallowed.

OTHER INFORMATION:
Widely and commonly used for dry itchy eyes.

Medications

Famciclovir

TRADE NAME:
Famvir.

DRUG CLASS:
Antiviral.

USES:
Treatment and prevention of genital herpes, shingles.

DOSAGE:

Treatment: 250mg three times a day.
Prevention: 125mg twice a day.

FORMS:
Tablets (white) of 125 and 250mg.

PRECAUTIONS:
Use with caution in pregnancy (B1), breast feeding and children.
Use with caution in serious kidney disease.

SIDE EFFECTS:
Common: Headache.
Unusual: Nausea, fatigue.

INTERACTIONS:
Other drugs:
- Probenecid, diuretics (fluid tablets).

PRESCRIPTION:
Yes.

PBS:
Yes (authority required – restricted to shingles and genital herpes only).

PERMITTED IN SPORT:
Yes.

OVERDOSE:
Exacerbation of side effects likely.

OTHER INFORMATION:
Introduced in 1996. Very safe and effective medication that has a very high success rate in treating Herpes infections. Chickenpox and shingles are caused by Herpes zoster, and cold sores and genital herpes by Herpes simplex. It is vital that any patient who suspects they have shingles must see their doctor immediately as medication only works if started within 72 hours of onset of rash.
See also Aciclovir.

Famotidine

TRADE NAMES:
Amfamox, Pepcid, Pepcidine.

DRUG CLASS:
H^2 Receptor antagonist.

USES:
Treatment and prevention of ulceration and inflammation of the stomach, duodenum (upper small intestine) and oesophagus (gullet).
Zollinger-Ellison syndrome (a rare cause of severe stomach ulceration).

DOSAGE:

20 to 40mg once a day at night. Higher doses with Zollinger-Ellison syndrome and severe ulceration.

FORMS:
Tablets of 20mg and 40mg, injection.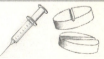

Home Guide to Medication

PRECAUTIONS:
Caution required in pregnancy (B1), with children and while breast feeding.
Use with caution in kidney disease.
Assess stomach with gastroscopy if not effective rapidly.

Do not take if:
 suffering from stomach cancer, significant kidney disease.

SIDE EFFECTS:
Common: Headache, dizziness, irregular bowel habits.
Unusual: Dry mouth, nausea, loss of appetite, bloating, tiredness, itchy skin, arthritis.

INTERACTIONS:
Herbs:
- Alfalfa, capsicum, eucalyptus, senega.

PRESCRIPTION:
Yes.

PBS:
Yes.

PERMITTED IN SPORT:
Yes.

OVERDOSE:
No serious adverse effects expected.

OTHER INFORMATION:
An effective and safe medication for rapidly easing the pain of peptic ulcers, and curing them. May be used safely long term.

FATTY ACIDS

TRADE and GENERIC NAMES:
Bioglan Evening Primrose Oil, Maxepa & EPO (Gammalinoleic acid and other fatty acids).
Bioglan Primrose Micelle, Blackmores Evening Primrose Oil, Naudicelle (Linoleic acid, gammalinoleic acid and other fatty acids).
Bioglan Maxepa, Blackmores Fish Oil, Fishaphos, Himega, Maxepa (Docosahexaenoic acid and other fatty acids).
Alfare, Calogen, Duocal, Liquigen, MCT Oil, Pepti-Junior, Portagen, Pregestimil, Ultracal (Triglycerides).
Efacal (Gammalinoleic acid, calcium and other fatty acids).
Evening Primrose Oil (Gammalinoleic acid).
Fatty acids are also found in numerous other nutritional, vitamin and mineral supplements.

USES:
Fatty acid (triglyceride) deficiency, premenstrual tension (gammalinoleic acid).

DOSAGE:
 Capsules: One or two capsules, two or three times a day with food.
Liquid: Dilute or mix and use as directed.
Powder: As directed by doctor.

FORMS:
Capsules, liquid, oil, powder to mix with water.

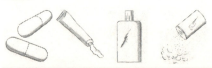

PRECAUTIONS:
Safe in pregnancy, breast feeding and children.
Not to be used long term.
Use with caution in hyperactive children and asthma.
Never inject liquid forms.

SIDE EFFECTS:
Common: Increased bleeding time, nausea.
Unusual: Vomiting.

INTERACTIONS:
Other drugs:
- Anticoagulants.

PRESCRIPTION:
No.

PBS:
Most forms: No.
Alfare, Duocal, MCT Oil, Pepti-Junior, Portagen, Pregestimil: Yes (some require an authority prescription).

PERMITTED IN SPORT:
Yes.

OVERDOSE:
Unlikely to have serious effects.

OTHER INFORMATION:
Does not cause addiction or dependence.

Felodipine

TRADE NAMES:
Agon SR, Felodur ER, Plendil ER

DRUG CLASS:
Calcium channel blocker (calcium antagonist).

USES:
High blood pressure.

DOSAGE:
 2.5 to 20mg once a day.

FORMS:
Tablets of 2.5, 5 and 10mg.

PRECAUTIONS:
Should only be used in pregnancy (C) and breast feeding if medically essential.
Not designed for use in children.
Do not take if:
 suffering from severe heart failure, low blood pressure, atrial flutter or fibrillation.

SIDE EFFECTS:
Common: Constipation, tiredness, headache, dizziness, indigestion, swelling of feet and ankles.
Unusual: Flushing, palpitations, slow heart rate, scalp irritation, depression, flushes, nightmares, excess wind.
Severe but rare (stop medication, consult doctor): Fainting.

INTERACTIONS:
Other drugs:
- Beta blockers (eg. propranolol), cyclosporin, digoxin, cimetidine, barbiturates, diazepam, amiodarone, quinidine, rifampicin, phenytoin, cisapride, theophylline, terbutaline, salbutamol, diltiazem.
- Additive effect with other medications for high blood pressure.

Herbs:
- Goldenseal, guarana, hawthorn, Korean ginseng, liquorice.

Other substances:
- Smoking may aggravate conditions that these medications are treating.
- Grapefruit juice.

PRESCRIPTION:
Yes.

PBS:
Yes.

PERMITTED IN SPORT:
Yes.

OVERDOSE:
May continue to be absorbed for up to 48 hours after overdose. Administer activated charcoal or induce vomiting. Purging should be encouraged to eliminate drug from gut. Overdose may cause low blood pressure, irregular heart rhythm, difficulty in breathing, heart attack and death. Obtain urgent medical attention.

OTHER INFORMATION:
Commonly used as a first line medication in high blood pressure.
See also Amlodipine, Diltiazem, Lercanidipine, Nifedipine, Nimodipine, Verapamil.

Fenoterol

TRADE NAME:
Berotec.

DRUG CLASS:
Bronchodilator (Beta-2 agonist).

USES:
Asthma.

DOSAGE:

Two inhalations every four to six hours.

FORMS:
Inhaler.

PRECAUTIONS:
Safe to use in pregnancy (A), breast feeding and children.
Not designed for long term constant use. Use with care in high blood pressure, heart disease, overactive thyroid gland, diabetes, liver and kidney disease.
Lower doses necessary in elderly.
Seek urgent medical assistance if no response to medication.

SIDE EFFECTS:
Common: Tremor, rapid heart rate, palpitations, headache.
Unusual: Nausea, flush, mouth irritation.

INTERACTIONS:
Other drugs:
- Sympathomimetics, beta blockers, theophyllines, steroids, diuretics, digoxin, MAOI, tricyclic antidepressants.

PRESCRIPTION:
Yes.

PBS:
No.

PERMITTED IN SPORT:
No.

OVERDOSE:
Exacerbation of side effects likely. May be dangerous in patients with heart disease or high blood pressure.

OTHER INFORMATION:
Designed for intermittent occasional use, and not to be taken regularly. Other medication should be used to prevent asthma if repeated doses of this medication are needed. Does not cause dependence or addiction. First introduced in the 1960s, beta-agonists have revolutionised life for asthmatics, but since deregulation in the mid 1980s, they have often been used excessively and inappropriately.
See also Salbutamol, Salmeterol, Terbutaline.

Fentanyl

TRADE NAMES:
Durogesic, Fentanyl Injection, Sublimaze.
Naropin with Fentanyl (with ropivacaine).

DRUG CLASS:
Narcotic analgesic.

USES:
Relief of severe pain.

DOSAGE:

Durogesic: One patch applied every three days.
Injection: Intramuscular or intravenous as determined by doctor.

FORMS:
Skin patch (25, 50, 75 and 100µg), injection.

PRECAUTIONS:
Not for use in pregnancy (C).
Use with caution in breast feeding and children.
Initial dose of patch should not exceed 25µg.
Use with caution in head injuries, fevers, severe lung, kidney, liver and heart disease.
Lower doses required in elderly.

Do not take if:

- suffering from intermittent or postoperative pain.
- history of drug abuse.

SIDE EFFECTS:
Common: Tolerance requiring higher doses, addiction to medication, tiredness, constipation, dry mouth, nausea, sweating.
Unusual: Vomiting, confusion, abdominal pain, hallucinations, reduced breath volume, low blood pressure, itchy rash, local skin reactions at site of patch application, excessive happiness (euphoria).
Severe but rare (stop medication, consult doctor): Retention of urine, irregular heartbeat, chest pain (angina).

INTERACTIONS:
Other drugs:
- Monoamine oxidase inhibitors (MAOI – used for severe depression), sedatives, ritonavir.

Other substances:
- Alcohol, marijuana.

PRESCRIPTION:
Yes.

PBS:
Most forms: Yes (restricted).
Naropin with Fentanyl: No.

PERMITTED IN SPORT:
No.

OVERDOSE:
Excessive use of patches may result in worsening of side effects to the point of life threatening lung and heart complications. The effects will persist for up to 24 hours after patches removed. Antidote available. Seek urgent medical attention.

OTHER INFORMATION:
Patches introduced in 2000 for the treatment of persistent cancer pain with less constipation and sedation than narcotic painkillers taken by mouth or injection. Injection usually used only during a general anaesthetic.

See also Alfentanil, Buprenorphine, Codeine Phosphate, Dextromoramide, Dextropropoxyphene, Heroin, Hydromorphone, Methadone, Morphine, Oxycodone, Pentazocine, Pethidine.

Fenugreek
(Trigonella)

USES:
Poor appetite, skin inflammation.

DOSAGE:
2g three times a day.

FORMS:
Capsules, powder for tea preparation.

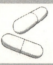

PRECAUTIONS:
Do not use in pregnancy or breast feeding.

SIDE EFFECTS:
Common: Minimal.
Unusual: Skin sensitisation.

INTERACTIONS:
Other drugs:
- Hypoglycaemics (used to treat diabetes).

PRESCRIPTION:
No.

PERMITTED IN SPORT:
Yes.

OTHER INFORMATION:
Not used in orthodox medicine.

Ferrous salts
(Ferric Pyrophosphate, Ferrous fumarate, Ferrous gluconate, Ferrous phosphate, Ferrous sulfate)
See IRON.

Feverfew
(Tanacetum parthenium)

USES:
Prevention of migraine.

DOSAGE:
 200mg to 250mg a day.

FORMS:
Capsules, tablets.

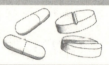

PRECAUTIONS:
Use with caution in pregnancy, breast feeding and children.
Avoid skin contact.
Rebound effects possible after cessation include headache, insomnia, muscle pains and stiffness, joint pain and tiredness.

SIDE EFFECTS:
Common: Minimal.
Unusual: Heartburn, belly pains, mouth irritation, anal irritation.
Severe but rare (stop medication, consult doctor): Severe diarrhoea.

INTERACTIONS:
Other drugs:
- Anticoagulants (eg. warfarin).

Herbs:
- Tansy, yarrow, aster, sunflower, laurel, liverwort.

PRESCRIPTION:
No.

PERMITTED IN SPORT:
Yes.

OTHER INFORMATION:
Not used in orthodox medicine.

Fexofenadine

See ANTIHISTAMINES, NON-SEDATING.

FIBRE

See Frangula, Ispaghula, Methylcellulose, Pectin, Psyllium, Sterculia.

FIBRINOLYTICS

TRADE and GENERIC NAMES:
Actilyse (Alteplase).
Streptase (Streptokinase).
Varidase (Streptokinase and streptodornase).

USES:
Lysis (destruction) of blood clots in veins and arteries, particularly in heart, lungs and brain.

DOSAGE:
 As administered by doctor.

FORMS:
Injection, solution.

PRECAUTIONS:
Only used in pregnancy (C) if medically essential. Breast feeding should be ceased if medication used.
Not designed for use in children, but may be necessary medically.
Do not take if:
 recent surgery performed.

SIDE EFFECTS:
Common: Minor unusual bleeding, fever.
Unusual: Significant unusual bleeding, allergy reaction.

INTERACTIONS:
Other drugs:
- Anticoagulants (eg. warfarin).

PRESCRIPTION:
Yes (injectable forms – restricted to treatment of acute heart attack in hospital).

PBS:
Injectable forms: Yes (very restricted).
Solution: No

PERMITTED IN SPORT:
Yes, but no vigorous activity should be undertaken for some time after use.

OVERDOSE:
Serious, but antidote available.

OTHER INFORMATION:
Injection used only in hospital for seriously ill patients. Topical forms used to clean up wound exudates.
See also Aprotinin.

Finasteride

TRADE NAMES:
Propecia, Proscar.

USES:
Benign enlargement of prostate gland (Proscar).
Increase hair growth in male pattern baldness (Propecia).

DOSAGE:
 One tablet a day for six to 12 months.

FORMS:
Tablets of 1mg (tan) and 5mg (blue).

PRECAUTIONS:
Must never be used in pregnancy (X) as severe damage may be caused to foetus. Must never be used in breast feeding or children.
Must never be used in women.
Pregnant women whose male partner is using finasteride must avoid sex during pregnancy as contact with semen may cause deformities in foetus.

SIDE EFFECTS:
Common: Impotence, decreased libido.
Unusual: Breast enlargement in men, rash.

INTERACTIONS:
None significant.

PRESCRIPTION:
Yes.

PBS:
No. Expensive.

PERMITTED IN SPORT:
Yes.

OVERDOSE:
No serious consequences expected.

OTHER INFORMATION:
Released in Australia in 1993. Extremely dangerous in pregnancy, otherwise safe and effective. May take some months for improvement in symptoms. Does not cause dependence or addiction.
See also Minoxidil.

Flecainide

TRADE NAMES:
Flecatab, Tambocor.

DRUG CLASS:
Antiarrhythmic.

USES:
Control and prevention of certain types of heartbeat irregularity.

DOSAGE:
 One to three tablets twice a day.

FORMS:
Tablets (white) of 50mg and 100mg, injection.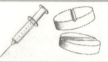

PRECAUTIONS:
Should be used only if essential and with caution in pregnancy (B3). Should only be used if medically essential in breast feeding and children.
Use with caution in heart failure, if pacemaker implanted, kidney or liver disease.
Do not take if:
 suffering from recent heart attack, or certain types of heart nerve conduction defects.

SIDE EFFECTS:
Common: Noises in ears, palpitations, fainting, chest pains, dizziness, rash, nausea, constipation, diarrhoea, belly pains, visual disturbances, shortness of breath.
Unusual: Angina, slow heart rate, high blood pressure, swelling of tissues, vomiting, fever, sweating, impotence, discomfort on urination, arthritis, leg cramps, muscle aches, dry mouth, twitches, double vision, anxiety, confusion, tiredness.
Severe but rare (stop medication, consult doctor): Jaundice, continued angina, severe shortness of breath, marked tissue swelling.

Medications

INTERACTIONS:
Other drugs:
- Digoxin, disopyramide, verapamil, amiodarone.

PRESCRIPTION:
Yes.

PBS:
Yes (restricted to treatment of serious cardiac arrhythmias where treatment is started in hospital).

PERMITTED IN SPORT:
Yes.

OVERDOSE:
Low blood pressure and rapid heart rate likely. Administer activated charcoal or induce vomiting if tablets taken recently. Seek medical assistance.

See also Amiodarone, Disopyramide, Mexiletine, Procainamide, Quinidine, Sotalol, Verapamil.

Flucloxacillin

TRADE NAMES:
Flopen, Floxapen, Floxsig, Flucil, Staphylex.

DRUG CLASS:
Penicillin antibiotic.

USES:
Treatment of infections caused by susceptible bacteria.

DOSAGE:

One or two capsules every six hours 30 minutes before food. Course (usually 7 days) should be completed.

FORMS:
Capsules, mixture (store in door of refrigerator), injection.

PRECAUTIONS:
May be used in pregnancy (B1), children and breast feeding if medically indicated. Use with caution in kidney failure, liver disease, premature infants and leukaemia. Not for use in eyes.

Do not take if:

 allergic to penicillin

- suffering from glandular fever or severe liver disease.

SIDE EFFECTS:
Common: Diarrhoea, nausea, vomiting.
Unusual: Genital itch or rash.
Severe but rare (stop medication, consult doctor): Itchy rash, hives, severe diarrhoea, yellow skin (jaundice), unusual bleeding or bruising.

INTERACTIONS:
Other drugs:
- Probenecid, oral contraceptives.

PRESCRIPTION:
Yes.

PBS:
Yes.

PERMITTED IN SPORT:
Yes.

OVERDOSE:
Vomiting and diarrhoea only likely effects.

OTHER INFORMATION:
Used for more severe infections. Some bacteria can break down simpler forms of penicillin. Cloxacillin, dicloxacillin and flucloxacillin are not able to be broken down this way and so can be effective when other penicillins fail. Does not cause dependence or addiction.

Fluconazole

TRADE NAME:
Diflucan.

DRUG CLASS:
Imidazole antifungal.

USES:
Fungal infections of vagina (thrush), skin, mouth, oesophagus, brain and other areas.

DOSAGE:

Vaginal thrush: 150mg tablet taken once.
More severe infections: Up to 400mg a day for up to a month.

FORMS:
Capsules of 50mg (light blue/white), 100mg (blue/white), 150mg (light blue) and 200mg (purple/white); suspension; infusion.

PRECAUTIONS:
Not to be used in pregnancy (D) or children unless medically essential. Cease breast feeding before use.
Use with caution in kidney disease and dehydration.
Ensure adequate fluid intake.

SIDE EFFECTS:
Common: Nausea, acne.
Unusual: Headache, rash, vomiting, diarrhoea, belly discomfort.
Severe but rare (stop medication, consult doctor): Liver damage, allergy.

INTERACTIONS:
Other drugs:
- Never use with cisapride.
- Warfarin, astemizole, phenytoin, cyclosporin, diazepam, hypoglycaemics, rifampicin, theophylline, zidovudine, oral contraceptives.

PRESCRIPTION:
Yes.

PBS:
Yes (authority required – restricted to patients with severe and life threatening fungal infections). Expensive.

PERMITTED IN SPORT:
Yes.

OVERDOSE:
Hallucinations and mental disturbance may occur. Administer activated charcoal or induce vomiting if medication taken recently. Seek medical attention.

OTHER INFORMATION:
Introduced in early 1990s. A single dose by mouth will cure most forms of thrush (Candidiasis) in the vagina, mouth or elsewhere in the body. Very useful in the treatment of fungal complications in AIDS. Very expensive.
See Clotrimazole, Econazole, Griseofulvin, Itraconazole, Ketoconazole, Miconazole.

Flucytosine

TRADE NAME:
Ancotil.

DRUG CLASS:
Antifungal.

USES:
Generalised fungal infections.

DOSAGE:

Infusion as determined by doctor.

FORMS:
Infusion.

PRECAUTIONS:
Not to be used in pregnancy (B3) unless clinically essential. Breast feeding should be ceased before use. May be used with caution in children.
Use with caution in bone marrow disease and kidney disease.

SIDE EFFECTS:
Common: Nausea.
Unusual: Vomiting, rash, diarrhoea.
Severe but rare: Liver and blood cell damage, irregular heartbeat.

INTERACTIONS:
Other drugs:
- Amphotericin B, cytarabine, corticosteroids.

PRESCRIPTION:
Yes.

PBS:
No.

PERMITTED IN SPORT:
Yes.

OVERDOSE:
May cause kidney, liver and blood cell damage.

OTHER INFORMATION:
Extremely expensive, and so reserved for the most severe fungal infections.

Fludrocortisone

TRADE NAME:
Florinef.

DRUG CLASS:
Corticosteroid.

USES:
Addison's disease, adrenogenital syndrome.

DOSAGE:
 One or two tablets a day as directed by doctor.

FORMS:
Tablets of 0.1mg (pink).

PRECAUTIONS:
Should be used in pregnancy (C), breast feeding and children only on specific medical advice.
Use with caution if under stress, and in patients with under-active thyroid gland, liver disease, diverticulitis, high blood pressure, heart failure, psychoses, myasthenia gravis, or kidney disease. Medication should not be ceased abruptly, but dosage should be slowly reduced.

Do not use if:
 suffering from any form of infection.
- having a vaccination

SIDE EFFECTS:
Common: May cause bloating, weight gain, rashes and intestinal disturbances.
Unusual: Biochemical disturbances of blood, muscle weakness, bone weakness, impaired wound healing, skin thinning, tendon weakness, peptic ulcers, gullet ulcers, bruising, increased sweating, loss of fat under skin, premature ageing, excess facial hair growth in women, pigmentation of skin and nails, acne, convulsions, headaches, dizziness, growth

suppression in children, aggravation of diabetes, worsening of infections, cataracts, aggravation of glaucoma, blood clots in veins and sleeplessness.
Most significant side effects occur only with prolonged use of tablets.
Severe but rare (stop medication, consult doctor): Any significant side effect should be reported to a doctor immediately.

INTERACTIONS:
Other drugs:
- Oral contraceptives, barbiturates, phenytoin, rifampicin, warfarin, isoniazid, amphotericin, diabetic medications, cyclosporin, digoxin, oestrogen, ketoconazole, NSAID.

PRESCRIPTION:
Yes.

PBS:
Yes.

PERMITTED IN SPORT:
Varies. Check with sports governing body.

OVERDOSE:
Medical treatment is required. Serious effects and death rare.

OTHER INFORMATION:
Extremely effective and useful medication if used correctly. Must be used with extreme care under strict medical supervision. Lowest dose possible should be used. Not addictive.

FLUID TABLETS
See DIURETICS.

Flumethasone

TRADE NAME:
Available in Australia only in combination with clioquinol.
Locacorten Vioform (with clioquinol).

DRUG CLASS:
Corticosteroid.

USES:
Eczema and inflammation of ear canal.

DOSAGE:

Two or three drops twice a day for no more than ten days.

FORMS:
Ear drops.

PRECAUTIONS:
Ear preparations safe in pregnancy, breast feeding and children over three years.
Avoid eye contact.
Use for shortest period of time possible.

SIDE EFFECTS:
Common: Minimal.
Unusual: Prolonged use – thinning of skin, itching, scarring of skin.

INTERACTIONS:
None significant.

PRESCRIPTION:
Yes.

PBS:
No.

PERMITTED IN SPORT:
Yes.

Flunitrazepam

TRADE NAMES:
Hypnodorm, Rohypnol (discontinued 2002).

DRUG CLASS:
Sedative/hypnotic, Benzodiazepine.

USES:
Severe insomnia (sleeplessness).

DOSAGE:

One or two at bedtime. Quarter to one tablet in elderly.

FORMS:
Tablet of 2mg

PRECAUTIONS:
Should be used with caution in pregnancy (C), but not at all if delivery of infant imminent as it may decrease desire to breathe in newborn infant. Should be used with caution in breast feeding. Not for use in children.
Lower dose required in elderly.
Should be used intermittently and not constantly as dependency may develop. Stopping suddenly after prolonged constant use may cause withdrawal symptoms.
Use with caution in glaucoma, myasthenia gravis, heart disease, low blood pressure, kidney or liver disease, psychiatric conditions, schizophrenia, depression and epilepsy.

Do not take if:
- suffering from severe lung disease, confusion.
- tendency to addiction or dependence.
- operating machinery, driving a vehicle or undertaking tasks that require concentration, coordination or alertness within next 12 hours.

SIDE EFFECTS:
Common: Confusion and falls in elderly, impaired alertness, dependency.
Unusual: Dizziness, incoordination, poor memory, headache, hangover in morning, slurred speech, nightmares.

INTERACTIONS:
Other drugs:
- Other medications that reduce alertness (eg. barbiturates, antihistamines, antianxiety drugs).
- Disulfiram, cimetidine, anticonvulsants, anticholinergics.

Herbs:
- Guarana, kava kava, passionflower, St John's wort, valerian, celery, camomile, goldenseal.

Other substances:
- Reacts with alcohol to cause excessive drowsiness.

PRESCRIPTION:
Yes.

PBS:
Yes (authority required, very restricted).

PERMITTED IN SPORT:
Yes.

OVERDOSE:
Seldom life threatening. May cause drowsiness, confusion and coma. Induce vomiting if tablets taken recently. Seek medical assistance.

OTHER INFORMATION:
One of the most powerful sleeping tablets available. Risk of dependency is high. Should be used only intermittently and for short periods except in exceptional cases.

See also BARBITURATES, Chlormethiazole, Midazolam, Nitrazepam, Temazepam, Triazolam, Zolpidem, Zopiclone.

Fluocortolone

TRADE NAME:
Ultraproct (with cinchocaine, clemizole).

DRUG CLASS:
Corticosteroid.

USES:
Severe inflammation of anus, piles, anal fissure.

DOSAGE:

Ointment: Apply two times a day.
Suppositories: Insert one into anus once a day after a bowel motion.

FORMS:
Ointment, suppositories.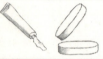

PRECAUTIONS:
Should be used with caution in early pregnancy (A).
May aggravate fungal infections of skin.
Use for shortest period of time possible.
Do not use if:
 suffering from any form of skin infection, anal ulcer or broken skin.

SIDE EFFECTS:
Common: Minimal.
Unusual: Thinning of skin, itching, burning, stinging, scarring of skin.

INTERACTIONS:
None significant

PRESCRIPTION:
Yes.

PBS:
No.

PERMITTED IN SPORT:
No.

OTHER INFORMATION:
Shortest possible course should be used. Not addictive. One of the older types of steroid cream.

Fluoride
(Sodium fluoride)

TRADE NAME:
NeutraFluor.
Fluoride is found naturally in water, and in numerous nutritional supplements and medications, all of which are available without prescription. It is also added artificially to some water supplies.

DRUG CLASS:
Mineral.

USES:
Prevention of tooth decay, in addition to calcium and vitamin D in the treatment of osteoporosis, multiple myeloma, Paget's disease.

DOSAGE:
 One to three times a day as directed by packaging or doctor.

FORMS:
Tablets, mixture, drops, capsules, toothpaste.

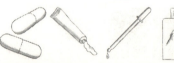

PRECAUTIONS:
Not to be used in pregnancy and breast feeding. May be used with caution in children.
Fluoride supplements should only be used where local water supply is low in fluoride.
Do not exceed recommended dose.
Do not take if:
 suffering from severe kidney disease.

SIDE EFFECTS:
Common: Nil at correct dose.
Uncommon: Excess dosage for a long period may cause white flecks or brown stains on teeth.

INTERACTIONS:
None significant.

PRESCRIPTION:
No.

PBS:
No.

PERMITTED IN SPORT:
Yes.

OVERDOSE:
Deliberate or accidental overdosage with a large number of tablets may cause significant poisoning. Administer activated charcoal or induce vomiting if taken recently. Symptoms of acute poisoning include vomiting, diarrhoea, convulsions, rapid weak pulse, difficulty in breathing, coma and possibly death. Seek urgent medical assistance.

OTHER INFORMATION:
Since the introduction of fluoride to water supplies, as a supplement, and in tooth paste, the incidence of tooth decay in children has dropped dramatically. In areas with fluoride in the water supply additional supplements are not required.

Fluorometholone

TRADE NAMES:
Flarex, Flucon, FML.

DRUG CLASS:
Corticosteroid.

USES:
Inflammation of eye, iritis.

DOSAGE:

Insert one or two drops two to four times a day.

FORMS:
Eye drops.

PRECAUTIONS:
May be used with caution in pregnancy, breast feeding and children.
Use with caution in bacterial eye infections.
Not designed for prolonged use.
Do not take if:
- suffering from any form of viral or fungal eye infection.
- suffering from tuberculosis of eye.

SIDE EFFECTS:
Common: Temporary blurred vision.
Severe but rare (stop medication, consult doctor): Glaucoma (halos around objects), eye pain, permanent blurred vision, weeping eye, pus in eye.

INTERACTIONS:
None significant.

PRESCRIPTION:
Yes.

PBS:
Yes.

PERMITTED IN SPORT:
Yes.

OTHER INFORMATION:

Must only be used strictly as directed by doctor. Infection must be excluded before use, or eye damage may result. Prolonged use may result in eye damage. Very useful in controlling severe eye inflammation.

Fluorouracil

TRADE NAMES:

Efudix, Fluorouracil.

USES:

Cream: Skin cancer and sun damaged skin, Bowen's disease.
Injection: Cancer of breast, colon, rectum, stomach and pancreas.

DOSAGE:

Cream: Apply to affected skin once or twice a day with a metal applicator or using a rubber glove for four to six weeks.

FORMS:

Cream, injection.

PRECAUTIONS:

Should not be used in pregnancy (D) unless mother's life is at risk as the safety of this medication (including lotion and cream) in pregnancy has not been established. Breast feeding should be ceased before use of injection. Should be used in children only if medically essential.
Cream must not be allowed to come into contact with eyes, mouth, lips, nose, anus or vagina.
Do not use cream on normal skin.
Avoid using cosmetics or other skin preparations on areas of skin being treated.
Avoid sun exposure to areas of skin being treated.
Regular blood tests to check blood cells and liver function essential for patients receiving injections.
Ensure adequate contraception while using fluorouracil.

Do not use injection if:

 suffering from poor nutrition, serious infection, bone marrow damage.

SIDE EFFECTS:

Common: Skin preparations – redness, itch, burning, pigmentation.
Injection – sore mouth, pain on swallowing, diarrhoea, loss of appetite, vomiting, hair loss, itch, rash.
Unusual: Skin preparations – scarring, dermatitis, soreness.
Injection – Dry skin, pigmentation, sun sensitivity, disorientation, nail changes.

INTERACTIONS:

Other drugs:
- Injection – Methotrexate, amphotericin, polymyxin.

PRESCRIPTION:

Yes.

PBS:

Cream: No. Available for some Veteran Affairs pensioners.
Injection: Yes.

PERMITTED IN SPORT:

Yes.

OVERDOSE:

Cream – inflammation and soreness of skin.
Injection – very serious. Seek urgent medical assistance.

OTHER INFORMATION:

Very effective and useful in many forms of skin cancer but must be used carefully. Despite serious side effects from injection, may save or prolong life in patients with some types of cancer.

Fluoxetine

TRADE NAMES:
Auscap, Fluohexal, GenRx Fluoxetine, Healthsense Fluoxetine, Lovan, Prozac, Zactin.

DRUG CLASS:
SSRI antidepressant.

USES:
Depression.

DOSAGE:

20 to 40mg, once or twice a day. Maximum 80mg a day.

FORMS:
Capsules and tablets of 20mg.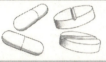

PRECAUTIONS:
Should be used in pregnancy (C), breast feeding and children with considerable caution.
Should be used with caution in epilepsy, diabetes, liver and kidney disease.
Use with caution after shock treatment. Lower doses necessary in elderly.

Do not take if:

MAOI antidepressants taken recently.

SIDE EFFECTS:
Common: Generally minimal. Nausea, drowsiness, sweating, tremor, tiredness, dry mouth, sleeplessness, impotence, weight loss.
Unusual: Headache, fever, palpitations, sweating, rash, blurred vision.
Severe but rare (stop medication, consult doctor): Convulsions.

INTERACTIONS:
Other drugs:
- MAOI, lithium, diazepam, flecainide, warfarin, anticoagulants (eg. warfarin), phenytoin, tryptophan, tramadol, sumatriptan.

Herbs:
- St John's wort, ma huang.

Other substances:
- Use of alcohol is not advised.

PRESCRIPTION:
Yes.

PBS:
Yes.

PERMITTED IN SPORT:
Yes.

OVERDOSE:
Symptoms may include nausea, tremor, dilated pupils, dry mouth and irritability. Death or serious effects unlikely. Administer activated charcoal or induce vomiting if tablets taken recently. Seek medical attention.

OTHER INFORMATION:
One of a group of antidepressants released in the early 1990s that has dramatically improved the treatment of depression because of their safety and lack of side effects. May take up to two weeks for patient to notice any improvement in depression.

See also Citalopram, Fluvoxamine, Paroxetine, Sertraline, Venlafaxine.

Flupenthixol

TRADE NAME:
Fluanxol.

DRUG CLASS:
Antipsychotic.

USES:
Schizophrenia.

DOSAGE:

One injection every two to four weeks.

FORMS:
Injection.

PRECAUTIONS:
Use in pregnancy (C) only if medically essential. Use with caution in breast feeding.
Not to be used in children.
Use lower doses in elderly.
Use with caution if taking anti-vomiting drugs.
Use with caution in glaucoma, extreme heat, epilepsy, agitation states, Parkinson's disease, hardening of arteries, heart disorders, stroke, liver and kidney disease.

Do not use if:
 suffering from depression, brain damage, blood abnormalities, phaeochromocytoma.
- sensitive to phenothiazines.
- having surgery.

SIDE EFFECTS:
Common: Confusion, twitches, tremors, muscle spasms, dry mouth.

INTERACTIONS:
Other drugs:
- Tricyclic antidepressants, phenobarbitone, carbamazepine, hypnotics, lithium, medications that lower blood pressure, levodopa, MAOI, metoclopramide.

Herbs:
- Evening primrose (linoleic acid).

Other substances:
- Organophosphate insecticides.
- Alcohol.

PRESCRIPTION:
Yes.

PBS:
Yes.

PERMITTED IN SPORT:
Yes.

OVERDOSE:
Causes sedation preceded by agitation, confusion and convulsions. May proceed to collapse, failure of breathing and death. Seek urgent medical attention. Support in hospital necessary.

OTHER INFORMATION:
Used long term to prevent symptoms of schizophrenia.

See also Amisulpride, Droperidol, Haloperidol, Lithium Carbonate, Olanzapine, PHENOTHIAZINES, Pimozide, Quetiapine, Risperidone, Thiothixene, Zuclopenthixol.

Fluphenazine
See PHENOTHIAZINES.

Flurbiprofen

TRADE NAMES:
Ocufen, Strepfen.

DRUG CLASS:
NSAID (Nonsteroidal anti-inflammatory drug).

USES:
Eye drops: Prevention of miosis (eye contraction) during eye surgery.
Lozenges: Relief of throat pain.

DOSAGE:
 Eye drops: As directed by eye doctor.
Lozenges: Dissolve one in mouth every three to six hours.

FORMS:
Eye drops, lozenges.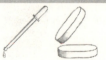

Medications

PRECAUTIONS:
Use with caution in pregnancy (C), breast feeding and children.
Care with eye drops in presence of eye infection.
Use lozenges with care in kidney, liver and heart disease.

Do not take if:
 (eye drops) suffering from viral eye infection (eg. Herpes).
- (lozenges) suffering from peptic ulcer, asthma, hay fever.
- sensitive to aspirin.

SIDE EFFECTS:
Common: Eye drops – Eye burning and stinging, delayed healing of eye wounds, increased bleeding tendency in eye.
Lozenges – Abnormal taste, nausea, diarrhoea.
Unusual: Lozenges – Stomach ulcer.

INTERACTIONS:
Eye drops: None significant.
Lozenges: Frusemide, other NSAIDs, warfarin, methotrexate, blood pressure medications.

PRESCRIPTION:
Lozenges: No.
Eye drops: Yes.

PBS:
Eye drops: Yes.
Lozenges: No.

PERMITTED IN SPORT:
Yes.

See also Aspirin, Bufexamac, Celecoxib, Diclofenac, Diflunisal, Ibuprofen, Indomethacin, Ketoprofen, Ketorolac trometanol, Mefenamic Acid, Naproxen, Piroxicam, Rofecoxib, Salicylic acid, Sulindac, Tenoxicam, Tiaprofenic Acid.

Flutamide

TRADE NAMES:
Eulexin, Flutamin, Fugerel.

DRUG CLASS:
Antiandrogen (acts against testosterone).

USES:
Cancer of prostate gland in combination with other medication.

DOSAGE:
 One tablet three times a day.

FORMS:
Tablets (cream) of 250mg.

PRECAUTIONS:
Not to be used by women or children.
Regular blood tests to check liver function essential.

Do not take if:
suffering from severe liver disease.

SIDE EFFECTS:
Common: Hot flushes, decreased libido, impotence, diarrhoea, nausea, vomiting, breast enlargement and tenderness.
Severe but rare (stop medication, consult doctor): Yellow skin (jaundice).

INTERACTIONS:
Other drugs:
- Warfarin, Paracetamol, Narcotics.

PRESCRIPTION:
Yes.

PBS:
Yes (authority required – restricted to severe prostate cancer).

OVERDOSE:
Exacerbation of side effects only likely result.

Medications

OTHER INFORMATION:
Usually not used alone, but in combination with other medication for prostate gland cancer.
See also Cyproterone, Nilutamide.

Fluticasone propionate

TRADE NAMES:
Beconase Allergy, Flixotide.
Seretide (with salmeterol).

DRUG CLASS:
Corticosteroid.

USES:
Prevention of asthma and hay fever.

DOSAGE:

Inhalation: One to four inhalations twice a day.
Nose spray: Two sprays in each nostril twice a day.

FORMS:
Inhaler, nasal spray, nebules.
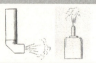

PRECAUTIONS:
Use with caution in pregnancy (B3), breast feeding and children over 4 years. Not to be used in children under 4 years. Use with caution in lung or throat infection and tuberculosis.
Lung function should be checked regularly to ensure adequate dose is received.

Do not take nose spray if:
suffering from nose infection.

SIDE EFFECTS:
Common: Fungal (thrush) infections of mouth, sore throat and mouth, dry mouth.
Unusual: Hoarseness, unusual bleeding and bruising, slowed growth.
Severe but rare (stop medication, consult doctor): Glaucoma (blurred vision).

INTERACTIONS:
Other drugs:
- Ritonavir, ketoconazole.

Herbs:
- Liquorice.

PRESCRIPTION:
Inhalations: Yes.
Nose spray: No

PBS:
Inhalations: Yes.
Nose spray: No

PERMITTED IN SPORT:
Yes.

OVERDOSE:
Unlikely to have any serious effects.

OTHER INFORMATION:
Introduced in 1994 as an advanced form of asthma treatment. Does not cause dependence or addiction.
See also Beclomethasone, Budesonide.

Fluvastatin

TRADE NAMES:
Lescol, Vastin.

DRUG CLASS:
Hypolipidaemic.

USES:
Treatment of high blood cholesterol level.

DOSAGE:

20 to 40mg once or twice a day.

FORMS:
Capsules of 20mg and 40mg.

PRECAUTIONS:
Not for use in pregnancy (C) unless medically essential. Use with caution in children.
Use with caution in muscle, liver and kidney disease.
Use with caution in alcoholics.
Regular blood tests to check cholesterol level and liver function necessary.

Do not take if:

- suffering from liver infection, myopathy.
- breast feeding.

SIDE EFFECTS:
Common: Nausea, diarrhoea.
Unusual: Liver damage, joint and muscle pain, muscle damage.

INTERACTIONS:
Other drugs:
- Cimetidine, cyclosporin, erythromycin, gemfibrizol, glibenclamide, nicotinic acid, omeprazole, ranitidine, rifampicin, tolbutamide, warfarin, cholestyramine.

Other substances:
- Excess alcohol.

Herbs:
- Alfalfa, fenugreek, garlic, ginger.

PRESCRIPTION:
Yes.

PBS:
Yes.

PERMITTED IN SPORT:
Yes.

OVERDOSE:
Induce vomiting or administer activated charcoal if taken recently. Seek medical attention.

OTHER INFORMATION:
Introduced in 1996 as an effective means of lowering cholesterol when combined with a low cholesterol diet.

See also Atorvastatin, Cholestyramine, Colestipol, Gemfibrizol, Nicotinic acid, Pravastatin, Probucol, Simvastatin.

Fluvoxamine

TRADE NAMES:
Faverin, Luvox, Movox.

DRUG CLASS:
SSRI antidepressant.

USES:
Depression, obsessive compulsive disorder.

DOSAGE:

Half to three tablets a day. Increase dose very slowly.

FORMS:
Tablets of 100mg.

PRECAUTIONS:
Use with caution in pregnancy (B2) and children.
Use with caution in epilepsy, bleeding disorders, liver and kidney disease.
Use lower doses in elderly.
Reduce dose slowly before stopping.

Do not take if:

- breast feeding.
- taking MAOI.

SIDE EFFECTS:
Common: Generally minimal.
Nausea, drowsiness, sweating, tremor, tiredness, dry mouth, sleeplessness, impotence.
Unusual: Headache, fever, palpitations, sweating, rash, blurred vision.

INTERACTIONS:
Other drugs:
- MAOI, other SSRI, tryptophan, tricyclic antidepressants, lithium, sumatriptan, anticoagulants (eg. warfarin), theophylline, clozapine, propranolol, cisapride, benzodiazepines (eg. diazepam).

Medications

Herbs:
- St John's wort, ma huang.

Other substances:
- Alcohol.

PRESCRIPTION:
Yes.

PBS:
Yes.

PERMITTED IN SPORT:
Yes.

OVERDOSE:
Symptoms may include nausea, tremor, dilated pupils, dry mouth and irritability. Death or serious effects unlikely. Administer activated charcoal or induce vomiting if tablets taken recently. Seek medical attention.

OTHER INFORMATION:
Introduced in 1997 as an effective treatment for depression.

See also Citalopram, Fluoxetine, Paroxetine, Sertraline, Venlafaxine.

Folic acid

TRADE NAMES:
Blackmores For Women Folic Acid, Megafol, Nature's Own Folic Acid. Fefol, FGF (with iron).
Folic acid is found in numerous other vitamin and mineral preparations.

DRUG CLASS:
Vitamin.

USES:
Some types of anaemia, prevention of anaemia in pregnancy, aids iron absorption.

DOSAGE:

Tablets and capsules: One or two a day.
Injection: One injection a day.

FORMS:
Capsules, tablets, injection.

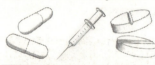

PRECAUTIONS:
Safe to use in pregnancy (A), breast feeding and children.
Use with caution in some types of tumours.

Do not take if:
 suffering from vitamin B12 deficiency.

SIDE EFFECTS:
Common: Minimal.
Unusual: Nausea, passing excess wind, diarrhoea, irritability, sleep disturbances.
Severe but rare (stop medication, consult doctor): Rash, asthma.

INTERACTIONS:
Other drugs:
- Anticonvulsants (drugs treating epilepsy), methotrexate, trimethoprim, pyrimethamine, sulfasalazine, gold.

Other substances:
- Reacts with alcohol.

PRESCRIPTION:
No.

PBS:
FGF, Megafol: Yes.
Other forms: No.

PERMITTED IN SPORT:
Yes.

OVERDOSE:
No serious effects likely.

OTHER INFORMATION:
Folic acid is essential for the formation of certain proteins in the body that are used in the manufacture of haemoglobin.
A lack of folic acid causes anaemia.
It is found naturally in liver, dark green leafy vegetables, peanuts, beans, whole grain wheat and yeast. It may be considered to be a vitamin.
See also IRON, VITAMINS.

Follicle stimulating hormone
(FSH, Follitropin)

TRADE NAMES:
Gonal-F, Puregon.

DRUG CLASS:
Sex hormone.

USES:
Female and male infertility.

DOSAGE:
 As determined by doctor for each patient.

FORMS:
Injection.

PRECAUTIONS:
Not to be used in pregnancy (B2), breast feeding and children.
Unlikely to be serious effects if used by mistake in pregnancy.
Do not take if:
suffering from ovarian cysts or enlargement, tumours of the ovaries or other sexual organs, testicular tumours, or undiagnosed vaginal bleeding.
- over 50 years of age.

SIDE EFFECTS:
Common: Nausea, diarrhoea, headache.
Unusual: Multiple pregnancies, breast tenderness and/or enlargement, acne, weight gain.
Severe but rare: Lung and heart effects, vein blood clots.

INTERACTIONS:
Other drugs:
- Clomiphene.

PRESCRIPTION:
Yes (restricted to infertility experts).

PBS:
Yes (very restricted).

PERMITTED IN SPORT:
Yes.

OTHER INFORMATION:
Widely used and effective medication to assist patients with specific types of infertility.
See also Clomiphene.

Follitropin

See Follicle Stimulating Hormone.

Fosfestrol

TRADE NAME:
Honvan.

USES:
Cancer of prostate gland.

DOSAGE:

Must be determined individually for each patient by doctor depending on response to medication.

FORMS:
Tablets (white) of 120mg.

PRECAUTIONS:
Not to be used by women or children. Use with caution in epilepsy, migraine, asthma, depression, diabetes, bone disease, heart or kidney disease.

Do not take if:
 suffering from liver disease, blood clots.

SIDE EFFECTS:
Common: Nausea, vomiting, belly cramps, bloating, loss of appetite, fluid retention, breast tenderness and enlargement, headache.
Unusual: Rash, loss of libido, depression, hair loss.
Severe but rare (stop medication, consult doctor): Yellow skin (jaundice), blood clot.

INTERACTIONS:
None significant.

PRESCRIPTION:
Yes.

PBS:
Yes.

PERMITTED IN SPORT:
Yes.

OVERDOSE:
Causes vomiting, diarrhoea, belly cramps, headache and dizziness.

OTHER INFORMATION:
Often used in combination with castration and radiotherapy.

Fosinopril
See ACE INHIBITORS.

Framycetin

TRADE NAMES:
Soframycin Ear, Soframycin Eye, Sofra-Tulle.
Otodex, Sofradex (with dexamethasone and gramicidin).
Soframycin Topical Ointment (with gramicidin).

DRUG CLASS:
Antibiotic.

USES:
Skin, ear and eye infections.

DOSAGE:

Eye drops: Insert six times a day.
Ear drops: Insert three times a day.
Eye and ear ointment: Insert or apply two or three times a day.
Tulle and topical ointment: Apply to clean wound daily.

FORMS:
Eye drops, eye ointment, ear drops, ear ointment, skin ointment, tulle (netting).

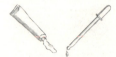

PRECAUTIONS:
Must be used with caution in pregnancy (D), but damage to foetus unlikely if used only on body surface. May be used in breast feeding and children.
Do not use ear applications if:
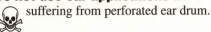 suffering from perforated ear drum.

SIDE EFFECTS:
Minimal.

INTERACTIONS:
None significant.

PRESCRIPTION:
Yes.

PBS:
Most forms: Yes.
Skin ointment, tulle: No.

PERMITTED IN SPORT:
Yes.

OTHER INFORMATION:
Very widely used for treatment of swimmer's ear and conjunctivitis.
Tulle useful for infected grazes and ulcers.

Frangula

TRADE NAMES:
Granocol, Normacol Plus (with sterculia).
Also found in other fibre supplements.

DRUG CLASS:
Fibre, laxative.

USES:
Constipation, firm bowel motions.

DOSAGE:
 Take required amount with water two or three times a day.

FORMS:
Granules, powder.

PRECAUTIONS:
Safe in pregnancy.
Not for use in breast feeding and children under 12 years.
Avoid at bedtime.
Not for prolonged use.
Do not take if:
 on a salt, potassium or sugar restricted diet
- suffering from severe constipation with impacted faeces.
- suffering from belly pain, nausea or vomiting.
- suffering from ulcerative colitis or acute diverticulitis.

SIDE EFFECTS:
Common: Minimal.
Unusual: Diarrhoea, belly discomfort.

INTERACTIONS:
Other drugs:
- Thiazide diuretics, steroids.

Other substances:
- Liquorice, high sugar content sweets.

PRESCRIPTION:
No.

PBS:
Yes (restricted).

PERMITTED IN SPORT:
Yes.

OVERDOSE:
Take additional water. Belly discomfort and passing excess wind only effects.

See also Bisacodyl, Docusate sodium, FIBRE, Glycerol, Lactulose, Paraffin, Poloxamer, Psyllium, Senna, Sodium phosphate, Sodium picosulfate, Sorbitol, Sterculia.

Fructose

TRADE NAME:
Emetrol (with glucose).

DRUG CLASS:
Sugar.

USES:
Nausea.

DOSAGE:
 20mLs to 40mLs every 15 minutes until nausea eases to a maximum of five doses.
Do not dilute, or take with other fluids.

FORMS:
Solution.

PRECAUTIONS:
Safe in pregnancy, breast feeding and children.
Do not take if:
 suffering from diabetes.

SIDE EFFECTS:
Nil.

INTERACTIONS:
Nil.

PRESCRIPTION:
No.

PBS:
No.

PERMITTED IN SPORT:
Yes.

OVERDOSE:
No serious consequences.
Vomiting likely.

OTHER INFORMATION:
Fructose is the form of sugar found in fruit. Works within a couple of minutes after taking by mouth.

Frusemide
(Furosemide)

TRADE NAMES:
Frusehexal, Frusid, GenRx Frusemide, Lasix, Uremide, Urex.

DRUG CLASS:
Loop diuretic (increases production of urine).

USES:
Excess fluid in body, high blood pressure, heart failure causing build up of fluid in lungs.

DOSAGE:
 One or more tablets in morning to a maximum of 1500mg a day.

FORMS:
Tablets of 20mg, 40mg and 500mg; solution, injection.

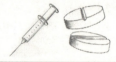

PRECAUTIONS:
Should only be used in pregnancy (C) if medically essential. Will reduce production of breast milk, and may be used to assist in drying of breast milk in women who have stopped breast feeding.
Safe in children and infants.
Should be used with caution in diabetes, diarrhoea and gout.
Regular blood tests to assess levels of chemicals (electrolytes) in blood are recommended.
Use with caution if sensitive to sulpha drugs.
Blood tests to check electrolyte levels advisable.
Do not take if:
 suffering from severe kidney failure, liver failure, jaundice, low blood pressure, difficulty in passing urine, low potassium or salt levels.

Medications

SIDE EFFECTS:
Common: Passing increased amounts of urine.
Unusual: Weakness, dizziness, thirst, muscle cramps, flushing.
Severe but rare (stop medication, consult doctor): Dehydration, blood clots, deafness, jaundice (yellow skin).

INTERACTIONS:
Other drugs:
- Digoxin, aspirin, steroids, salicylates, lithium, antibiotics, ethacrynic acid, NSAID, sucralfate.
- Medications that lower blood pressure (eg. ACE inhibitors).

Herbs:
- Celery, dandelion, uva ursi.

PRESCRIPTION:
Yes.

PBS:
Yes.

PERMITTED IN SPORT:
No (acts as masking agent for other illegal drugs).

OVERDOSE:
Severe dehydration may result. Induce vomiting if tablets taken recently. Give extra fluids. Seek medical assistance.

OTHER INFORMATION:
Widely used, safe, and extremely effective medication that has been available since the 1960s. Potassium supplements may be needed.

See also Amiloride, Bumetanide, Ethacrynic Acid, Spironolactone, **THIAZIDE DIURETICS**.

FSH
See Follicle stimulating hormone.

Furosemide
See Frusemide.

Fusidic Acid
See Sodium fusidate.

Medications

Gabapentin

TRADE NAMES:
Gantin, GenRx Gabapentin, Neurontin, Pendine.

DRUG CLASS:
Anticonvulsant.

USES:
Epilepsy, particularly epilepsy that affects only part of the body; nerve pain.

DOSAGE:
 Slowly increasing dosage until desired result obtained. Taken in two or more doses a day. Maximum 2400mg a day.

FORMS:
Capsules of 100mg, 300mg and 400mg.

PRECAUTIONS:
Use with caution in pregnancy (B1), breast feeding and children under 12 years.
Use with caution in kidney disease.
Do not stop suddenly, but reduce dosage slowly.

SIDE EFFECTS:
Common: Tiredness, drowsiness, incoordination, nausea, dizziness.
Unusual: Vomiting, blurred vision, tremor, weight gain.

INTERACTIONS:
Other drugs:
- Antacids, cimetidine.

Herbs:
- Evening primrose (linoleic acid), Gingko biloba.

Other substances:
- Borage.

PRESCRIPTION:
Yes.

PBS:
Yes (authority required).

PERMITTED IN SPORT:
Yes.

OVERDOSE:
Unlikely to be lethal. Symptoms may include double vision, slurred speech, drowsiness and diarrhoea.

OTHER INFORMATION:
One of the newer medications for poorly controlled epilepsy that was introduced in the late 1990s. Also very effective in treating intractable nerve pain.
See also BARBITURATES, BENZODIAZEPINES, Carbamazepine, Clonazepam, Ethosuximide, Lamotrigine, Levetiracetam, Oxcarbazepine, Phenytoin, Primidone, Sodium valproate, Sulthiame, Tiagabine, Topiramate, Vigabatrin.

Galantamine

TRADE NAME:
Reminyl.

USES:
Alzheimer's disease.

DOSAGE:
 4mg to 12mg twice a day. Increase dose slowly.

FORMS:
Tablets of 4mg (off-white), 8mg (pink) and 12mg (orange).

PRECAUTIONS:
Not designed for use in pregnancy (B1), breast feeding and children.
Use with caution with heart rhythm irregularities, peptic ulcer, recent surgery, epilepsy, severe asthma, emphysema, poor urinary flow and liver disease.
Take adequate fluids with medication.
Do not take if:
 suffering severe liver or kidney disease.

SIDE EFFECTS:
Common: Nausea, diarrhoea, weight loss, tiredness, poor appetite.
Unusual: Low blood pressure, low blood potassium levels, urinary infection, watery nasal discharge.
Severe but rare (stop medication, consult doctor): Irregular heartbeat, abnormal bleeding.

INTERACTIONS:
Other drugs:
- Anticholinergics, digoxin, beta blockers, paroxetine, ketoconazole, erythromycin, quinidine, fluoxetine, fluvoxamine.

PRESCRIPTION:
Yes.

PBS:
Yes (authority required – very restricted).

PERMITTED IN SPORT:
Yes.

OTHER INFORMATION:
Introduced in 2001. Assists memory and reasoning power in only some patients with Alzheimer's disease. Regular mental tests necessary to assess effectiveness.
See also Donepezil, Rivastigmine, Tacrine.

Gamma Globulin
(Immunoglobulin, Normal Human)

TRADE NAMES:
Intragram, Intraglobulin, Normal Immunoglobulin, Sandoglobulin.

DRUG CLASS:
Immunoglobulin.

USES:
Prevention and treatment of hepatitis, polio and measles; adjunctive treatment for bacterial infections; low natural levels of immunoglobulin; some types of leukaemia; Wiskott-Aldrich syndrome; multiple myeloma and congenital AIDS.

DOSAGE:
 For injection as determined by doctor for each patient.

FORMS:
Injection.

PRECAUTIONS:
Safe in pregnancy, breast feeding and children.
Use with caution in idiopathic thrombocytopenia, kidney disease, and severe bacterial infections.
Do not use high doses.
Do not take if:
 suffering from IgA deficiency.

SIDE EFFECTS:
Common: Headache, fever, anxiety, flushing, itch.
Unusual: Brain irritation, change in blood pressure, chills, muscle aches, belly pains.
Severe but rare (stop medication, consult doctor): Allergy reaction.

INTERACTIONS:
Other drugs:
- Live virus vaccines (eg. Sabin polio).

Medications

PRESCRIPTION:
Yes.

PBS:
No.

PERMITTED IN SPORT:
Yes.
See also IMMUNOGLOBULINS.

Gammalinoleic acid
(Evening Primrose oil)
See FATTY ACIDS.

Ganciclovir

TRADE NAMES:
Cymevene, Vitrasert Implant.

DRUG CLASS:
Antiviral.

USES:
Treatment or prevention of cytomegalovirus (CMV) infections of eyes or lungs in patients with AIDS, immunosuppression or transplants.

DOSAGE:
 Four tablets three times a day, or by drip into a vein.

FORMS:
Tablets, injection, eye implant.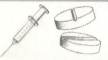

PRECAUTIONS:
Not to be used in pregnancy (D) or breast feeding.
Not for use in infants. Use with caution in children.
Only use in severe cases of CMV.
Use with caution in poor hydration, kidney disease, and elderly.
Regular blood tests to check blood cell levels essential.

SIDE EFFECTS:
Common: Low blood white cell count, low blood platelet count (causes abnormal bleeding), anaemia, nausea, diarrhoea, damage to foetus during pregnancy.
Unusual: Vomiting, reduced fertility long term.
Severe but rare (stop medication, consult doctor): Inflamed pancreas (severe belly pain), blood infection.

INTERACTIONS:
Other drugs:
- Probenecid, didanosine, zidovudine, cilastin, imipenem.

PRESCRIPTION:
Yes.

PBS:
Capsules: Yes (authority required – very restricted).
Other forms: No.

PERMITTED IN SPORT:
Yes.

OVERDOSE:
Highly toxic and may cause severe organ damage. Induce vomiting if taken recently. Seek urgent medical attention.

Gatifloxacin

TRADE NAME:
Tequin.

DRUG CLASS:
Aminoglycoside antibiotic.

USES:
Severe bacterial infections such as pneumonia, sinusitis, bronchitis and gonorrhoea.

DOSAGE:
 One tablet a day.

FORMS:
Tablets (white) of 400mg, infusion, injection.

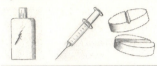

PRECAUTIONS:
Use with caution in pregnancy (B3), breast feeding and children.
Use with caution in irregular heart rhythm, hardening of arteries (arteriosclerosis), epilepsy, and kidney disease.

SIDE EFFECTS:
Common: Nausea, diarrhoea, vaginal irritation, headache, dizziness.
Unusual: Irritability, weakened tendons.
Severe but rare (stop medication, consult doctor): Irregular heart rhythm, severe diarrhoea (pseudomembranous colitis), worsening infection.

INTERACTIONS:
Other drugs:
- Oral contraceptives, cisapride, erythromycin, antipsychotics, tricyclic antidepressants, digoxin, probenecid, iron, zinc, antacids.

PRESCRIPTION:
Yes.

PBS:
Yes (authority required).

PERMITTED IN SPORT:
Yes.

OVERDOSE:
Ear and kidney damage possible. Give copious fluids to increase excretion through kidneys.

OTHER INFORMATION:
Introduced in 2001 for the treatment of resistant infections.
See also Amikacin, Gentamicin, Neomycin, Tobramycin.

Gemfibrizol

TRADE NAMES:
Ausgem, Gemhexal, GenRx Gemfibrizol, Jezil, Lipazil, Lopid.
Other locally produced brands of Gemfibrizol exist.

DRUG CLASS:
Hypolipidaemic.

USES:
Reducing excessive blood levels of cholesterol and triglyceride.

DOSAGE:

One tablet twice daily 30 minutes before meals.

FORMS:
Tablet of 600mg.

PRECAUTIONS:
Use in pregnancy (B3) only if medically essential. Not for use in breast feeding and children.
Patients must remain on a low fat diet.
Use with caution with irregular heartbeat, liver disease.
Regular blood tests to check blood fat levels, liver enzymes and blood cells are necessary.
Do not persist for more than three months if ineffective.

Do not take if:
 suffering from severe liver or kidney disease, gall stones.
- trying to get pregnant as drug may reduce fertility.

SIDE EFFECTS:
Common: Heartburn, belly pains, diarrhoea, tiredness, nausea, muscle pain.
Unusual: Vomiting, eczema, rash, dizziness, constipation, headache.
Severe but rare (stop medication, consult doctor): Yellow skin (jaundice), gall stones, disabling muscle pain.

INTERACTIONS:
Other drugs:
- Anticoagulants (eg. warfarin), cerivastatin, colestipol.

Herbs:
- Alfalfa, fenugreek, garlic, ginger.

PRESCRIPTION:
Yes.

PBS:
Yes.

PERMITTED IN SPORT:
Yes.

OVERDOSE:
No significant problems likely.

OTHER INFORMATION:
Medication introduced in 1995 that is particularly effective and safe in the treatment of excess blood levels of triglycerides and cholesterol.

See also Atorvastatin, Cholestyramine, Colestipol, Fluvastatin, Nicotinic acid, Pravastatin, Probucol, Simvastatin.

Gentamicin

TRADE NAMES:
Genoptic, Gentamicin, Minims Gentamicin, Septopal.
Celestone VG (with betamethasone).

DRUG CLASS:
Aminoglycoside antibiotic.

USES:
Severe infections, particularly bone, lung, kidney, soft tissue, uterus, eye and belly infections; infected burns.

DOSAGE:

Injection: Every eight hours, or by continuous drip infusion.
Eye drops: Two drops every four hours.
Ointment and cream: Apply three or four times a day.

FORMS:
Injection, eye drops, ointment, cream, beads for implantation.

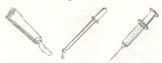

PRECAUTIONS:
Not to be used in pregnancy (D) unless absolutely essential for mother's well being. Breast feeding must be ceased before use.
Use with caution and only when essential in children.
Eye drops and skin preparations may be used with caution in pregnancy and breast feeding.
Use injection with caution in kidney disease.
Blood tests to check that correct dose is being administered are recommended.

SIDE EFFECTS:
Common: Eye drops and skin preparations – Minimal.
Injection – Rash, nausea, headache.
Unusual: Ear and kidney damage (dose related), vomiting.
Severe but rare (stop medication, consult doctor): Ear noises or deafness, unusual bleeding or bruising.

INTERACTIONS:
Other drugs:
- Penicillin, cephalosporins, ethacrynic acid, frusemide, other aminoglycoside antibiotics, vitamin K, narcotics, some general anaesthetics.

PRESCRIPTION:
Yes.

PBS:
Injection, eye drops: Yes.
Other forms: No.

PERMITTED IN SPORT:
Yes.

OVERDOSE:
Ear and kidney damage possible.
Give copious fluids to increase excretion through kidneys.

OTHER INFORMATION:
Very useful for the treatment of severe infections. Little risk of serious side effects if dose monitored by blood tests.

See Amikacin, Gatifloxacin, Neomycin, Tobramycin.

Gestodene
See ORAL CONTRACEPTIVES.

Gestrinone

TRADE NAME:
Dimetriose.

DRUG CLASS:
Sex hormone.

USES:
Endometriosis.

DOSAGE:
 One capsule twice a week for six months.

FORMS:
Capsules (white) of 2.5mg.

PRECAUTIONS:
Must not be used in pregnancy (D), breast feeding or children.
Use with caution in elderly.
Use with caution in diabetes and high blood fat (cholesterol or triglycerides) levels.
Do not take if:
- suffering from significant heart, kidney, liver or metabolic diseases.
- suffering from blood vessel disorders.
- male.

SIDE EFFECTS:
Common: Acne, oily skin, hair growth on face, ankle and foot swelling, excess sweating, low libido, leg cramps, headache, nausea, vomiting, loss of appetite, excess hunger, dizziness, tiredness, rash, hot flushes, reduced breast size.
Unusual: Deepening voice, fainting, blurred vision, anxiety, flashing lights in vision, indigestion, diarrhoea, belly pain, weight loss, thirst, muscle cramps, numbness, red face, breast lumps.

INTERACTIONS:
Other drugs:
- Epilepsy medications, rifampicin.

PRESCRIPTION:
Yes.

PBS:
Yes (authority required. Restricted to endometriosis proven by surgery).

PERMITTED IN SPORT:
No.

OVERDOSE:
Serious exacerbation of side effects likely. Induce vomiting and seek urgent medical attention.

Ginkgo
(Ginkgo biloba)

USES:
Poor circulation, dizziness, ringing in ears (tinnitus), dementia.

DOSAGE:

40mg to 80mg three times a day.

FORMS:
Capsules, tablets, liquid.

PRECAUTIONS:
Do not use in pregnancy or if trying to become pregnant.
Use with caution in high blood pressure.

SIDE EFFECTS:
Common: Nausea, diarrhoea.
Unusual: High blood pressure, vein inflammation (phlebitis).
Severe but rare (stop medication, consult doctor): Skin hypersensitivity, abnormal bleeding, infertility, stroke.

INTERACTIONS:
Other drugs:
- Anticoagulants (eg. warfarin), aspirin, NSAIDs.

PRESCRIPTION:
No.

PERMITTED IN SPORT:
Yes.

OVERDOSE:
Muscle spasms and cramps, weakness and incoordination may occur. Seek medical assistance.

OTHER INFORMATION:
Not used in orthodox medicine.

Ginseng

USES:
Fatigue.

DOSAGE:

1g to 2g of root a day, divided into three or four doses.

FORMS:
Capsules, tablets, liquid, cream.

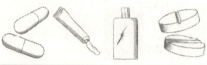

PRECAUTIONS:
Do not use in pregnancy and breast feeding (masculisation of female foetus and baby possible).
Use with caution in heart disease, diabetes and high blood pressure.

SIDE EFFECTS:
Common: Sleeplessness, nose bleeds, headache, nervousness, vomiting.
Unusual: Breast tenderness and lumps, vaginal bleeding, high blood pressure.

INTERACTIONS:
Other drugs:
- Insulin, hypoglycaemics (for diabetes), warfarin, NSAIDs, aspirin, MAOI, frusemide.

Other substances:
- Caffeine.

PRESCRIPTION:
No.

PBS:
No.

OVERDOSE:
High blood pressure, insomnia, increased muscle tone, fluid retention and tissue swelling occur.

OTHER INFORMATION:
Not used in orthodox medical practice.

GLAUCOMA MEDICATIONS

See Acetazolamide, Apraclonidine, Betaxolol, Bimatoprost, Brimonidine tartrate, Brinzolamide, Carbachol, Dipivefrine hydrochloride, Dorzolamide hydrochloride, Latanoprost, Levobunolol, Phenylephrine, Pilocarpine, Timolol, Travoprost.

Glibenclamide

TRADE NAMES:
Daonil, Glimel.

DRUG CLASS:
Hypoglycaemic.

USES:
Diabetes not requiring insulin injections.

DOSAGE:
One or two tablets, one to three times a day before meals. Maximum four tablets a day. Do not vary from prescribed dose without reference to a doctor.

FORMS:
Tablets of 2.5 and 5mg.

PRECAUTIONS:
Not to be used in pregnancy (C), breast feeding or children.
Use with caution if operating machinery or driving a vehicle.
Use with caution in all forms of kidney disease.
Illness, changes in diet, exercise and stress may change dosage requirements.
Lower doses required in elderly and debilitated patients.
Strict control of carbohydrates and sugars in diet essential.
Do not take if:
- suffering from severe liver or kidney disease.
- insulin dependent diabetic.

SIDE EFFECTS:
Common: Minimal.
Unusual: Blurred vision, drowsiness, nausea, heartburn, belly discomfort, rash.
Severe but rare (stop medication, consult doctor): Low blood sugar (see Overdose below), yellow skin (jaundice), unusual bleeding or bruising.

INTERACTIONS:
Other drugs:
- ACE inhibitors, beta blockers, other hypoglycaemics, chloramphenicol, clofibrate, clonidine, warfarin, probenecid, MAOI, miconazole, salicylates, tetracycline, sulphonamides, diazoxide, corticosteroids, nicotinic acid, oestrogens, progestogens, phenothiazines, phenytoin, thyroid hormones, laxatives.

Other substances:
- Reacts adversely with alcohol.

Herbs:
- Alfalfa, celery, eucalyptus, fenugreek, garlic, ginger, ginseng, karela.

PRESCRIPTION:
Yes.

PBS:
Yes.

PERMITTED IN SPORT:
Yes.

OVERDOSE:
Serious. Symptoms of low blood sugar (hypoglycaemia) may include tiredness, confusion, chills, palpitations, sweating, vomiting, dizziness, hunger, blurred vision and fainting. Significant overdosage can lead to coma and death. Give sugary drinks or sweets if conscious. Seek emergency medical assistance.

OTHER INFORMATION:
Used mainly in elderly patients who develop maturity onset diabetes that is not severe enough to require insulin injections.
See also Acarbose, Gliclazide, Glimepride, Glipizide, INSULINS, Metformin, Repaglinide, Rosiglitazone, Tolbutamide.

Gliclazide

TRADE NAMES:
Diamicron, GenRx Gliclazide, Glyade, Nidem.

DRUG CLASS:
Hypoglycaemic.

USES:
Diabetes not requiring insulin injections.

DOSAGE:

Half to two tablets, one or two times a day before meals. Maximum four tablets a day.
Do not vary from prescribed dose without reference to a doctor.

FORMS:
Tablets (white) of 80mg.

PRECAUTIONS:
Not to be used in pregnancy (C), breast feeding or children.
Illness, changes in diet, exercise and stress may change dosage requirements.
Lower doses required in elderly and debilitated patients.
Strict control of carbohydrates and sugars in diet essential.

Do not take if:

- suffering from severe liver or kidney disease.
- an insulin dependent diabetic.

SIDE EFFECTS:
Common: Uncommon.
Unusual: Blurred vision, drowsiness, nausea, heartburn, belly discomfort, rash.
Severe but rare (stop medication, consult doctor): Low blood sugar (see Overdose below), yellow skin (jaundice), unusual bleeding or bruising.

INTERACTIONS:
Other drugs:
- ACE inhibitors, beta blockers, other hypoglycaemics, chloramphenicol, clofibrate, clonidine, warfarin, probenecid, MAOI, miconazole, salicylates, tetracycline, sulphonamides, diazoxide, corticosteroids, nicotinic acid, oestrogens, progestogens, phenothiazines, phenytoin, thyroid hormones, laxatives.

Other substances:
- Reacts adversely with alcohol.

Herbs:
- Alfalfa, celery, eucalyptus, fenugreek, garlic, ginger, ginseng, karela.

PRESCRIPTION:
Yes.

PBS:
Yes.

PERMITTED IN SPORT:
Yes.

OVERDOSE:
Serious. Symptoms of low blood sugar (hypoglycaemia) may include tiredness, confusion, chills, palpitations, sweating, vomiting, dizziness, hunger, blurred vision and fainting. Significant overdosage can lead to coma and death. Give sugary drinks or sweets if conscious. Seek emergency medical assistance.

OTHER INFORMATION:
Used mainly in elderly patients who develop maturity onset diabetes that is not severe enough to require insulin injections.

See also Acarbose, Glibenclamide, Glimepride, Glipizide, INSULINS, Metformin, Repaglinide, Rosiglitazone, Tolbutamide.

Glimepride

TRADE NAME:
Amaryl.

DRUG CLASS:
Hypoglycaemic.

USES:
Maturity onset (type 2) diabetes.

DOSAGE:
 Start with 1mg a day with breakfast, swallowed whole with plenty of water.
Increase by 1mg every week or two until diabetes controlled. Unusual to go above 4mg a day.

FORMS:
Tablets of 1mg (pink), 2mg (green) and 4mg (blue).

PRECAUTIONS:
Not to be used in pregnancy (C), breast feeding and children.
Use with caution with recent surgery, significant infection, poor diet, or other physical stress.
Use with care in elderly.
Regular blood tests of sugar levels and liver function necessary.

Do not take if:
 suffering from juvenile (type 1) diabetes, severe kidney or liver disease.

SIDE EFFECTS:
Common: Vision disturbances, nausea, diarrhoea.
Unusual: Liver damage, blood chemistry disturbances, low blood sugar.

INTERACTIONS:
Other drugs:
- Other hypoglycaemics (used to treat diabetes), beta blockers, ACE inhibitors, clofibrate, MAOI, probenecid.

Other substances:
- Alcohol.

Herbs:
- Alfalfa, celery, eucalyptus, fenugreek, garlic, ginger, ginseng, karela.

PRESCRIPTION:
Yes.

PBS:
Yes.

PERMITTED IN SPORT:
Yes.

OVERDOSE:
Severe life threatening drop in blood sugar levels may occur. Seek urgent medical attention. Give glucose-rich drinks and sweets. Recurrences of effects may occur after apparent recovery and patient must be observed closely for several days.

OTHER INFORMATION:
Introduced in 2000.

See also Acarbose, Glibenclamide, Gliclazide, Glipizide, INSULINS, Metformin, Repaglinide, Rosiglitazone, Tolbutamide.

Glipizide

TRADE NAMES:
Melizide, Minidiab.

DRUG CLASS:
Hypoglycaemic.

USES:
Diabetes not requiring insulin injections.

DOSAGE:

One or two tablets, one to three times a day before meals. Maximum eight tablets a day.
Do not vary from prescribed dose without reference to a doctor.

FORMS:
Tablets of 5mg.

PRECAUTIONS:
Not to be used in pregnancy (C), breast feeding or children.
Use with caution in all forms of kidney and liver disease.
Illness, changes in diet, exercise and stress may change dosage requirements.
Strict control of carbohydrates and sugars in diet essential.

Do not take if:
 suffering from severe thyroid, liver or kidney disease.
- uncontrolled infection present.
- an insulin dependent diabetic.
- allergic to sulphas.

SIDE EFFECTS:
Common: Nausea, diarrhoea, constipation.
Unusual: Blurred vision, drowsiness, dizziness, headache, heartburn, belly discomfort, rash.
Severe but rare (stop medication, consult doctor): Low blood sugar (see Overdose below), yellow skin (jaundice), unusual bleeding or bruising.

INTERACTIONS:
Other drugs:
- ACE inhibitors, beta blockers, other hypoglycaemics, chloramphenicol, clofibrate, clonidine, warfarin, probenecid, MAOI, miconazole, salicylates, tetracycline, sulphonamides, diazoxide, corticosteroids, nicotinic acid, oestrogens, progestogens, phenothiazines, phenytoin, thyroid hormones, laxatives.

Herbs:
- Alfalfa, celery, eucalyptus, fenugreek, garlic, ginger, ginseng, karela.

Other substances:
- Reacts adversely with alcohol.

PRESCRIPTION:
Yes.

PBS:
Yes.

PERMITTED IN SPORT:
Yes.

OVERDOSE:
Serious. Symptoms of low blood sugar (hypoglycaemia) may include tiredness, confusion, chills, palpitations, sweating, vomiting, dizziness, hunger, blurred vision and fainting. Significant overdosage can lead to coma and death. Give sugary drinks or sweets if conscious. Seek emergency medical assistance.

OTHER INFORMATION:
Used mainly in elderly patients who develop maturity onset diabetes that is not severe enough to require insulin injections.

See also Acarbose, Glibenclamide, Gliclazide, Glimepride, INSULINS, Metformin, Repaglinide, Rosiglitazone, Tolbutamide.

Glucagon

TRADE NAMES:
Glucagen.

USES:
Low blood sugar in diabetics.

DOSAGE:

Inject contents of ampoule if patient suffers acute low blood sugar not responding to sugar by mouth.

FORMS:
Injection.

PRECAUTIONS:
May be used with caution in pregnancy (B2). Safe to use in breast feeding and children.
Use repeatedly only with caution.
Use with caution in blood clots, heart attack, liver and kidney disease.

Do not take if:
 suffering from phaeochromocytoma, insulinoma.

SIDE EFFECTS:
Common: Nausea, vomiting.

INTERACTIONS:
Other drugs:
- Warfarin, beta blockers (eg. propranolol).

PRESCRIPTION:
Yes.

PBS:
Yes.

PERMITTED IN SPORT:
Yes.

OVERDOSE:
Exacerbation of side effects likely.

OTHER INFORMATION:
May be life saving. Family members and associates should be instructed in use. Diabetics who use too much insulin or eat too little may suffer from sudden low blood sugar that can cause them to rapidly lose consciousness. An injection of Glucagon will revive them rapidly by releasing sugar stored in body.

Glucose

TRADE NAMES:
Glucose, Insta Glucose.
Dexsal, Gastrolyte, Gluco-lyte, Pedialyte, Repalyte (with electrolytes).
Dynamo (with vitamin B and caffeine).
Emetrol (with fructose).
Used as an additive or sweetener in many medications.

DRUG CLASS:
Sugar.

USES:
Correction of severe nutritional loss, nausea, diuretic (increasing production of urine), correction of insulin overdose, reduction of excessive pressure in brain fluid.

DOSAGE:

Depends on use. Follow instructions on label, or use as directed by doctor.
Do not dilute, or take with other fluids.

FORMS:
Lozenges, tablets, solution, injection.

PRECAUTIONS:
Safe in pregnancy, breast feeding and children.
Do not take if:
 suffering from diabetes, unless suffering insulin overdose.

SIDE EFFECTS:
Minimal.

INTERACTIONS:
None significant.

PRESCRIPTION:
No.

PBS:
Injection: Yes.
Other forms: No.

PERMITTED IN SPORT:
Injection: No.
Orally: Yes (beware of added caffeine).

OVERDOSE:
No serious consequences.
Vomiting likely.

OTHER INFORMATION:
Glucose is a common form of sugar. Works within a couple of minutes after being taken by mouth.

Glutaraldehyde

TRADE NAME:
Diswart.

DRUG CLASS:
Keratolytic.

USES:
Removal of warts.

DOSAGE:
 Apply twice a day to wart.

FORMS:
Liquid.

PRECAUTIONS:
Safe to use in pregnancy, breast feeding and children.
Avoid warts on face, anus, genitals and other areas of sensitive skin.

SIDE EFFECTS:
Common: Skin inflammation and soreness, skin staining.

INTERACTIONS:
None significant.

PRESCRIPTION:
No.

PBS:
No.

PERMITTED IN SPORT:
Yes.

OVERDOSE:
Serious if swallowed. Seek urgent medical attention.
See also KERATOLYTICS, PODOPHYLLUMS.

Glycerol

TRADE NAMES:
Glycerin Suppositories, Glycerol Suppositories, Hamilton Body Lotion, QV Wash.
Aci-Jel (with acetic acid, ricinoleic acid, hydroxyquinolone).
Anusol Wipes, Egozite, Gentlees, Hamilton Cleansing Lotion, QV Cream, Replens, Solosite Wound Gel (with paraffin and other ingredients).
Used in many different preparations as a lubricant and base ingredient.

Medications

DRUG CLASS:
Lubricant, laxative.

USES:
Constipation, vaginal dryness, skin dryness.

DOSAGE:

Suppository: One suppository rectally as required.
Vaginal gel: Insert every second day as needed.
Skin creams: As required.

FORMS:
Suppository, vaginal gel (store in cool place), skin preparations.
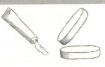

PRECAUTIONS:
Safe in pregnancy, breast feeding, infants and children.
Should not be used repeatedly for prolonged periods.

SIDE EFFECTS:
Minimal.

INTERACTIONS:
None significant.

PRESCRIPTION:
No.

PBS:
No. Some forms available to Veterans Affairs pensioners.

PERMITTED IN SPORT:
Yes.

OVERDOSE:
Causes diarrhoea only.

OTHER INFORMATION:
Very safe ancient remedy.
See also Bisacodyl, Docusate sodium, FIBRE, Frangula, Lactulose, Paraffin, Poloxamer, Psyllium, Senna, Sodium phosphate, Sodium picosulfate, Sorbitol, Sterculia.

Glyceryl Trinitrate
(GTN, Nitroglycerine)

TRADE NAMES:
Anginine, Minitran, Nitro-Dur, Nitrolingual Spray, Rectogesic, Transiderm Nitro.

DRUG CLASS:
Antiangina.

USES:
Relief or prevention of angina, anal fissures and tears.

DOSAGE:

Tablets: One tablet under tongue every ten minutes as required to a maximum of six a day starting immediately any chest pain experienced. Should not be swallowed.
Spray: One spray under tongue every five minutes as required to a maximum of two sprays per attack starting immediately any chest pain experienced.
Patches: Apply to skin of trunk, upper arms or thighs once a day for 16 hours a day.
Anal ointment: Insert 1 to 1.5cm into anus three times a day.

FORMS:
Tablets, mouth spray, skin patches, anal ointment, injection.

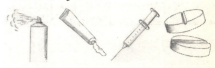

Tablets must not be exposed to light. Should be stored below 25°C. Discard bottle three months after opening.

PRECAUTIONS:
Should be used with caution in pregnancy (B2) and breast feeding.
Use with caution with strokes, anaemia, severe arteriosclerosis, lung disease, glaucoma, overactive thyroid gland and in the elderly.
Apply patches to different areas with each

application.
Tolerance may develop if used constantly.
Do not take if:
 suffering from head injury, recent stroke, cardiomyopathy.

SIDE EFFECTS:
Common: Headache, flushing, rapid heart rate.
Unusual: Dizziness, fainting.

INTERACTIONS:
Other drugs:
- Silandafel (Viagra), tadalafil (Cialis) – potentially fatal interaction.

Other substances:
- Reacts with alcohol. Smoking may exacerbate disease process.

PRESCRIPTION:
Yes.

PBS:
Most forms: Yes.
Rectogesic: No.

PERMITTED IN SPORT:
Yes.

OVERDOSE:
Fainting and low blood pressure occur. Red blood cells may be damaged. Administer activated charcoal or induce vomiting if tablets taken recently. Remove patches and ointment. Seek medical assistance.

OTHER INFORMATION:
Tablets under tongue have been used successfully for many decades, but in the last decade better delivery systems in the form of patches and sprays have been developed. Sprays are more convenient, more stable and easier to use than tablets which can deteriorate with time. Nitroglycerine is an incorrect technical name.

See also Isosorbide nitrate, Nicorandil, Perhexiline.

Glycyrrhizin
See Liquorice.

GOLD
See Auranofin, Sodium aurothiomalate.

Gonadotrophin, menopausal, human
See Menopausal gonadotrophin, human.

Goserelin acetate

TRADE NAME:
Zoladex.

DRUG CLASS:
Cytotoxic.

USES:
Metastatic and severe prostate cancer. Advanced breast cancer. Fibroids of the uterus. Endometriosis.

DOSAGE:
 Implant inserted every one to three months.

FORMS:
Implants of 3.6mg and 10.8mg.

PRECAUTIONS:
Not to be used in pregnancy (D), breast feeding or children.
Use with caution in osteoporosis, spinal or ureter disease, polycystic ovarian syndrome.

SIDE EFFECTS:
Common: Infertility, impotence, decreased libido, hot flushes, headaches, dry vagina, cessation of menstrual periods, changes in blood pressure, breast formation in males,

temporary increase in bone pain.
Unusual: Breast pain, joint pain, rash, reactions at site of implant or injection, decrease in bone density (osteoporosis).

INTERACTIONS:
Other drugs:
- Sex hormones.

PRESCRIPTION:
Yes.

PBS:
Yes (authority required – restricted to advanced breast and prostate cancer, and proven endometriosis).

PERMITTED IN SPORT:
Yes.

Gramicidin

TRADE NAMES:
Available in Australia only in combination with other medications.
Kenacomb, Otocomb (with triamcinolone, neomycin, nystatin).
Neosporin (with polymyxin B, neomycin and other ingredients).
Otodex, Sofradex (with framycetin and dexamethasone).
Soframycin (with framycetin).

DRUG CLASS:
Antibiotic.

USES:
Infections of skin, eyes and ears.

DOSAGE:

Ear ointment: Insert twice a day.
Ear drops: Insert two or three times a day (may be used in conjunction with wick in ear).
Cream, ointment: Apply three times a day.
Eye drops: Insert every three or four hours.
Eye ointment: Insert three times a day.

FORMS:
Eye ointment,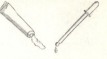
eye drops
(keep cool).
Ointment,
cream, ear drops, ear ointment.

PRECAUTIONS:
Use with caution in pregnancy. May be used in breast feeding and children.
Do not use if:
 suffering from viral skin infections or tuberculosis.

SIDE EFFECTS:
Minimal. Tissue damage possible with prolonged use.

INTERACTIONS:
None significant.

PRESCRIPTION:
Yes.

PBS:
Most forms: Yes.
Kenacomb skin cream: No.

PERMITTED IN SPORT:
Yes.

OTHER INFORMATION:
Gramicidin is a constituent in some of the most widely used and effective combinations for treating eye, ear and skin infections.
See also Neomycin.

Griseofulvin

TRADE NAMES:
Griseostatin, Grisovin.

DRUG CLASS:
Antifungal.

USES:
Fungal infection of skin, hair and nails that do not respond to creams and lotions.

DOSAGE:
 One tablet a day after food for several weeks or months.

FORMS:
Tablets (white) of 500mg.

PRECAUTIONS:
Should not be used in pregnancy (B3) unless medically essential. Breast feeding should be ceased before use. May be used in children.
Use with care in liver disease.
Avoid sunlight while using medication.
Use with care if operating machinery or driving a vehicle.
Use with care if allergic to penicillin.

Do not take if:
 suffering from severe liver disease, porphyria, systemic lupus erythematosus (SLE).
- trying to fall pregnant.
- planning to father a child within six months (sperm abnormalities possible).

SIDE EFFECTS:
Common: Headache, nausea, sunburn.
Unusual: Dizziness, confusion, tiredness, vomiting, sore mouth, furry tongue, rash.

INTERACTIONS:
Other drugs:
- Anticoagulants (eg. warfarin), barbiturates, sedatives, hypnotics, oral contraceptives.
- Cross reacts with penicillin.

Other substances:
- Reacts adversely with alcohol.

PRESCRIPTION:
Yes.

PBS:
Yes.

PERMITTED IN SPORT:
Yes.

OVERDOSE:
Unlikely to cause serious effects.

OTHER INFORMATION:
Widely and commonly used for fungal infections, but more effective (and expensive) medications have been recently introduced.

See also Amphotericin, Fluconazole, Itraconazole, Ketoconazole, Terbinafine.

Growth Hormone
See Somatropin.

GTN
See Glyceryl trinitrate.

Guaiphenesin

TRADE NAMES:
Lemsip Chesty Cough, Robitussin EX, Vicks Chesty Cough.
Actifed Chesty (with pseudoephedrine and triprolidine).
Benadryl for the Family Chesty, Logicin Congested Chesty Cough, Nyal Plus Chesty Cough, Robitussin PS (with pseudoephedrine).
Brondecon Expectorant (with choline theophyllinate).
Dimetapp Cold Cough and Flu Liquid Capsules (with pseudoephedrine, paracetamol and dextromethorphan).
Dimetapp Cold Cough and Sinus Liquid Capsules, Sigma Relief (with pseudoephedrine and dextromethorphan).

Logicin Expectorant, Robitussin ME, Tussinol Expectorant (with bromhexine).
Nyal Chesty Cough (with other ingredients).
Robitussin DM (with dextromethorphan). Also found in numerous locally produced cough mixtures.

DRUG CLASS:
Expectorant (assists coughing up phlegm).

USES:
Moist chesty cough.

DOSAGE:
 Take every four hours.

FORMS:
Mixture, syrup, capsules.

PRECAUTIONS:
Safe to use in pregnancy (A), breast feeding and children.
Use with caution under 2 years.
Not for long term use.
Does not reduce mucus production.

SIDE EFFECTS:
Common: Dizziness, nausea, diarrhoea.
Unusual: Drowsiness.

INTERACTIONS:
Other drugs: MAOI antidepressants (serious interaction).

PRESCRIPTION:
No.

PBS:
No.

PERMITTED IN SPORT:
Yes (provided not combined with pseudoephedrine).

OVERDOSE:
Unlikely to have any serious effects.

OTHER INFORMATION:
Widely used and safe medication.
See also Ammonium bicarbonate, Bromhexine, Camphor, Senega.

Guanethidine

TRADE NAME:
Ismelin.

DRUG CLASS:
Vasodilator.

USES:
Dilating small arteries in areas where circulation is poor, lowering blood pressure.

DOSAGE:
 Injection as determined by doctor.

FORMS:
Injection.

PRECAUTIONS:
Safe in pregnancy (A), breast feeding and children.
Use with caution in peptic ulcers, low blood pressure tendency, asthma, kidney disease and diabetes.
Do not take if:
☠ suffering from phaeochromocytoma, heart block or abnormal heart rhythm, congestive heart failure.

SIDE EFFECTS:
Common: Drowsiness, low blood pressure, faintness, dizziness, slow heart rate.
Unusual: Angina, heart failure, nausea, diarrhoea, asthma, impotence, dermatitis, hair loss.
Severe but rare (stop medication, consult doctor): Blood cell abnormalities.

INTERACTIONS:
Other drugs:
- MAOI antidepressants (serious interaction), anticoagulants (eg. warfarin – serious interaction), antiarrhythmics, beta blockers, digoxin, antihypertensives, sympathomimetics, antipsychotics, tricyclic antidepressants, oral contraceptives, some anaesthetics.

Other substances:
- Alcohol

PRESCRIPTION:
Yes.

PBS:
No.

PERMITTED IN SPORT:
Yes.

See also Betahistine, Diazoxide, Nicotinic Acid, Phenoxybenzamine.

Guarana
(Paullinia cupana)

USES:
Tonic, stimulant.

DOSAGE:

1g a day.

FORMS:
Tablets, capsules, liquid.

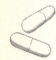

PRECAUTIONS:
Not for use in pregnancy. Use with caution in breast feeding and children. Use with caution in heart disease, kidney disease, anxiety states, hyperthyroidism (over-active thyroid gland), psychoses and muscle spasms (eg. spasticity).

SIDE EFFECTS:
Common: Insomnia (sleeplessness), agitation, increased urine production.
Unusual: Low blood potassium levels (hypokalaemia), abnormal bleeding.

INTERACTIONS:
Other drugs:
- Digoxin, theophylline.

Other substances:
- Caffeine.

PRESCRIPTION:
No.

PERMITTED IN SPORT:
No.

OVERDOSE:
Vomiting, painful and frequent passing of urine, intestinal spasms, irritability and irrational behaviour may occur. Seek medical advice.

OTHER INFORMATION:
Not used in orthodox medicine. Its clinical effects can be explained by the caffeine content of the herb. 250mg of guarana contains about 100mg of caffeine.

H² RECEPTOR ANTAGONISTS

DISCUSSION:

Peptic ulcers have caused belly pains for millennia, and were poorly treated until a significant advance in medication occurred in the late 1970s with the introduction of cimetidine, the first of the H2 receptor antagonists. These drugs are distantly related to antihistamines and act to cure ulcers by reducing the amount of acid secreted into the stomach. This also enables them to control reflux oesophagitis, which may accompany a hiatus hernia. Treatment is usually rapidly effective, but must be continued for weeks or months to prevent relapses.

See Cimetidine, Famotidine, Nizatadine, Ranitidine.

Haemophilus influenzae B vaccine
(HiB vaccine)

TRADE NAMES:
Hiberix, Pedvax HiB.
Comvax (with hepatitis B vaccine).

DRUG CLASS:
Vaccine.

USES:
Prevention of meningitis and epiglottitis (throat infection) caused by the bacteria Haemophilus influenzae B in children under 5 years.

DOSAGE:
 Three or four doses, two months apart.

FORMS:
Injection.

PRECAUTIONS:
Not recommended for use in pregnancy (B2) or adults, but unlikely to cause problems if given accidentally during pregnancy or breast feeding. Designed for use in children and infants.
Use with caution in fever, acute infection or immune system problems.
Do not inject into a vein.

SIDE EFFECTS:
Common: Redness and soreness at injection site.
Unusual: Irritability, tiredness, sleeplessness, diarrhoea, rash.

INTERACTIONS:
None significant.

PRESCRIPTION:
Yes.

PBS:
No, but provided free to doctors by state governments.

PERMITTED IN SPORT:
Yes.

OTHER INFORMATION:
Introduced in early 1990s to prevent one type of meningitis, and a rare but potentially fatal infection that can attack the epiglottis at the back of the throat and block the airway preventing breathing. All children should start a course of this vaccine at two months of age, and have two or three follow-up injections (depending on formulation). Older children need a shorter course, but greatest risk occurs under 12 months.

HAEMOSTATIC AGENTS

TRADE and GENERIC NAMES:
Konakion (Phytomenadione – vitamin K).
K-Thrombin (Menadione – vitamin K analogue – mimics action of vitamin K).

USES:
Treatment and prevention of excessive bleeding (particularly in newborn infants), overdose of anticoagulants.

DOSAGE:
 Depends on severity of bleeding.

FORMS:
Tablets, injection.

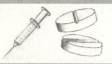

PRECAUTIONS:
Should be used with caution in pregnancy, breast feeding and children.
Use with caution in severe liver disease and the elderly.
Inject into vein only, do not inject into muscle.

Do not take if:
 suffering from severe allergy tendency.

SIDE EFFECTS:
Common: Minimal.
Uncommon: Vein inflammation, flushing, sweating, abnormal taste.
Severe but rare (stop medication, consult doctor): Yellow skin (jaundice), allergy reaction.

INTERACTIONS:
Other drugs:
- Warfarin, anticonvulsants.

PRESCRIPTION:
No.

PBS:
No.

PERMITTED IN SPORT:
Yes.

OVERDOSE:
No serious effects, except in infants where anaemia may occur.

OTHER INFORMATION:
Vitamin K is a fat soluble group of compounds essential for the formation of the factors that clot blood. It is found in most foods (particularly green leafy vegetables) and is also made by bacteria that live in the gut. The adequate daily allowance is 1mg A lack of vitamin K is rare, but may occur if fat absorption from the gut is abnormal. Newborn infants can be low on vitamin K and are often given vitamin K at birth to prevent excessive bleeding.

See also Aminocaproic Acid, Tranexamic acid.

Haloperidol

TRADE NAMES:
Haldol, Serenace.

DRUG CLASS:
Antipsychotic.

USES:
Psychotic disorders, mania, acute alcoholism, hallucinations, Tourette syndrome, severe vomiting, addition to painkillers.

DOSAGE:
 Individualised to patients' requirements. Follow doctor's instructions carefully.

FORMS:
Tablets of 0.5mg, 1.5mg and 5mg; liquid; injection.

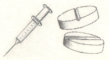

Medications

PRECAUTIONS:

Should not be used in pregnancy (C) unless medically essential. Breast feeding should be ceased before use. Not for use in children under 3 years.

Should be used with caution in epilepsy, over-active thyroid gland, glaucoma, irregular heart rhythm, liver disease, kidney disease, severe heart disease and hardening of arteries.

Lower doses necessary in elderly. Use for shortest time possible.

Do not take if:
- suffering from depression, Parkinson's disease, in a coma.
- operating machinery, driving a vehicle or undertaking tasks that require concentration and coordination.

SIDE EFFECTS:

Common: Minimal in low doses. Incoordination, drowsiness, muscle spasms, tremor.
Unusual: Depression, anxiety, restlessness, headache, sleeplessness, confusion, dizziness, loss of appetite, rapid heart rate, enlarged breasts (both sexes), increase or decrease in libido.
Severe but rare (stop medication, consult doctor): Repetitive unwanted movements of face, rigid muscles, fever, coma.

INTERACTIONS:

Other drugs:
- Narcotics, analgesics, barbiturates, sedatives, anticoagulants (eg. warfarin), tricyclic antidepressants, quinidine, buspirone, fluoxetine, fluvoxamine, nefazodone, paroxetine, venlafaxine, propranolol, lithium.

Herbs:
- Evening primrose (linoleic acid), sparteine (Cytisus scoparius).

Other substances:
- Reacts adversely with alcohol and cigarette smoking.

PRESCRIPTION:
Yes.

PBS:
Yes.

PERMITTED IN SPORT:
Yes.

OVERDOSE:

May cause sedation, muscle spasms, twitching, convulsions, coma, reduced breathing and death. Administer activated charcoal or induce vomiting if taken recently and patient alert. Seek urgent medical assistance.

See also **Amisulpride, Droperidol, Flupenthixol, Lithium Carbonate, Olanzapine, PHENOTHIAZINES, Pimozide, Quetiapine, Risperidone, Thiothixene, Zuclopenthixol.**

HCG

See Chorionic gonadotrophin, human.

Heparin

TRADE NAMES:
Calciparine, Heparin.

DRUG CLASS:
Anticoagulant.

USES:
Prevention and treatment of blood clots.

DOSAGE:

As determined by doctor.

FORMS:
Injection, infusion.

PRECAUTIONS:

Should only be used in pregnancy (C) if medically essential. Breast feeding should be ceased if Heparin treatment necessary. May be used in children.
Lower doses required in elderly.
Use with caution in asthma, kidney and

liver disease, high blood pressure, eye retina disease.
Regular blood tests to monitor blood clotting time essential.

Do not take if:

 suffering from bleeding disorders, threatened abortion, heart infection, peptic ulcer, severe high blood pressure, severe liver or kidney disease.
- due for surgery.

SIDE EFFECTS:

Common: Excessive bleeding, bruising.
Unusual: Nose bleeds, vomiting blood, blood in faeces, rash, itch, asthma.

INTERACTIONS:

Other drugs:
- Other anticoagulants (eg. warfarin), aspirin, NSAID, corticosteroids, hydroxychloroquine, ethacrynic acid, sulfinpyrazone, vitamin K, antihistamines, tetracyclines, digoxin, vitamin C, insulin, nicotine.

Herbs:
- Goldenseal.

PRESCRIPTION:
Yes.

PBS:
Yes.

PERMITTED IN SPORT:
Yes, but not advised in any active sport.

OVERDOSE:
Extremely serious. Massive bleeding may occur. Antidote available.

OTHER INFORMATION:
Only administered by doctors by injection or infusion (drip) in hospital, or strictly controlled outpatient basis. Used for many years to very effectively control life threatening blood clots. Once stabilised, patient is usually switched to an anticoagulant tablet such as warfarin. Available in two forms that vary in their speed and method of action.

See also Dalteparin, Enoxaparin.

Heparinoid

TRADE NAMES:
Hirudoid.
Lasonil (with hyaluronidase).
Movelat Sportz (with Salicylic acid).

USES:
Blood clots in veins close to skin, inflammation of veins, softening of hard scars, bruises, swelling caused by injury to tissue, sprains, haematomas (blood collections under skin).

DOSAGE:
 Apply and massage in once or twice a day.

FORMS:
Cream, ointment.

PRECAUTIONS:
Safe in pregnancy, breast feeding and children.

Do not use on:

 bleeding areas, infected areas and eye.

SIDE EFFECTS:
Common: Skin redness.

INTERACTIONS:
Other drugs:
- Heparin, anticoagulants (eg. warfarin).

PRESCRIPTION:
No.

PBS:
No.

PERMITTED IN SPORT:
Yes.

OTHER INFORMATION:
Useful and effective medication. Do not use excessive amounts.

Hepatitis A vaccine

TRADE NAME:
Avaxim, Havrix 1440, Havrix Junior, VAQTA.
Twinrix (with hepatitis B vaccine).
Vivaxim (with typhoid vaccine).

DRUG CLASS:
Vaccine.

USES:
Prevention of hepatitis A.

DOSAGE:

Twinrix: Three injections at intervals of one month and six to 12 months give at least five years, and possibly far longer, protection.
Havrix 1440, Havrix Junior, VAQTA: Two injections, 6 to 12 months apart, give at least five years protection.

FORMS:
Injection.

PRECAUTIONS:
Not designed to be used in pregnancy (B2), but unlikely to cause serious adverse effects if given inadvertently. May be given with caution in breast feeding and children under 5 years. May be given to children over 5 years.
First injection takes effect after 14 days, and lasts for at least six months. Booster gives long term protection.
Use with caution if exposed to hepatitis A.

Do not take if:
 suffering from significant fever.

SIDE EFFECTS:
Common: Local reaction at injection site.
Unusual: Headache, fever, tiredness, nausea, loss of appetite, general unwellness.

INTERACTIONS:
Other drugs:
- Immunoglobulin.

PRESCRIPTION:
Yes.

PBS:
No.

PERMITTED IN SPORT:
Yes.

OVERDOSE:
An inadvertent additional vaccination is unlikely to have any serious effects.

OTHER INFORMATION:
Hepatitis A causes liver damage and is caught from eating contaminated food or poor personal hygiene. It is very common in some developing countries.

See also Salmonella typhi vaccine.

Hepatitis B vaccine

TRADE NAMES:
Engerix-B, H-B-Vax II.
Comvax (with HiB vaccine).
Infanrix HepB (with tetanus, diphtheria and whooping cough vaccines).
Twinrix (with hepatitis A vaccine).

DRUG CLASS:
Vaccine.

USES:
Prevention of Hepatitis B.

DOSAGE:

Three injections at intervals of one month and six months gives at least five years protection.

FORMS:
Injection.

PRECAUTIONS:
Should not be used during pregnancy (B2) unless essential. Accidental vaccination during pregnancy is unlikely to cause any significant problem. Use with caution in breast feeding. May be used in children. Use with caution if immune system damaged, recently exposed to hepatitis B, or severely ill.

Do not take if:
 suffering from severe infection or fever.

SIDE EFFECTS:
Common: Local soreness, swelling, redness and hardness.
Unusual: Headache, dizziness, fever, muscle aches, tiredness, nausea, diarrhoea, joint pain, rash.

INTERACTIONS:
None significant.

PRESCRIPTION:
Yes.

PBS:
No. Some forms supplied free to doctors for use in children by state governments.

PERMITTED IN SPORT:
Yes.

OVERDOSE:
No adverse effects likely from an inadvertent additional dose.

OTHER INFORMATION:
Hepatitis B is endemic (widely spread) in Aborigines and southeast Asians. It is spread by sex, blood, sharing needles, blood splashes into eye, and possibly by close contact of open wounds. Now a routine vaccination in Australia.

Heroin

DRUG CLASS:
Narcotic.

USES:
No current recognised medical uses in Australia.
Used overseas for relief of severe pain.
Used illegally as a psychoactive drug to cause euphoria (abnormal happiness).

FORMS:
Injection.

PRECAUTIONS:
Should never be used in pregnancy, breast feeding or children.

Do not use if:
suffering from liver disease, kidney disease, epilepsy, head injury, diabetes, alcoholism, lung disease (eg. asthma), prostate disease.
- driving a car, operating machinery, swimming or undertaking any activity that requires concentration.

SIDE EFFECTS:
Common: Constipation, confusion, sweating, contracted pupils, difficulty passing urine, dry mouth, flushing, euphoria (artificial happiness), dizziness, slow heart rate, irregular heart rate, sedation, mood change, rash.
Unusual: Itch, blurred vision, low blood pressure, difficulty in breathing, convulsions.

INTERACTIONS:
Other drugs:
- Hypnotics, sedatives, marijuana, MAOI, cocaine.

Other substances:
- Increases the effect of alcohol.

PRESCRIPTION:
Illegal.

Medications

PERMITTED IN SPORT:
No.

OVERDOSE:
Very serious. May cause convulsions, irregular heartbeat, difficulty in breathing, coma and death. Seek emergency medical assistance. Antidote available.

OTHER INFORMATION:
Illegal drug of dependence. Highly addictive. Toleration may develop quickly (higher dose required to obtain same effect). Possession may lead to criminal charges. Heroin is closely related to Morphine. It may be preferred to Morphine when available because it is said to produce more calming effects.

See also Alfentanil, Buprenorphine, Codeine Phosphate, Dextromoramide, Dextropropoxyphene, Fentanyl, Hydromorphone, Methadone, Morphine, Oxycodone, Pentazocine, Pethidine.

Hexamethylmelamine

See Altretamine.

Hexamine hippurate

TRADE NAME:
Hiprex.

DRUG CLASS:
Urinary antiseptic.

USES:
Prevention of recurrent urine infections.

DOSAGE:
One tablet twice a day.

FORMS:
Tablet (white) of 1g.

PRECAUTIONS:
Safe for use in pregnancy (A), breast feeding and children.
Use with caution in vegetarians.
Do not take if:
suffering from severe liver or kidney disease, dehydration, severe kidney infection (without other antibiotic).

SIDE EFFECTS:
Common: Nausea, burning urine.
Unusual: Vomiting, rash, stomach discomfort.

INTERACTIONS:
Other drugs:
• Urinary alkalinisers, sulfonamides.

PRESCRIPTION:
No.

PBS:
Yes.

PERMITTED IN SPORT:
Yes.

OVERDOSE:
Exacerbation of side effects likely.

OTHER INFORMATION:
Used mainly in women who have recurrent attacks of cystitis, and in patients with a urinary catheter.

Hexylresorcinol

TRADE NAME:
Strepsils Extra.

DRUG CLASS:
Anaesthetic.

USES:
Sore throat and mouth.

DOSAGE:
 Use lozenges every two hours as required.

FORMS:
Lozenges.

PRECAUTIONS:
Safe in pregnancy and breast feeding. Not for use in children under 7 years.

SIDE EFFECTS:
Common: Mouth numbness.

INTERACTIONS:
None significant.

PRESCRIPTION:
No.

PBS:
No.

PERMITTED IN SPORT:
Yes.

OVERDOSE:
Unlikely to have any serious consequences if swallowed.
See also ANAESTHETICS, LOCAL.

HiB vaccine
See Haemophilus influenzae B Vaccine.

Homatropine hydrobromide
See MYDRIATICS.

HORMONE REPLACEMENT THERAPY (HRT)

DISCUSSION:

Concerns about the safety of hormone replacement therapy (HRT) relate to long term (greater than five years) use of combined (oestrogen and progestogen) HRT. Short term use for up to five years is still apparently safe and is used to control the symptoms of menopause (eg. hot flushes, dry vagina, aching).

Long term use needs to be weighed for each individual woman according to her risk factors for heart disease, osteoporosis, breast cancer, stroke and blood clot.

Every woman should assess her needs and risks on an individual basis after a discussion with her doctor.

BENEFITS:
- Improved sense of well being.
- Improved libido and vaginal lubrication.
- Breast shape retained for longer without drooping.
- Reduced risk of bowel cancer (risk decreases from 1.6 women in every 1000 developing bowel cancer in any one year to 1.0).
- Significantly reduced risk of osteoporosis (risk decreases from 1.5 women in every 1000 having a hip fracture from osteoporosis in any one year to 0.9).
- Improved skin quality and tone (fewer wrinkles).
- Improves mood and reduces irritability.

DISADVANTAGES:
- Increased risk of breast cancer if taken for more than four years (risk rises from

3.1 women in every 1000 developing breast cancer in any one year to 3.9).
- Increased risk of heart attacks if taken for more than four years (risk rises from 2.4 women in every 1000 having a heart attack in any one year to 3.1).
- Increased risk of blood clots in veins (leg blood clots) (risk rises from 1.1 women in every 1000 developing a blood clot in any one year to 2.9).
- Increased risk of stroke (risk rises from 1.9 women in every 1000 developing a stroke in any one year to 2.7).
- Breast tenderness and breakthrough bleeding in early stages of use.

Statistics are for postmenopausal women on combined oestrogen and progestogen HRT.

See Oestradiol; Oestriol; Oestrogen.

HORMONES, SEX

See Chorionic gonadotrophin, Cyproterone acetate, Danazol, Dydrogesterone, Ethinyloestradiol, Follicle stimulating hormone, Gestrinone, HORMONE REPLACEMENT THERAPY, Medroxyprogesterone acetate, Menopausal gonadotrophin, Mesterolone, Nafarelin, Oestradiol, Oestriol, Oestrogen, ORAL CONTRACEPTIVES, Oxandrolone, Piperazine oestrone sulfate, Testosterone.

HRT

See HORMONE REPLACEMENT THERAPY.

Human chorionic gonadotrophin

See Chorionic gonadotrophin, human.

Hyaluronidase

TRADE NAMES:

Hyalase.
Lasonil (with heparinoid).

USES:

Ointment: Blood clots in superficial veins, bruises, varicose ulcers, sprains and strains.
Injection: Aids diffusion of fluids through tissue.

DOSAGE:

Ointment: Two or three times a day.
Injection: As determined by doctor for each patient.

FORMS:

Ointment, injection.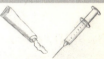

PRECAUTIONS:

Safe in pregnancy, breast feeding and children.

Do not use if:
 suffering from infection or cancer.
- do not use on bleeding wounds.
- not to be injected into a vein.

SIDE EFFECTS:

Minimal.

INTERACTIONS:

None significant.

PRESCRIPTION:

No.

PBS:

No.

PERMITTED IN SPORT:

Yes.

Hydralazine

TRADE NAMES:
Alphapress, Apresoline.

DRUG CLASS:
Antihypertensive.

USES:
High blood pressure, often in combination with other medications.
Particularly useful in the high blood pressure associated with pre-eclampsia of pregnancy.

DOSAGE:
One to four tablets twice a day to a maximum of 200mg per day.

FORMS:
Tablets of 25 and 50mg
Injection.

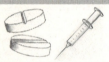

PRECAUTIONS:
Should not be used in first seven months of pregnancy (C), and only if medically necessary later in pregnancy. Safe in breast feeding. Should not be used in children.
Take with care if suffering from angina, recent heart attack, other heart diseases, recent stroke, kidney or liver disease.
Not for prolonged use.

Do not take if:
 Suffering from SLE (systemic lupus erythematosus), very rapid pulse, aortic aneurysm, heart failure, corpulmonale.

SIDE EFFECTS:
Common: Slowed reactions, rapid heart rate, palpitations, dizziness, flushing, low blood pressure, angina.
Unusual: Headaches, joint pains and swelling, muscle aches, nasal congestion, stomach upsets.
Severe but rare (stop medication, consult doctor): Unusual bleeding, irregular heartbeat.

INTERACTIONS:
Other drugs:
- Vasodilators, calcium channel blockers, ACE inhibitors, diuretics, other medications for high blood pressure, diazoxide, tricyclic antidepressants, tranquillisers, beta blockers, adrenaline, MAOI (monoamine oxidase inhibitors).

Other substances:
- Reacts adversely with alcohol.

PRESCRIPTION:
Yes.

PBS:
Yes.

PERMITTED IN SPORT:
Yes.

OVERDOSE:
Results in rapid heart rate, low blood pressure, dizziness, nausea, sweating, irregular heart rate, angina, heart attack and death. If taken recently induce vomiting. Seek urgent medical assistance.

OTHER INFORMATION:
Only used in the most severe and difficult forms of high blood pressure. Interacts with a wide range of other medications.

Hydrochlorothiazide

See THIAZIDE DIURETICS.

Hydrocortisone
(Cortisol)

TRADE NAMES:
Colifoam, Cortaid, Cortef, Cortic, Derm-Aid, Egocort, Hycor Eye Drops, Hysone, Sigmacort, Siguent Hycor Eye Ointment.
Ciproxin HC (with ciprofloxacin).
Fungocort (with miconazole).
Hydroform (with clioquinol).
Hydrozole (with clotrimazole).
Proctosedyl, Rectinol HC (with cinchocaine).
Solu-Cortef (Hydrocortisone sodium succinate).
Xyloproct (with lignocaine, aluminium acetate, zinc oxide).

DRUG CLASS:
Corticosteroid.

USES:
Inflammation of skin (eczema, dermatitis etc), anus (piles), rectum (ulcerative colitis), mouth (mouth ulcers), eyes and other tissues.

DOSAGE:

Cream and ointment: Apply three or four times a day.
Rectal foam: Insert twice a day initially, then every two days.
Suppositories: Insert up to three times a day initially, then reduce to once a day for up to three weeks.
Eye drops: Insert every two to four hours.
Eye ointment: Insert two to four times a day.
Ear drops: Three drops twice a day for one week.
Tablets: As directed by doctor.

FORMS:
Cream, ointment, foam, suppository, eye drops, eye ointment, ear drops, tablets, injection.

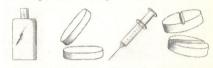

PRECAUTIONS:
Tablets, injections and rectal preparations should be used in pregnancy (C), breast feeding and children only on specific medical advice.
Skin and eye preparations safe in pregnancy, breast feeding and children over three years.
Use tablets, injections and rectal preparations with caution if under stress, and in patients with under-active thyroid gland, liver disease, diverticulitis, high blood pressure, myasthenia gravis, or kidney disease.
Avoid eyes with all forms except eye drops and ointment.
Do not use skin preparations for long periods in children.
Medication should not be ceased abruptly, but dosage should be slowly reduced.

Do not take if:
 suffering from infections, peptic ulcer, osteoporosis.
- having a vaccination.

Do not apply to:
- infected, fungally affected or ulcerated skin or other tissue unless combined with an antibiotic or antifungal.

SIDE EFFECTS:
Most significant side effects occur only with prolonged use of tablets, injections or rectal preparations.
Common: Tablets, injections and rectal preparations – Bloating, weight gain, rashes and intestinal disturbances.
Creams and ointments – Rarely cause adverse reactions.
Unusual: Tablets, injections and rectal

forms – Biochemical disturbances of blood, muscle weakness, bone weakness, impaired wound healing, skin thinning, tendon weakness, peptic ulcers, gullet ulcers, bruising, increased sweating, loss of fat under skin, premature ageing, excess facial hair growth in women, pigmentation of skin and nails, acne, convulsions, headaches, dizziness, growth suppression in children, aggravation of diabetes, worsening of infections, cataracts, aggravation of glaucoma, blood clots in veins and sleeplessness.
Severe but rare (stop medication, consult doctor): Any significant side effect should be reported to a doctor immediately.

INTERACTIONS:
Other drugs:
- Creams do not interact with other drugs.
- Tablets, injections and rectal preparations of hydrocortisone may be affected by oral contraceptives, barbiturates, phenytoin, and rifampicin.

Herbs:
- Liquorice.

PRESCRIPTION:
Yes.
Some weak strength creams and ointments do not require a prescription.

PBS:
Low strength creams, ointments, rectal preparations and combined preparations: No.
Medium and high strength creams and ointments, tablets and injections: Yes.

PERMITTED IN SPORT:
Rectal preparations, creams and ointments: Yes.
Other forms: No.

OVERDOSE:
Medical treatment is required. Serious effects and death rare.

OTHER INFORMATION:
Extremely effective and useful medication if used correctly. Safe to use on skin, but other forms must be used with extreme care under strict medical supervision. Lowest dose and shortest possible course should be used. Not addictive.

See also Betamethasone, Desonide, Methylprednisolone, Mometasone, Triamcinolone.

Hydrogen peroxide

TRADE NAMES:
Available under numerous locally produced trade names, and in combination with many other antiseptics.

DRUG CLASS:
Disinfectant.

USES:
Minor skin and mouth infections, removing slough from a wound, cleaning surgical instruments and contact lenses.

DOSAGE:

Apply or gargle three or four times a day.

FORMS:
Lotion, mouthwash, sterilising solution.

PRECAUTIONS:
Safe to use in pregnancy, breast feeding and children.
Avoid eyes.
Do not use for more than one month.

SIDE EFFECTS:
Minimal.

INTERACTIONS:
Other drugs: Iodine, permanganate.

PRESCRIPTION:
No.

Medications

PBS:
No.

PERMITTED IN SPORT:
Yes.

OVERDOSE:
Vomiting and diarrhoea only likely effects if swallowed.

OTHER INFORMATION:
Very old-fashioned, but still effective.

Hydromorphone

TRADE NAME:
Dilaudid.

DRUG CLASS:
Narcotic.

USES:
Relief of severe pain.

DOSAGE:

2 to 4mg every four hours as required.

FORMS:
Tablets of 2mg (orange), 4mg (yellow) and 8mg (white), liquid, injection.

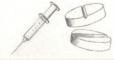

PRECAUTIONS:
Not for use in pregnancy, breast feeding and children.
Use with caution in under-active thyroid gland, severe lung disease, kidney or adrenal gland disease, and enlarged prostate gland.
Reduce dose in elderly.

Do not take if:
 suffering from poor lung function, in a coma, severe undiagnosed abdominal disease, head injury, convulsions, alcoholism.

SIDE EFFECTS:
Common: Constipation, nausea, vomiting, drowsiness.
Unusual: Tolerance and dependence, low blood pressure.
Severe but rare (stop medication, consult doctor): Reduced ability to breathe.

INTERACTIONS:
Other drugs:
- MAOI, sedatives, phenothiazines, some general anaesthetics.

Other substances:
- Alcohol.

PRESCRIPTION:
Yes.

PBS:
Yes (restricted)

PERMITTED IN SPORT:
No.

OVERDOSE:
Serious. Sedation, convulsions, coma and death may occur. Administer activated charcoal or induce vomiting if medication taken recently and patient alert. Seek emergency medical assistance. Antidote available.

OTHER INFORMATION:
Highly addictive if used inappropriately. Very effective and unlikely to cause addiction if used appropriately for severe pain. Patients with terminal diseases (eg. cancer) should use dose adequate to control pain, and not be concerned about possibility of addiction. Derived from opium poppy and closely related to heroin.

See also Alfentanil, Buprenorphine, Codeine Phosphate, Dextromoramide, Dextropropoxyphene, Fentanyl, Heroin, Methadone, Morphine, Oxycodone, Pentazocine, Pethidine.

Hydroquinone

TRADE NAME:
Only available in Australia in combination with other medications.
Superfade (with salicylic acid and other ingredients).

USES:
Fades dark skin blemishes, excessive skin pigmentation.

DOSAGE:

After testing on small patch for one day to check for sensitivity, apply twice a day.

FORMS:
Cream.

PRECAUTIONS:
Safe for use in pregnancy, breast feeding and children over 6 years.
Avoid eye contact.
Do not expose treated area to bright sun light.
Use with care on sensitive skin.
Apply to pigmented area only.
Seek medical advice if no response in ten days.

Do not use on:
 skin cancers, melanoma, moles, irritated or damaged skin.
- skin near eyes.

SIDE EFFECTS:
Minimal. Occasional skin sensitivity.

INTERACTIONS:
None significant.

PRESCRIPTION:
No.

PBS:
No.

PERMITTED IN SPORT:
Yes.

OTHER INFORMATION:
Important not to treat moles that may be cancerous. If a dark spot or patch fails to respond it may be a cancerous area. If in doubt, seek medical advice.

Hydroxocobalamin
(Vitamin B12)

TRADE NAME:
Neo-Cytamen.
A large number of other preparations include various forms of Vitamin B12 alone or in combination with other medications.

DRUG CLASS:
Vitamin.

USES:
Pernicious anaemia, pins and needles sensation of feet, some eye disorders (optic neuropathy).

DOSAGE:

Injection: Once every three months, or as determined by doctor.
Recommended daily allowance: 2µg a day.

FORMS:
Tablets, capsules, mixture, drops, injection.
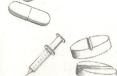

PRECAUTIONS:
Safe in pregnancy, breast feeding and children.
Do not take in high doses or for prolonged periods of time.
Use with caution in polycythaemia vera.

Medications

SIDE EFFECTS:
Common: Minimal.
Unusual: Low blood potassium, diarrhoea, itch, swelling sensation.
Severe but rare (stop medication, consult doctor): Blood clot in vein.

INTERACTIONS:
Other drugs:
- Oral contraceptives, chloramphenicol, folic acid.

PRESCRIPTION:
No.

PBS:
Injection: Yes.
Other forms: No.

PERMITTED IN SPORT:
Yes.

OVERDOSE:
Unlikely to cause any serious effects.

OTHER INFORMATION:
Several chemical variations of Vitamin B12 exist including Cyanocobalamin and Hydroxycobalamin. They are identical in their actions and use. Cyanocobalamin was the original form of Vitamin B12 used medically. Vitamin B12 is a water soluble vitamin found in animal products. It is essential for the formation of red blood cells, normal growth, and normal fat and sugar metabolism. In pernicious anaemia, the body loses the ability to absorb vitamin B12 from the stomach. Remember, vitamins are merely chemicals that are essential for the functioning of the body, and if taken to excess, act as a drug.
See also Cyanocobalamin.

Hydroxychloroquine

TRADE NAME:
Plaquenil.

DRUG CLASS:
Antirheumatic, antimalarial.

USES:
Rheumatoid arthritis, systemic lupus erythematosus (SLE), prevention and treatment of malaria.

DOSAGE:
 Rheumatoid and SLE: One tablet two or three times a day with meals.
Malaria prevention: Two tablets a week.
Malaria treatment: Four tablets at once, two tablets eight hours later, then two tablets a day for a further two days.

FORMS:
Tablets (white) of 200mg.

PRECAUTIONS:
Not to be used in pregnancy (D) as the foetus may be damaged. Use with caution in breast feeding and children.
Do not use long term in children.
Use with caution in severe brain disease, severe intestinal disease, porphyria, psoriasis, liver disease and alcoholism.
Exposure to sunlight while taking higher doses may cause excessive sunburn or rash.
Regular eye checks for damage to cornea or retina required if used long term.

Do not take if:
 suffering from macular eye damage.

SIDE EFFECTS:
Common: Rash, itching, dry skin, nausea.
Unusual: Vomiting, loss of appetite, belly cramps.
Severe but rare (stop medication, consult doctor): Blurred vision, unusual bleeding or bruising.

INTERACTIONS:
Other drugs:
- MAOI, digoxin.

PRESCRIPTION:
Yes.

PBS:
Yes.

PERMITTED IN SPORT:
Yes.

OVERDOSE:
Very serious. Causes severe liver damage. Symptoms include headache, blurred vision, convulsions, heart failure and death. Administer activated charcoal or induce vomiting if medication taken recently. Seek emergency medical treatment.

OTHER INFORMATION:
Quinine from the bark of the South American chincona tree has been used to treat malaria for centuries. Hydroxychloroquine is derived from quinine. Found serendipitously to control some rheumatoid conditions, and with most forms of malaria now being resistant to Quinine derivatives, it is now used for this purpose far more often than for malaria. Does not cause addiction or dependence.

See also Artemether and Lumefantrine, Atovaquone, Chloroquine, Doxycycline, Mefloquine, Primaquine, Proguanil, Pyrimethamine, Quinine, Sulfadoxine.

Hydroxyethylcellulose
See EYE LUBRICANTS.

Hydroxyethylrutosides

TRADE NAME:
Paroven.

USES:
Poor arterial and venous circulation, swelling of ankles and other tissue, varicose veins, tired aching legs.

DOSAGE:

500 to 1000mg a day in divided doses.

FORMS:
Tablets of 500mg (green/yellow), capsules of 250mg (yellow).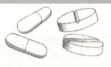

PRECAUTIONS:
Safe in all but first three months of pregnancy. Use with caution in breast feeding.
Eat diet high in fibre and protein.

SIDE EFFECTS:
Common: Nausea, indigestion.
Unusual: Constipation, diarrhoea, headache, light headedness, flushing, rash.

INTERACTIONS:
Other drugs:
- Calcium channel blockers (used for high blood pressure and heart disease).

PRESCRIPTION:
No.

PBS:
No.

PERMITTED IN SPORT:
Yes.

OVERDOSE:
Constipation only likely effect.

Medications

OTHER INFORMATION:
Successfully used for tired aching legs, particularly in women who must stand for a long period of time in their work. Very safe. Does not cause dependence.

Hydroxypropylcellulose
See EYE LUBRICANTS.

Hydroxyquinolone
See Acetic acid.

Hydroxyurea

TRADE NAME:
Hydrea.

USES:
Leukaemia, melanoma, cancer of the ovary.

DOSAGE:
 Must be individualised by doctor for each patient depending on disease, severity and weight of patient.

FORMS:
Capsules (aqua/pink) of 500mg.

PRECAUTIONS:
Must not be used in pregnancy (D) unless mother's life is at risk as damage to foetus may occur. Breast feeding must be ceased before use. May be used in children if medically essential.
Regular blood and bone marrow tests to check levels of blood and marrow cells and liver function essential.
Adequate contraception must be used by women while hydroxyurea is being taken. Use with caution in AIDS, kidney and liver disease.

Do not take if:
 suffering from anaemia or bone marrow damage.

SIDE EFFECTS:
Common: Mouth soreness and ulcers, nausea, loss of appetite, vomiting, diarrhoea, rash.
Unusual: Hair loss.
Severe but rare (stop medication, consult doctor): Yellow skin (jaundice).

INTERACTIONS:
Other drugs:
• Other treatments for cancer, allopurinol.

PRESCRIPTION:
Yes.

PBS:
Yes.

PERMITTED IN SPORT:
Yes.

OVERDOSE:
Serious. Induce vomiting if medication taken recently. Seek urgent medical assistance.

Hylan

TRADE NAME:
Synvisc.

USES:
Adds to level of synovial fluid in knee joint to give pain relief in osteoarthritis of the knee.

DOSAGE:
 Weekly injections into knee for three weeks, followed by top up injections every one to six months as necessary.

FORMS:
Injection.

PRECAUTIONS:
Use with caution in pregnancy and children.
To be injected into joint space only.
Use with caution if blood supply to leg poor and severe varicose veins.

Do not take if:

 suffering from poor lymphatic or blood drainage from leg, infected or inflamed joint, large fluid collection in knee joint.
- allergic to birds.

SIDE EFFECTS:
Common: Temporary pain and swelling of knee joint.
Severe but rare: Joint infection.

INTERACTIONS:
None significant.

PRESCRIPTION:
No.

PBS:
No (expensive).

PERMITTED IN SPORT:
Yes.

OTHER INFORMATION:
Expensive artificial joint fluid released onto market in 1999.

Hyoscine and Hyoscyamine

TRADE NAMES:
Buscopan, Kwells, Setacol, Travacalm HO.
Atrobel, Donnalix, Donnatab (with atropine).
Donnagel (with kaolin, pectin, atropine, ethanol, hydroxybenzoate and other ingredients).
Travacalm (with caffeine, dimenhydrinate).

DRUG CLASS:
Anticholinergic (dries secretions).
Spasmolytic (eases intestinal spasms).
Antiemetic (prevents nausea and vomiting).

USES:
Irritable bowel syndrome, gut spasms and colic, prevents motion sickness, dries excess nasal secretions.

DOSAGE:
10 to 20mg two to four times a day.

FORMS:
Tablets, capsules, mixture and injection.

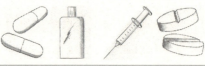

PRECAUTIONS:
Should be used with caution in pregnancy (B2) and breast feeding.
Use with caution in eye diseases that cause vision problems.

Do not take if:

 suffering from glaucoma, myasthenia gravis, megacolon, enlarged prostate, porphyria, rapid irregular heart rhythm.

SIDE EFFECTS:
Common: Drowsiness, dry mouth, reduced sweating.
Unusual: Rapid heart rate, difficulty in passing urine, dilated pupil, drowsiness.
Severe but rare (stop medication, consult doctor): Hallucinations, confusion, muscle spasm.

INTERACTIONS:
Other drugs:
- Dry mouth and drowsiness worsen if used with tricyclic antidepressants, amantadine, quinidine, antihistamines, phenothiazines and monoamine oxidase inhibitors (MAOI).
- Rapid heart rate worsens if used with beta blockers.

Other substances:
- Reacts with alcohol to cause excessive drowsiness.

PRESCRIPTION:
No.

PBS:
No.

PERMITTED IN SPORT:
Yes.

OVERDOSE:
No serious effects reported. Induce vomiting. Doctors would use stomach washout and activated charcoal.
See also Atropine, Dicyclomine, Mebeverine, Propantheline.

Hypericum perforatum
See Saint John's Wort.

HYPNOTICS AND SEDATIVES
(Sedate and induce sleep)
See BARBITURATES, Chlormethiazole, Flunitrazepam, Midazolam, Nitrazepam, Temazepam, Triazolam, Zolpidem, Zopiclone.

HYPOGLYCAEMICS

DISCUSSION:
Hypoglycaemics are drugs that lower the level of sugar (glucose) in the bloodstream of diabetics by allowing the sugar to cross the membrane surrounding a cell and to enter the interior of the cell. They are used mainly in the maturity onset (type 2) form of diabetes. Alteration to the dosage of all types of hypoglycaemics may be required with changes in exercise, or diet, surgery or the occurrence of other illnesses, particularly if a fever is present. A doctor should be consulted immediately in these situations. As well as treatment with hypoglycaemics, all diabetics must remain on an appropriate diet for the rest of their lives. Regular blood tests and urine tests are essential for the adequate control of all forms of diabetes. Some patients now use small machines the size of a thick credit card to test their own blood sugar.

Hypoglycaemics fall into two main groups – tablets and injections. Insulin, which is normally produced by the pancreas to transport sugar across the cell membrane, can only be given by injection, and is invariably required in type 1 diabetes which has its onset in children and young adults. Maturity onset (type 2) diabetes has its onset in the middle-aged and elderly, and is normally treated by hypoglycaemic tablets and diet, but sometimes insulin is also required.

See Acarbose, Glibenclamide, Gliclazide, Glimepride, Glipizide, INSULINS, Metformin, Pioglitazone, Repaglinide, Rosiglitazone, Tolbutamide.

HYPOLIPIDAEMIC

DISCUSSION:
The term 'hypo' means low (as opposed to 'hyper', meaning high), lipids are fats, and the term 'aemia' refers to the blood (compare 'anaemia' – lack of blood), so a hypolipidaemic is a drug that lowers fat in the blood. The fats include both cholesterol and triglycerides. An excess of either, or both, of these in the bloodstream can cause serious diseases such as strokes and heart attacks. A combination of diet and drugs are used to control excess levels of fat in the bloodstream. Diet alone may be sufficient in many patients.

See Atorvastatin, Cholestyramine, Colestipol, Fluvastatin, Gemfibrizol, Nicotinic acid, Pravastatin, Probucol, Simvastatin.

Hypromellose
See EYE LUBRICANTS.

Ibuprofen

TRADE NAMES:
Act-3, Actiprofen, Brufen, Bugesic, Nurofen, Rafen, Tri-Profen.
Dimetapp Headcold and Flu, Nurofen Cold & Flu, Sudafed Congestion and Sinus Pain, Triprofen Cold and Flu (with pseudoephedrine).

DRUG CLASS:
NSAID (Nonsteroidal anti-inflammatory drug).

USES:
All forms of arthritis, back pain, period pain, migraine, general pain relief, fevers.

DOSAGE:

Tablets and capsules: One or two tablets, one to four times a day with food.
Gel: Rub into affected area three or four times a day for up to two weeks.

FORMS:
Tablets, capsules, mixture, gel.

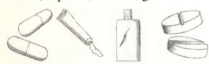

PRECAUTIONS:
Use with caution in pregnancy (C) and breast feeding.
May be used in children.
Gel safe in pregnancy.
Use tablets and capsules with caution in asthma, dehydration, high blood pressure, severe infection, heart failure and kidney disease.
Lower doses required in elderly, who may suffer more side effects.

Do not take if:

suffering from peptic ulcer at present or in recent past.
- sensitive to anti-inflammatories or aspirin.
- due for surgery (including dental surgery).
- suffering from bleeding disorder or anaemia.

SIDE EFFECTS:
Common: Stomach discomfort, diarrhoea, constipation, heartburn, nausea, headache, dizziness.
Unusual: Blurred vision, stomach ulcer, ringing noise in ears, retention of fluid, swelling of tissue, drowsiness, itch, rash, shortness of breath.
Severe but rare (stop medication, consult doctor): Vomiting blood, passing blood in faeces, other unusual bleeding, asthma induced by medication.

INTERACTIONS:
Other drugs:
- Must never be used with anticoagulants (eg. warfarin).
- Probenecid, diuretics, lithium, methotrexate, beta blockers, ACE inhibitors.
- Gel has minimal interactions.

PRESCRIPTION:
Low strength preparations and skin applications: No.
High strength preparations: Yes.

PBS:
Prescription tablets: Yes.
Gel: No.
Low strength non-prescription forms: No.

PERMITTED IN SPORT:
Yes.

OVERDOSE:
Causes nausea, vomiting, severe headache, dizziness, confusion and convulsions. Administer activated charcoal or induce vomiting if taken recently. Seek medical assistance.

OTHER INFORMATION:

Extensively used to give excellent relief to a wide variety of inflammatory and pain conditions. Significant side effects (particularly on the stomach) in about 5% of patients limit their use. Specially coated forms reduce side effects. Minimal side effects with gel, but less effective.

See also Aspirin, Bufexamac, Celecoxib, Diclofenac, Diflunisal, Flurbiprofen, Indomethacin, Ketoprofen, Ketorolac trometanol, Mefenamic Acid, Naproxen, Piroxicam, Rofecoxib, Salicylic acid, Sulindac, Tenoxicam, Tiaprofenic Acid.

Ichthammol

TRADE NAMES:
Egoderm Cream, Ichthammol Ointment.
Egoderm Ointment (with zinc oxide, allantoin and other ingredients).

USES:
Skin inflammation, eczema.

DOSAGE:
Apply two or three times a day.

FORMS:
Cream, ointment.

PRECAUTIONS:
Safe in pregnancy, breast feeding and children.

SIDE EFFECTS:
Minimal.

INTERACTIONS:
None significant

PRESCRIPTION:
No.

PBS:
No.

PERMITTED IN SPORT:
Yes.

Idarubicin

TRADE NAME:
Zavedos.

DRUG CLASS:
Cytotoxic.

USES:
Leukaemia.

DOSAGE:
 As determined for each patient by doctor.

FORMS:
Capsules of 5mg (red/orange), 10mg (red/orange) and 25mg (white). Injection.

PRECAUTIONS:
Not to be used in pregnancy (D). Use with caution in breast feeding. May be used in children.
Use with caution in heart disease and bone marrow suppression.
Use with caution if receiving radiotherapy.
Regular blood tests essential to check liver, kidney and blood cell function.
Use with care if driving or operating machinery.

Do not take if:
 suffering from severe liver or kidney disease, uncontrolled infection, recent heart attack, or irregular heart rhythm.

SIDE EFFECTS:
Common: Nausea, vomiting, mouth inflammation, belly pain, diarrhoea, loss of hair, rash.
Unusual: Heart damage, itch, redness of palms and soles, kidney and liver damage, ankle swelling.
Severe but rare (stop medication, consult doctor): Abnormal bleeding, abnormal heart rhythm, significant infection.

Medications

INTERACTIONS:
Other drugs:
- Other medications used to treat leukaemia.

PRESCRIPTION:
Yes.

PBS:
Yes.

PERMITTED IN SPORT:
Yes.

OVERDOSE:
Significant heart damage possible, aggravation of side effects likely. Induce vomiting or administer activated charcoal if capsules taken recently. seek urgent medical attention.

Idoxuridine

TRADE NAMES:
Stoxil.
Virasolve (with lignocaine and benzalkonium).

DRUG CLASS:
Antiviral.

USES:
Cold sores.

DOSAGE:
 Apply every one to four hours.

FORMS:
Cream, solution, ointment.

PRECAUTIONS:
Use with caution in pregnancy (B3), breast feeding and infants. May be used in children.
 Do not take internally or use in eyes.
Use with caution if sore has a secondary bacterial infection.

SIDE EFFECTS:
Common: Minimal.
Unusual: Irritation of skin.

INTERACTIONS:
Other drugs:
- Boric acid.

PRESCRIPTION:
No.

PBS:
No.

PERMITTED IN SPORT:
Yes.

OTHER INFORMATION:
Very effective medication, but must be used on cold sores immediately any sign of infection present.
See also Aciclovir.

Imatinib

TRADE NAME:
Glivec.

DRUG CLASS:
Antineoplastic.

USES:
Chronic myeloid leukaemia.

DOSAGE:
 Complex. Determined by doctor for each patient.

FORMS:
Capsules of 100mg (grey/white).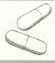

PRECAUTIONS:
Not for use in pregnancy (D) or breast feeding. Use with caution in children.
Use with caution in liver and kidney disease. Regular blood tests necessary to check for toxic effects.

SIDE EFFECTS:
Common: Nausea, diarrhoea, muscle pains and cramps, bloating.
Unusual: Fluid retention, rash, headache, tiredness, joint pains, fever.
Severe but rare (stop medication, consult doctor): Gut bleeding, stroke, blood cell damage.

INTERACTIONS:
Other drugs:
- Ketoconazole, erythromycin, clarithromycin, itraconazole, antivirals, dexamethasone, phenytoin, carbamazepine, rifampicin, phenobarbitone, warfarin.

Other substances:
- Grapefruit juice.

PRESCRIPTION:
Yes.

PBS:
Yes (authority required – very restricted).

PERMITTED IN SPORT:
Yes.

OVERDOSE:
Serious, but minimal information available. Induce vomiting or give activated charcoal if taken recently. Seek urgent medical attention.

IMIDAZOLES
See Clotrimazole, Econazole, Fluconazole, Itraconazole, Ketoconazole, Miconazole.

Imipenem
See Cilastin and Imipenem.

Imipramine
See TRICYCLIC ANTIDEPRESSANTS.

Imiquimod

TRADE NAME:
Aldara.

DRUG CLASS:
Immunomodifier.

USES:
Treatment of genital and anal warts, and condylomata accuminata.
Unapproved use includes treatment of basal cell carcinomas (skin cancer).

DOSAGE:

Apply three times a week at night and leave on for six to 10 hours.

FORMS:
Cream.

PRECAUTIONS:
Use with caution in pregnancy (B1), breast feeding and children.
Use with care in vagina and anal canal. Avoid inflamed skin.
Remove cream before sexual contact.
Uncircumcised men should wash under foreskin daily.
Do not cover treated warts with a bandage.
Use for no more than four months.

Do not take if:
 suffering from HIV, AIDS or impaired immunity.

SIDE EFFECTS:
Common: Skin irritation and redness, swelling of tissue.
Unusual: Ulceration and scabbing of skin, burning skin pain, headache.

INTERACTIONS:
Condoms and diaphragms.

PRESCRIPTION:
Yes.

PBS:
No.

PERMITTED IN SPORT:
Yes.

OTHER INFORMATION:
Released in 1999 as a radical and effective new way to treat a very distressing problem that previously often required minor surgery. Being used experimentally to treat some forms of skin cancer.

IMMUNOGLOBULINS

GENERIC NAMES:
Immunoglobulins against cytomegalovirus (CMV), hepatitis B, rabies, rhesus factor (anti-D), rotavirus (causes diarrhoea), tetanus and zoster (chickenpox and shingles) are available as well as pooled normal human immunoglobulin (see gamma globulin).

USES:
Prevention and treatment of specific diseases or as a boost to patients with a deficient immune system.

DOSAGE:

Depends on disease and individual patient requirements.

FORMS:
Injection.

PRECAUTIONS:
May be used in pregnancy, breast feeding and children.
Should only be used when strictly medically indicated.
Caution must be used with repeat doses.

SIDE EFFECTS:
Common: Tenderness at injection site.
Unusual: Fever, tiredness, belly discomfort, flush, headache, rash, itch, shortness of breath, nausea.

INTERACTIONS:
Other drugs:
• Vaccines.

PRESCRIPTION:
Yes.

PBS:
No. Only available through blood banks or hospitals.

PERMITTED IN SPORT:
Yes.

OVERDOSE:
Inadvertent additional dose may cause allergy reaction (sometimes serious) or exacerbation of side effects.

OTHER INFORMATION:
Purified from blood donations.
See also Gamma Globulin.

IMMUNOMODIFIERS

DISCUSSION:
Immunomodifiers are used to suppress (control or reduce) the immune reaction that occurs after the transplantation of foreign tissue into a body. They may also be used in the treatment of some types of cancer and defects in immunity that allow a few rare diseases to arise within the body. They are the drugs that have made kidney, liver, heart and other transplants possible, as the body normally uses its immune system to reject these donated organs.

See Azathioprine, Cyclosporin, Imiquimod, Interferon, Sirolimus.

IMPOTENCE DRUGS

See Alprostadil, Sildenafil, Tadalafil.

Indapamide

TRADE NAMES:
Dapa-Tabs, GenRx Indapamide, Indahexal, Insig, Napamide, Natrilix. Coversyl Plus (with perindopril).

DRUG CLASS:
Diuretic (increases urine production).

USES:
High blood pressure.

DOSAGE:
 One tablet in morning.

FORMS:
Tablets.

PRECAUTIONS:
Should only be used in pregnancy (C) and breast feeding if medically essential. Not for use in children.
Use with caution in systemic lupus erythematosus (SLE), kidney and liver disease. Regular blood tests necessary to check for irregularities in blood chemistry (electrolytes).

Do not take if:
 suffering from severe kidney or liver disease.

SIDE EFFECTS:
Common: Tiredness, dizziness, headache, muscle cramps, diarrhoea.
Unusual: Rash, impotence, sleeplessness, nausea, gout.
Severe but rare (stop medication, consult doctor): Fainting.

INTERACTIONS:
Other drugs: Barbiturates, narcotics, lithium, other diuretics.
Herbs: Celery, dandelion, uva ursi.
Other substances: Reacts adversely with alcohol.

PRESCRIPTION:
Yes.

PBS:
Yes.

PERMITTED IN SPORT:
No (acts as masking agent for other illegal drugs).

OVERDOSE:
No serious effect. Induce vomiting if taken recently.

OTHER INFORMATION:
Often used in combination with other blood pressure medications to increase their effect. Work by increasing output of urine.
See also Amiloride, Bumetanide, Ethacrynic Acid, Frusemide, Spironolactone, THIAZIDE DIURETICS.

Indinavir

TRADE NAME:
Crixivan.

DRUG CLASS:
Antiviral.

USES:
AIDS, HIV infection.

DOSAGE:
 Up to 800mg three times a day. Often combined with other therapy.

FORMS:
Capsules (white) of 100mg, 200mg and 400mg.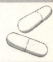

PRECAUTIONS:
Use with considerable caution in pregnancy (B3), breast feeding and children.
Use lower dose in elderly.
Use with caution in liver disease and diabetes.
Ensure adequate fluid intake.

SIDE EFFECTS:

Common: Nausea, diarrhoea, headache and others.
Unusual: Vomiting, kidney stones, liver damage causing jaundice.
Severe but rare (stop medication, consult doctor): Anaemia.

INTERACTIONS:

Other drugs:
- Serious interaction with astemizole, alprazolam, cisapride, triazolam, midazolam, pimozide.
- Calcium channel blockers, didanosine, erythromycin, ketoconazole, itraconazole, efavirenz, sildenafil, rifabutin, rifampicin, SSRI.

Herbs:
- St John's wort.

Other substances:
- Grapefruit.

PRESCRIPTION:
Yes.

PBS:
Yes (authority required – very restricted).

PERMITTED IN SPORT:
Yes.

See **Abacavir, Delavirdine, Didanosine, Efavirenz, Lamivudine, Nelfinavir, Nevirapine, Ritonavir, Saquinavir, Stavudine, Tenofovir, Zidovudine.**

Indomethacin

TRADE NAMES:
Arthrexin, Indocid.

DRUG CLASS:
NSAID (Nonsteroidal anti-inflammatory drug).

USES:
All forms of arthritis, inflammatory disorders, gout, back pain, ankylosing spondylitis, bone pain, period pain, correction of heart defect (patent ductus arteriosus) in premature infants.

DOSAGE:
 50 to 200mg a day in divided doses.

FORMS:
Capsules, injection.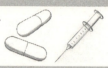

PRECAUTIONS:
Should not be used in pregnancy (C) unless medically essential. Breast feeding should be ceased if necessary to use NSAID. Not for use in children under 2. Use tablets and capsules with caution in psychiatrically disturbed patients, epilepsy, severe infection, heart failure and kidney disease.
Lower doses required in elderly, who may suffer more side effects.

Do not take if:
 suffering from peptic ulcer at present or in recent past.
- due for surgery (including dental surgery).
- suffering from bleeding disorder or anaemia.

SIDE EFFECTS:

Common: Stomach discomfort, diarrhoea, constipation, heartburn, nausea, headache, dizziness.
Unusual: Blurred vision, stomach ulcer, ringing noise in ears, retention of fluid, swelling of tissue, drowsiness, itch, rash, shortness of breath.
Severe but rare (stop medication, consult doctor): Vomiting blood, passing blood in faeces, other unusual bleeding, asthma induced by medication.

INTERACTIONS:

Other drugs:
- Must never be used with anticoagulants (eg. warfarin).
- Probenecid, diuretics, lithium, methotrexate, beta blockers, ACE inhibitors.

Herbs:
- Feverfew.

Medications

PRESCRIPTION:
Yes.

PBS:
Yes.

PERMITTED IN SPORT:
Yes.

OVERDOSE:
Causes nausea, vomiting, severe headache, dizziness, confusion and convulsions. Administer activated charcoal or induce vomiting if taken recently. Seek medical assistance.

OTHER INFORMATION:
One of the original NSAIDs, and available for nearly 50 years. Extensively used to give excellent relief to a wide variety of inflammatory conditions. Significant side effects (particularly on the stomach) in about 5% of patients limit their use.

See also Aspirin, Bufexamac, Celecoxib, Diclofenac, Diflunisal, Flurbiprofen, Ibuprofen, Ketoprofen, Ketorolac trometanol, Mefenamic Acid, Naproxen, Piroxicam, Rofecoxib, Salicylic acid, Sulindac, Tenoxicam, Tiaprofenic Acid.

Influenza virus vaccine

TRADE NAMES:
Fluarix, Fluvax, Fluvirin, Influvac, Vaxigrip.

DRUG CLASS:
Vaccine.

USES:
Prevention of influenza.

DOSAGE:

One injection in autumn every year. Two injections a month apart for first vaccination if under 18 years.

FORMS:
Injection.

PRECAUTIONS:
Not designed to be used in pregnancy (B2), but no adverse effects expected if vaccination given inadvertently. May be used in breast feeding. Use in children only if specifically indicated.
Use with caution in Guillain-Barré syndrome and AIDS.

Do not take if:
 suffering from fever.
- allergic to eggs, poultry products, neomycin, polymyxin or gentamicin.

SIDE EFFECTS:
Common: Local discomfort and redness at injection site.
Unusual: Fever, muscle pain.
Severe but rare: Vomiting, dizziness, rash, blood vessel inflammation, arthritis.

INTERACTIONS:
Other drugs:
- Theophylline, warfarin, phenytoin.

PRESCRIPTION:
Yes.

PBS:
Yes (seasonal).

PERMITTED IN SPORT:
Yes.

OVERDOSE:
An inadvertent additional dose is unlikely to cause any serious effects.

OTHER INFORMATION:
Influenza vaccine gives only limited protection, but this increases with subsequent doses. It should be given to persons over 65 years, persons with debilitating illness, persons with chronic diseases (eg. of the lung, heart, kidneys etc.), persons undergoing immunotherapy, and health and medical personnel. Formulation varies every year to match the strains of flu virus present in the community.

INSULINS

TRADE and GENERIC NAMES:
ASPART INSULIN – Onset of action, 30–60 minutes; peak action, four hours; duration, 6–10 hours.
NovoMix 30, NovoRapid.
NEUTRAL INSULIN – Onset of action, 30–60 minutes; peak action, four hours; duration, 6–10 hours.
Actrapid, Actrapid Novolet, Actrapid Penfill, Hypurin Neutral, Humulin R.
ISOPHANE INSULIN – Onset of action, 2–4 hours; peak action, 4–12 hours; duration, 24 hours.
Humulin NPH, Hypurin Isophane, Protaphane.
LENTE INSULIN (INSULIN zinc SUSPENSION) – Onset of action, three hours; peak action, 6–10 hours; duration, 24 hours.
Humulin L, Monotard.
ULTRALENTE INSULIN (CRYSTALLINE INSULIN ZINC SUSPENSION) – Onset of action, 4–6 hours; peak action, 10–30 hours; duration, 24–36 hours.
Humulin UL, Ultratard.
LISPRO INSULIN – Onset of action, 15 minutes; peak action, 1 hour; duration, 3.5–4.5 hours.
Humalog, Humalog Mix25.
BIPHASIC INSULIN (mixture of neutral insulin and isophane insulin) – Onset of action, 30–60 min.; peak action, 4–12 hours; duration, 24 hours.
Humulin 20/80, Humulin 30/70, Humulin 50/50, Mixtard 20/80, Mixtard 30/70, Mixtard 50/50.

USES:
Diabetes mellitus.

DOSAGE:

As determined by doctor or patient depending on blood sugar levels. Varies from one individual to another, and depends on food intake and exercise.

FORMS:
Injection, injection pens.

PRECAUTIONS:
Safe to use in pregnancy (A), breast feeding and children.
Pregnancy, illness, infections, change in diet, exercise and stress may cause change in insulin requirements.
Regular monitoring of blood sugar levels essential.
Knowledge of dietary requirements by patient essential.
Vary site of insulin injection.
Relatives and close friends should be made aware of symptoms of hypoglycaemia (low blood sugar) and first aid requirements.
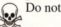 Do not inject into vein.

SIDE EFFECTS:
Common: Minimal.
Unusual: Low blood sugar, loss of fat at site of regular injection.

INTERACTIONS:

Other drugs:
- Corticosteroids, thiazides, frusemide, ethacrynic acid, protamine, isoniazid, phenothiazines, salbutamol, phenytoin, anabolic steroids, ACE inhibitors, sulfonamides, oral contraceptives, thyroxine, MAOI, salicylates, beta blockers.

Herbs:
- Ginseng, karela.

Other substances:
- Alcohol may increase need for insulin.

PRESCRIPTION:
Yes.

PBS:
Yes.

PERMITTED IN SPORT:
Yes.

OVERDOSE:
Very serious. Symptoms of low blood sugar (hypoglycaemia) may include tiredness, confusion, palpitations, sweating, vomiting, dizziness, hunger, blurred vision and fainting. Significant overdosage can lead rapidly to coma and death. Give sugary drinks or sweets if conscious. Seek emergency medical assistance.

OTHER INFORMATION:
Insulin is a natural hormone that is essential for the transport of sugar from the blood stream into the cells of the body. It is produced in the pancreas, which lies in the centre of the belly. For the past 70 years, insulin has been derived from the pancreas of cattle or pigs since it was originally identified and isolated by the Canadian doctors, Banting and Best. Because it was derived from animals, there were occasional reactions to the foreign animal protein present in the insulin. In the last few years, genetically engineered human insulin has almost totally replaced the animal insulin. The new form causes virtually no adverse reaction after injection.

Interferon

TRADE NAMES:
Avonex, Betaferon, Imukin, Intron A, Rebif, Roferon A.
Rebetron (with ribavirin).

DRUG CLASS:
Immunomodifier.

USES:
Some types of leukaemia, genital warts, some skin cancers, multiple myeloma, multiple sclerosis, AIDS, hepatitis B and C and several other rare diseases.

DOSAGE:

Depends on disease and patient's condition. Must be individualised by doctor.

FORMS:
Injection.

PRECAUTIONS:
Should not be used in pregnancy (C) unless medically essential as risk of miscarriage increased. Breast feeding should be ceased before use. Use with considerable caution in children.
Use with caution in heart disease, liver and kidney disease, psychiatric conditions and psoriasis.
Ensure adequate fluid intake.
Regular medical check-ups essential.

Do not take if:
- suffering from severe liver disease or some autoimmune disease (check with doctor).
- if a transplanted organ recipient.

SIDE EFFECTS:
Common: Fever, fatigue, headache, muscle pain, chills, loss of appetite, nausea, backache, joint pains, rash.
Unusual: Dry mouth, altered taste, low blood pressure, vomiting, diarrhoea, dizziness, confusion, sleeplessness, depression, hair loss, sweating.

Medications

INTERACTIONS:
Other drugs:
- Narcotics, hypnotics, sedatives, theophylline.

Other substances:
- Alcohol.

PRESCRIPTION:
Yes.

PBS:
Yes (authority required – restricted to specific diseases).

PERMITTED IN SPORT:
Yes.

OVERDOSE:
Exacerbation of side effects likely.

OTHER INFORMATION:
Wide range of uses from serious exotic diseases to use by general practitioners to treat skin cancers. Once hailed as a miracle cure-all drug when introduced in the early 1980s. Very useful when prescribed appropriately.

INTRA-UTERINE DEVICE
See Levonorgestrel.

IODINE

TRADE and GENERIC NAMES:
Betadine, EDP, Hexal PI, Microshield PVP, Minidine, Savlon Antiseptic Powder, Viodine (povidone-iodine). Other forms of iodine are found in numerous non-prescription antiseptics, mineral and vitamin supplements.

DRUG CLASS:
Antiseptic, mineral.

USES:
Prevention and treatment of minor bacterial, viral and fungal infections of skin, mouth and vagina.
Iodine deficiency.

DOSAGE:

Recommended daily allowance: 120 to 150µg a day.
Skin preparations: Apply several times a day as needed.

FORMS:
Iodine: Capsules, tablets, mixture.

Povidone-iodine: Cream, gargle, lotion, ointment, pads, paint, powder, scrub, spray, swabs.

PRECAUTIONS:
Safe for use in pregnancy, breast feeding and children.
Not for use on premature infants.
Do not use if:
 sensitive to Iodine

SIDE EFFECTS:
None significant.

Medications

INTERACTIONS:
None significant.

PRESCRIPTION:
No.

PBS:
No. Some forms available to Veteran Affairs pensioners.

PERMITTED IN SPORT:
Yes.

OVERDOSE:
May cause diarrhoea and stomach upsets if significant amount swallowed.

OTHER INFORMATION:
Widely used, safe and effective. Small number of people are excessively sensitive to Iodine.

See also Sodium iodide.

Ipratropium bromide

TRADE NAMES:
Apoven, Atrovent, Ipratrin, Ipravent. Combivent (with salbutamol).
Numerous locally produced and marketed forms of ipratropium also exist.

DRUG CLASS:
Bronchodilator.

USES:
Prevention of asthma and hay fever, chronic lung disease.

DOSAGE:

Asthma spray: Two inhalations three or four times a day.
Nose spray: Two sprays into each nostril two to four times a day.

FORMS:
Inhaler, nebuliser solution, nasal spray.

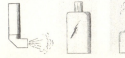

PRECAUTIONS:
May be used in pregnancy (B1), breast feeding and children.
Use with caution in glaucoma, enlarged prostate gland, difficulty in passing urine, cystic fibrosis, constipation and irregular heartbeat.
Avoid contact with eyes.

Do not take if:
 sensitive to soy beans or peanuts.

SIDE EFFECTS:
Common: Dry mouth, throat irritation.
Unusual: Blurred vision, difficulty in passing urine, cough, headache, nausea.
Severe but rare (stop medication, consult doctor): Eye pain or halos seen around objects.

INTERACTIONS:
Other drugs:
• Sodium cromoglycate.

PRESCRIPTION:
Yes.

PBS:
Yes.

PERMITTED IN SPORT:
Yes.

OVERDOSE:
Exacerbation of side effects only likely consequence.

OTHER INFORMATION:
Commonly used in conjunction with other medication for severe asthma, emphysema and chronic bronchitis. May be used alone in some forms (eg. exercise induced) of asthma. Very useful and safe medication.

See also Tiotropium.

Irbesartan

See ANGIOTENSIN II RECEPTOR ANTAGONISTS.

IRON

TRADE and GENERIC NAMES:
Blackmores Iron Compound (Ferrous phosphate).
Calvita (Ferrous sulfate with calcium, vitamins).
FAB Iron and B (Iron amino acid chelate with vitamin B).
Fefol, FGF (Ferrous sulfate with Folic acid).
Fergon (Ferrous gluconate).
Ferrograd C (Ferrous sulfate with vitamin C).
Ferro-Gradumet (Ferrous sulfate).
Ferrosig, Ferrum H (Iron polymaltose).
Numerous other vitamin and mineral supplements also contain various forms of iron (eg. ferric ammonium citrate, ferric pyrophosphate, ferrous fumarate).
NB: Iron compounds underlined.

DRUG CLASS:
Mineral.

USES:
Iron deficiency, some types of anaemia.

DOSAGE:
 One tablet or capsule a day on an empty stomach.
Recommended daily intake: 12 to 16mg a day.

FORMS:
Tablets, capsules, mixture, injection.

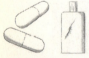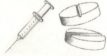

PRECAUTIONS:
Safe in pregnancy (A), breast feeding and children.
Cause of any anaemia should be determined before use.
Do not use excessive dose.
Do not take if:
 suffering from haemochromatosis, ulcerative colitis, ileostomy or colostomy, anaemia not due to iron deficiency.

SIDE EFFECTS:
Common: Slight stomach upsets, dark coloured faeces.
Unusual: Temporary tooth staining.

INTERACTIONS:
Other drugs:
- Tetracycline, penicillamine, antacids, calcium, methyldopa, levodopa, chloramphenicol, cimetidine, thyroxine, phenytoin, cholestyramine.

Herbs:
- St John's wort.

PRESCRIPTION:
No.

PBS:
Fergon, FGF: Yes.
Other forms: No.

PERMITTED IN SPORT:
Yes.

OVERDOSE:
Constipation and stomach cramps only likely effects.

OTHER INFORMATION:
Iron is absorbed from the gut at a set rate, and using higher doses is unlikely to have any clinical effect. Iron is found in red meats (particularly liver) and green vegetables. Pregnant women are at risk of iron deficiency because the developing baby absorbs iron to build muscle and blood cells.

See also Folic acid.

Isoniazid

TRADE NAME:
Isoniazid.

USES:
Tuberculosis (TB).

DOSAGE:
 One tablet, two or three times a day. Dosage adjusted carefully to match weight of patient.

FORMS:
Tablets of 100mg (white).

PRECAUTIONS:
May be used safely in pregnancy (A), breast feeding and children.
Use with caution in liver and kidney disease.
Regular checks of eyes recommended.
Regular blood tests to check liver and kidney function recommended.
Use only in combination with other medications for treatment of tuberculosis.

Do not take if:
 suffering from severe liver disease.

SIDE EFFECTS:
Common: Pins and needles, nausea.
Unusual: Vomiting, diarrhoea, belly discomfort, fever, rash.
Severe but rare (stop medication, consult doctor): Eye damage, unusual bruising or bleeding, yellow skin (jaundice).

INTERACTIONS:
Other drugs:
- Phenytoin, carbamazepine, rifampicin, paracetamol.

Other substances:
- Reacts with alcohol.
- Glucose test strips.

PRESCRIPTION:
Yes.

PBS:
Yes.

PERMITTED IN SPORT:
Yes.

OVERDOSE:
Serious. May cause vomiting, dizziness, blurred vision, slurred speech, hallucinations, difficulty in breathing, convulsions and coma. Administer activated charcoal or induce vomiting if medication taken recently. Seek urgent medical assistance.

See also **Clofazimine, Cycloserine, Ethambutol, Pyrazinamide, Rifabutin, Rifampicin.**

Isophane Insulin

See **INSULINS.**

Isoprenaline

TRADE NAME:
Isuprel.

USES:
Heart diseases due to the blockage of nerve conduction within the heart and resulting in irregular heart rhythm or stopping of the heart.
Severe lung spasm (bronchospasm – similar to asthma) during surgery.
Sudden severe drop in blood pressure, shock.

DOSAGE:
 As determined by doctor.

FORMS:
Injection.

Medications

PRECAUTIONS:
Safe in pregnancy (A) and breast feeding.
Use with caution in some types of heart disease, high blood pressure, diabetes, over-active thyroid gland.
Use lower doses in elderly and children.
Patient should be connected to a heart monitor during administration.

Do not take if:
 suffering from rapid heart rate, overdose of digoxin, recent heart attack or angina.

SIDE EFFECTS:
Common: Irregular heartbeat, nervousness, headache, dizziness, restlessness.
Unusual: Hot flushes, tremor, weakness, muscle tension.
Severe but rare (stop medication, consult doctor): Very high blood pressure.

INTERACTIONS:
Other drugs:
- Adrenaline, digoxin, chlorpromazine, MAOI.

PRESCRIPTION:
Yes.

PBS:
No.

PERMITTED IN SPORT:
No.

OVERDOSE:
Very serious. Urgent medical attention necessary.
See also Adrenaline.

Isopropyl alcohol

TRADE NAMES:
Aquaear, Ear Clear for Swimmer's Ear (with acetic acid).
Also available in numerous other preparations.

USES:
Drying water in ears to prevent swimmer's ear.
Cleaning contact lenses.

DOSAGE:
 Ear drops: four to six drops in each ear after swimming.

FORMS:
Ear drops, solution.

PRECAUTIONS:
Safe in pregnancy.
Not to be swallowed.

Do not use ear drops if:
 suffering from ear infection, ear discharge, blocked ear canals, perforated ear drum.
- grommets inserted.

SIDE EFFECTS:
Ear canal irritation.

INTERACTIONS:
None.

PRESCRIPTION:
No.

PBS:
No.

PERMITTED IN SPORT:
Yes.

OVERDOSE:
Not likely to be harmful if swallowed in small quantities.

Isosorbide nitrate

TRADE NAMES:
Duride, Imdur Durules, Imtrate SR, Monodur (Isosorbide mononitrate).
Isordil, Sorbidin (Isosorbide dinitrate).

DRUG CLASS:
Antiangina.

USES:
Prevention and treatment of angina, some types of heart failure, poor blood supply to heart.

DOSAGE:

Duride, Imdur Durules, Imtrate SR, Monodur: One or two tablets once a day.
Sublingual Isordil: One or two tablets under tongue every two or three hours.
Isordil and Sorbidin tablets: One to three tablets three times a day.

FORMS:
Tablets, sublingual (under tongue) tablets, long acting tablets.

PRECAUTIONS:
Should be used with caution in pregnancy (B1, B2) and breast feeding. Not for use in children.
Tolerance may develop if used long term. Duride, Monodur & Imdur not designed for use in acute angina.
Duride, Monodur & Imdur should not be ceased suddenly, but withdrawn slowly. Use with caution in kidney and liver disease, reduced brain blood flow and low blood pressure.

Do not take if:
suffering from right heart failure, low blood pressure, constrictive pericarditis, severe anaemia, increased brain pressure.

SIDE EFFECTS:
Common: Headache, low blood pressure, rapid heart rate, dizziness, poor appetite, nausea, sleep disturbances.
Unusual: Flushing, swelling of tissues, rash, vomiting, anaemia.
Severe but rare (stop medication, consult doctor): Slow heart rate.

INTERACTIONS:
Other drugs:
- Severe interaction with sildenafil, tadalafil.
- Phenothiazines, tricyclics, anticholinergics, beta blockers.
- Drugs that lower blood pressure.

PRESCRIPTION:
Yes.

PBS:
Yes.

PERMITTED IN SPORT:
Yes.

OVERDOSE:
Headache, severe low blood pressure, rapid heart rate and collapse may occur. Administer activated charcoal or induce vomiting if tablets taken recently. Seek urgent medical attention.

OTHER INFORMATION:
Used for several decades for treatment and prevention of angina. Slow release forms (Duride, Imdur Durules, Imtrate SR, Monodur) have far fewer side effects and have dramatically improved the life of patients with angina.
See also Glyceryl trinitrate, Nicorandil, Perhexiline.

Isotretinoin

TRADE NAMES:
Accure, Isohexal, Isotrex, Oratane, Roaccutane.

USES:
Severe acne not responding to other medication.

DOSAGE:
Capsules: One or two capsules once or twice a day with food for up to 16 weeks.
Gel: Apply sparingly once a day at night.

FORMS:
Capsules of 10mg and 20mg, gel.

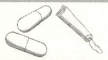

PRECAUTIONS:
Absolutely forbidden in pregnancy (X), breast feeding and children under 12.
Must be used with caution in all patients.
Adequate contraception essential for all women using isotretinoin.
Regular blood tests recommended.
Use with caution in diabetes.
Avoid sun exposure during use.
Never exceed recommended dose or length of course.

Do not take if:
 suffering from liver disease, any form of cancer, high cholesterol or triglycerides, hypervitaminosis A.
- taking tetracyclines.

SIDE EFFECTS:
Common: Sore mouth and lips, dry eyes, dry mouth, dry skin, nose bleeds, muscle pain, joint pain, joint stiffness, hair thinning, peeling of palms and soles, sun sensitivity.
Unusual: Tiredness, headache, depression, gout, diarrhoea, initial worsening of acne, altered blood test results.
Severe but rare (stop medication, consult doctor): Severe headache, intractable vomiting, visual disturbances.

INTERACTIONS:
Other drugs:
- Tetracycline, minocycline.

Other substances:
- Reacts with alcohol.
- Vitamin A.

PRESCRIPTION:
Yes (capsules restricted to specialist dermatologists and consultant physicians only).

PBS:
Capsules: Yes (restricted to severe acne uncontrolled by other methods and must be prescribed by a dermatologist or consultant physician).
Gel: No.

PERMITTED IN SPORT:
Yes.

OVERDOSE:
May cause headache, vomiting, flushing, mouth soreness and dryness, abdominal pain and incoordination. Seek medical assistance.

OTHER INFORMATION:
A very potent and potentially dangerous drug, but if used correctly can dramatically and often permanently cure severe chronic acne. Use in pregnancy will always cause severe damage to foetus.

Ispaghula

TRADE NAME:
Fybogel.

DRUG CLASS:
Fibre.

USES:
Constipation.

DOSAGE:
 Take required amount with water twice a day.

FORMS:
Granules.

PRECAUTIONS:
Safe in pregnancy and breast feeding. Use with caution in phenylketonuria.
Do not take if:
 on a salt restricted diet.
- suffering from megacolon or gut obstruction.

SIDE EFFECTS:
Common: Minimal.
Unusual: Diarrhoea, belly discomfort, excess wind.

INTERACTIONS:
None significant.

PRESCRIPTION:
No.

PBS:
No. Available to some Veterans Affairs pensioners.

PERMITTED IN SPORT:
Yes.

OVERDOSE:
Take additional water.
Belly discomfort and passing excess wind only effects.

OTHER INFORMATION:
Widely used, natural fibre supplement.
See Frangula, Ispaghula, Methylcellulose, Pectin, Psyllium, Sennosides, Sterculia.

Itraconazole

TRADE NAME:
Sporanox.

DRUG CLASS:
Antifungal.

USES:
Severe fungal infections of mouth (thrush), skin, vagina and eye.

DOSAGE:
 Capsules: One or two, once or twice a day with food.
Mouth wash: Rinse mouth once a day with 20mLs solution.

FORMS:
Capsules (blue/pink) of 100mg, mouth wash.

PRECAUTIONS:
Not to be used in pregnancy (B3) unless medically essential. Cease breast feeding before use. Use with caution in children. Not to be used long term.
Use capsules with caution in liver and kidney disease, heart failure.

SIDE EFFECTS:
Common: Nausea, diarrhoea, headache, dizziness.
Unusual: Swelling of tissue, pins and needles sensation.
Severe but rare (stop medication, consult doctor): Yellow skin (jaundice), heart failure.

INTERACTIONS:
Other drugs:
- Severe interaction with cisapride, astemizole, mizolastine, quinidine, pimozide, simvastatin, midazolam, triazolam.
- Digoxin, cyclosporin, phenytoin, rifampicin, H^2 antagonists, anticoagulants (eg. warfarin), isoniazid, hypoglycaemics, norethisterone.

Other substances:
- Reacts with alcohol.

PRESCRIPTION:
Yes.

PBS:
Yes (very restricted, on authority only).

PERMITTED IN SPORT:
Yes.

OVERDOSE:
May cause liver damage. Administer activated charcoal or induce vomiting if taken recently. Seek medical assistance.

OTHER INFORMATION:
Introduced 1994. Expensive.
See Clotrimazole, Econazole, Fluconazole, Griseofulvin, Ketoconazole, Miconazole.

Ivermectin

TRADE NAME:
Stromectol.

DRUG CLASS:
Anthelmintic.

USES:
Onchocerciasis, strongyloidiasis (intestinal worms).

DOSAGE:

Single dose that depends on body weight of patient.

FORMS:
Tablets of 3mg (white).

PRECAUTIONS:
Use with considerable caution in pregnancy (B3). Use with caution in breast feeding and children under 5 years. Use with caution if liver involved. Use only if infestation positively diagnosed.

SIDE EFFECTS:
Common: Diarrhoea, nausea, dizziness, itch, enlarged lymph nodes, rash, fever.
Unusual: Eye effects, facial swelling, foot and hand swelling, rapid heart rate.

INTERACTIONS:
None significant.

PRESCRIPTION:
Yes.

PBS:
Yes (authority required – restricted to onchocerciasis and strongyloidiasis).

PERMITTED IN SPORT:
Yes.

OTHER INFORMATION:
Onchocerciasis and strongyloidiasis are worm infestations of the body encountered only in areas of tropical countries with poor hygiene and mainly in central Africa.

Japanese encephalitis virus vaccine

TRADE NAME:
Je-Vax.

DRUG CLASS:
Vaccine.

USES:
Prevention of Japanese encephalitis infection.

DOSAGE:
 Three injections given one and three weeks apart.

FORMS:
Injection.

PRECAUTIONS:
May be used with caution in pregnancy (B2), breast feeding and children.
Use with caution with history of urticaria, asthma, hay fever and allergies.
Avoid alcohol for two days after vaccination.

Do not take if:
 sensitive to specific preservatives (thiomersal).

SIDE EFFECTS:
Common: Allergy reaction, swelling of tissue.
Unusual: Asthma-like reaction, fever, headache, tiredness, rash, dizziness, muscle pain, nausea, vomiting.

INTERACTIONS:
Other drugs:
- Other vaccines.

Other substances:
- Alcohol.

PRESCRIPTION:
Yes.

PBS:
No.

PERMITTED IN SPORT:
Yes.

OTHER INFORMATION:
Travellers to primitive areas of east and southeast Asia may be exposed to this mosquito-borne virus. Vaccine takes at least 10 days to become effective.

Kaolin

TRADE NAMES:
Bispectin (with codeine, aluminium hydroxide, pectin).
DeWitt's Antacid Powder (with antacids).
Donnagel (with atropine and other ingredients).
Kaomagma with Pectin (with pectin and aluminium hydroxide).

Available alone and in combination with other medications in numerous other antidiarrhoeal preparations.

DRUG CLASS:
Antidiarrhoeal.

USES:
Diarrhoea.

DOSAGE:
 30mLs initially, then 15 to 30mLs every two to four hours as required for condition.
Take at least an hour away from other medications.

FORMS:
Suspension.

PRECAUTIONS:
Safe in pregnancy, breast feeding and children over 3 years.
Do not take if:
 suffering from kidney disease.
- for prolonged periods.

SIDE EFFECTS:
Common: Minimal.
Unusual: Constipation.

INTERACTIONS:
Other drugs:
- Kaolin markedly affects the absorption of many other drugs including antibiotics, anticoagulants (eg. warfarin), H2 antagonists (used for stomach ulcers), iron, isoniazid, phenothiazines and aspirin.

PRESCRIPTION:
No.

PBS:
No.

PERMITTED IN SPORT:
Yes.

OVERDOSE:
Causes constipation, nausea and vomiting.

OTHER INFORMATION:
Kaolin is a form of clay that has been used for thousands of years to treat diarrhoea. Also used in making fine china.

See also Atropine, Attapulgite, Codeine Phosphate, Diphenoxylate, Loperamide, Pectin.

Medications

KERATOLYTICS

TRADE and GENERIC NAMES:
Acnederm Lotion, Skinoren (azelaic acid).
Benzac, Brevoxyl, Clearasil Ultra, Oxy, Panoxyl (benzoyl peroxide).
Calmurid (lactic acid with urea).
Clearasil Medicated Foam (triclosan and salicylic acid).
Clearaway Wart Remover, Clearasil Medicated Wipes, Duofilm Gel, Egozite Cradle Cap Lotion, Ionil (salicylic acid).
Cornkil (salicylic acid and lactic acid with benzocaine end ether).
Curaderm (salicylic acid and linoleic acid with Urea and other ingredients).
DermaDrate (lactic acid with urea and other ingredients).
Dermatech, Duofilm (salicylic acid and lactic acid).
Dermaveen Acne Bar (salicylic acid with oatmeal).
Ionil T (salicylic acid with coal tar).
Isophyl (salicylic acid with cetrimide).
Movelat Sportz (salicylic acid with heparinoid).
Mycoderm (salicylic acid with antifungals).
Mycozol (salicylic acid and benzoic acid with chlorbutol and other ingredients).
Posalfilin (salicylic acid with podophyllum resin).
Psor-Asist Cream (salicylic acid with coal tar and sulfur).
Psor-Asist Scalp Lotion (salicylic acid with urea).
Pyralvex (salicylic acid with anthraquinone).
Retin-A, Retrieve, Stieva-A, Vesanoid (tretinoin).
Sebitar (salicylic acid with coal tar, pine tar and undecylenamide).
Seborrol (salicylic acid with resorcinol, undecylenamide and other ingredients).
SM-33 (salicylic acid with lignocaine and other ingredients).
SOOV Prickly Heat Powder (salicylic acid with zinc oxide, paraffin and hydroxybenzoate).
SP Cream (salicylic acid with urea and other ingredients).
Superfade (salicylic acid with hydroxyquinoline and padimate).
Available in numerous other creams and lotions.
NB: Keratolytics are underlined. Isotretinoin and etretinate (see separate entries) are also keratolytics.

DRUG CLASS:
Keratolytics remove keratin from skin to thin, dry and soften the skin. Keratin is a protein that creates the horny, hard layers of the skin. Triclosan and azelaic acid also have antiseptic properties.

USES:
Acne, minor skin infections, psoriasis, thickened skin, corns, warts.

DOSAGE:

Follow directions on packaging, as directions vary with composition, form and strength.

FORMS:
Gel, cream, ointment, liquid, wash, foam, wipes, solution, face mask, bar, soap.

PRECAUTIONS:
Tretinoin should not be used in pregnancy. Other keratolytics may be used in with caution in pregnancy, breast feeding and children. Not designed for use in young children.
Avoid eyes, nostrils, mouth, vagina and anus with all preparations.
Avoid open wound contact.
Avoid sun exposure after use.
Do not exceed recommended dose.

Do not take if:
 suffering from eczema or sunburn.

Home Guide to Medication

SIDE EFFECTS:
Common: Stinging, warmth, skin redness.
Unusual: Swelling, peeling, sun sensitivity.
Severe but rare (stop medication, consult doctor): Skin pain, marked swelling, severe peeling.

INTERACTIONS:
Other drugs:
- Other keratolytics, abrasives.

Other substances:
- Many cosmetics.

PRESCRIPTION:
Tretinoin: Yes.
Others: No.

PBS:
No.

PERMITTED IN SPORT:
Yes.

OVERDOSE:
Excessive use may lead to skin damage, burning and pain. Wash off any excess from skin immediately.

OTHER INFORMATION:
Keratolytics are skin preparations that are designed to remove the outermost layer of the skin (the keratin layer) and therefore act as the ultimate skin cleanser. They are used to treat diseases such as acne, psoriasis and some forms of dermatitis. Excessive or inappropriate use may cause reddening, burning and discolouration of the skin, particularly on the face. It is wise to make a test application on an area of skin that is not cosmetically important before applying a keratolytic to the face. Tretinoin is a vitamin A derivative. All Keratolytics must be used carefully, but if correctly used, may markedly improve acne and other skin diseases.

See also Acitretin, Aluminium Oxide, Glutaraldehyde, Isotretinoin, Salicylic acid.

Ketoconazole

TRADE NAMES:
Daktagold, Nizoral, Sebizole.

DRUG CLASS:
Antifungal.

USES:
Significant fungal infections of skin and internal organs, severe dandruff, tinea.

DOSAGE:

Tablets: One tablet a day with food.
Cream: Apply once or twice a day.
Shampoo: Apply to wet scalp for five minutes twice a week for four weeks.

FORMS:
Tablets (white) of 200mg, cream, shampoo.

PRECAUTIONS:
Tablets should not be used in pregnancy (B3) unless medically essential, and breast feeding should be ceased before use.
Tablets not to be used in children.
Shampoo and cream may be used in pregnancy, breast feeding and children with caution.
Should not be used long term.
Use with caution in older women.
Use with caution in adrenal disease, if griseofulvin taken recently.
Avoid eye contact with cream and shampoo.

Do not take tablets if:
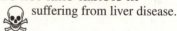 suffering from liver disease.
- allergic to griseofulvin or penicillin.

SIDE EFFECTS:

Common: Tablets – Nausea.
Shampoo and cream – Skin irritation, itch, rash and redness.
Unusual: Vomiting, diarrhoea, belly pain, rash, itch, headache, dizziness.
Severe but rare (stop medication, consult doctor): Yellow skin (jaundice).

INTERACTIONS:

Other drugs:
- Serious interaction with astemizole, mizolastine, cisapride, midazolam, triazolam, pimozide, quinidine, simvastatin.
- Tablets – Isoniazid, rifampicin, griseofulvin, antacids, ritonavir, warfarin, cyclosporin, sildenafil, digoxin, verapamil, phenytoin.
- Shampoo – Corticosteroid scalp applications.

Herbs:
- Echinacea.

Other substances:
- Tablets – Alcohol.

PRESCRIPTION:
Yes.

PBS:
Tablets: Yes (authority required – restricted to severe or recurrent fungal infections).
Shampoo and cream: No.

PERMITTED IN SPORT:
Yes.

OVERDOSE:
Induce vomiting if medication taken recently. Seek medical assistance.

OTHER INFORMATION:
Introduced in mid 1980s. Very effective, but may cause liver damage if used inappropriately or for long periods.
See Clotrimazole, Econazole, Fluconazole, Griseofulvin, Itraconazole, Miconazole.

Ketoprofen

TRADE NAMES:
Orudis, Oruvail

DRUG CLASS:
NSAID (Nonsteroidal anti-inflammatory drug).

USES:
All forms of arthritis, inflammatory disorders, gout, back pain, bone pain.

DOSAGE:
 100 to 200mg once a day

FORMS:
Capsules of 100 and 200mg, gel.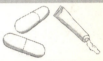

PRECAUTIONS:
Should not be used in pregnancy (C) unless medically essential. Breast feeding should be ceased if necessary to use NSAID. Not for use in children under two. Gel safe in pregnancy.
Use tablets and capsules with caution in psychiatrically disturbed patients, epilepsy, severe infection, heart failure and kidney disease.
Lower doses required in elderly, who may suffer more side effects.

Do not take if:
 suffering from peptic ulcer at present or in recent past.
- due for surgery (including dental surgery).
- suffering from bleeding disorder or anaemia.

SIDE EFFECTS:
Common: Gel – Minimal.
Other forms – Stomach discomfort, diarrhoea, constipation, heartburn, nausea, headache, dizziness.
Unusual: Blurred vision, stomach ulcer, ringing noise in ears, retention of fluid,

swelling of tissue, drowsiness, itch, rash, shortness of breath.
Severe but rare (stop medication, consult doctor): Vomiting blood, passing blood in faeces, other unusual bleeding, asthma induced by medication.

INTERACTIONS:
Other drugs:
- Must never be used with anticoagulants (eg. warfarin).
- Probenecid, diuretics, lithium, methotrexate, beta blockers, ACE inhibitors, diuretics.
- Gel has minimal interactions.

PRESCRIPTION:
Gel: No.
Capsules: Yes.

PBS:
Capsules: Yes.
Gel: No.

PERMITTED IN SPORT:
Yes.

OVERDOSE:
Causes nausea, vomiting, severe headache, dizziness, confusion and convulsions. Administer activated charcoal or induce vomiting if taken recently. Seek medical assistance.

OTHER INFORMATION:
Extensively used to give excellent relief to a wide variety of inflammatory conditions. Significant side effects (particularly on the stomach) in about 5% of patients limit their use. Specially coated forms reduce side effects. Minimal side effects with gel, but less effective.

See also Aspirin, Bufexamac, Celecoxib, Diclofenac, Diflunisal, Flurbiprofen, Ibuprofen, Indomethacin, Ketorolac trometanol, Mefenamic Acid, Naproxen, Piroxicam, Rofecoxib, Salicylic acid, Sulindac, Tenoxicam, Tiaprofenic Acid.

Ketorolac trometanol

TRADE NAMES:
Acular, Toradol

DRUG CLASS:
NSAID (Nonsteroidal anti-inflammatory drug).

USES:
Post operative pain, allergic conjunctivitis, inflammation during eye surgery.

DOSAGE:

Tablets: One every four to six hours.
Injection: Every four to six hours.
Eye drops: One or two drops four times a day.

FORMS:
Tablets of 10mg, injection (Toradol); eye drops (Acular).

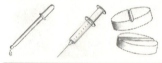

PRECAUTIONS:
Should not be used in pregnancy (C) unless medically essential.
Breast feeding should be ceased if necessary to use NSAID.
Not for use in children under 2 years.
Use tablets and injection with caution in psychiatrically disturbed patients, epilepsy, severe infection, heart failure and kidney disease.
Lower doses required in elderly, who may suffer more side effects.

Do not take if:
 suffering from peptic ulcer at present or in recent past.
- due for surgery (including dental surgery).
- suffering from bleeding disorder or anaemia.

SIDE EFFECTS:

Common: Eye drops – Stinging, burning, red eye, droopy eyelids, dry eyes. Injection and tablets – Stomach discomfort, diarrhoea, constipation, heartburn, nausea, headache, dizziness.
Unusual: Blurred vision, stomach ulcer, ringing noise in ears, retention of fluid, swelling of tissue, drowsiness, itch, rash, shortness of breath.
Severe but rare (stop medication, consult doctor): Vomiting blood, passing blood in faeces, other unusual bleeding, asthma induced by medication, glaucoma.

INTERACTIONS:

Other drugs:
- Must never be used with anticoagulants (eg. warfarin).
- Probenecid, diuretics, lithium, methotrexate, beta blockers, ACE inhibitors.

PRESCRIPTION:
Yes.

PBS:
No.

PERMITTED IN SPORT:
Yes.

OVERDOSE:
Causes nausea, vomiting, severe headache, dizziness, confusion and convulsions. Administer activated charcoal or induce vomiting if taken recently. Seek medical assistance.

OTHER INFORMATION:
Used to give excellent relief to a wide variety of inflammatory conditions.

See also Aspirin, Bufexamac, Celecoxib, Diclofenac, Diflunisal, Flurbiprofen, Ibuprofen, Indomethacin, Ketoprofen, Mefenamic Acid, Naproxen, Piroxicam, Rofecoxib, Salicylic acid, Sulindac, Tenoxicam, Tiaprofenic Acid.

L

Labetalol

TRADE NAMES:
Presolol, Trandate.

DRUG CLASS:
Alpha-Beta Blocker, Antihypertensive.

USES:
High blood pressure.

DOSAGE:
 One to three tablets, two to four times a day to a maximum of 2400mg per day.

FORMS:
Tablets of 100mg and 200mg.

PRECAUTIONS:
Should not be used in pregnancy (C) unless medically essential. Should be used with caution in breast feeding and elderly. Not recommended in children. Should not be stopped suddenly, but dosage should be slowly reduced over several days.

Do not take if:
☠ suffering from heart disease, narrowed arteries, Prinzmetal angina, diabetes, overactive thyroid gland, phaeochromocytoma or liver failure.
- having a general anaesthetic. Discuss with doctor.

SIDE EFFECTS:
Common: Minimal.
Unusual: Slow heart rate, dizziness, headache, tiredness, blurred vision, eye irritation, asthma, rash, difficulty in passing urine.

INTERACTIONS:
Other drugs:
- Beta agonists, calcium channel blockers, drugs for treatment of irregular heartbeat.
- Tremor with tricyclic antidepressants.
- Cimetidine increases blood levels of labetalol.
- Clonidine, methyldopa, NSAIDs.

PRESCRIPTION:
Yes.

PBS:
Yes.

PERMITTED IN SPORT:
No.

OVERDOSE:
Low blood pressure and slow heart rate. Lay patient flat and raise legs. Administer charcoal or induce vomiting if tablets taken recently. Seek medical assistance.

See also Carvedilol, Esmolol, Labetalol, Metoprolol, Oxprenolol, Pindolol, Propranolol, Sotalol.

Lactic acid
See KERATOLYTICS.

Lactulose

TRADE NAMES:
Actilax, Duphalac, Genlac, Lac-Dol.

DRUG CLASS:
Laxative.

USES:
Severe constipation. Also used in rare form of brain inflammation.

DOSAGE:

30 to 45mLs three or four times a day.

FORMS:
Syrup.

PRECAUTIONS:
Safe in pregnancy, breast feeding and children.
Should be used with caution in diabetics. Use with caution if lactose intolerant.
Should not be used for more than six months without medical check-up.

Do not take if:
 suffering from galactosaemia, bowel obstruction.

SIDE EFFECTS:
Common: Intestinal cramps, bloating, passing wind.
Unusual: Diarrhoea, nausea, loss of appetite, increased thirst.

INTERACTIONS:
Other drugs:
- Interacts with neomycin and other antibiotics given by mouth.
- Antacids.

PRESCRIPTION:
No.

PBS:
Yes.

PERMITTED IN SPORT:
Yes (almost guaranteed to result in failure in any sport!).

OVERDOSE:
Diarrhoea and intestinal cramps only problem.

OTHER INFORMATION:
Normally only used for severe constipation when other medications ineffective.

See also Bisacodyl, Docusate sodium, FIBRE, Frangula, Paraffin, Poloxamer, Psyllium, Senna, Sodium phosphate, Sodium picosulfate, Sorbitol, Sterculia.

Lamivudine

TRADE NAMES:
3TC, Zeffix.
Combivir (with zidovudine).
Trizivir (with abacavir, zidovudine).

DRUG CLASS:
Antiviral.

USES:
HIV infection, AIDS, chronic hepatitis B.

DOSAGE:
 Depends on condition being treated. Usually 100mg a day.

FORMS:
Tablets, mixture.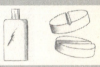

PRECAUTIONS:
Use with considerable caution in pregnancy (B3) and children. Use with caution in breast feeding.
Use with caution in kidney and liver disease, diabetes and pancreas disease.

Do not use for HIV/AIDS unless combined with other antivirals.

SIDE EFFECTS:
Common: Nausea, headache, tiredness, inability to sleep, rashes.
Unusual: Lung and throat infection.
Unusual: Pancreatitis.

INTERACTIONS:
Other drugs:
- Trimethoprim, zalcitabine.

PRESCRIPTION:
Yes.

PBS:
Yes (very restricted).

PERMITTED IN SPORT:
Yes.

See Abacavir, Delavirdine, Didanosine, Efavirenz, Indinavir, Nelfinavir, Nevirapine, Ritonavir, Saquinavir, Stavudine, Tenofovir, Zalcitabine, Zidovudine.

Lamotrigine

TRADE NAME:
Lamictal.

DRUG CLASS:
Anticonvulsant.

USES:
Epilepsy, particularly seizures that affect only one part of the body and are not controlled by other anticonvulsants.

DOSAGE:

Gradually increase dose until control obtained, usually between 200mg and 400mg a day taken in two doses. Lower doses used in combination with other anticonvulsants.

FORMS:
Tablets (white) of 2mg, 5mg, 25mg, 50mg, 100mg and 200mg.

PRECAUTIONS:
Use with great caution in pregnancy (B3), breast feeding and children under 12 years.
Use with caution in kidney and liver disease.
☠ Do not stop suddenly, but reduce dosage slowly.

SIDE EFFECTS:
Common: Dizziness, headache, double vision, incoordination, tiredness, nausea, blurred vision, vomiting.
Severe but rare (stop medication, consult doctor): Rash (Stevens-Johnson syndrome or toxic epidermal necrolysis – may be severe and life threatening).

INTERACTIONS:
Other drugs:
- Other anticonvulsants, sodium valproate.

Herbs:
- Evening primrose (linoleic acid), Gingko biloba.

Other substances:
- Borage.

PRESCRIPTION:
Yes.

PBS:
Yes (authority required – restricted to epilepsy uncontrolled by other medication).

PERMITTED IN SPORT:
Yes.

OVERDOSE:
Sedation, incoordination, double vision and vomiting may occur. Administer charcoal or induce vomiting if taken recently. Seek medical assistance.

OTHER INFORMATION:
Introduced in 1993 to assist the most severe and difficult to control forms of epilepsy. Unfortunately, cost and side effects limit its usefulness.

See also BARBITURATES, BENZODIAZEPINES, Carbamazepine, Clonazepam, Ethosuximide, Gabapentin, Levetiracetam, Oxcarbazepine, Phenytoin, Primidone, Sodium valproate, Sulthiame, Tiagabine, Topiramate, Vigabatrin.

Lansoprazole

See PROTON PUMP INHIBITORS.

Latanoprost

TRADE NAMES:
Xalantan.
Xalacom (with timolol).

USES:
Glaucoma.

DOSAGE:

One drop in affected eye(s) once a day. Apply pressure to tear duct at inner corner of eye for five minutes after application.

FORMS:
Eye drops.

PRECAUTIONS:
Use with considerable caution in pregnancy (B3). Use with caution in breast feeding and children.
Use with caution in eye inflammation, pigmentary and hereditary glaucoma.

Do not use if:
 wearing contact lenses.

SIDE EFFECTS:
Common: Change in eye colour, irritation of eye surface, redness of eye, blurred vision, eye burning and itching.
Unusual: Swelling of eye surface, ulceration of eye surface.

INTERACTIONS:
Other drugs:
- Thiomersal drops, acetazolamide.

PRESCRIPTION:
Yes.

PBS:
Yes.

PERMITTED IN SPORT:
Yes.

OVERDOSE:
Eye irritation and exacerbation of side effects likely.

OTHER INFORMATION:
Introduced in 1998 for treatment of glaucoma unresponsive to other medications.
See Acetazolamide, Apraclonidine, Betaxolol, Bimatoprost, Brimonidine tartrate, Brinzolamide, Carbachol, Dipivefrine, Dorzolamide hydrochloride, Levobunolol, Phenylephrine, Pilocarpine, Timolol, Travoprost.

LAXATIVES

DISCUSSION:
When you've just got to go, but you can't go, a laxative may be the answer to a large bowel's prayer. Constipation is a relative matter, as some people consider it normal to pass faeces three times a day, while others consider once a week to be normal. If retained faeces and the attempts to pass them cause pain or discomfort, then constipation needs treatment. Laxatives should be the last resort in the treatment of constipation, after increased fluid intake and alterations to increase the bulk residue of the food in your diet have been tried.

Laxatives vary from simple lubricants, such as paraffin, to bulking agents that contain senna and other fibres, different sugars that draw fluid into the gut (eg. lactulose), and gut stimulants (eg. bisacodyl) that actually increase the contractions of the gut. They are available as tablets, mixtures, granules, suppositories and enemas (the last two for anal use). All are available without prescription.

The main complication with laxatives is their overuse. Patients may use laxatives to pass faeces excessively, and become dependent upon them for the natural functioning of the bowel. Patients trying to

Medications

lose weight by increasing the rate of faeces output may create this type of dependence, and it is a practice to be deplored. Laxatives should never be used if there is any suspicion of more sinister disease in the gut. Many patients have treated a pain in the abdomen with laxatives, only to find that they have worsened a case of appendicitis. Laxatives should be used with great caution in children and during pregnancy. Many other substances, foods and fibres (eg. senna) are used as laxatives.

See Bisacodyl, Docusate sodium, FIBRE, Frangula, Glycerol, Lactulose, Paraffin, Poloxamer, Psyllium, Sennosides, Sodium lauryl sulfoacetate, Sodium phosphate, Sodium picosulfate, Sorbitol, Sterculia, Tegaserod.

L-Dopa

See LEVODOPA COMPOUNDS.

Leflunomide

TRADE NAME:
Arava.

USES:
Treatment of rheumatoid arthritis.

DOSAGE:

100mg a day for three days, then 10mg to 20mg once a day.

FORMS:
Tablets of 10mg (white) and 20mg (yellow).

PRECAUTIONS:
Never to be used in pregnancy (X) and breast feeding.
May be used with caution in children and the elderly.
Regular blood tests to check liver function and blood cell count necessary.
Use with caution in generalised infection, bone marrow damage, tuberculosis and kidney damage.

Do not take if:
☠ suffering from immunodeficiency, low platelet or white cell count, severe infection, Stevens-Johnson syndrome, liver disease or erythema multiforme.
- female partner is pregnant (may be transferred during sex).

SIDE EFFECTS:
Common: Skin reactions, nausea, diarrhoea, hair loss.
Unusual: High blood pressure, sore mouth, belly pain, liver and blood cell damage, tendon and muscle pain, headache, dizziness, weight loss, pins and needles sensation, allergy reaction.
Severe but rare (stop medication, consult doctor): Severe skin reaction, blistering and loss of skin.

INTERACTIONS:
Other drugs:
- Methotrexate, phenytoin, warfarin, tolbutamide, some vaccines, rifampicin, charcoal, cholestyramine, NSAID, celecoxib, rofecoxib, methotrexate.

Other substances:
- Alcohol.

PRESCRIPTION:
Yes.

PBS:
Yes (authority required – restricted to severe rheumatoid arthritis in which other medications are ineffective).

PERMITTED IN SPORT:
Yes.

OVERDOSE:
Likely to be serious, but no information available. Seek urgent medical attention.

OTHER INFORMATION:
Introduced in 1999 as a last resort, but effective treatment, for the most severe forms of rheumatoid arthritis.

Lente insulin

See INSULINS.

Lercanidipine

TRADE NAME:
Zanidip.

DRUG CLASS:
Antihypertensive, calcium channel blocker.

USES:
Treatment of high blood pressure (hypertension).

DOSAGE:
 One or two tablets once a day.

FORMS:
Tablets of 10mg (yellow).

PRECAUTIONS:
Not to be used in pregnancy (C), breast feeding or children.
Use with caution in the elderly, angina, aortic stenosis, heart failure, recent heart attack, kidney and liver disease.
Do not take if:
 suffering from severe liver or kidney disease.

SIDE EFFECTS:
Common: Constipation, tiredness, headache, dizziness, indigestion, swelling of feet and ankles.
Unusual: Flushing, palpitations, slow heart rate, scalp irritation, depression, flushes, nightmares, excess wind.
Severe but rare (stop medication, consult doctor): Fainting.

INTERACTIONS:
Other drugs:
- Cyclosporin (severe reaction).
- Ketoconazole, itraconazole, erythromycin, ritonavir, fluoxetine, phenytoin, carbamazepine, rifampicin, amiodarone, quinidine, metoprolol, propranolol, digoxin, cimetidine, simvastatin.

Other substances:
- Alcohol, grapefruit juice.

PRESCRIPTION:
Yes.

PBS:
Yes.

PERMITTED IN SPORT:
Yes.

OVERDOSE:
Administer activated charcoal or induce vomiting. Purging should be encouraged to eliminate drug from gut. Overdose may cause low blood pressure, irregular heart rhythm, difficulty in breathing, heart attack and death. Obtain urgent medical attention.

OTHER INFORMATION:
Introduced in 2001 for the management of hypertension.

See also Amlodipine, Diltiazem, Felodipine, Nifedipine, Nimodipine, Verapamil.

Letrozole

TRADE NAME:
Femara.

DRUG CLASS:
Antineoplastic.

USES:
Some types of advanced breast cancer in postmenopausal women.

DOSAGE:
 One tablet a day.

FORMS:
Tablets of 2.5mg (dark yellow).

PRECAUTIONS:
Not to be used in pregnancy (D), breast feeding or children.
Use with caution in kidney and liver disease.

Do not take if:
 still having menstrual periods.

SIDE EFFECTS:
Common: Headache, nausea, diarrhoea, swelling of hands and feet, tiredness, hot flushes, hair thinning, rash, vaginal discharge.
Unusual: Weight change, muscle pain, vaginal bleeding, sweating, dizziness, tiredness, increased appetite, joint pain, urgent desire to pass urine, acne, breast enlargement.
Severe but rare (stop medication, consult doctor): Blood clot in vein (thrombosis).

INTERACTIONS:
Other drugs:
- Tamoxifen.

PRESCRIPTION:
Yes.

PBS:
Yes.

PERMITTED IN SPORT:
Restricted for use in sport to women only.

OVERDOSE:
Effect unknown. Induce vomiting or administer activated charcoal if tablets taken recently. Seek medical attention.

OTHER INFORMATION:
Introduced in 1998 for treatment of severe relapses of some types of breast cancer.
See also Tamoxifen, Toremifene.

LEUKOTRENE RECEPTOR ANTAGONISTS

DISCUSSION:
New group of oral medications that prevent and treat asthma.
See Montelukast, Zafirlukast.

Leuprorelin

TRADE NAME:
Lucrin.

DRUG CLASS:
Antineoplastic.

USES:
Prostate cancer, endometriosis, fibroids of the uterus prior to surgery.

DOSAGE:
 Daily, monthly or quarterly injection depending on formulation of injection.

FORMS:
Injection, depot injection.

Medications

PRECAUTIONS:
Not to be used in pregnancy (D), breast feeding and children.
Use with caution with metastatic cancer involving the spine, urinary tract obstruction.

Do not take if:

 suffering from osteoporosis, undiagnosed bleeding from the vagina.

SIDE EFFECTS:
Common: Hot flushes, sweats, swelling of hands and feet, nausea, diarrhoea, pins and needles sensation.
Unusual: Pain at cancer or fibroid sites, shortness of breath, tiredness, headache, emotional instability, palpitations, breast tenderness.
Severe but rare (stop medication, consult doctor): High blood pressure, osteoporosis.

INTERACTIONS:
None significant.

PRESCRIPTION:
Yes.

PBS:
Yes (restricted to advanced prostate cancer).

PERMITTED IN SPORT:
Yes.

Levamisole

TRADE NAME:
Ergamisol.

USES:
Cancer of the colon.

DOSAGE:
 As determined for each patient by doctor. Always taken in conjunction with other medication for cancer.

FORMS:
Tablets of 50mg (white).

PRECAUTIONS:
Use with considerable caution in pregnancy (B3). Use with caution in breast feeding and elderly.
Use with caution in rheumatoid arthritis and other autoimmune diseases, liver disease and the elderly.
Do not exceed recommended dose.
Regular blood tests necessary to assess blood cell numbers.

Do not take if:

 suffering from significant kidney disease.

SIDE EFFECTS:
Common: Nervousness, sleeplessness, nausea, vomiting, loss of appetite, altered bowel habits, depression, mouth inflammation, altered taste and smell, flu-like symptoms.
Unusual: Rash, dermatitis, muscle pains, joint pains, white blood cell damage.
Severe but rare (stop medication, consult doctor): Blood white cell damage.

INTERACTIONS:
Other drugs:
- Phenytoin, warfarin.

Other substances:
- Alcohol.

Medications

PRESCRIPTION:
Yes.

PBS:
Yes.

PERMITTED IN SPORT:
Yes.

OVERDOSE:
Very serious. Exacerbation of side effects leading to severe organ damage and death may occur. Induce vomiting or give activated charcoal if taken recently. Seek urgent medical assistance.

OTHER INFORMATION:
Introduced in 1997.

SIDE EFFECTS:
Common: Tiredness, dizziness.
Unusual: Aggression, confusion, psychiatric disturbances.

INTERACTIONS:
Other drugs:
- Probenecid.

PRESCRIPTION:
Yes.

PBS:
No (expensive).

PERMITTED IN SPORT:
Yes.

OTHER INFORMATION:
Introduced in 2003.

See also BARBITURATES, BENZODIAZEPINES, Carbamazepine, Clonazepam, Ethosuximide, Gabapentin, Lamotrigine, Oxcarbazepine, Phenytoin, Primidone, Sodium valproate, Sulthiame, Tiagabine, Topiramate, Vigabatrin.

Levetiracetam

TRADE NAME:
Keppra.

DRUG CLASS:
Anticonvulsant.

USES:
Partial seizures of epilepsy.

DOSAGE:
 500 to 1500mg twice a day.

FORMS:
Tablets of 250mg (blue), 500mg (yellow) and 1000mg (white).

PRECAUTIONS:
Use with caution in pregnancy (B3) and children under 16 years. Not to be used if breast feeding.
Do not stop tablets suddenly, but reduce dose slowly.
Use with caution with kidney and liver disease.

Levobunolol

TRADE NAME:
Betagan.

DRUG CLASS:
Beta blocker.

USES:
Glaucoma.

DOSAGE:
 One drop twice a day.

FORMS:
Eye drops.

PRECAUTIONS:
Should be used with caution in pregnancy (C), but eye drops unlikely to cause problems.
Safe to use in breast feeding.
May be used with caution in children.
Use with care if suffering from alcoholism, liver or kidney failure or about to have surgery.
Use with caution in diabetes, shock, slow heart rate, or enlarged right heart.

Do not take if:
 suffering from heart failure, asthma, slow heart rate, or allergic conditions.

SIDE EFFECTS:
Common: Low blood pressure, slow heart rate, burning eyes, stinging, asthma.
Severe but rare (stop medication, consult doctor): Severe asthma.

INTERACTIONS:
Other drugs:
- Calcium channel blockers, disopyramide, clonidine, adrenaline, other medications for irregular heartbeat, lignocaine, ergotamine, indomethacin, chlorpromazine, beta blocker tablets.

PRESCRIPTION:
Yes.

PBS:
Yes.

PERMITTED IN SPORT:
Yes.

OVERDOSE:
Unlikely to be serious effects if eye drops swallowed.

See also Betaxolol, Bimatroprost, Pilocarpine, Timolol.

Levocabastine

TRADE NAME:
Livostin.

DRUG CLASS:
Antihistamine.

USES:
Allergic conjunctivitis, hay fever.

DOSAGE:
 Eye drops: One drop in eye twice a day.
Nose spray: Two sprays in each nostril two to four times a day.

FORMS:
Eye drops, nose spray.

PRECAUTIONS:
Do not use in pregnancy (B3).
Use with caution in breast feeding and kidney disease.
Use with caution if wearing contact lenses.
Do not use continuously for more than eight weeks.

SIDE EFFECTS:
Common: Local irritation, headaches.
Unusual: Tiredness, nose bleed.

INTERACTIONS:
None significant.

PRESCRIPTION:
No.

PBS:
No (available for some Veteran Affairs beneficiaries).

PERMITTED IN SPORT:
Yes.

OVERDOSE:
Unlikely to be serious.

LEVODOPA COMPOUNDS
(L-dopa)

TRADE and GENERIC NAMES:

Madopar (levodopa and benserazide).
Kinson, Sinemet (levodopa and carbidopa).

DRUG CLASS:

Antiparkinsonian.

USES:

Parkinson's disease.

DOSAGE:

 Individualised depending on patient's response. Follow doctor's instructions carefully.

FORMS:

Capsules, tablets.

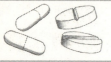

PRECAUTIONS:

Should be used in pregnancy (B3) only if medically essential. Breast feeding should be ceased before use. Not for use in children.
Use with caution in psychiatric conditions, heart disease, peptic ulcers, epilepsy, osteoporosis, glaucoma and osteomalacia. Do not undertake sudden increases in exercise levels.

Do not take if:

suffering from glaucoma, glandular disease, severe lung disease, liver or kidney disease, psychoses, melanoma, tremor, Huntington's chorea.
- under 30 years of age.

SIDE EFFECTS:

Common: Nausea, loss of appetite, palpitations, weight gain, constipation, incoordination, twitching, depression, tiredness, hiccups, sleeplessness, muscle cramps, excess excitability, tissue swelling, drowsiness.
Unusual: Vomiting, angina, shortness of breath, reduced libido, irregular heart rhythm, diarrhoea, leg pain, fainting, hallucinations, confusion.
Severe but rare (stop medication, consult doctor): Significant psychiatric disturbances.

INTERACTIONS:

Other drugs:
- Drugs acting on the heart (eg. some antihypertensives).
- Tricyclic antidepressants, phenothiazines, risperidone, isoniazid, phenytoin, MAOI, selegiline.
- Drugs used in general anaesthetics.

Herbs:
- Kava kava.

PRESCRIPTION:

Yes.

PBS:

Yes (some dosage combinations restricted to more severe forms of Parkinson's disease).

PERMITTED IN SPORT:

Yes.

OVERDOSE:

Symptoms include all side effects above, but exaggerated in severity. Administer activated charcoal or induce vomiting if patient alert and medication taken recently. Seek urgent medical assistance.

OTHER INFORMATION:

Despite their significant side effects, these medications have dramatically improved the quality of life for many patients with Parkinson's disease. Hailed as a miracle cure when introduced in the late 1960s, Levodopa is now accepted as one part of the treatment for this disease. Unfortunately, its effect tends to decrease the longer it is used. An important brain hormone, Dopamine is depleted in Parkinson's disease. Providing extra material from which the brain can make Dopamine improves the condition for many years.

See also Amantadine, Biperiden, Selegiline.

Levonorgestrel

TRADE NAMES:
Mirena (intra-uterine device – IUD).
Postinor (tablets).
Also in numerous oral contraceptives – see separate entry.

DRUG CLASS:
Sex hormone.

USES:
IUD: Contraception.
Tablets: Emergency post coital contraception ('morning after' pill).

DOSAGE:

Intrauterine device: Replaced every five years.
Tablets: One tablet as soon as possible after sex, then second tablet 12 hours later. Only two tablets in course. Not effective more than 72 hours after sex.

FORMS:
Intrauterine device, tablet of 750µg.

PRECAUTIONS:
Not for use in pregnancy (D), breast feeding or children.
Not for use in males.
Use IUD with caution in women who have not had children.
Use IUD with care in heart disease, migraine sufferers, liver disease, breast cancer, heart anatomy abnormalities, and with history of sexually transmitted diseases.
Use tablets with caution in severe high blood pressure, severe diabetes, heart disease, stroke, Crohn's disease, diarrhoea.
Do not use tablets repeatedly.
Tablets may not be effective if vomiting occurs soon after being taken – see doctor again.

Do not use IUD if:

suffering from genital or uterine infection, genital cancer, recent abortion, undiagnosed uterine bleeding, abnormal shape of uterus and significant liver disease.

Do not take tablets if:
suffering from unexplained vaginal bleeding or breast cancer.

SIDE EFFECTS:
IUD – *Common:* Pain low in belly and back, headache, breast tenderness.
Unusual: Nausea, acne, abnormal menstrual bleeding, infection of uterus.
Severe but rare (stop medication, consult doctor): Perforation of uterus, blood clot (calf pain, short of breath, chest pain).
Tablets – *Common:* Nausea, tiredness, belly pains, diarrhoea, dizziness, headache, breast tenderness, unusual vaginal bleeding.
Unusual: Increased bleeding tendency, vomiting.

INTERACTIONS:
Other drugs:
- Other sex hormones, primidone, barbiturates, phenytoin, carbamazepine, rifampicin, griseofulvin, phenylbutazone, ritonavir, ampicillin and other antibiotics, hypoglycaemics (treat diabetes), insulin.

PRESCRIPTION:
Yes.

PBS:
IUD: Yes
Tablets: No.

PERMITTED IN SPORT:
Yes.

OTHER INFORMATION:
IUD introduced in 2001 as a totally new type of contraception. Tablets introduced in 2002 as the first officially recognised form of 'morning after' pill (previously contrived by doctors from potent oral contraceptives).
See also **ORAL CONTRACEPTIVES**.

Medications

Lignocaine
See ANAESTHETICS, LOCAL.

Lincomycin

TRADE NAME:
Lincocin.

DRUG CLASS:
Antibiotic.

USES:
Serious bacterial infections of lung, skin and bone.

FORMS:
Injection.

PRECAUTIONS:
Safe in pregnancy (A), breast feeding and children. Not to be used under three months of age.
Use with caution in gut inflammation, asthma, meningitis and liver disease.
Not to be used long term.
Lower doses necessary in elderly.

SIDE EFFECTS:
Common: Sore mouth, nausea.
Unusual: Diarrhoea, rash.
Severe but rare (stop medication, consult doctor): Severe or bloody diarrhoea, worsening infection, unusual bleeding or bruising, yellow skin (jaundice).

INTERACTIONS:
Other drugs:
• Erythromycin.

PRESCRIPTION:
Yes.

PBS:
Yes.

PERMITTED IN SPORT:
Yes.

OVERDOSE:
Exacerbation of side effects likely.

OTHER INFORMATION:
Serious rare side effects have led to this otherwise safe and effective medication being restricted to only serious infections.

Linezolid

TRADE NAME:
Zyvox.

DRUG CLASS:
Antibiotic.

USES:
Severe bacterial infections resistant to other antibiotics.

DOSAGE:
 One tablet twice a day.

FORMS:
Tablets (white) of 600mg, suspension, injection.

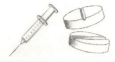

PRECAUTIONS:
Use with caution in pregnancy (B3), breast feeding and children.
Use with caution in chronic infections.
Not for long term use.
Regular blood tests necessary to check blood cells.

SIDE EFFECTS:
Common: Headache, nausea, diarrhoea.
Unusual: Abnormal taste, fungal infections (eg. thrush).
Severe but rare (stop medication, consult doctor): White blood cell damage, worsening infection, pseudomembranous colitis (bloody diarrhoea), liver damage (jaundice), vision changes.

INTERACTIONS:
Other drugs:
- Pseudoephedrine, phenylpropanolamine, dopamine, adrenaline.

Other substances:
- Yeast containing foods (eg. Vegemite).

PRESCRIPTION:
Yes.

PBS:
No.

PERMITTED IN SPORT:
Yes.

OTHER INFORMATION:
Introduced in 2002.

Liniments

DISCUSSION:
Liniments are creams or lotions that are rubbed into the skin to create local warmth and skin redness. There are scores of liniments available from chemists to treat bruises, sprains, fibrositis and arthritic conditions (eg. camphor, menthol, alcohol, salicylates). They should not be used on the face, near body openings (eg. anus, vagina), or on grazes or cuts. Many NSAIDs (see separate entry) are also available as creams and gels.

See **Benzydamine hydrochlorine, Camphor, Capsaicin, Heparinoid, Menthol, SALICYLATES.**

Linoleic acid
(Evening primrose oil)
See **FATTY ACIDS.**

Liothyronine

TRADE NAME:
Tertroxin (T3).

USES:
Severely under-active thyroid gland (myxoedema), thyroiditis.

DOSAGE:

One or two tablets a day on an empty stomach.
Start with low initial dose and slowly increase to a dose determined by doctor after regular blood tests.

FORMS:
Tablets of 20µg (white).

PRECAUTIONS:
Safe to use in pregnancy (A), breast feeding and children.
Use with caution in heart disease and high blood pressure.

Do not take if:
 suffering from angina, Addison's disease.

SIDE EFFECTS:
Only occur with overdosage.

INTERACTIONS:
Other drugs:
- Coumarin anticoagulants (eg. warfarin), barbiturates, narcotics, insulin, catecholamines, tricyclic antidepressants, digoxin, corticosteroids, colestipol, phenytoin, cholestyramine, oral contraceptives.

PRESCRIPTION:
Yes.

PBS:
Yes (authority required).

PERMITTED IN SPORT:
Yes.

OVERDOSE:

Serious. May cause rapid heart rate, irregular heartbeat, angina, restlessness, anxiety, tremor, headache, diarrhoea, vomiting, rapid breathing, fever, heart attack and death. Administer activated charcoal or induce vomiting if medication taken recently. Seek urgent medical assistance.

OTHER INFORMATION:

Widely used to counter the slowly progressive effects of thyroid underactivity, a problem that is common in middle aged women. Does not cause addiction or dependence, but lifelong treatment usually necessary.

See also Thyroxine

Liquorice
(Glycyrrhizin, Licorice)

USES:
Cough, gastritis (stomach inflammation).

DOSAGE:
5g to 15g of root a day (200mg to 600mg of glycyrrhizin extract).

FORMS:
Capsules, extract for tea preparation.

PRECAUTIONS:
Do not use in pregnancy and breast feeding. Do not use long term (over six weeks) as low blood potassium and high blood sodium levels may occur.
Use with caution in fluid retention disorders, high blood pressure and heart disease.

Do not take if:
 suffering from hepatitis, gall bladder disease, cirrhosis, severe kidney disease, diabetes, irregular heart rhythm, untreated high blood pressure, excess muscle tone.
- under other circumstances

SIDE EFFECTS:
Common: Retention of fluid, weight gain.
Unusual: High blood pressure.
Severe but rare (stop medication, consult doctor): Irregular heart rhythm.

INTERACTIONS:
Other drugs:
- Frusemide, thiazide diuretics, digoxin, procainamide, quinidine, steroids.

Other substances:
- Smoking tobacco.

PRESCRIPTION:
No.

PBS:
No.

OVERDOSE:
Blood chemistry disorders may occur, leading to irregular heart rhythm and high blood pressure.

OTHER INFORMATION:
Not used in orthodox medical practice.

Lisinopril
See ACE INHIBITORS.

Lithium carbonate

TRADE NAMES:
Lithicarb, Quilonum SR.

DRUG CLASS:
Antipsychotic.

USES:
Manic-depressive psychoses, other psychiatric conditions.

DOSAGE:
 One or two tablets, two or three times a day.
Dosage must be individualised for each patient.
Follow doctor's instructions carefully.

FORMS:

Tablets (white) of 250mg and 450mg.

PRECAUTIONS:

Lithium must not be used in pregnancy (D) except under exceptional circumstances as it may cause malformations of the heart and damage to the thyroid gland of the foetus. Breast feeding must be ceased if Lithium is taken. Not for use in children.
Diet should remain regular during dosage with lithium as changes in diet and fluid intake can affect blood levels of Lithium. Regular blood tests to check dosage of lithium recommended.

Do not take if:

suffering from significant heart and kidney disease, Addison's disease, under-active thyroid gland.

SIDE EFFECTS:

Common: Weight gain, goitre, swelling of tissues (oedema), dermatitis, loss of appetite, nausea, belly discomfort, diarrhoea, tiredness, slurred speech.
Unusual: Vomiting, tremor, agitation.

INTERACTIONS:

Other drugs:
- Steroids, appetite suppressants, other psychotropic drugs, NSAID, ACE inhibitors, calcium channel blockers, urea, xanthine, methyldopa, diuretics, antidepressants.

Herbs:
- Evening primrose (linoleic acid), psyllium.

PRESCRIPTION:
Yes.

PBS:
Yes.

PERMITTED IN SPORT:
Yes.

OVERDOSE:

Extremely serious. Symptoms may include diarrhoea, vomiting, weakness, incoordination, drowsiness, twitching, disorientation, coma and death. Administer activated charcoal or induce vomiting if taken recently and patient alert. Seek emergency medical assistance.

OTHER INFORMATION:

Widely used and effective treatment developed in Melbourne, Australia. Used for some specific types of mental illness. Does not cause addiction or dependence.

See also **Amisulpride, Droperidol, Flupenthixol, Haloperidol, Olanzapine, PHENOTHIAZINES, Pimozide, Quetiapine, Risperidone, Thiothixene, Zuclopenthixol.**

LOCAL ANAESTHETICS

See ANAESTHETICS, LOCAL.

Lodoxamide

TRADE NAME:
Lomide.

USES:

Allergic conjunctivitis, keratoconjunctivitis.

DOSAGE:

 One drop in eye four times a day.

FORMS:

Eye drops.

PRECAUTIONS:

May be used with caution in pregnancy (B1), breast feeding and children under 4 years.
Use with caution if wearing contact lenses. Do not persist with use if symptoms continue.

SIDE EFFECTS:
Common: Eye discomfort, eye itch, blurred vision.
Unusual: Crusting of lid margins, dry eye, red eye, excess tears.

INTERACTIONS:
None significant.

PRESCRIPTION:
Yes.

PBS:
Yes (authority required).

PERMITTED IN SPORT:
Yes.

OVERDOSE:
Unlikely to be serious.

OTHER INFORMATION:
Introduced in 1997 as an effective treatment for allergic reaction in the eye unrelieved by simpler medications.

Lomustine

TRADE NAME:
CeeNU.

DRUG CLASS:
Alkylater.

USES:
Brain tumours, Hodgkin's disease.

DOSAGE:
 As determined for each patient by doctor. Take on an empty stomach.

FORMS:
Capsules of 10mg (white), 40mg (white/green) and 100mg (green).

PRECAUTIONS:
Must not be used in pregnancy (D) or breast feeding.
Not for long term use.
Regular blood tests essential to check function of liver, kidney and blood cells.
Potential to aggravate other undetected cancers.

Do not take if:
 suffering from bone marrow suppression.

SIDE EFFECTS:
Common: Decreased fertility, liver and kidney damage, brain disturbances.
Unusual: Bone marrow damage.
Severe but rare (stop medication, consult doctor): Jaundice (liver damage).

INTERACTIONS:
Other drugs:
- Other medications that suppress bone marrow function.

PRESCRIPTION:
Yes.

PBS:
No (very expensive).

PERMITTED IN SPORT:
Yes.

OVERDOSE:
Extremely toxic. Serious organ damage may occur. Induce vomiting or give activated charcoal if taken recently. Seek emergency medical assistance.

LOOP DIURETICS

DISCUSSION:
Subgroup of diuretics that work in a specific way in the kidney (on the loop of Henle apparatus). All diuretics act to increase the production of urine and remove fluid from the body.

See Bumetanide, Ethacrynic Acid, Frusemide.

Loperamide

TRADE NAMES:
Gastro Stop, Harmonise, Imodium. Imodium Advanced (with simethicone).

DRUG CLASS:
Antidiarrhoeal.

USES:
Diarrhoea.

DOSAGE:

Two capsules at once, then one capsule after each episode of diarrhoea to a maximum of eight capsules a day.

FORMS:
Capsules.

PRECAUTIONS:
Should be used in pregnancy (B3) and breast feeding only on medical advice. Not approved for use in children under 12 years.
Do not use for more than 48 hours without medical advice.
Use with caution in ulcerative colitis, Crohn's disease, glaucoma, liver and kidney disease.

Do not take if:
 suffering from cirrhosis of liver or severe kidney disease.
- suffering from glaucoma or difficulty in passing urine.
- constipated.

SIDE EFFECTS:
Common: Excess passage of wind, constipation, nausea, belly pain.
Unusual: Giddiness, rash, vomiting, metallic taste, decreased sexual drive, headache, weakness, tiredness, dry mouth, blurred vision.

INTERACTIONS:
Other drugs:
- Interacts with tranquillisers in some patients.
- May interact with monoamine oxidase inhibitors (MAOI).

Other substances:
- Do not take with alcohol.

PRESCRIPTION:
Up to eight capsules no prescription required. Prescription required for larger quantities.

PBS:
Yes.

PERMITTED IN SPORT:
Yes.

OVERDOSE:
Constipation and vomiting only likely effects.

OTHER INFORMATION:
Widely used and relatively safe medication. Acts to sedate bowel muscles without any effect on the brain.

See also Atropine, Attapulgite, Codeine Phosphate, Diphenoxylate hydrochloride, Kaolin, Pectin.

Lopinavir

See Ritonavir.

Loratadine

See ANTIHISTAMINES, NON-SEDATING.

Lorazepam

TRADE NAME:
Ativan.

DRUG CLASS:
Benzodiazepine (Anxiolytic).

USES:
Relief of anxiety, anxiety associated with depression, preoperative sedation.

DOSAGE:

One to four tablets a day in one or more doses. Do not exceed dose directed by doctor.

FORMS:
Tablets of 1mg (white) and 2.5mg (yellow).

PRECAUTIONS:
Should be used with caution in pregnancy (C), but not at all if delivery of infant imminent as it may decrease desire to breathe in newborn infant. Should be used with caution in breast feeding. Not for use in children.
Lower dose required in elderly.
Should be used intermittently and not constantly as dependency may develop. Use with caution in glaucoma, myasthenia gravis, heart disease, kidney or liver disease, psychiatric conditions, schizophrenia, depression and epilepsy.

Do not take if:
 suffering from severe lung disease, confusion.
- tendency to addiction or dependence.
- operating machinery, driving a vehicle or undertaking tasks that require concentration and alertness.

SIDE EFFECTS:
Common: Reduced alertness, dependence.
Unusual: Incoordination, tremor, confusion, increased risk of falls in elderly, rash, low blood pressure, nausea, muscle weakness.
Severe but rare (stop medication, consult doctor): Jaundice (yellow skin).

INTERACTIONS:
Other drugs:
- Sedatives, other anxiolytics, disulfiram, cimetidine, anticonvulsants, anticholinergics.

Herbs:
- Guarana, kava kava, passionflower, St John's wort, valerian.

Other substances:
- Reacts with alcohol to cause sedation and confusion.

PRESCRIPTION:
Yes.

PBS:
No.

PERMITTED IN SPORT:
Yes.

OVERDOSE:
Seldom life threatening. May cause drowsiness, confusion and coma. Induce vomiting if tablets taken recently. Seek medical assistance.

OTHER INFORMATION:
Dependency becoming a significant problem, particularly in elderly, due to overuse.

See also **Alprazolam, Bromazepam, Buspirone, Clobazam, Diazepam, Oxazepam**.

Losartan

See **ANGIOTENSIN II RECEPTOR ANTAGONISTS**.

LUBRICANTS, EYE

See **EYE LUBRICANTS**.

Lumefantrine

See **Artemether and Lumefantrine**.

Medications

Macrogol 400
See EYE LUBRICANTS

MACROLIDES

DISCUSSION:
Macrolides are antibiotics that act against bacteria by interfering with the way their internal chemical reactions occur. They are most commonly used in chest, sinus and ear infections. They can interact with theophylline, which is used by asthmatics and in some cough mixtures. Some people who are allergic to penicillin are also allergic to macrolides.

See Azithromycin, Clarithromycin, Erythromycin, Roxithromycin.

PRECAUTIONS:
Safe to use in pregnancy, breast feeding and children.

SIDE EFFECTS:
Minimal.

INTERACTIONS:
None significant.

PRESCRIPTION:
No.

PBS:
No.

PERMITTED IN SPORT:
Yes.

OVERDOSE:
Stomach and bowel upsets likely.

Magnesium

TRADE NAMES:
Magnesium, in various forms, is found in numerous vitamin and mineral supplements.

DRUG CLASS:
Mineral.

USES:
Magnesium deficiency.

DOSAGE:

Recommended daily intake:
Females – 270mg a day;
Males – 320mg a day.

FORMS:
Tablets, capsules.

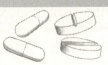

Magnesium Salts
See ANTACIDS, ELECTROLYTES.

Magnesium sulfate

TRADE NAME:
Magnoplasm (with glycerol).
Also found in numerous vitamin and mineral supplements.

DRUG CLASS:
Mineral.

USES:
By mouth: Magnesium deficiency.
Paste: Boils, abscesses, carbuncles.

DOSAGE:
 Paste: Apply thickly on lint (cloth) and bandage over affected area.

FORMS:
Paste, tablets, capsules.

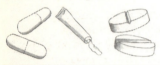

PRECAUTIONS:
Safe to use in pregnancy, breast feeding and children.
Avoid using paste on healing wounds.

SIDE EFFECTS:
Minimal.

INTERACTIONS:
None.

PRESCRIPTION:
No.

PBS:
No.

PERMITTED IN SPORT:
Yes.

OTHER INFORMATION:
Magnesium sulfate paste is an ancient and superseded medication that works by drawing fluid out of tissue. Better treatments now exist for boils etc.

Maldison

TRADE NAME:
Lice Rid.

DRUG CLASS:
Antiparasitic.

USES:
Head lice.

DOSAGE:
 Apply 20mLs to dry hair, leave 12 hours, wash and fine comb.

FORMS:
Liquid.

PRECAUTIONS:
Safe to use in pregnancy (B2), breast feeding and children over six months.
Avoid contact with eyes, nostrils and mouth.
Wash hands thoroughly after use.
Not for use for body lice.
Do not wear hats or shower caps for an hour after use.
Do not use electric hair dryer or smoke for one hour after use (flammable).

SIDE EFFECTS:
Common: Minimal.
Unusual: Skin irritation.

INTERACTIONS:
None significant.

PRESCRIPTION:
No.

PBS:
No.

PERMITTED IN SPORT:
Yes.

Medications

OVERDOSE:
Toxic if swallowed. Administer activated charcoal or induce vomiting and seek urgent medical advice.

OTHER INFORMATION:
Treat all members of family and other close contacts at same time. Use fine comb on hair repeatedly to remove egg cases. Repeat after five to seven days in case any eggs remain to hatch later.
See also Permethrin, Piperonyl butoxide.

MAOI
(Monoamine oxidase inhibitors)

TRADE and GENERIC NAMES:
Nardil (Phenelzine).
Parnate (Tranylcypromine).

DRUG CLASS:
Antidepressant.

USES:
Severe depression, phobias (fears).

DOSAGE:

One or two tablets, two or three times a day.

FORMS:
Tablets.

PRECAUTIONS:
Should be used in pregnancy (B3) only if medically essential. Not for use in breast feeding or children.
Use with caution in kidney disease. Occasional blood tests to check liver function are recommended.
Regular blood pressure checks to detect low blood pressure are recommended. Possible serious interactions with food and medication. Read literature supplied by doctor or pharmacist carefully and do not take drug unless you understand instructions completely.

Do not take if:
☠ suffering from epilepsy, heart disease, stroke, high blood pressure, severe headaches or liver disease.
- over 60 years of age.
- you are unsure of interactions with foods and medications.

SIDE EFFECTS:
Common: Dizziness, constipation, dry mouth, low blood pressure, drowsiness, weakness, fatigue, swelling of tissues (oedema), nausea.
Unusual: Blurred vision, sweating, glaucoma, inability to pass urine.
Severe but rare (stop medication, consult doctor): Agitation.

INTERACTIONS:
Other drugs:
- Intcracts with a very wide range of medications. Do not take any medication, including non-prescription and supermarket items without consulting a doctor.

Herbs:
- Aniseed, capsicum, ginseng, ma huang, parsley.

Other substances:
- Reacts adversely with alcohol, particularly wine and beer.
- Reacts adversely with cheese, broad beans, pickled herrings, yeast extracts (eg. Vegemite, Marmite), soy sauce, and beef extracts.

PRESCRIPTION:
Yes.

PBS:
Yes (restricted).

PERMITTED IN SPORT:
Yes.

OVERDOSE:
Very serious. Faintness, chest pain, headache, low blood pressure, agitation, clammy skin, fits, coma and death may

occur. Administer activated charcoal or induce vomiting if tablets taken recently and patient alert. Seek urgent medical assistance.

OTHER INFORMATION:
A very useful medication in severely depressed patients, but its usefulness is limited by its side effects and severe potential to interact with other drugs and foods. MAOI are potent antidepressants that are only used in severe and chronic cases of depression. They are slow to become effective, and their effects may persist for a couple of weeks after they are stopped. Any patient on MAOI should be given by their doctor a list of foods and drugs they must avoid. This list must be observed carefully, or serious side effects may occur. If taken correctly, they can dramatically improve a depressed patient's life.
See also Selegiline.

Marijuana

OTHER NAMES:
Pot, cannabis, grass, hash, dope, charas, THC (tetrahydrocannabinol).

DRUG CLASS:
Cannabinoid.

USES:
No recognised medical uses in Australia. Used experimentally for nausea, vomiting, pain relief, intestinal spasm, sedation, epilepsy, glaucoma, high blood pressure and muscle spasm.
Used illegally as a psychoactive drug to cause euphoria (artificial happiness).

FORMS:
Used experimentally as a tablet or mixture.
Used illegally in many forms including smoke, and cooked in soup or biscuits.

PRECAUTIONS:
Should never be used in pregnancy, breast feeding or children. Marijuana may damage the foetus.
Do not use if:
 suffering from psychiatric disturbances, asthma, chronic lung disease.
- driving a car, operating machinery, swimming or undertaking any activity that requires concentration.

SIDE EFFECTS:
Common: Unwanted flashbacks, sexual disinhibition, drowsiness, palpitations, rapid pulse, dry mouth, sore and red eyes, dizziness, poor concentration, nausea, poor coordination.
Unusual: Hallucinations, vomiting, panic attacks, blackouts, perceptual changes, impotence, infertility.
Long term: Increased risk of lung cancer (greater risk than with tobacco smoking) and emphysema. Can bring on certain serious mental illnesses (eg. schizophrenia).

INTERACTIONS:
Other drugs:
- Hypnotics, sedatives, heroin.
Other substances:
- Increases the effect of alcohol.
- May lead to desire for stronger psychoactive drugs.

PRESCRIPTION:
Illegal.

PERMITTED IN SPORT:
No.

OVERDOSE:
May be serious if swallowed in large quantities. Exacerbation of side effects, convulsions and coma may lead rarely to death. Seek urgent medical attention.

OTHER INFORMATION:
Illegal drug of dependence. Toleration may develop quickly (higher dose required to obtain same effect).

Possession may lead to criminal charges. Derived from the Indian Hemp plant. Used at least once by about one third of all Australians. Metabolised slowly by the liver, and stored in fat. Complete elimination of a single dose may take up to six weeks.
See also Heroin.

Measles vaccine

TRADE NAMES:
MMR II, Priorix (with mumps and rubella vaccines).
Only available in Australia combined with other vaccines.

DRUG CLASS:
Vaccine.

USES:
Prevention of measles (morbilli).

DOSAGE:
 Two injections, one at 12 months and the second at 4 to 5 years of age.

FORMS:
Injection.

PRECAUTIONS:
Should not be used in pregnancy (B2), but unintentional use during pregnancy unlikely to have any serious effect. May be used in breast feeding and children. Use with caution if history of febrile convulsions or head injury.

Do not take if:
 suffering from active infection or tuberculosis.
- suffering from AIDS, immune deficiency or bone marrow disease.
- taking drugs for cancer or leukaemia.
- recent blood transfusion or globulin injection.
- sensitivity to hen eggs or neomycin.

SIDE EFFECTS:
Common: Redness, soreness and lump at injection site; fever.
Unusual: Rash.

INTERACTIONS:
Other drugs:
- Some other vaccines.

PRESCRIPTION:
Yes.

PBS:
No, but available free to doctors from state governments or local councils in combination with rubella and mumps vaccines.

PERMITTED IN SPORT:
Yes.

OVERDOSE:
An unintentional additional dose is unlikely to have any serious effect.

OTHER INFORMATION:
Measles has been eradicated in most countries by immunisation, but a flare up could still occur if immunisation levels in the community drop. In most cases it is a mild disease, but occasionally it can cause brain damage and death. All children should be vaccinated at 1 and 5 years of age. An attenuated live virus vaccine.
See also Mumps vaccine, Rubella vaccine.

Mebendazole

TRADE NAMES:
DeWorm, Combantrin Mebendazole, Vermox.

DRUG CLASS:
Anthelmintic (kills worms).

USES:
Threadworm, roundworm, whipworm and hookworm infestations of the intestine.

DOSAGE:

Threadworm: One tablet as a single dose, repeated in two to four weeks.
Other infestations: One tablet twice a day for three days.

FORMS:
Tablets, suspension.

PRECAUTIONS:
Not for use in pregnancy (B3) unless medically necessary. Breast feeding should be ceased before use. May be used in children over 2 years.

SIDE EFFECTS:
Common: Minimal.
Unusual: Diarrhoea, vomiting, belly pains, drowsiness, itch, headache, dizziness.
Severe but rare (stop medication, consult doctor): Rash, itch.

INTERACTIONS:
Other drugs:
• Cimetidine.

PRESCRIPTION:
No.

PBS:
No. Available to some Veteran Affairs pensioners.

PERMITTED IN SPORT:
Yes.

OVERDOSE:
Exacerbation of side effects plus possible liver damage. Seek medical attention.

OTHER INFORMATION:
Widely, safely and effectively used.
See also Pyrantel embonate.

Mebeverine

TRADE NAMES:
Colese, Colofac.

DRUG CLASS:
Antispasmodic.

USES:
Spasms of the intestine. Irritable bowel syndrome.

DOSAGE:

One tablet three times a day with or before food.

FORMS:
Tablets (white) of 135mg.

PRECAUTIONS:
Use with caution in pregnancy (B2) and breast feeding.
Use with caution if suffering from irregular heartbeat, angina, severe liver disease, severe kidney disease, or lactose intolerance.

SIDE EFFECTS:
Common: Minimal.
Unusual: Indigestion, heartburn, dizziness, sleeplessness, loss of appetite, constipation, slow pulse.

INTERACTIONS:
None significant.

PRESCRIPTION:
Yes.

Medications

PBS:
No. Available to some Veteran Affairs pensioners.

PERMITTED IN SPORT:
Yes.

OVERDOSE:
No significant problems reported.

OTHER INFORMATION:
Very safe, long established and widely used medication.
See also Alverine Citratel, Dicyclomine.

Medroxyprogesterone acetate (MPA)

TRADE NAMES:
Depo Provera, Depo Ralovera, Medroxyhexal, Provera, Ralovera. Menoprem (deleted 2002)**, Premia, Provelle** (with oestrogen).

DRUG CLASS:
Sex hormone.

USES:
Endometriosis, cessation of menstrual periods, abnormal bleeding from uterus, breast cancer, cancer of lining of uterus, some types of kidney cancer.
In combination with oestrogen in the treatment of menopause.
Injection used for contraception.

DOSAGE:
 Tablets: Half to three or more tablets a day, depending on diagnosis.
Injection: One injection every three months for contraception.

FORMS:
Tablets, capsules, injection.

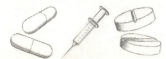

PRECAUTIONS:
Not to be used in pregnancy (D), breast feeding or children.
Use with caution with a history of blood clots in veins, eye disease, diabetes, depression, high blood pressure, heart failure or fluid retention.
Gynaecological and physical examination before prescription necessary.
Do not exceed prescribed dose.

Do not take if:
suffering from blood clot or tendency to form clots, stroke, liver disease, undiagnosed breast disease, undiagnosed uterine bleeding, or severe hypertension.
• recent abortion performed.

SIDE EFFECTS:
Common: Abnormal vaginal bleeding, headache, reduced fertility.
Unusual: Sleeplessness, nervousness, dizziness, tremor, rash, sweating, nausea, breast tenderness, weight gain.
Severe but rare (stop medication, consult doctor): Blood clot, calf pain, chest pain, yellow skin (jaundice).

INTERACTIONS:
Other drugs:
• Anticoagulants, hypoglycaemics, insulin.
• May interfere with laboratory tests.

PRESCRIPTION:
Yes.

PBS:
Yes.

PERMITTED IN SPORT:
Yes.

OVERDOSE:
Exacerbation of side effects likely.

OTHER INFORMATION:
Injection used in Europe and New Zealand for contraception since late 1960s, but only approved for general use as a contraceptive in Australia in 1994. Tablets very useful for controlling menstrual period problems, and delaying periods that may be due at an awkward time.

See Cyproterone acetate, Danazol, Dydrogesterone, Ethinyloestradiol, Etonogestrel, HORMONE REPLACEMENT THERAPY, Oestradiol, Oestriol, Oestrogen, ORAL CONTRACEPTIVES, Oxandrolone, Piperazine oestrone sulfate.

Mefenamic Acid

TRADE NAMES:
Mefic, Ponstan.

DRUG CLASS:
NSAID (Nonsteroidal anti-inflammatory drug).

USES:
Period pain, migraine, general pain relief.

DOSAGE:

Two capsules three times a day with food.

FORMS:
Capsules of 250mg.

PRECAUTIONS:
Should not be used in pregnancy (C) unless medically essential. Breast feeding should be ceased if necessary to use NSAID. Not for use in children under 2 years.
Use with caution in psychiatrically disturbed patients, epilepsy, severe infection, heart failure and kidney disease. Lower doses required in elderly, who may suffer more side effects.

Do not take if:
 suffering from peptic ulcer at present or in recent past.
- due for surgery (including dental surgery).
- suffering from bleeding disorder or anaemia.

SIDE EFFECTS:
Common: Stomach discomfort, diarrhoea, constipation, heartburn, nausea, headache, dizziness.
Unusual: Blurred vision, stomach ulcer, ringing noise in ears, retention of fluid, swelling of tissue, drowsiness, itch, rash, shortness of breath.
Severe but rare (stop medication, consult doctor): Vomiting blood, passing blood in faeces, other unusual bleeding, asthma induced by medication.

INTERACTIONS:
Other drugs:
- Must never be used with anticoagulants (eg. warfarin).
- Probenecid, diuretics, lithium, methotrexate, beta blockers, ACE inhibitors.

PRESCRIPTION:
Yes.

PBS:
Yes.

PERMITTED IN SPORT:
Yes.

OVERDOSE:
Causes nausea, vomiting, severe headache, dizziness, confusion and convulsions. Administer activated charcoal or induce vomiting if taken recently. Seek medical assistance.

OTHER INFORMATION:
Gives excellent relief to many women with period pain. Significant side effects (particularly on the stomach) in about 5% of patients limit their use.

See also Aspirin, Bufexamac, Celecoxib, Diclofenac, Diflunisal, Flurbiprofen, Ibuprofen, Indomethacin, Ketoprofen, Ketorolac trometanol, Naproxen, Piroxicam, Rofecoxib, Salicylic acid, Sulindac, Tenoxicam, Tiaprofenic Acid.

Mefloquine

TRADE NAME:
Lariam.

DRUG CLASS:
Antimalarial.

USES:
Prevention and treatment of malaria.

DOSAGE:

Prevention: One tablet a week for one week before entering, and two weeks after leaving malarious country.
Treatment: Three tablets at once, then two tablets six hours later.

FORMS:
Tablets (white) of 250mg.

PRECAUTIONS:
May be used in pregnancy (B3) if medically necessary. Breast feeding should be ceased before use. Not designed for use in children under 14 years.
Use with caution in heart disease and epilepsy.

Do not take if:
 suffering from liver or kidney disease, convulsions, psychiatric disturbances.

SIDE EFFECTS:
Common: Dizziness, vomiting.
Unusual: Giddiness, faints, pins and needles, muscle pain, fever.
Severe but rare (stop medication, consult doctor): Psychiatric disturbances.

INTERACTIONS:
Other drugs:
- Quinine, chloroquine, anticonvulsants, beta blockers, beta blockers (eg. propranolol, atenolol), calcium channel blockers (eg. verapamil, nifedipine), antihistamines, tricyclic antidepressants, phenothiazines, typhoid oral vaccine.

PRESCRIPTION:
Yes.

PBS:
No. Expensive.

PERMITTED IN SPORT:
Yes.

OVERDOSE:
Exacerbation of side effects likely. Administer activated charcoal or induce vomiting if medication taken recently. Seek medical assistance.

OTHER INFORMATION:
Introduced in the late 1980s to combat the increasing incidence of Chloroquine-resistant malaria. Effective, easy to use and safe.

See also Atovaquone, Artemether and Lumefantrine, Chloroquine, Doxycycline, Hydroxychloroquine, Primaquine, Proguanil, Pyrimethamine, Quinine, Sulfadoxine.

Megestrol

TRADE NAME:
Megace.

USES:
Breast cancer.

DOSAGE:

One tablet four times a day.

FORMS:
Tablet (white) of 40mg.

PRECAUTIONS:
Not to be used in pregnancy (D) unless mother's life at risk as damage to foetus possible. Breast feeding must be ceased before use. Not for use in children. Women must use adequate contraception

while taking Megestrol.
Regular blood tests to check blood sugar level recommended.
Use with caution in blood clots and diabetes.

SIDE EFFECTS:
Common: Nausea, weight gain, fluid retention, abnormal vaginal bleeding.
Unusual: Vomiting, tumour pain, bone pain, hot flushes.
Severe but rare (stop medication, consult doctor): Blood clot in vein.

INTERACTIONS:
None significant.

PRESCRIPTION:
Yes.

PBS:
Yes.

OVERDOSE:
Not likely to be serious. Exacerbation of side effects probable. Seek medical attention.

OTHER INFORMATION:
Used to slow the progress of breast cancer as a last resort after it has spread to other organs.

Meloxicam

TRADE NAME:
Mobic.

DRUG CLASS:
Cox-2 inhibitor.

USES:
Osteoarthritis.

DOSAGE:
 7.5mg to 15mg a day.

FORMS:
Tablets of 7.5mg and 15mg.

PRECAUTIONS:
Use with caution in pregnancy (C) and breast feeding.
Not for use in children.
Use with considerable caution with history of peptic ulcer or stomach bleed.
Use with caution with heart failure, liver disease (eg. cirrhosis), kidney disease (eg. nephrotic syndrome), high blood pressure, and the elderly.

Do not take if:
suffering from asthma, urticaria from aspirin, peptic ulcer disease, severe liver or kidney disease.
• under 18 years of age

SIDE EFFECTS:
Common: Nausea.
Unusual: Dizziness, headache, mouth ulcers.
Severe but rare (stop medication, consult doctor): Stomach pain, ulceration or bleeding

INTERACTIONS:
Other drugs:
• Severe interaction with fluconazole, sulfaphenazone, sulfinpyrazone.
• Ketoconazole, itraconazole,

erythromycin, astemizole, cyclosporin, amiodarone, quinidine, diuretics, other NSAIDs, anticoagulants (eg. warfarin), methotrexate, oral contraceptives, hypoglycaemics (used for diabetes), cholestyramine.

PRESCRIPTION:
Yes.

PBS:
Yes.

PERMITTED IN SPORT:
Yes.

OVERDOSE:
Exacerbation of side effects likely. Induce vomiting or give activated charcoal if swallowed recently. Seek medical attention.
See also Celecoxib, Rofecoxib.

Melphalan

TRADE NAME:
Alkeran.

USES:
Cancer of breast and ovary, sarcoma, melanoma, multiple myeloma, polycythaemia vera.

DRUG CLASS:
Alkylater.

DOSAGE:

Must be individualised by doctor for each patient depending on disease, severity, age and weight of patient.

FORMS:
Tablets of 2mg (white), injection.

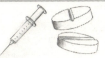

PRECAUTIONS:
Must not be used in pregnancy (D) unless medically essential for the life of the woman. Breast feeding must be ceased before use. Not for use in children unless essential for the life of the child.
Use with caution in kidney disease and if given radiation or cytotoxic treatment recently.
Regular blood tests to check blood cells essential.

SIDE EFFECTS:
Common: Damage to bone marrow and white blood cells, nausea, vomiting, diarrhoea, sore mouth.
Unusual: Hair loss, anaemia, lung damage.
Severe but rare (stop medication, consult doctor): Severe abnormal bleeding or bruising.

INTERACTIONS:
Other drugs:
• Cyclosporin, nalidixic acid.

PRESCRIPTION:
Yes.

PBS:
Tablets: Yes.
Injection: No.

PERMITTED IN SPORT:
Yes.

OVERDOSE:
Very serious. Destruction of bone marrow possible, which may lead to fatal infections. Seek urgent medical attention.

Menadione

See HAEMOSTATIC AGENTS.

Meningococcal vaccine

TRADE NAMES:
Mencevax ACWY, Meningitec, Menjugate, Menomune, NeisVac-C.

DRUG CLASS:
Vaccine.

USES:
Prevention of meningococcal meningitis caused by Neisseria meningitidis. There are more than a dozen strains of the disease. Mencevax ACWY and Menomune protect against strains A, C, W and Y and are mainly used for short term protection in travellers to poorer countries and during epidemics. Meningitec, Menjugate and NeisVac-C protect only against strain C, which is the strain most likely to cause death, and are used for long term prevention of infection in population-based programs.

DOSAGE:

Under 1 year of age – three injections a month apart.
Over 1 year of age – one injection.

FORMS:
Injection.

PRECAUTIONS:
Not designed to be used in pregnancy (B2), but inadvertent administration is unlikely to cause any serious adverse effect.
Use with caution in malaria, bleeding disorders or impaired immunity.

Do not take if:
 suffering from significant fever.

SIDE EFFECTS:
Common: Injection site pain and redness.
Unusual: Headache, rash, muscle pains, irritability, diarrhoea.

INTERACTIONS:
Other drugs:
- Other vaccines (administer in different limb).

PRESCRIPTION:
Yes.

PBS:
No, but supplied free through government supplies to doctors and vaccination clinics for some age groups.

PERMITTED IN SPORT:
Yes.

OVERDOSE:
An inadvertent additional vaccination is unlikely to have any serious side effects.

OTHER INFORMATION:
Widespread vaccination of children began in Australia during 2003.

Menopausal gonadotrophin, human
(Menotrophin)

TRADE NAME:
Humegon.

DRUG CLASS:
Trophic hormone.

USES:
Male and female infertility. Stimulates production of sperm and eggs.

DOSAGE:
 As determined by doctor for each patient.

FORMS:
Injection.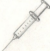

Medications

PRECAUTIONS:
Not for use in pregnancy (B2), breast feeding and children.
Only for use in specific types of female infertility caused by failure of egg release from the ovaries.
Regular blood tests to measure hormone levels essential.
Regular ultrasound scans to assess size of ovaries essential.

Do not use if:
 suffering from tumour of ovary, testes or pituitary gland.

SIDE EFFECTS:
Common: Ovarian pain, multiple pregnancy, injection site pain.

INTERACTIONS:
Other drugs:
- Sex hormones.

PRESCRIPTION:
Yes.

PBS:
Yes.

PERMITTED IN SPORT:
Yes.

Menotrophin
See Menopausal gonadotrophin, human.

Menthol

TRADE NAMES:
Dencorub Arthritis Ice, Ice Gel. APR Cream, Biosal, Deep Heat, Dencorub Pain Cream, Metsal, Radian B, Rubesal, Seda-Gel, SM-33 Gel, Vicks Inhaler (with salicylic acid and other ingredients).
Avil Decongestant (with pheniramine and ammonium chloride).
Karvol, Logicin Chest Rub, Nyal Cold Sore Cream, Sarna Lotion, Vicks Vaporub (with other ingredients).
Bonnington's Irish Moss (with camphor).
Vasylox, Vicks Sinex (with oxymetazoline).
SOOV Bite (with lignocaine and cetrimide).
Also found in numerous other lotions, creams, ointments, decongestants etc.

USES:
Relief of muscular pain, relief of nasal congestion, disguising unwanted aromas.

DOSAGE:
 Varies with form. As directed on packaging.

FORMS:
Gel, cream, ointment, powder, inhaler, mixture, lotion, spray.

PRECAUTIONS:
Nil.

SIDE EFFECTS:
Minimal.

INTERACTIONS:
None significant.

PRESCRIPTION:
No.

PBS:
No.

PERMITTED IN SPORT:
Yes.

OVERDOSE:
Not a problem.

OTHER INFORMATION:
Used primarily for its aroma and ability to dissolve other medications. Clinical effects probably minimal.

Mepivacaine
See ANAESTHETICS, LOCAL.

Mepyramine
See ANTIHISTAMINES, SEDATING.

Mercaptopurine

TRADE NAME:
Puri-Nethol.

USES:
Leukaemia.

DOSAGE:
 Must be individualised for each patient by doctor depending on response.

FORMS:
Tablets (yellow) of 50mg.

PRECAUTIONS:
Must not be used in pregnancy (D) unless the mother's life is at risk as the foetus may be damaged. Breast feeding must be ceased before use. May be used with caution in children.
Adequate contraception must be used by women taking Mercaptopurine.
Regular blood tests to check blood cells and liver function essential.

SIDE EFFECTS:
Common: Liver and bone marrow damage.
Unusual: Loss of appetite, nausea, vomiting, mouth ulcers.
Severe but rare (stop medication, consult doctor): Yellow skin (jaundice), unusual bleeding or bruising.

INTERACTIONS:
Other drugs:
- Allopurinol, warfarin, sulfonamides, tranquillisers.

PRESCRIPTION:
Yes.

PBS:
Yes.

PERMITTED IN SPORT:
Yes.

OVERDOSE:
May cause fatal damage to liver or bone marrow. Administer activated charcoal or induce vomiting if medication taken recently. Seek urgent medical assistance.

OTHER INFORMATION:
Despite serious side effects, Mercaptopurine may save or prolong life in patients with leukaemia.
See also **VINCA ALKALOIDS**.

Meropenem

TRADE NAME:
Merrem.

DRUG CLASS:
Antibiotic.

USES:
Serious bacterial infections.

DOSAGE:
500mg to 1000mg by drip into a vein every eight hours.

FORMS:
Injection.

PRECAUTIONS:
Use with caution in pregnancy (B2), breast feeding and infants.
Use with caution in Pseudomonas infections, liver and kidney disease.

SIDE EFFECTS:
Common: Injection site redness and pain, diarrhoea.
Unusual: Liver damage, large bowel damage, growth of resistant bacteria, damage to white blood cells.
Severe but rare (stop medication, consult doctor): Unusual bleeding or bruising.

INTERACTIONS:
Other drugs:
• Probenecid, valproic acid.

PRESCRIPTION:
Yes.

PBS:
No.

PERMITTED IN SPORT:
Yes.

OTHER INFORMATION:
Used only in hospital.

Mesalazine

TRADE NAMES:
Mesasal, Salofalk.

DRUG CLASS:
Bowel anti-inflammatory.

USES:
Ulcerative colitis, Crohn's disease, other forms of bowel inflammation.

DOSAGE:
 One or two tablets, or half to one sachet of granules, 30 minutes before meals three times a day with plenty of fluid.
Enemas used at night immediately before retiring.

FORMS:
Tablets of 250mg (tan), granules, enema.

PRECAUTIONS:
Should not be used in pregnancy (C).
Should not be used in breast feeding.
Use with caution in patients with liver disease and kidney disease, asthma and phenylketonuria.
Regular blood tests necessary to check for cell damage, liver and kidney function.
Do not take if:
 allergic to aspirin or salicylates.
• suffering from severe kidney or liver disease, peptic ulcer or bleeding disorder.

SIDE EFFECTS:
Common: Headache, nausea, rash, belly pains, diarrhoea.
Unusual: Kidney damage, pancreas inflammation.
Severe but rare (stop medication, consult doctor): Blood cell damage.

INTERACTIONS:
Other drugs:
- Do not use with lactulose or anticoagulants.
- Interacts with sulfonylureas, methotrexate, warfarin, frusemide, spironolactone, rifampicin, azathioprine and probenecid.

PRESCRIPTION:
Yes.

PBS:
Yes (authority required – restricted to colitis where sulfasalazine ineffective).

PERMITTED IN SPORT:
Yes.

OTHER INFORMATION:
Very effective medication for a number of uncommon diseases.

See also Olsalazine.

Mesna

TRADE NAME:
Uromitexan.

USES:
Prevents damage to lining of urinary tract and kidney that may be caused by powerful anticancer (cytotoxic) drugs.

DOSAGE:

As determined by doctor individually for each patient.

FORMS:
Injection, tablets (white) of 400 and 600mg.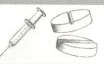

PRECAUTIONS:
May be used in pregnancy (B1), breast feeding and children.
Use with care in autoimmune diseases.

SIDE EFFECTS:
Common: Nausea, diarrhoea.
Unusual: Allergy reactions, headache, tiredness.

INTERACTIONS:
Adversely effects laboratory tests on urine.

PRESCRIPTION:
Yes.

PBS:
Injection: Yes.
Tablets: No.

PERMITTED IN SPORT:
Yes.

OVERDOSE:
Unlikely to be serious.

Mesterolone

TRADE NAME:
Proviron.

DRUG CLASS:
Sex hormone.

USES:
Male infertility, male impotence.

DOSAGE:

One tablet, one to three times a day.

FORMS:
Tablets of 25mg (white).

PRECAUTIONS:
Not to be used in women or children.
Use with caution in prostate disease.
Do not take if:
 suffering from prostate cancer or liver tumour.

SIDE EFFECTS:
Common: Minimal
Unusual: Prolonged penile erection.

INTERACTIONS:
None significant.

PRESCRIPTION:
Yes.

PBS:
No.

PERMITTED IN SPORT:
No.

OVERDOSE:
Painful, damaging, prolonged penile erection possible. Induce vomiting or administer activated charcoal if taken recently. Seek medical attention.
See also Testosterone.

Mestranol

See ORAL CONTRACEPTIVES.

Metformin

TRADE NAMES:
Diabex, Diaformin, GenRx Metformin, Glucohexal, Glucomet, Glucophage.

DRUG CLASS:
Hypoglycaemic.

USES:
Diabetes not requiring insulin injections.

DOSAGE:

One or two tablets, two or three times a day before meals.
Do not vary from prescribed dose without reference to a doctor.

FORMS:
Tablets of 500 and 850mg.

PRECAUTIONS:
Not to be used in pregnancy (C), breast feeding or children.
Annual blood tests to check for pernicious anaemia recommended. Blood tests every three to six months to check long term sugar levels and acidosis recommended. Illness, changes in diet, exercise and stress may change dosage requirements.
Use with caution if dehydrated, recent significant injury, suffering from liver or kidney disease. Lower doses required in elderly and debilitated patients.
Strict control of carbohydrates and sugars in diet essential.
Do not take if:
suffering from type 1 diabetes, severe heart disease, blood clot in lungs, pancreatitis, alcoholism, severe liver or kidney disease, recent surgery, severe infection.
• using insulin.

SIDE EFFECTS:

Common: Uncommon.
Unusual: Nausea, vomiting, belly discomfort, weakness.
Severe but rare (stop medication, consult doctor): Low blood sugar (see Overdose below), yellow skin (jaundice), unusual bleeding or bruising, rash.

INTERACTIONS:

Other drugs:
- Cimetidine, other hypoglycaemics, beta blockers, diclofenac, ACE inhibitors, corticosteroids, anticoagulants (eg. warfarin), thiazide diuretics, thyroxine.

Herbs:
- Alfalfa, celery, eucalyptus, fenugreek, garlic, ginger, ginseng, karela.

Other substances:
- Reacts adversely with alcohol.

PRESCRIPTION:
Yes.

PBS:
Yes.

PERMITTED IN SPORT:
Yes.

OVERDOSE:
Serious. Symptoms of low blood sugar (hypoglycaemia) may include tiredness, confusion, chills, palpitations, sweating, vomiting, dizziness, hunger, blurred vision and fainting. Significant overdosage can lead to coma and death. Give sugary drinks or sweets if conscious. Seek emergency medical assistance.

OTHER INFORMATION:
Used mainly in elderly patients who develop maturity onset diabetes that is not severe enough to require insulin injections.

See also Acarbose, Glibenclamide, Glicalazide, Glimepride, Glipizide, INSULINS, Repaglinide, Rosiglitazone, Tolbutamide.

Methadone

TRADE NAMES:
Biodone Forte, Methadone, Physeptone.

DRUG CLASS:
Narcotic, Analgesic.

USES:
Severe pain, narcotic addiction.

DOSAGE:

One or two tablets every six to eight hours. 2mLs to 10mLs of syrup a day.

FORMS:
Tablets (white) of 5mg and 10mg, syrup, injection.

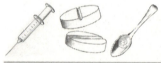

PRECAUTIONS:
Not to be used in the last stages of pregnancy (C) as methadone may cause the newborn infant to have difficulty in breathing. Use with caution in breast feeding and children.
Not designed for prolonged use.
Use with caution in hypothyroidism (under-active thyroid gland), adrenal gland disease, enlarged prostate gland, diabetes, kidney and liver disease.

Do not take if:
suffering from severe lung disease, acute asthma, alcoholism, recent head injury, kidney or gall stones, ulcerative colitis, severe liver disease.
- operating machinery or driving a vehicle.
- addictive tendency unless under supervision.

SIDE EFFECTS:
Common: Dizziness, drowsiness, vomiting, mood changes.
Unusual: Difficulty in breathing, dependence.

INTERACTIONS:
Other drugs:
- MAOI, rifampicin, phenytoin, carbamazepine, propranolol.

Other substances:
- Alcohol should not be used with methadone.

PRESCRIPTION:
Yes (very restricted).

PBS:
Tablets, injection: Yes.
Syrup: No.

PERMITTED IN SPORT:
No.

OVERDOSE:
Serious. Symptoms may not appear for some hours after medication taken, and may include drowsiness, difficulty in breathing, and coma. Administer activated charcoal or induce vomiting if medication taken recently and patient alert. Seek urgent medical attention. Antidote available.

OTHER INFORMATION:
Used in a slowly reducing dose to ease heroin addicts off their addiction. May itself be addictive if used inappropriately.

See also Alfentanil, Buprenorphine, Codeine Phosphate, Dextromoramide, Dextropropoxyphene, Fentanyl, Heroin, Hydromorphone, Morphine, Oxycodone, Pentazocine, Pethidine.

Methdilazine
See ANTIHISTAMINES, SEDATING.

Methenolone

TRADE NAME:
Primobolan.

DRUG CLASS:
Anabolic steroid.

USES:
Osteoporosis, uncontrolled breast cancer.

DOSAGE:
 One or two tablets twice a day.

FORMS:
Tablets of 5mg (white), injection.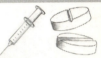

PRECAUTIONS:
Must not be used in pregnancy (D), breast feeding, adolescents or children.
Use with caution in diabetes, high blood calcium.
Not for long term use.

Do not take if:
 suffering from prostate disease, liver tumour.

SIDE EFFECTS:
Common: Nausea, headache, altered libido, fluid retention, premature cessation of growth in adolescents.
Menstrual irregularities and increased body hair in women.
Infertility, impotence, shrinking of testes and breast enlargement in men.
Severe but rare (stop medication, consult doctor): Yellow skin (jaundice).

INTERACTIONS:
Other drugs:
- Anticoagulants (eg. warfarin), corticosteroids, insulin, hypoglycaemics.

Herbs:
- Echinacea.

PRESCRIPTION:
Yes.

PBS:
Tablets: Yes (authority required. Restricted to osteoporosis and for patients on long term corticosteroids).
Injection: No.

PERMITTED IN SPORT:
No. Very strictly enforced.

OVERDOSE:
Exacerbation of side effects likely.

OTHER INFORMATION:
Does not cause dependence or addiction. Short term gains in muscle bulk when used inappropriately by body builders, may result in long term permanent body damage that may lead to early heart attacks, infertility, bone weakness, liver disease and premature death. Bottom line is – don't use it except under strict medical supervision when indicated for specific diseases.

See also Nandrolone decanoate.

Methionine

TRADE NAME:
Methnine.

DRUG CLASS:
Antidote.

USES:
Counteracts overdosage with paracetamol, liver damage.

DOSAGE:

Paracetamol overdose: Five tablets at once, repeated at four hour intervals for a total of four doses.

FORMS:
Tablets (white) of 500mg.

PRECAUTIONS:
May be used in pregnancy, breast feeding and children.
Administer activated charcoal or induce vomiting if paracetamol overdose taken recently.
Treatment must be undertaken immediately after vomiting has been successfully induced, before any signs of poisoning are evident.
Medication does not replace hospital care and other treatments.
Hospitals usually measure levels of paracetamol before starting specific treatment.

SIDE EFFECTS:
Minimal.

INTERACTIONS:
None significant.

PRESCRIPTION:
No.

PBS:
No.

PERMITTED IN SPORT:
Yes.

OTHER INFORMATION:
Overdosage with paracetamol may cause fatal liver damage. Methionine may prevent this damage if given within ten hours of the overdose being taken.

Methotrexate

TRADE NAMES:
Ledertrexate, Methoblastin, Methotrexate.

USES:
Numerous types of cancer including cancer of breast and uterus, leukaemia, severe psoriasis, severe rheumatoid arthritis.

DOSAGE:
 Must be individualised for each patient by doctor depending on disease, severity and weight of patient. Often given once a week.

FORMS:
Tablets of 2.5 and 10mg, injection.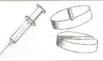

PRECAUTIONS:
Must not be used in pregnancy (D) unless mother's life is at risk, as the foetus may be damaged. Breast feeding must be ceased before use. May be used in children if medically essential.
Regular blood tests to check blood cells and liver function are essential.
Adequate contraception must be used by women while methotrexate is being taken. Use with caution in infection, active infection, peptic ulcer and ulcerative colitis.

Do not take if:
suffering from severe liver or kidney disease, significant infection, bone marrow disease, low level of white blood cells, low level of blood platelets, significant anaemia, immune deficiency (eg. AIDS), alcoholism.

SIDE EFFECTS:
Common: Mouth ulcers, nausea, belly pains, diarrhoea.
Unusual: Tiredness, chills, dizziness, reduced resistance to infection, rash, infertility.
Severe but rare (stop medication, consult doctor): Yellow skin (jaundice), unusual bleeding or bruising, bone marrow damage, vision changes.

INTERACTIONS:
Other drugs:
- NSAID, aspirin, sulfonamides, phenytoin, tetracyclines, chloramphenicol, folic acid, probenecid, co-trimoxazole, NSAIDs, drugs used to lower cholesterol levels, other cytotoxics.

Herbs:
- Echinacea, willow bark.

PRESCRIPTION:
Yes.

PBS:
Yes.

PERMITTED IN SPORT:
Yes.

OVERDOSE:
Serious. Administer activated charcoal or induce vomiting if medication taken recently. Seek urgent medical assistance. Antidote available.

OTHER INFORMATION:
Despite risk of significant side effects, Methotrexate may save the life, or improve the quality of life, of many patients.

See also Hydroxyurea, Thioguanine.

Methoxsalen

TRADE NAME:
Oxsoralen.

DRUG CLASS:
Psoralen.

USES:
Vitiligo (depigmentation of skin).

DOSAGE:

Lotion: Apply to lesions and expose to measured amount of ultraviolet light once a week.
Capsules: Take two with food two hours before exposure to measured amount of ultraviolet light.

FORMS:
Capsules (pink) of 10mg, lotion.

PRECAUTIONS:
Not to be used in pregnancy (B2), breast feeding and children under 12 years.
Avoid exposure to sunlight.
Protect eyes and lips for 24 hours after use.

SIDE EFFECTS:
Common: Stomach upset.
Unusual: Skin burning and blistering, allergy reactions.

INTERACTIONS:
Other drugs:
• Tetracyclines, phenothiazines.
Other substances:
• Reacts with figs, limes, parsley, parsnips, mustard, carrots, celery.

PRESCRIPTION:
Yes.

PBS:
No.

PERMITTED IN SPORT:
Yes.

OVERDOSE:
Avoidance of all sunlight essential or severe skin burning may result. Seek urgent medical advice.

OTHER INFORMATION:
Psoralens have no action in or on the body unless the skin is exposed to ultraviolet (UV) or sunlight. Psoralens sensitise the skin to UV and sunlight to cause a reaction that helps to add pigment to areas of skin that have lost pigment. Must be used strictly according to doctor's instructions. Skin should be exposed to measured amount of artificial UV light after use of Psoralen and sunlight should be avoided.
See also Dihydroxyacetone.

Methylcellulose

TRADE NAMES:
Numerous brands of fibre supplements.

DRUG CLASS:
Fibre.

USES:
Constipation, fibre supplementation, appetite suppression, diverticulitis.

DOSAGE:

Two to five tablets three times a day with water before meals.

FORMS:
Tablets.

PRECAUTIONS:
Safe in pregnancy and breast feeding.
Not recommended in children.
Ensure adequate fluid intake.
Do not take if:
 suffering from bowel blockage.

SIDE EFFECTS:
Common: Loose bulky motions.

INTERACTIONS:
Other drugs:
- May affect the absorption of a wide range of medications.

PRESCRIPTION:
No.

PBS:
No.

PERMITTED IN SPORT:
Yes.

OVERDOSE:
No adverse effects likely.

OTHER INFORMATION:
Totally inactive in body, and merely acts to add bulk to faeces.
See also Frangula, Ispaghula, Pectin, Psyllium, Sterculia.

Methyldopa

TRADE NAMES:
Aldomet, Hydopa.

DRUG CLASS:
Antihypertensive.

USES:
High blood pressure.

DOSAGE:
 One or two tablets two or three times a day to a maximum of 3000mg a day.

FORMS:
Tablets of 250mg.

PRECAUTIONS:
Safe in pregnancy (A), breast feeding and children.
Should be used with caution in patients with a history of depression and those on dialysis.
Do not take if:
 suffering from liver disease.

SIDE EFFECTS:
Common: Fever, sedation, headache.
Unusual: Aggravation of angina, swelling of tissues.
Severe but rare (stop medication, consult doctor): Unusual bleeding, severe tiredness.

INTERACTIONS:
Other drugs:
- Significant interaction with MAOI.
- Interacts with some anaesthetics, lithium and other medications that lower blood pressure.

Other substances:
- Smoking aggravates high blood pressure.

PRESCRIPTION:
Yes.

PBS:
Yes.

PERMITTED IN SPORT:
Yes.

OVERDOSE:
Causes low blood pressure, sedation, weakness, dizziness, slow heart rate, diarrhoea, nausea and vomiting. Rarely fatal. If taken recently, administer activated charcoal or induce vomiting. If taken more than two hours earlier, give patient additional fluids. Seek medical assistance.

OTHER INFORMATION:
An oldie but a goodie. One of the first really effective treatments for high blood pressure.

Methylphenidate

TRADE NAMES:
Attenta, Ritalin.

DRUG CLASS:
Stimulant.

USES:
Attention deficit hyperactivity disorder (ADHD), narcolepsy.

DOSAGE:
 Individualised. Start with low dose and gradually increase as determined by doctor until adequate response obtained.

FORMS:
Tablets of 10mg (white).

PRECAUTIONS:
Not for use in pregnancy (B3) unless medically essential. Not for use in breast feeding. Not for use in children under 6 years.
Use with caution in high blood pressure and epilepsy.
If possible, should not be used for prolonged periods of time.

Do not take if:
suffering from depression, psychoses, anxiety, agitation, twitches, Tourette syndrome, glaucoma, over-active thyroid gland, irregular heartbeat or angina.

SIDE EFFECTS:
Common: Sleeplessness, irritability, drowsiness, loss of appetite, belly pains, nausea, tolerance and dependency.
Unusual: Vomiting, irregular heartbeat, rash, growth retardation, blurred vision, psychiatric disturbances, angina, fever, hair loss, liver damage.

INTERACTIONS:
Other drugs:
- Tricyclic antidepressants, MAOI, anticoagulants (eg. warfarin), anticonvulsants, phenylbutazone, guanethidine, medications for treatment of high blood pressure.

Other substances:
- Alcohol.

PRESCRIPTION:
Yes (restricted to specific doctors only in some states).

PBS:
No.

PERMITTED IN SPORT:
No.

OVERDOSE:
Very serious. May cause vomiting, agitation, tremors, twitching, confusion, hallucinations, convulsions, coma and death. Administer activated charcoal or induce vomiting if tablets taken recently. Seek urgent medical attention.

OTHER INFORMATION:
May cause dependence and addiction if used inappropriately. May make a dramatic improvement in the quality of life for some hyperactive children and their parents, but use is still controversial as correct diagnosis of ADHD is difficult to determine.

Methylphenobarbitone

See BARBITURATES.

Methylprednisolone

TRADE NAMES:

Advantan (Methylprednisolone aceponate).
Depo-Medrol, Depo-Nisolone (Methylprednisolone acetate).
Solu-Medrol (Methylprednisolone sodium succinate).
Neo-Medrol Acne Lotion (Methylprednisolone acetate with neomycin, aluminium chlorohydrate, sulfur).

DRUG CLASS:
Corticosteroid.

USES:
Severe inflammation of skin (eg. acne, eczema).
Severe asthma, rheumatoid and other forms of severe arthritis, autoimmune diseases (eg. Sjögren Syndrome), severe allergy reactions, and other severe and chronic inflammatory diseases.

DOSAGE:

Tablets: Strictly as directed by doctor.
Lotion: Apply twice a day to affected skin.
Cream and ointment: Apply once a day.

FORMS:
Tablets, lotion, cream, ointment, fatty ointment, injection.

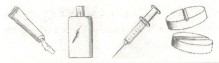

PRECAUTIONS:
Should be used in pregnancy (C), breast feeding and children only on specific medical advice.
Skin preparations safe in pregnancy, breast feeding and children over four months.
Use tablets and injection with caution if under stress, and in patients with underactive thyroid gland, liver disease, diverticulitis, high blood pressure, myasthenia gravis or kidney disease.
Avoid eyes with skin preparations.
Use for shortest period of time possible.
Tablets should not be ceased abruptly, but dosage should be slowly reduced.
Use skin preparations with caution on infected skin.

Do not use tablets or injection if:
 suffering from any form of infection, peptic ulcer, or osteoporosis.
- having a vaccination.

SIDE EFFECTS:
Most significant side effects occur only with prolonged use of tablets or injections.
Common: Skin preparations – Minimal.
Tablets – May cause bloating, weight gain, rashes and intestinal disturbances.
Unusual: Skin preparations – Thinning of skin, premature ageing, red skin.
Tablets – Biochemical disturbances of blood, muscle weakness, bone weakness, impaired wound healing, skin thinning, tendon weakness, peptic ulcers, gullet ulcers, bruising, increased sweating, loss of fat under skin, premature ageing, excess facial hair growth in women, pigmentation of skin and nails, acne, convulsions, headaches, dizziness, growth suppression in children, aggravation of diabetes, worsening of infections, cataracts, aggravation of glaucoma, blood clots in veins and sleeplessness.
Severe but rare (stop medication, consult doctor): Any significant side effect should be reported to a doctor immediately.

INTERACTIONS:
Other drugs:
- Tablets – Oral contraceptives, barbiturates, phenytoin, rifampicin.

PRESCRIPTION:
Yes.

PBS:
Neo-Medrol: No.
Other forms: Yes.

PERMITTED IN SPORT:
Tablets and injection: No.
Skin preparations: Yes.

OVERDOSE:
Medical treatment is required. Serious effects and death rare.

OTHER INFORMATION:
Extremely effective and useful medication if used correctly. Tablets must be used with extreme care under strict medical supervision. Lowest dose and shortest possible course should be used. Not addictive.

See also Betamethasone, Desonide, Hydrocortisone, Mometasone, Triamcinolone.

Methysergide

TRADE NAME:
Deseril.

DRUG CLASS:
Antimigraine.

USES:
Prevention of migraine and cluster headaches.

DOSAGE:

One or two tablets two or three times a day with food.

FORMS:
Tablets of 1mg (off-white).

PRECAUTIONS:
Should not be used in pregnancy (C), breast feeding or children.
Sudden cessation may cause rebound migraine – reduce dosage slowly when ceasing.
Use with caution if suffering from poor circulation to arms and legs.

Do not take if:
☠ suffering from poor circulation to heart, hardening of arteries, vein inflammation, severe infections, high blood pressure, collagen diseases, severe kidney or liver disease, urinary tract disease.

SIDE EFFECTS:
Common: Nausea, vomiting.
Unusual: Sleeplessness, dizziness, rash, tissue swelling, chest pain, belly pain, pins and needles sensation.
Severe but rare (stop medication, consult doctor): Difficulty in producing urine, backache, pain on passing urine, poor blood supply to legs.

INTERACTIONS:
None significant.

PRESCRIPTION:
Yes.

PBS:
Yes.

PERMITTED IN SPORT:
Yes.

OVERDOSE:
Administer activated charcoal or induce vomiting if tablets taken recently. Symptoms include vomiting, diarrhoea, thirst, cold skin, itch, rapid weak pulse, tingling, confusion. Seek medical assistance.

OTHER INFORMATION:
One of several medications that may be used to prevent migraines. Trial and error between these medications if often necessary to find the best one. Because of very rare but serious complications with long term use (retroperitoneal fibrosis – scar tissue forming at back of belly around kidneys), Methysergide is often towards the bottom of the list of medications considered.

See also Pizotifen.

Metoclopramide

TRADE NAMES:
Maxolon, Pramin.

DRUG CLASS:
Antiemetic.

USES:
Nausea, vomiting, during investigative procedures.

DOSAGE:

One tablet three times a day.

FORMS:
Tablets of 10mg, syrup, injection.

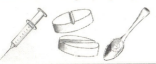

PRECAUTIONS:
Safe in pregnancy (A), breast feeding and children.
Use with caution in epilepsy, liver and kidney disease.
Lower doses required in elderly.
Do not persist with medication if vomiting continues, but seek further medical assessment.

Do not take if:
 suffering from phaeochromocytoma.

SIDE EFFECTS:
Common: Drowsiness, restlessness, tiredness.
Unusual: Sleeplessness, headache, dizziness, diarrhoea.
Severe but rare (stop medication, consult doctor): Incoordination, twitching, muscle spasms.

INTERACTIONS:
Other drugs:
- Narcotics, sedatives, anticholinergics, tetracycline, L-dopa, digoxin.

Other substances:
- Reacts adversely with alcohol.

PRESCRIPTION:
Yes.

PBS:
Yes.

PERMITTED IN SPORT:
Yes.

OVERDOSE:
Abnormal muscle twitching, muscle spasms and incoordination may occur. Seek medical advice.

OTHER INFORMATION:
Very widely used, safe and effective medication. Does not cause addiction or dependence.

See also Domperidone, Prochlorperazine, Promethazine.

Metoprolol

TRADE NAMES:
Betaloc, Lopresor, Metohexal, Metolol, Minax.
Numerous locally produced brands also exist.

DRUG CLASS:
Beta blocker.

USES:
High blood pressure, angina, rapid heart rate, irregular heartbeat, paroxysmal atrial tachycardia, heart attack, prevention of migraine.

DOSAGE:
 50 to 400mg a day in divided doses.

FORMS:
Tablets of 50 and 100mg, injection.

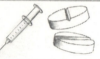

PRECAUTIONS:
Should be used in pregnancy (C) only if medically essential.
Safe to use in breast feeding.
May be used with caution in children.
Use with care if suffering from alcoholism, diabetes, prinzmetal angina, over-active thyroid gland, liver or kidney failure or about to have surgery.

Do not take if:
 suffering from asthma or allergic conditions.
- suffering from heart failure, shock, slow heart rate, enlarged right side of heart or phaeochromocytoma.
- if undertaking prolonged fast.

SIDE EFFECTS:
Common: Low blood pressure, slow heart rate, cold hands and feet, asthma.
Unusual: Loss of appetite, nausea, diarrhoea, impotence, tiredness, sleeplessness, nightmares, rash, loss of libido, hair loss, noises in ears.
Severe but rare (stop medication, consult doctor): Severe asthma.

INTERACTIONS:
Other drugs:
- Calcium channel blockers, prazosin, MAOI, disopyramide, clonidine, adrenaline, other medications for irregular heartbeat, lignocaine, ergotamine, indomethacin, chlorpromazine.

PRESCRIPTION:
Yes.

PBS:
Yes.

PERMITTED IN SPORT:
No.

OVERDOSE:
Slow heart rate, low blood pressure, asthma and heart failure may result. Administer activated charcoal or induce vomiting if tablets taken recently. Use Salbutamol or other asthma sprays for difficulty in breathing. Seek medical assistance.

OTHER INFORMATION:
Except for asthmatics, very safe and effective. First released in 1970s.

See also Atenolol, Carvedilol, Esmolol, Labetalol, Oxprenolol, Pindolol, Propranolol, Sotalol.

Metronidazole

TRADE NAMES:
Flagyl, Metrogyl, Metronide, Rozex.

DRUG CLASS:
Antibiotic.

USES:
Bacterial infections of gut and vagina, particularly Giardiasis of gut and Trichomonal infections of vagina. Acne rosacea.

DOSAGE:

Tablets: One or two tablets three times a day.
Gel and ointment: Apply thinly twice daily after washing.

FORMS:
Tablets, suppository, ointment, gel, suspension, infusion.

PRECAUTIONS:
Use with caution in pregnancy (B2) and breast feeding. Safe to use in children.
Avoid eyes, nostrils, mouth, vagina and anus with skin preparations.
Not designed for long term use.
Use with caution in kidney and liver disease.

Do not take if:

suffering from brain disease, blood cell abnormalities.

SIDE EFFECTS:
Common: Tablets – Bad taste, nausea, diarrhoea, headache.
Skin preparations – Redness, dryness, burning, irritation.
Unusual: Vomiting, loss of appetite, belly discomfort.

INTERACTIONS:
Other drugs:
- Warfarin, cyclophosphamide, phenytoin, phenobarbitone, cimetidine, lithium, cyclosporin, 5-fluorouracil.

Other substances:
- Reacts adversely with alcohol.
- May affect some laboratory blood test results.

PRESCRIPTION:
Yes.

PBS:
Yes.

PERMITTED IN SPORT:
Yes.

OVERDOSE:
With tablet overdosage disorientation and vomiting only likely effects.

OTHER INFORMATION:
Widely used. Very safe and effective. Often used in combination with other antibiotics for infections of female pelvic organs. Most effective treatment for the unusual skin condition of acne rosacea. Bad taste with tablets occurs in virtually every patient, as drug comes to taste buds on tongue through blood stream, and not from mouth, and so <u>cannot</u> usually be removed by sucking pleasantly flavoured sweets.

See also Tinidazole.

Metyrapone

TRADE NAME:
Metopirone.

USES:
Diagnosis of adrenal gland dysfunction, hyperaldosteronism, Cushing syndrome.

DOSAGE:
 Strictly as directed and determined by doctor.

FORMS:
Capsules (cream) of 250mg.

PRECAUTIONS:
Use with care (B2) in pregnancy, breast feeding and children.
Use with care in liver, pituitary gland and thyroid disease.
Do not take if:
 suffering from adrenocortical insufficiency.

SIDE EFFECTS:
Common: Nausea, diarrhoea, dizziness, sedation, headache.
Unusual: Low blood pressure, belly pain, excess hair growth.

INTERACTIONS:
Other drugs:
- May interact with numerous medications.

PRESCRIPTION:
Yes.

PBS:
No.

PERMITTED IN SPORT:
Yes.

OVERDOSE:
Very serious damage to numerous glands may occur.

OTHER INFORMATION:
Normally only used in hospitals as a diagnostic tool.

Mexiletine

TRADE NAME:
Mexitil.

DRUG CLASS:
Antiarrhythmic.

USES:
Serious heartbeat irregularities in the heart ventricles.

DOSAGE:
 Variable from one patient to another. Usually about 200mg three times a day.

FORMS:
Capsules of 50mg (red/purple) and 200mg (red), injection.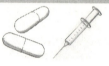

PRECAUTIONS:
Should be used with caution in pregnancy (B1) and breast feeding. Not designed for use in children.
Use with caution with low blood pressure, slow heart rate, liver or kidney failure.
Should not be stopped suddenly, but dose should be slowly decreased over several days.
Do not take if:
 suffering from recent heart attack or heart block.
- you are hypersensitive to local anaesthetics.

SIDE EFFECTS:
Common: Usually only on commencement of medication due to blood concentrations being too high. Minimal on long term use.
Unusual: Nausea, vomiting, hiccups, bad tastes, drowsiness, confusion, dizziness, double vision, tremor, blurred vision, palpitations.

INTERACTIONS:

Other drugs:
- Other medications that treat heart rhythm irregularities.
- Theophylline, warfarin, narcotics.

Other substances:
- Reacts with alcohol and caffeine.

PRESCRIPTION:
Yes.

PBS:
Yes.

PERMITTED IN SPORT:
Yes.

OVERDOSE:
Very serious. Administer activated charcoal or induce vomiting if tablets taken recently. Seek urgent medical assistance. Symptoms may include vomiting, drowsiness, confusion, slow heart rate, heart attack and death.

See also Amiodarone, Disopyramide, Flecainide, Procainamide, Quinidine, Sotalol, Verapamil.

Mianserin

TRADE NAMES:
Lumin, Tolvon.

DRUG CLASS:
Tetracyclic antidepressant.

USES:
Depression.

DOSAGE:
 One or two tablets, three times a day between meals but with fluid. Do not chew tablet.

FORMS:
Tablets of 10mg and 20mg.

PRECAUTIONS:
Should be used with caution in pregnancy (B2). Breast feeding should be stopped if it is necessary to use Mianserin. Not for use in children.

Use with caution in epilepsy, jaundice (yellow skin), glaucoma, enlarged prostate gland, diabetes, tissue swelling (oedema), heart disease, kidney and liver disease.

Potentially suicidal patients must be observed closely.

Lower doses necessary in elderly.

Do not take if:

 suffering from mania or severe liver disease.

SIDE EFFECTS:
Common: Drowsiness, tiredness, dry mouth, dizziness, faintness, weakness, tremor, headache.

Unusual: Swelling of tissues, changes in blood pressure, rapid heart rate, sweating, constipation, weight gain, muscle pains, blurred vision.

Severe but rare (stop medication, consult doctor): Unusual bleeding or bruising, yellow skin (jaundice).

INTERACTIONS:

Other drugs:
- MAOI cause serious reaction.
- Anticonvulsants, barbiturates, phenytoin, medications that lower blood pressure.

Herbs:
- Ma huang.

Other substances:
- Reacts adversely with alcohol.

PRESCRIPTION:
Yes.

PBS:
Yes.

PERMITTED IN SPORT:
Yes.

OVERDOSE:
Serious. Symptoms include drowsiness, high blood pressure, rapid heart rate, coma and death. Administer activated charcoal or induce vomiting if tablets taken recently and patient alert. Seek urgent medical assistance. Patients are often observed in intensive care units.

See also TRICYCLIC ANTIDEPRESSANTS.

Miconazole

TRADE NAMES:
Daktarin, Fungo Powder, Eulactol, Fungo Solution, Leuko Fungex, Monistat.
Daktozin (with zinc).
Fungo Cream, Fungo Vaginal (with dimethicone).
Fungo Soothing Balm (with bufexamac, dimethicone).
Fungocort (with hydrocortisone).
Numerous locally produced creams also exist.

USES:
Treatment of fungal infections of skin (tinea, athlete's foot, pityriasis versicolor), vagina (thrush), mouth, nails and scalp.

DOSAGE:

Skin: Apply two or three times a day.
Vagina: Insert once a day at night.

FORMS:
Cream, vaginal cream, vaginal pessary, gel, lotion, solution, tincture, powder, spray.

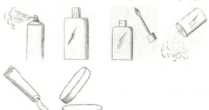

PRECAUTIONS:
Safe to use in pregnancy (A), breast feeding and children.
Should not be swallowed or used in eyes.
Use with care on open wounds.

SIDE EFFECTS:
Common: Nil.
Unusual: Skin irritation, rash.

INTERACTIONS:
None significant.

PRESCRIPTION:
No.

PBS:
No. Some forms available to Veterans Affairs pensioners.

PERMITTED IN SPORT:
Yes.

OTHER INFORMATION:
This class of medication dramatically improved the treatment of fungal infections when introduced in the early 1970s. Very safe and effective.

See Clotrimazole, Econazole, Fluconazole, Itraconazole, Ketoconazole.

Midazolam

TRADE NAME:
Hypnovel.

DRUG CLASS:
Sedative/Hypnotic, Benzodiazepine.

USES:
Short acting sedation for procedures (eg. gastroscopy), continuous sedation of acutely ill patients, sedation prior to anaesthesia.

DOSAGE:
 As given by doctor.

FORMS:
Injection.

PRECAUTIONS:
Should be used with caution in pregnancy (C), but not at all if delivery of infant imminent as it may decrease desire to breathe in newborn infant. Should be used with caution in breast feeding and children.

Do not take if:
 suffering from myasthenia gravis, shock, alcoholism or glaucoma.

SIDE EFFECTS:
Common: Reduces lung and heart activity.
Rare: Hiccups, nausea, vomiting, memory loss of events immediately before and after injection.

INTERACTIONS:
Other drugs:
- Cimetidine, erythromycin, other sedatives, sodium valproate.

Herbs:
- Guarana, kava kava, passionflower, St John's wort, valerian, celery, camomile, goldenseal.

Other substances:
- Reacts adversely with alcohol.

PRESCRIPTION:
Yes.

PBS:
No.

OTHER INFORMATION:
Excellent medication to allow many non-painful but uncomfortable and frightening procedures to be performed with minimal risk.

See also BARBITURATES, Chlormethiazole, Flunitrazepam, Nitrazepam, Temazepam, Triazolam, Zolpidem, Zopiclone.

MINERALS

DISCUSSION:
Minerals are inorganic substances (i.e. not vegetable or animal in origin) that are necessary for the normal functioning of the body.

See Calcium, Copper, Fluoride, Iodine, Iron, Magnesium sulphate, Phosphorus, Potassium, Selenomethionine (Selenium), Zinc.

Minocycline

TRADE NAMES:
Akamin, Minomycin.

DRUG CLASS:
Tetracycline antibiotic.

USES:
Infections caused by susceptible bacteria, acne.

DOSAGE:
 Treatment: 200mg at once, then 100mg a day.
Prevention of acne: 50mg a day.

FORMS:

Capsules of 100mg, tablets of 50mg, injection.

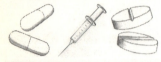

PRECAUTIONS:

Not to be used in pregnancy (D) or children under 12 as Minocycline may cause permanent staining of teeth of foetus or child. Use with caution in breast feeding.
Use with caution in kidney disease.

Do not take if:
suffering from severe kidney disease, systemic lupus erythematosus (SLE), Staphylococcal infection.

SIDE EFFECTS:

Common: Loss of appetite, nausea, sore mouth, diarrhoea, difficulty in swallowing, inflamed colon.
Unusual: Vomiting, inflamed pancreas, rash, secondary fungal infection (thrush).
Severe but rare (stop medication, consult doctor): Severe belly pain, severe diarrhoea, tooth discolouration.

INTERACTIONS:

Other drugs:
- Anticoagulants (eg. warfarin), penicillin, antacids, iron, oral contraceptives, diuretics (fluid tablets).

Other substances:
- Milk may reduce absorption from gut.

PRESCRIPTION:
Yes.

PBS:
Yes.

PERMITTED IN SPORT:
Yes.

OVERDOSE:
Exacerbation of side effects only likely effect.

OTHER INFORMATION:

Used for a wide range of infections in general practice, including prevention of acne. Does not cause dependence or addiction.

See also **Demeclocycline, Doxycycline, Tetracycline.**

Minoxidil

TRADE NAMES:
Loniten, Regaine Topical.

DRUG CLASS:
Antihypertensive.

USES:
Severe high blood pressure, baldness.

DOSAGE:

 Tablets: One to four tablets a day as a single dose.
Lotion: Apply twice a day to scalp.

FORMS:
Tablets of 10mg, scalp solution, gel.

PRECAUTIONS:

Use in pregnancy (C) and breast feeding only if medically necessary.
Should not be used for mild high blood pressure.
Fluid intake must be controlled carefully.
May be necessary to check heart with regular cardiographs (ECG).
Use lotion only on scalp.

Do not take if:
 suffering from recent heart attack.

SIDE EFFECTS:

Common: Excess hair growth on face and scalp, darkening and thickening of fine body hair, weight gain, fluid retention,

increased heart rate.
Unusual: Low blood pressure, breast tenderness, rash, nausea, diarrhoea.

INTERACTIONS:
Other drugs:
- Lotion reacts with steroid creams and acne preparations.

PRESCRIPTION:
Yes.

PBS:
Tablets: Yes (authority required – restricted to severe refractory high blood pressure where treatment started in hospital).
Lotion: No.

PERMITTED IN SPORT:
Yes.

OVERDOSE:
Low blood pressure only likely effect.

OTHER INFORMATION:
Ability to reverse male baldness found by accident in patients taking drug for blood pressure. Success in baldness varies greatly between patients, and long term use is required. Used for only most severe forms of high blood pressure.

MIOTICS

DISCUSSION:
Medications that are used to contract the pupil in the eye, usually for the treatment of glaucoma.
See Acetylcholine chloride, Carbachol.

Mirtazapine

TRADE NAMES:
Avanza, Mirtazon, Remeron.

DRUG CLASS:
Antidepressant.

USES:
Severe depression.

DOSAGE:
 15mg to 60mg at night.

FORMS:
Tablets of 30mg.

PRECAUTIONS:
Use with caution in pregnancy (B3), breast feeding and children.
Use with caution in epilepsy, kidney and heart disease, low blood pressure, jaundice, difficulty in passing urine, glaucoma, diabetes, psychoses and mania.

SIDE EFFECTS:
Common: Increased appetite and subsequent weight gain, swelling, dizziness.
Unusual: Headache, drowsiness (eases with time), nausea, joint and muscle pain.
Severe but rare (stop medication, consult doctor): Rash, bone marrow damage.

INTERACTIONS:
Other drugs:
- Severe interaction with MAOI.
- Benzodiazepines (eg. diazepam), erythromycin, clotrimazole, econazole, fluconazole, itraconazole, ketoconazole, miconazole, erythromycin, nefazodone, carbamazepine, rifampicin, phenytoin, cimetidine.

Herbs:
- Ma huang.

Other substances:
- Reacts with alcohol.

PRESCRIPTION:
Yes.

PBS:
Yes.

PERMITTED IN SPORT:
Yes.

OVERDOSE:
Induce vomiting or administer activated charcoal if tablets taken recently. Seek medical attention.

OTHER INFORMATION:
Introduced in 2002 as an additional effective treatment for most types of depression.
See also Citalopram, Fluoxetine, Fluvoxamine, MAOI, Mianserin, Moclobemide, Nefazodone, Paroxetine, Sertraline, TRICYCLIC ANTIDEPRESSANTS, Venlafaxine.

Misoprostol

TRADE NAMES:
Cytotec.
Arthrotec (with diclofenac).

DRUG CLASS:
Antiulcerant, Prostaglandin analogue.

USES:
Treatment of ulcers of the stomach and duodenum (upper small intestine). Prevention of ulcers in patients who are likely to develop them.

DOSAGE:

Up to 800µg a day divided into two to four doses.

FORMS:
Tablets.

PRECAUTIONS:
Extremely dangerous in pregnancy (X). Pregnancy must be prevented in any woman using this medication by adequate contraception. May cause miscarriage and serious damage to the foetus. Not recommended in children and breast feeding.
Use with caution in epilepsy, low blood pressure and asthma.

SIDE EFFECTS:
Common: Diarrhoea, belly pains.
Unusual: Belly cramps, menstrual disorders, nausea, headache, passing wind, constipation.

INTERACTIONS:
None significant.

PRESCRIPTION:
Yes.

PBS:
Cytotec: Yes (authority required. Restricted to use in proven stomach and duodenal ulcers).
Arthrotec: No.

PERMITTED IN SPORT:
Yes.

OVERDOSE:
The effects of an overdose are unknown.

OTHER INFORMATION:
A very potent and effective form of treatment for ulcers that have failed to heal by other methods. Widely used in severely injured or ill patients to prevent stomach ulcers. Must never be used in pregnancy.
See also PROTON PUMP INHIBITORS.

Moclobemide

TRADE NAMES:
Arima, Aurorix, Clobemix, Maosig, Mohexal.
Other locally produced and marketed forms of moclobemide exist.

DRUG CLASS:
Antidepressant, RIMA (reversible inhibitor of monoamine oxidase type A).

USES:
Depression.

DOSAGE:

One or two tablets, once or twice a day after a meal.

FORMS:
Tablets of 150 and 300mg.

PRECAUTIONS:
Should be used in pregnancy (B3) and breast feeding only with great caution. Not for use in children.
Use with caution in excited and agitated patients, schizophrenia, high blood pressure, thyroid disease, liver and kidney disease.
Lower doses should be used in elderly. Use with caution in agitated state, high blood pressure, liver and kidney disease, thyrotoxicosis (over-active thyroid gland), phaeochromocytoma and if suicidal.

Do not take if:
 suffering from schizophrenia and similar psychiatric conditions.

SIDE EFFECTS:
Common: Usually minimal. Dizziness, nausea, sleeplessness, headache.
Unusual: Dry mouth, constipation, diarrhoea, anxiety, restlessness.

INTERACTIONS:
Other drugs:
- Metoprolol, cimetidine, pethidine, selegiline, clomipramine, SSRI antidepressants (citalopram, fluoxetine, fluvoxamine, paroxetine, sertraline, venlafaxine), dextromethorphan.

Herbs:
- Ma huang, sparteine (Cytisus scoparius).

PRESCRIPTION:
Yes.

PBS:
Yes.

PERMITTED IN SPORT:
Yes.

OVERDOSE:
Drowsiness, low blood pressure and rapid heart rate may occur. Not serious. Seek medical advice.

OTHER INFORMATION:
One of the newer antidepressants released in Australia in the early 1990s that has improved the treatment of depression because of its safety and lack of side effects. May take up to two weeks for patient to notice any improvement in depression.

See Citalopram, Fluoxetine, Fluvoxamine, MAOI, Mianserin, Mirtazapine, Nefazodone, Paroxetine, Sertraline, TRICYCLIC ANTIDEPRESSANTS, Venlafaxine.

Modafinil

TRADE NAME:
Modavigil.

USES:
Narcolepsy (excessive sudden sleep).

DOSAGE:

200mg to 400mg a day, usually taken in the morning.

FORMS:
Tablets of 100mg.

PRECAUTIONS:
Not for use in pregnancy (B3).
Use with caution in breast feeding and children under 16 years.
Use with caution with significant anxiety disorder, high blood pressure, heart failure, angina, recent heart attack, severe liver and kidney disease. Beware of tendency for dependency to develop.

SIDE EFFECTS:
Common: Headache, nausea, depression.
Unusual: Nervousness, diarrhoea, dry mouth, loss of appetite, watery nose, dizziness, sore throat.

INTERACTIONS:
Other drugs: Oral contraceptives, methylphenidate, triazolam, MAOI, diazepam, phenytoin, propranolol, tricyclic antidepressants, cyclosporin, rifampicin, ketoconazole, itraconazole, warfarin.
Herbs: Ma huang.

PRESCRIPTION:
Yes.

PBS:
No.

PERMITTED IN SPORT:
No.

See also Methylphenidate.

Mometasone

TRADE NAMES:
Elocon, Novasone (skin preparations).
Allermax, Nasonex (nasal sprays).

DRUG CLASS:
Corticosteroid.

USES:
Severe inflammation of skin (eczema, dermatitis etc.).
Treatment and prevention of persistent hay fever (allergic rhinitis).

DOSAGE:

Use once a day.

FORMS:
Cream, ointment, lotion, nose spray.

PRECAUTIONS:
Should be used with caution in pregnancy (B3), breast feeding and children.
Avoid eyes.
Use for shortest period of time possible.
Do not use:
 if suffering from any form of skin or nose infection.
- nose sprays with nose bleeding tendency.

SIDE EFFECTS:
Common: Minimal.
Unusual: Skin preparations – thinning of skin, itching, burning, stinging, scarring of skin.
Nasal spray – nose and throat irritation, nose bleed, headache.
Severe but rare (stop medication, consult doctor): Perforation of nasal septum (nose spray).

Medications

INTERACTIONS:
None significant.

PRESCRIPTION:
Yes.

PBS:
Skin preparations: Yes.
Nose sprays: No.

PERMITTED IN SPORT:
Yes.

OTHER INFORMATION:
Extremely effective and useful medication, that is just as effective as other steroid creams that are used two or three times a day. Lowest dose and shortest possible course should be used. Not addictive. Introduced 1993.

See also Betamethasone, Desonide, Hydrocortisone, Methylprednisolone, Triamcinolone.

Montelukast

TRADE NAME:
Singulair.

USES:
Prevention and treatment of chronic asthma.

DOSAGE:

5 to 10mg at bedtime.

FORMS:
Tablets of 4mg (pink), 5mg (pink) and 10mg (beige).

PRECAUTIONS:
May be used with care in pregnancy (B1), breast feeding and children.
Not for treatment of acute asthma.
Two 5mg tablets are NOT equivalent to one 10mg tablet.

SIDE EFFECTS:
Common: Minimal.
Unusual: Nausea, diarrhoea, headache, belly ache, rash, insomnia, dizziness, joint and muscle pains, tiredness.

INTERACTIONS:
Other drugs:
- Aspirin, NSAID, phenobarbitone, phenytoin, rifampicin.

PRESCRIPTION:
Yes.

PBS:
Yes (authority required – restricted to children under 14 years).

PERMITTED IN SPORT:
Yes.

OVERDOSE:
Exacerbation of side effects likely.

OTHER INFORMATION:
Released 1999 for the management of more difficult cases of persistent asthma. A remarkably effective an easy to use form of asthma prevention with virtually no side effects. May also be used (without approval) for hay fever and other allergy conditions.

See Zafirlukast.

'MORNING AFTER' PILL

See Levonorgestrel.

Morphine

TRADE NAMES:
**Anamorph, Kapanol, Morphine, MS-Contin, MS Mono, Ordine.
Morphalgin** (with aspirin).

DRUG CLASS:
Narcotic.

USES:
Severe pain.

DOSAGE:
Depends on form and level of pain. Follow doctor's directions strictly.

FORMS:
Tablets, slow release capsules or tablets (Kapanol, MS-Contin, MS Mono), mixture, injection.

 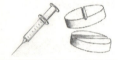

PRECAUTIONS:
Should only be used during pregnancy (C) if medically essential. Use with caution in breast feeding.
May be used in children.
Use with caution in colic caused by gall stones, pancreatitis, ulcerative colitis, underactive thyroid gland, enlarged prostate gland, head injury and shock.

Do not take if:
 suffering from heart failure, severe head injury, acute diabetes, severe liver disease, severe alcoholism, poor lung function or convulsions.
- do not operate machinery, drive a vehicle or undertake tasks requiring concentration after use of morphine.

SIDE EFFECTS:
Common: Sedation, constipation, confusion, sweating, nausea, loss of appetite.
Unusual: Vomiting, difficulty passing urine, flushing, dizziness, slow heart rate, irregular heart rate, fainting, mood changes.
Severe but rare (stop medication, consult doctor): Difficulty in breathing, convulsions.

INTERACTIONS:
Other drugs:
- MAOI, sedatives, cimetidine, warfarin, zidovudine, pentazocine, thiopentone, diazepam, barbiturates, phenothiazines, amphetamines, chlorpromazine, beta blockers (eg. propranolol).

Other substances:
- Should not be used with alcohol.

PRESCRIPTION:
Yes (tightly restricted).

PBS:
Yes.

PERMITTED IN SPORT:
No.

OVERDOSE:
Serious. Sedation, convulsions, coma and death may occur. Administer activated charcoal or induce vomiting if medication taken recently and patient alert. Seek emergency medical assistance. Antidote available.

OTHER INFORMATION:
Highly addictive if used inappropriately. Very effective and unlikely to cause addiction if used appropriately for severe pain. Patients with terminal diseases (eg. cancer) should use dose adequate to control pain, and not be concerned about possibility of addiction. Derived from opium poppy and closely related to heroin, but not as addictive. The drug gets its name from the Greek god of sleep, Morpheus.

See also Alfentanil, Buprenorphine, Codeine Phosphate, Dextromoramide, Dextropropoxyphene, Fentanyl, Heroin, Hydromorphone, Methadone, Oxycodone, Pentazocine, Pethidine.

MPA

See Medroxyprogesterone acetate.

MUCOLYTICS

DISCUSSION:
Mucolytics liquefy and break down thick mucus. Mucus produced during colds, flu, bronchitis and other infections of the airways is often sticky and tenacious. Mucolytics make this phlegm watery and runny, so that coughing and sneezing can more easily clear it from the body. They are available as tablets and mixtures.

See Bromhexine.

Mumps vaccine

TRADE NAMES:
MMR II, Priorix (with measles and rubella vaccines).
Only available in Australia combined with other vaccines.

DRUG CLASS:
Vaccine.

USES:
Prevention of mumps.

DOSAGE:
 One injection at 12 months and a second one at 4 or 5 years of age.

FORMS:
Injection.

PRECAUTIONS:
Not designed for use in pregnancy (B2), but unlikely to cause adverse effects if given inadvertently. May be used in children and breast feeding.
Use with caution in history of febrile convulsions or brain injury.

Do not take if:
- suffering from allergy to eggs, poultry or neomycin.
- significant fever, immune system disease (eg. AIDS).
- blood transfusion within three months.
- suffering from TB, bone marrow disease, or leukaemia.

SIDE EFFECTS:
Common: Burning at site of injection.
Unusual: Fever, enlarged glands, itch, rash.
Severe but rare: Brain inflammation.

INTERACTIONS:
None significant.

PRESCRIPTION:
Yes.

PBS:
No, but supplied free to doctors by state health departments.

PERMITTED IN SPORT:
Yes.

OVERDOSE:
An additional inadvertent dose is unlikely to have any serious side effects.

OTHER INFORMATION:
Mumps is usually a mild disease, but may rarely cause infertility, brain damage and death. Only available in combination with measles and rubella vaccines. Vaccination with rubella, measles and mumps routine in Australia at 1 and 4 years of age.

Mupirocin

TRADE NAME:
Bactroban.

DRUG CLASS:
Antibiotic.

USES:
Bacterial skin infections, school sores (impetigo), infected wounds.

DOSAGE:
 Apply three times a day.

FORMS:
Ointment, cream.

PRECAUTIONS:
Safe to use in pregnancy (B1), breast feeding and children over 2 years. Not for use in eyes or mouth.

SIDE EFFECTS:
Common: Minimal.
Unusual: Skin irritation.

INTERACTIONS:
None significant.

PRESCRIPTION:
Yes.

PBS:
No. Available to some Veterans Affairs pensioners.

PERMITTED IN SPORT:
Yes.

OTHER INFORMATION:
Excellent and safe medication for treating minor skin infections. Introduced in late 1980s.

See also Chlorhexidine, Neomycin, Sodium fusidate.

MUSCLE RELAXANTS

DISCUSSION:
Muscle relaxants are used to relieve muscle cramps and the spasms associated with spasticity (cerebral palsy), paralysis (paraplegia and quadriplegia), multiple sclerosis and some rare brain diseases.

See Baclofen, Dantrolene, Orphenadrine.

Mycophenolate mofetil

TRADE NAME:
Cellcept.

DRUG CLASS:
Immune system modifier.

USES:
Prevention of rejection of kidney and other transplanted organs.

DOSAGE:
 1000mg twice a day.

FORMS:
Capsules of 250mg (blue/brown), tablet of 500mg (lavender), infusion.

PRECAUTIONS:
Must not be used in pregnancy (D). May be used with caution in children and breast feeding.
Regular blood tests to monitor blood cell function essential.
Use with caution in stomach, intestine and severe kidney disease.

SIDE EFFECTS:
Common: Skin cancer incidence increased, infection, low white blood cell count, diarrhoea, bleeding from intestine.

Unusual: Severe abdominal pain.
Severe but rare (stop medication, consult doctor): Cancer of lymph nodes, perforation of intestine.

INTERACTIONS:
Other drugs:
- Aciclovir, ganciclovir, iron, magnesium salts and aluminium salts (eg. in antacids), oral contraceptives, probenecid, drugs secreted in kidney, cholestyramine. Check with doctor before using any other medication.
- Live vaccines (eg. polio).

Other substances:
- Alcohol.

PRESCRIPTION:
Yes.

PBS:
Yes (under very specific authorised circumstances only).

PERMITTED IN SPORT:
Yes.

OVERDOSE:
Extremely serious organ damage may occur. Induce vomiting or administer activated charcoal if taken recently. Seek emergency medical attention.

OTHER INFORMATION:
Introduced in 1997.

MYDRIATICS

TRADE and GENERIC NAMES:
Cyclogyl (Cyclopentolate).
Isopto Homatropine (Homatropine hydrobromide).
Minims Mydriatics (Atropine, cyclopentolate, homatropine hydrobromide, phenylephrine, tropicamide).
Mydriacyl (Tropicamide).
Atropine is also a mydriatic – see separate entry.

DRUG CLASS:
Anticholinergic.

USES:
Dilates pupil for examination and surgery.

DOSAGE:
 Use drops as directed by doctor. Often used by doctors in their surgery or operating theatre.

FORMS:
Eye drops.

PRECAUTIONS:
May be used in pregnancy and breast feeding. Use with caution in children. Not designed for prolonged use.

Do not take if:
 suffering from glaucoma.

SIDE EFFECTS:
Common: Irritation of eye with prolonged use, sensitivity to bright light.
Unusual: Disorientation, blurred vision, dry mouth, incoordination, rapid heart rate.

INTERACTIONS:
None significant.

PRESCRIPTION:
Yes.

PBS:
Homatropine: Yes.
Others: No.

PERMITTED IN SPORT:
Yes.

OTHER INFORMATION:
Mainly used before eye examinations, and before and during eye surgery.
See also Atropine.

Nafarelin

TRADE NAME:
Synarel.

DRUG CLASS:
Sex hormone.

USES:
Treatment of endometriosis. Preliminary treatment to stimulate ovary before in vitro fertilisation (IVF).

DOSAGE:
One or two sprays into different nostrils, twice a day commencing two to four days after menstrual period starts.

FORMS:
Nasal spray.

PRECAUTIONS:
Must never be used in pregnancy (D), breast feeding or children.
Use with caution in osteoporosis, polycystic ovaries and hay fever.
Use with caution under 18 years.
Do not use if:
 suffering from unusual vaginal bleeding.
• male.

SIDE EFFECTS:
Common: Ovarian pain, ovarian cysts, belly pain, dry vagina, breast shrinkage, hot flushes, poor libido, headaches, acne.
Unusual: Emotional changes, muscle pains, nasal irritation.

INTERACTIONS:
Other drugs:
• Other sex hormones.

PRESCRIPTION:
Yes.

PBS:
Yes (authority required. Restricted to treatment of visually proven endometriosis).

PERMITTED IN SPORT:
No.

OVERDOSE:
Unlikely to be serious.

OTHER INFORMATION:
Introduced in 1996 as a radically new and effective treatment for endometriosis via a novel route that overcomes the necessity for injections, and side effects caused by swallowing tablets.

Naloxone

TRADE NAMES:
Naloxone, Narcan.

DRUG CLASS:
Antidote.

USES:
Reversal of effects of overdosage with narcotics (eg. morphine, heroin).

DOSAGE:
Repeated injections at intervals of two or three minutes until desired effect achieved.

FORMS:
Injection

Medications

PRECAUTIONS:
May be used in pregnancy (B1), breast feeding and children of all ages.
Use with caution in narcotic addicts, heart disease.
Exclude other poisons that may be responsible for symptoms.
Patient must be monitored closely by doctors.

SIDE EFFECTS:
Common: High blood pressure, irregular heartbeat, shortness of breath, convulsions.
Unusual: Heart attack.

INTERACTIONS:
None significant.

PRESCRIPTION:
Yes.

PBS:
Yes (supplied free to doctors for use in emergencies).

PERMITTED IN SPORT:
Yes.

OTHER INFORMATION:
Often life saving in addicts who take heroin overdose, or in newborn infants of mothers who are heroin addicts. May precipitate withdrawal in narcotic addicts.

Naltrexone

TRADE NAME:
Revia.

USES:
Narcotic drug and alcohol dependence.

DOSAGE:

50mg once or twice a day for three to 12 months. Half dose given initially in narcotic drug addiction.

FORMS:
Tablet of 50mg.

PRECAUTIONS:
Use with caution in pregnancy (B3) and breast feeding.
Use with caution in children.
Use with caution in liver and kidney disease.
Patients must have a negative urine test for narcotics before first dose given, and must never use narcotics.

Do not take if:
 taking any narcotic or opioid medications (eg. codeine, morphine) or illegal drugs (eg. heroin).
May result in fatal reaction.
- suffering from acute hepatitis or liver failure.

SIDE EFFECTS:
Common: Severe withdrawal effects if not previously completely withdrawn from alcohol or narcotics, diarrhoea, nausea, dizziness, tiredness.
Unusual: Liver damage (jaundice), nervousness, fatigue, anxiety, joint and muscle pains.

INTERACTIONS:
Other drugs:
- All narcotic drugs (eg. codeine, pethidine, morphine, heroin, opium – may result in death).
- Thioridazine.

Other substances:
- Alcohol.

PRESCRIPTION:
Yes.

PBS:
Yes (authority required – restricted to alcohol addiction only).

PERMITTED IN SPORT:
Yes.

OVERDOSE:
Exacerbation of side effects likely. Seek medical attention.

OTHER INFORMATION:
Must be combined with a drug or alcohol withdrawal program.
See also Acamprosate.

Nandrolone decanoate

TRADE NAME:
Deca Durabolin.

DRUG CLASS:
Anabolic steroid.

USES:
Kidney failure, inoperable breast cancer, severe osteoporosis, aplastic anaemia, suppression of white cells, in addition to corticosteroids used long term.
Used dangerously and in an unapproved manner by body builders and athletes.

DOSAGE:

As directed and determined by doctor. Usually one injection a week.

FORMS:
Injection

PRECAUTIONS:
Must not be used in pregnancy (D) or breast feeding. Use with caution in children as growth suppression may occur. Use with caution in heart disease, enlarged prostate gland, diabetes.
Do not take if:
suffering from prostate and testicular cancer, male breast cancer, heart failure, liver and kidney disease.

SIDE EFFECTS:
Common: Increased hairiness and decreased breast size in women, voice deepening in women, acne, frequent unwanted erections, infertility.
Unusual: Anaemia, enlargement of clitoris in women, cessation of menstrual periods, decrease in testicular size, impotence, breast enlargement in males, baldness in females, reduced libido.
Severe but rare (stop medication, consult doctor): Unusual bruising or bleeding, calcium deposits (lumps) in tissue, jaundice (yellow skin).

INTERACTIONS:
Other drugs:
- Insulin, warfarin, hypoglycaemics (used for diabetes).

Herbs:
- Echinacea.

PRESCRIPTION:
Yes.

PBS:
Yes (authority required. Restricted to specific disease states).

PERMITTED IN SPORT:
No – strictly prohibited. Although increasing muscle bulk, there is no evidence that this medication enhances athletic ability. Long term inappropriate use may cause permanent damage to the body.

Medications

OVERDOSE:
Exacerbation of side effects likely.

OTHER INFORMATION:
Does not cause dependence or addiction. Short term gains in muscle bulk when used inappropriately by body builders, may result in long term permanent body damage that may lead to early heart attacks, infertility, bone weakness, liver disease and premature death. Bottom line is – don't use it except under strict medical supervision when indicated for specific diseases.

See also Methenolone.

Naphazoline and Antazoline

TRADE NAMES:
Albalon, Clear Eyes, Naphcon Forte, Optazine (naphazoline).
Albalon-A, Anthistine-Privine (antazoline and naphazoline).
Murine Allergy (antazoline with xylometazoline).
Naphcon A, Visine Allergy with Antihistamine (naphazoline with pheniramine).
Optrex (naphazoline with other ingredients).

DRUG CLASS:
Vasoconstrictor.

USES:
Allergic conjunctivitis, inflamed eyes.

DOSAGE:
 One or two drops in eye, four to six times a day.

FORMS:
Eye drops.

PRECAUTIONS:
May be used in pregnancy and breast feeding. Use with caution in children. Not to be used for more than two weeks without medical review.
Use with caution in high blood pressure, irregular heart rhythm, diabetes, and an over-active thyroid gland (hyperthyroidism).

Do not take if:
 suffering from glaucoma.

SIDE EFFECTS:
Common: Stinging on inserting drops.

INTERACTIONS:
Other drugs:
- MAOI, tricyclic antidepressants.

PRESCRIPTION:
No.

PBS:
Some brands: Yes.
Most forms: No. These may be available to some Veterans Affairs pensioners.

PERMITTED IN SPORT:
Yes.

OTHER INFORMATION:
Widely used and effective treatment for tired, itchy, watery, red eyes. If symptoms do not settle rapidly, seek medical advice.

Naproxen

TRADE NAMES:
Aleve, Anaprox, Crysanal, Inza, Naprogesic, Naprosyn, Nurolasts, Proxen

DRUG CLASS:
NSAID (Nonsteroidal anti-inflammatory drug).

USES:
All forms of arthritis, inflammatory disorders, gout, back pain, ankylosing spondylitis, bone pain, period pain, migraine, general pain relief.

DOSAGE:
 250 to 1000mg a day with food. May be given in one or more doses.
Suppository: One or two inserted a day.
Mixture: 10mLs three or four times a day with food.

FORMS:
Tablets, capsules, mixture, suppository.

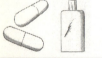 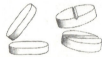

PRECAUTIONS:
Should not be used in pregnancy (C) unless medically essential. Breast feeding should be ceased if necessary to use NSAID. Not for use in children under two.
Use tablets and capsules with caution in psychiatrically disturbed patients, epilepsy, severe infection, heart failure and kidney disease.
Lower doses required in elderly, who may suffer more side effects.

Do not take if:
 suffering from peptic ulcer at present or in recent past.
- due for surgery (including dental surgery).
- suffering from bleeding disorder or anaemia.
- suffering from proctitis (suppository only).

SIDE EFFECTS:
Common: Stomach discomfort, diarrhoea, constipation, heartburn, nausea, headache, dizziness.
Unusual: Blurred vision, stomach ulcer, ringing noise in ears, retention of fluid, swelling of tissue, drowsiness, itch, rash, shortness of breath.
Severe but rare (stop medication, consult doctor): Vomit blood, pass blood in faeces, other unusual bleeding, asthma induced by medication.

INTERACTIONS:
Other drugs:
- Must never be used with anticoagulants (eg. warfarin).
- Probenecid, diuretics, lithium, methotrexate, beta blockers, ACE inhibitors.

Herbs:
- Feverfew.

PRESCRIPTION:
Low strength preparations: No.
High strength preparations: Yes.

PBS:
Most forms: Yes.
Low strength non-prescription forms: No.

PERMITTED IN SPORT:
Yes.

OVERDOSE:
Causes nausea, vomiting, severe headache, dizziness, confusion and convulsions. Administer activated charcoal or induce vomiting if taken recently. Seek medical assistance.

OTHER INFORMATION:

Extensively used to give excellent relief to a wide variety of inflammatory conditions. Significant side effects (particularly on the stomach) in about 5% of patients limit their use. Specially coated forms reduce side effects.

See also Aspirin, Bufexamac, Celecoxib, Diclofenac, Diflunisal, Flurbiprofen, Ibuprofen, Indomethacin, Ketoprofen, Ketorolac trometanol, Mefenamic Acid, Piroxicam, Rofecoxib, Salicylic acid, Sulindac, Tenoxicam, Tiaprofenic Acid.

Naratriptan

TRADE NAME:
Naramig.

DRUG CLASS:
Antimigraine.

USES:
Treatment of acute migraine.

DOSAGE:

Take one tablet at onset of migraine. Repeat after four hours if necessary.

FORMS:
Tablets of 2.5mg (green).

PRECAUTIONS:
May be used with caution in pregnancy (B3), breast feeding, the elderly and children.
Use with caution in paralysis and visual disturbances due to migraine (exclude other serious causes).
Use with caution in heart disease, kidney and liver disease.
May cross react in patients with a sulphur allergy.

Do not take if:
suffering from angina, heart attack, stroke, TIAs (transient ischaemic attacks), poor circulation, uncontrolled high blood pressure, severe liver or kidney disease.

SIDE EFFECTS:
Common: Tiredness, fatigue, dizziness, tingling, heat sensation.
Unusual: Chest heaviness, pressure, tightness, slow or rapid heart rate, disturbed vision.

INTERACTIONS:
Other drugs:
- Other migraine treatments, ergotamine, methysergide.

Herbs:
- St John's wort.

PRESCRIPTION:
Yes.

PBS:
Yes (authority required).

PERMITTED IN SPORT:
Yes.

OVERDOSE:
Causes high blood pressure and may affect heart. Recovery within eight hours usual unless heart damaged. Seek medical attention.

OTHER INFORMATION:
Introduced in 1998. Not addictive.

See also Ergotamine, Sumatriptan, Zolmitriptan.

NARCOTICS

DISCUSSION:
Narcotics are strong, addictive and effective painkillers derived from opium. They are highly restricted in their use, and must be kept in safes by chemists and doctors. If they are used appropriately, they give relief from severe pain to patients with acute injuries, and pain from diseases such as cancer and kidney stones. They are often used before, during and after operations to ease the pain of the procedure. If used in this way, it is unlikely that addiction will occur. If used excessively, a psychological and physical addiction can rapidly develop. Heroin is an infamous illegal narcotic that is broken down to morphine in the body. Narcotics not only relieve severe pain, they also reduce anxiety, stop coughs, sedate and cause euphoria (a 'high' – artificial happiness). They should be used with caution in asthma and other lung diseases, liver disease and after head injuries.

See Alfentanil, Buprenorphine, Codeine Phosphate, Dextromoramide, Dextropropoxyphene, Fentanyl, Heroin, Hydromorphone, Methadone, Morphine, Oxycodone, Pentazocine, Pethidine.

Nedocromil sodium

TRADE NAME:
Tilade.

USES:
Prevention of asthma.

DOSAGE:

Two puffs, two to four times a day.

FORMS:
Inhaler.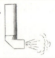

PRECAUTIONS:
Safe to use with caution in pregnancy (B1), breast feeding and children over 12 years.
Not to be used for the relief of acute asthma attacks.
Do not exceed recommended dose.

SIDE EFFECTS:
Common: Unpleasant taste.
Unusual: Headache, nausea, cough.

INTERACTIONS:
None significant.

PRESCRIPTION:
Yes.

PBS:
Yes.

PERMITTED IN SPORT:
Yes.

OVERDOSE:
Unlikely to cause any serious problems.

OTHER INFORMATION:
Introduced in 1996 as a very effective preventer of inflammation in the lungs.
See also Sodium cromoglycate.

Nefazodone

TRADE NAME:
Serzone.

DRUG CLASS:
Antidepressant.

USES:
Moderate to severe depression.

DOSAGE:

Start with 100mg twice a day, increase slowly until effective result obtained. Maximum dose 600mg a day.

FORMS:
Tablets of 50mg (pink), 100mg (white), 200mg (yellow) and 300mg (peach).

PRECAUTIONS:
May be used with caution in pregnancy (B3), breast feeding and children.
Use with caution in brain, kidney, liver, heart and blood vessel disease.
Use with caution in low blood pressure, recent heart attack, mania, epilepsy, suicidal tendencies, recent surgery and history of priapism (prolonged painful erection of penis).
Do not stop suddenly, but reduce dose slowly.

Do not take if:

- MAOI (phenelzine, tranylcypromine) used within two weeks.
- Suffering from active liver disease.

SIDE EFFECTS:
Common: Nausea, diarrhoea, low blood pressure, fainting, drowsiness.
Unusual: Vomiting, painful erection of penis.

INTERACTIONS:
Other drugs:
- Serious interaction with MAOI, astemizole, pimozide, cisapride.
- Medications that lower blood pressure, carbamazepine, propranolol, fluoxetine, alprazolam, atorvastatin, simvastatin, buspirone, digoxin, triazolam, cyclosporin.

Herbs:
- St John's wort, ma huang.

Other substances:
- Alcohol.

PRESCRIPTION:
Yes.

PBS:
Yes.

PERMITTED IN SPORT:
Yes.

OVERDOSE:
May be very serious. Induce vomiting or give activated charcoal if taken recently. Seek urgent medical attention.

OTHER INFORMATION:
Introduced in 1997 as an effective treatment for more difficult cases of depression. Not addictive or dependence forming.

See Citalopram, Fluoxetine, Fluvoxamine, MAOI, Mianserin, Mirtazapine, Moclobemide, Paroxetine, Sertraline, TRICYCLIC ANTIDEPRESSANTS, Venlafaxine.

Neisseria meningitidis vaccine

See Meningococcal Vaccine.

Nelfinavir

TRADE NAME:
Viracept.

DRUG CLASS:
Antiviral.

USES:
HIV (AIDS) infection.

DOSAGE:
 Three tablets, three times a day.

FORMS:
Tablets of 250mg (light blue).

PRECAUTIONS:
May be used with care in pregnancy (B2), breast feeding and children.
Use with caution in diabetes, kidney disease, liver disease and haemophilia.
Must be used in combination with other antivirals.

SIDE EFFECTS:
Common: Diarrhoea.
Unusual: Diabetes develops.

INTERACTIONS:
Other drugs:
- Serious interaction with astemizole, cisapride, midazolam, triazolam, ergotamine, amiodarone, quinidine.
- Rifampicin, rifabutin, simvastatin, atorvastatin, oral contraceptives and anticonvulsants.

Herbs:
- St John's wort.

PRESCRIPTION:
Yes.

PBS:
Yes (authority required).

PERMITTED IN SPORT:
Yes.

OTHER INFORMATION:
Always used in combination with other antivirals. Introduced in 2000.

See **Abacavir, Delavirdine, Didanosine, Efavirenz, Indinavir, Lamivudine, Nevirapine, Ritonavir, Saquinavir, Stavudine, Tenofovir, Zidovudine.**

Neomycin

TRADE NAMES:
Minims Neomycin, Neosulf, Siguent Neomycin.
Kenacomb, Otocomb (with triamcinolone, nystatin and gramicidin).
Cicatrin, Nemdyn (with bacitracin).
Neo Medrol Acne Lotion (with methylprednisolone, sulfur, aluminium chlorohydrate).
Neosporin (with polymyxin, gramicidin, thiomersal).

DRUG CLASS:
Aminoglycoside antibiotic.

USES:
Infections of eye, ear, skin and bowel.

DOSAGE:
 Tablets: Two tablets every four hours.
Skin: Apply two or three times a day.
Eye drops: Two drops four times a day.
Eye and ear ointment: Apply twice a day.

FORMS:
Tablets, irrigation solution, ear drops, ear ointment, eye drops, eye ointment, cream, lotion, powder.

PRECAUTIONS:
Skin, eye and ear preparations may be used with caution in pregnancy, breast feeding and children.
Tablets must not be used in pregnancy (D) or breast feeding.
Use tablets with caution in kidney disease and hearing damage.
Tablets are designed for very short term use.
Avoid eye contact with forms not designed for use in eye.
Skin preparations should not be used on viral infections.

Do not take tablets if:

 suffering from ulcerative colitis or bowel obstruction.

SIDE EFFECTS:
Common: Tablets – diarrhoea.
Other forms – minimal.
Unusual: Tablets – ear and kidney damage.

INTERACTIONS:
Other drugs:
- Tablets – Penicillin, cephalosporins, frusemide, warfarin. methotrexate, vitamin B12, digoxin.

PRESCRIPTION:
Yes.

PBS:
Tablets, eye and ear preparations: Yes.
Other forms: No.

PERMITTED IN SPORT:
Yes.

OVERDOSE:
Tablets may cause severe diarrhoea, ear and kidney damage.

OTHER INFORMATION:
Widely used for superficial mild infections. Available for over 40 years.
See Amikacin, Gatifloxacin, Gentamicin, Tobramycin.

Neostigmine

TRADE NAME:
Neostigmine.

DRUG CLASS:
Anticholinesterase.

USES:
Myasthenia gravis, inability to pass urine.

DOSAGE:
 As determined by doctor.

FORMS:
Injection.

PRECAUTIONS:
May be used in pregnancy (B2) with caution. Safe for use in breast feeding.
Use with caution in children.
Dosage must be carefully monitored by doctor.
Use with caution in epilepsy, slow heart rate, asthma, recent heart attack, irregular heartbeat, over-active thyroid gland, and peptic ulcer.

Do not take if:

 suffering from gut obstruction or peritonitis.

SIDE EFFECTS:
Common: Slow heart rate, headache, nausea, diarrhoea, excess salivation, cough, wheeze, bowel noises.
Unusual: Confusion, slurred speech, vomiting, belly cramps, desire to pass urine, muscle cramps, contracted pupils.
Severe but rare (stop medication, consult doctor): Difficulty breathing, chest pain.

INTERACTIONS:
Other drugs:
- Muscle relaxants, atropine, aminoglycosides, drugs used to treat irregular heartbeat, some anaesthetics.

PRESCRIPTION:
Yes.

PBS:
No.

PERMITTED IN SPORT:
Yes.

OVERDOSE:
Serious. May cause diarrhoea, vomiting, difficulty in breathing, weakness, low blood pressure, slow heart rate and heart attack. Seek urgent medical attention.

OTHER INFORMATION:
Old-fashioned drug only useful for the few patients with the distressing muscle disease of myasthenia gravis, and in severe cases of inability to pass urine.
See also Donepezil, Pyridostigmine.

Netilmicin

TRADE NAME:
Netromycin.

DRUG CLASS:
Antibiotic.

USES:
Severe bacterial infections.

DOSAGE:

By injection into a muscle, or slow infusion by a drip into a vein. Dosage as determined by doctor for each patient.

FORMS:
Injection.

PRECAUTIONS:
Must not be used in pregnancy (D) or breast feeding. Use with caution in children.
Use with caution in kidney disease, myasthenia gravis and low blood calcium levels.
Beware of dehydration.
Reduce dose in elderly.
Not for prolonged use.

SIDE EFFECTS:
Common: Adverse effects on ear, nerve and kidney function.
Unusual: Resistant infection.

INTERACTIONS:
Other drugs:
- Frusemide, other diuretics, anaesthetics, cephalosporins, numerous other medications.

Other substances:
- Some forms of blood transfusion.

PRESCRIPTION:
Yes.

PBS:
No.

PERMITTED IN SPORT:
Yes.

OTHER INFORMATION:
Introduced in 1996 for the treatment of more difficult and severe infections.

Neutral insulin

See INSULINS.

Nevirapine

TRADE NAME:
Viramune.

DRUG CLASS:
Antiviral.

USES:
AIDS, HIV infection.

DOSAGE:

One to two tablets, once a day in combination with other antiviral treatment.

FORMS:
Tablets of 200mg (white), powder for addition to fluid.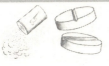

PRECAUTIONS:
Use with caution in pregnancy (B3), breast feeding and children.
Use with caution in kidney and liver disease.

SIDE EFFECTS:
Common: Rash, itch, fever, nausea, headache.
Unusual: Severe skin reactions, vomiting, liver damage.
Severe but rare (stop medication, consult doctor): Jaundice (yellow skin).

INTERACTIONS:
Other drugs:
- Rifampicin, rifabutin, sex hormones, oral contraceptives, methadone, prednisolone, saquinavir, ketoconazole.

Herbs:
- St John's wort.

PRESCRIPTION:
Yes.

PBS:
Yes (under very strictly regulated conditions).

PERMITTED IN SPORT:
Yes.

OVERDOSE:
May cause serious organ damage. Induce vomiting or give activated charcoal if taken recently. Seek urgent medical attention.

OTHER INFORMATION:
Introduced in 1997 as an additive medication for the management of HIV (Human Immunodeficiency Virus) infection.
See Abacavir, Delavirdine, Didanosine, Efavirenz, Indinavir, Lamivudine, Nelfinavir, Ritonavir, Saquinavir, Stavudine, Tenofovir, Zidovudine.

Niacin

See Nicotinic acid.

Nicorandil

TRADE NAME:
Ikorel.

DRUG CLASS:
Antiangina, vasodilator.

USES:
Angina (heart pain).

DOSAGE:

5mg to 20mg twice a day. Use minimum effective dose.

FORMS:
Tablets (white) of 10 and 20mg.

PRECAUTIONS:
Use with caution in pregnancy (B3), breast feeding and children.
Do not take if:
 suffering from low blood pressure or heart failure.
- sensitive to nicotinic acid.

SIDE EFFECTS:
Common: Headache, muscle pain, tiredness, palpitations, dizziness, nausea.
Unusual: High blood pressure, diarrhoea, shortness of breath.
Severe but rare (stop medication, consult doctor): Low blood pressure.

INTERACTIONS:
Other drugs:
- Other vasodilators, tricyclic antidepressants, sildenafil (Viagra), other medications that aid penile erection, medications that lower blood pressure.

Other substances
- Alcohol.

PRESCRIPTION:
Yes.

PBS:
Yes.

PERMITTED IN SPORT:
Yes.

OVERDOSE:
Low blood pressure, rapid heart rate and collapse may occur. Induce vomiting or administer activated charcoal if tablets taken recently. Seek medical assistance.

OTHER INFORMATION:
Introduced in 1998.
See also Glyceryl trinitrate, Isosorbide nitrate, Perhexiline.

Nicotinamide
See Nicotinic acid.

Nicotine

TRADE NAMES:
Nicabate, Nicorette, Nicotinell, QuitX.
Nicotine is also one of the active chemicals in tobacco.

DRUG CLASS:
Stimulant.

USES:
Assists in stopping smoking.

DOSAGE:
 Chewable tablets: Chew one or two at a time when urge to smoke is felt. Maximum 60mg a day. Reduce frequency of use over time.
Patches: Apply to different place on non-hairy skin of trunk or upper arm once a day in morning. Instructions vary with brands. Follow doctors directions. Progressively reduce strength of patch over 10 to 12 weeks.
Inhaler: Inhale as required for up to 20 minutes without a break.
Use six to 12 cartridges a day.

FORMS:
Chewable gum, skin patches, inhaler.

PRECAUTIONS:
Not to be used in pregnancy (D) (NB: Smoking is also harmful to the foetus in pregnancy).
Breast feeding should be ceased before use. Not designed for use in children under 14 years.
Not designed for long term use.
Use chewable tablets with caution if:
- wearing dentures or having dental work.
- suffering from mouth ulcers or inflammation,
- suffering from peptic ulcer or inflamed stomach.

Use all forms in caution with heart disease.
Use patches with caution in dermatitis and eczema.

Do not take if:
☠ suffering from recent heart attack, angina, irregular heart rate or recent stroke.
• continuing to smoke.

SIDE EFFECTS:
Common: Patches – Rash at application site.
Inhaler – Cough, headache, nausea.
Unusual: Dizziness, nausea, diarrhoea, sore mouth or throat (with gum and inhaler).

INTERACTIONS:
Other drugs:
• Cessation of smoking may result in altered availability of many medications, and may require alteration in their doses.
• Phenacetin, theophylline, imipramine, oxazepam, paracetamol, pentazocine, propranolol, frusemide, insulin.

Other substances:
• Continued smoking while using nicotine may cause significant serious adverse effects.
• Caffeine.

PRESCRIPTION:
No.

PBS:
No (available to some Veterans Affairs pensioners on authority).

PERMITTED IN SPORT:
Yes.

OVERDOSE:
Nausea and vomiting only likely effects.

OTHER INFORMATION:
Nicotine substitution works best if used with an appropriate smoking cessation program. Will only work if the patient wants to stop smoking, and is prepared to use nicotine as assistance to his or her own determination. Nicotine by itself will not stop someone from smoking. Nicotine medications may cause dependence. Nicotine is highly addictive.

See also Bupropion.

Nicotinic Acid
(Niacin and Nicotinamide)
(Vitamin B3)

TRADE NAMES:
Nicotinic Acid.
Dynamo (with caffeine, glucose).
NoDoz Plus (with caffeine, glucose, thiamine).
Also found in numerous vitamin and mineral supplements.

DRUG CLASS:
Vitamin, hypolipidaemic, vasodilator.

USES:
High levels of blood cholesterol and triglycerides, pellagra, poor circulation.

DOSAGE:

Pellagra: 500mg a day.
High cholesterol/triglyceride: 250mg to 1500mg three times a day after meals.
Poor circulation: 100mg to 150mg three or four times a day.

FORMS:
Tablets, capsules.
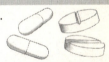

PRECAUTIONS:
Use with caution in pregnancy (B2) and breast feeding.
Blood tests to check liver function, uric acid levels and blood fat levels recommended.
Use with caution with low blood pressure and poor liver function.

Do not take if:
☠ suffering from peptic ulcer, stomach upsets, recent heart attack, severe liver disease, diabetes, gout, heart disease, gall bladder disease, glaucoma, tendency to bleed easily.

SIDE EFFECTS:
Common: Rashes, itchy skin, changes in heart function, stomach upsets,

nervousness.
Unusual: Dry skin, skin pigmentation.
Severe but rare (stop medication, consult doctor): Yellow skin.

INTERACTIONS:

Other drugs:
- Drugs used to treat high blood pressure.
- Steroids, hallucinogens, reserpine, chlordiazepoxide.

Herbs:
- Alfalfa, fenugreek, garlic, ginger.

Other substances:
- Other vitamins may affect nicotinic acid absorption.

PRESCRIPTION:

Nicotinic Acid, Tri-B3: Yes.
Others: No.

PBS:

Nicotinic Acid: Yes.
Others: No.

PERMITTED IN SPORT:

Yes.

OVERDOSE:

Causes flushing, itch, vomiting, diarrhoea, heartburn, belly cramps, fainting. Induce vomiting if tablets taken recently. Seek medical assistance.

OTHER INFORMATION:

Used as a starting point in the treatment of high cholesterol blood levels and poor circulation. Remember, vitamins are merely chemicals that are essential for the functioning of the body, and if taken to excess, act as a drug.

See also Atorvastatin, Cholestyramine, Colestipol, Fluvastatin, Gemfibrizol, Guanethidine, Pravastatin, Probucol, Simvastatin.

Nifedipine

TRADE NAMES:

Adalat, Adalat Oros, GenRx Nifedipine, Nifecard, Nifehexal, Nyefax.

DRUG CLASS:

Calcium channel blocker (calcium antagonist).

USES:

High blood pressure, angina.

DOSAGE:

10 to 40mg a day.
Do not vary dosage without medical advice.

FORMS:

Tablets, capsules, slow release tablets.
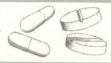

PRECAUTIONS:

Should only be used in pregnancy (C) and breast feeding if medically essential. Not designed for use in children.

Do not take if:

suffering from severe heart failure, low blood pressure, atrial flutter or fibrillation.

SIDE EFFECTS:

Common: Constipation, tiredness, headache, dizziness, indigestion, swelling of feet and ankles.
Unusual: Flushing, palpitations, slow heart rate, scalp irritation, depression, flushes, nightmares, excess wind.
Severe but rare (stop medication, consult doctor): Fainting.

INTERACTIONS:

Other drugs:
- Beta blockers (eg. propranolol), cyclosporin, digoxin, cimetidine, diazepam, amiodarone, quinidine, rifampicin, phenytoin, cisapride, theophylline, terbutaline, salbutamol, diltiazem.

- Additive effect with other medications for high blood pressure.

Herbs:
- Goldenseal, guarana, hawthorn, Korean ginseng, liquorice.

Other substances:
- Smoking may aggravate conditions that these medications are treating.
- Grapefruit juice.

PRESCRIPTION:
Yes.

PBS:
Yes.

PERMITTED IN SPORT:
Yes.

OVERDOSE:
May continue to be absorbed for up to 48 hours after overdose. Administer activated charcoal or induce vomiting. Purging should be encouraged to eliminate drug from gut. Overdose may cause low blood pressure, irregular heart rhythm, difficulty in breathing, heart attack and death. Obtain urgent medical attention.

OTHER INFORMATION:
Commonly used as a first line medication in high blood pressure and to prevent angina.

See also Amlodipine, Diltiazem, Felodipine, Nimodipine, Verapamil.

Nilutamide

TRADE NAME:
Anandron.

DRUG CLASS:
Antiandrogen (acts against testosterone), antineoplastic.

USES:
Cancer of prostate gland.

DOSAGE:
 One or two tablets a day.

FORMS:
Tablets of 150mg (off-white).

PRECAUTIONS:
Must not to be used by women or children.
Regular blood tests to check liver function essential.
Regular checks of lung function essential.
Use with caution if of Japanese ancestry.

Do not take if:
 suffering from liver damage, severe lung disease.

SIDE EFFECTS:
Common: Nausea, intolerance of changes in light, dizziness.
Unusual: Lung damage, liver damage, abnormal gland function.
Severe but rare (stop medication, consult doctor): Jaundice (yellow skin), very short of breath.

INTERACTIONS:
Other drugs:
- Anticoagulants, drugs affecting the liver.

Other substances:
- Alcohol.

PRESCRIPTION:
Yes.

Medications

PBS:
Yes (authority required. Restricted to certain types of prostate cancer).

PERMITTED IN SPORT:
Yes.

OVERDOSE:
Serious organ damage may occur. Induce vomiting or administer activated charcoal if taken recently. Seek urgent medical attention.

OTHER INFORMATION:
Introduced in 1997.
See also Bicalutamide.

Nimodipine

TRADE NAMES:
Nimotop.

DRUG CLASS:
Calcium channel blocker (calcium antagonist).

USES:
Poor blood supply to brain after haemorrhage into brain (stroke).

DOSAGE:
 As determined by doctor. Start within four days of stroke.

FORMS:
Tablets, injection.

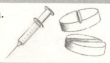

PRECAUTIONS:
Should only be used in pregnancy (C) and breast feeding if medically essential. Not designed for use in children.

Do not take if:
 suffering from severe heart failure, low blood pressure, atrial flutter or fibrillation.

SIDE EFFECTS:
Common: Constipation, tiredness, headache, dizziness, indigestion, swelling of feet and ankles, low blood pressure.
Unusual: Flushing, palpitations, slow heart rate, scalp irritation, depression, flushes, nightmares, excess wind.
Severe but rare (stop medication, consult doctor): Fainting.

INTERACTIONS:
Other drugs:
- Beta blockers (eg. propranolol), cyclosporin, digoxin, cimetidine, diazepam, amiodarone, quinidine, rifampicin, phenytoin, cisapride, theophylline, terbutaline, salbutamol, diltiazem.
- Additive effect with other medications for high blood pressure.

Herbs:
- Goldenseal, guarana, hawthorn, Korean ginseng, liquorice.

Other substances:
- Smoking may aggravate conditions that these medications are treating.
- Grapefruit juice.

PRESCRIPTION:
Yes.

PBS:
No.

PERMITTED IN SPORT:
Yes.

OVERDOSE:
May continue to be absorbed for up to 48 hours after overdose. Administer activated charcoal or induce vomiting. Purging should be encouraged to eliminate drug from gut. Overdose may cause low blood pressure, irregular heart rhythm, difficulty in breathing, heart attack and death. Obtain urgent medical attention.

See also Amlodipine, Diltiazem, Felodipine, Nifedipine, Verapamil.

Nitrazepam

TRADE NAMES:
Alodorm, Mogadon.

DRUG CLASS:
Sedative/hypnotic, Benzodiazepine.

USES:
Relieves insomnia (sleeplessness).

DOSAGE:

One or two at bedtime.

FORMS:
Tablet of 5mg.

PRECAUTIONS:
Should be used with caution in pregnancy (C), but not at all if delivery of infant imminent as it may decrease desire to breathe in newborn infant. Should be used with caution in breast feeding. Not for use in children.
Lower dose required in elderly.
Should be used intermittently and not constantly as dependency may develop.
Stopping suddenly after prolonged constant use may cause withdrawal symptoms.
Use with caution in glaucoma, myasthenia gravis, heart disease, kidney or liver disease, psychiatric conditions, depression and epilepsy.

Do not take if:
 suffering from severe lung disease, confusion.
- tendency to addiction or dependence.

SIDE EFFECTS:
Common: Confusion and falls in elderly, impaired alertness.
Unusual: Dizziness, incoordination, poor memory, headache, hangover in morning, slurred speech, nightmares.

INTERACTIONS:
Other drugs:
- Other medications that reduce alertness (eg. barbiturates, antihistamines, antianxiety drugs).
- Disulfiram, cimetidine, anticonvulsants, anticholinergics, antihistamines.

Herbs:
- Guarana, kava kava, passionflower, St John's wort, valerian, celery, camomile, goldenseal.

Other substances:
- Reacts with alcohol to cause excessive drowsiness.

PRESCRIPTION:
Yes.

PBS:
Yes.

PERMITTED IN SPORT:
Yes.

OVERDOSE:
Seldom life threatening. May cause drowsiness, confusion and coma. Administer activated charcoal or induce vomiting if tablets taken recently. Seek medical assistance.

OTHER INFORMATION:
In use for over 30 years. Very safe and effective, but dependence (inability to sleep or function without medication) a problem if used regularly.

See also BARBITURATES, Chlormethiazole, Flunitrazepam, Midazolam, Temazepam, Triazolam, Zolpidem, Zopiclone.

Nitrofurantoin

TRADE NAMES:
Furadantin, Macrodantin, Ralodantin.

DRUG CLASS:
Antibiotic.

USES:
Bacterial infections of urine.

DOSAGE:
 One or two capsules four times a day with food.

FORMS:
Capsules, suspension.

PRECAUTIONS:
Safe to use in pregnancy (A), breast feeding and children. Not for use during labour of pregnancy or if labour imminent. Not for use under one month of age.
Not designed for long term use.
Use with caution in kidney function disorders, diabetes, blood chemistry (electrolyte) disorders.

Do not take if:
 suffering from severe kidney failure.

SIDE EFFECTS:
Common: Nausea, vomiting.
Unusual: Brown urine.
Severe but rare (stop medication, consult doctor): Numbness or tingling, yellow skin (jaundice).

INTERACTIONS:
Other drugs:
- Barbiturates, antacids, urinary acidifiers and alkalinisers.

PRESCRIPTION:
Yes.

PBS:
Yes.

PERMITTED IN SPORT:
Yes.

OVERDOSE:
Exacerbation of side effects likely. Give additional fluids by mouth to increase rate of excretion.

OTHER INFORMATION:
Useful and effective medication.
See also Hexamine hippurate.

Nitroglycerine

See Glyceryl Trinitrate.

Nitromersol

OTHER INFORMATION:
Nitromersol is an antiseptic that is only available in Australia in combination with lignocaine as **Abbott Cold Sore Balm** and with butyl aminobenzoate as **Butesin Pictrate With Metaphen.**
See also ANAESTHETICS, LOCAL.

Nizatadine

TRADE NAME:
Tazac.

DRUG CLASS:
Antiulcerant, H2 receptor antagonist.

USES:
Prevention and treatment of ulcers of the stomach, oesophagus (gullet) and duodenum (upper small intestine). Prevention of acid reflux into the oesophagus (heartburn).

DOSAGE:
 300mg a day in one or two doses.

FORMS:
Capsules of 150mg (dark yellow, cream) and 300mg (brown, cream).

PRECAUTIONS:
Care should be taken with use in pregnancy (B3) and breast feeding. Safety in children not established.
Do not take if:
 suffering from severe kidney or liver disease or phenylketonuria.
- suffering from stomach cancer.

SIDE EFFECTS:
Common: Anaemia, tiredness, drowsiness, rash.
Unusual: Constipation, breast enlargement and tenderness (both sexes).
Severe but rare (stop medication, consult doctor): Hepatitis (jaundice), rapid or irregular heartbeat.

INTERACTIONS:
Other drugs:
- Aspirin.
Herbs:
- Alfalfa, capsicum, eucalyptus, senega.

PRESCRIPTION:
Yes.

PBS:
Yes.

PERMITTED IN SPORT:
Yes.

OVERDOSE:
No serious effects reported.

OTHER INFORMATION:
Introduced in 1992. H2 receptor antagonist that may be more effective in reflux oesophagitis than others in this class.
See also **Cimetidine, Famotidine, Ranitidine.**

Nonoxynol 9
See **SPERMICIDES**.

Norethisterone
(Norethindrone)

TRADE NAMES:
Locilan, Micronor, Noriday, Primolut-N.
Estalis, Estracombi, Kliogest, Kliovance, Trisequens (with oestradiol).
Used in numerous oral contraceptives (eg. **Brevinor, Improvil, Norimin, Norinyl, Synphasic**).

DRUG CLASS:
Sex hormone.

USES:
Added to oestrogen in menopausal hormone replacement therapy (HRT). Abnormal bleeding from uterus, failure of menstrual period, premenstrual tension, breast tenderness and endometriosis.
Contraception.

DOSAGE:

 Tablets: One or two tablets, one to three times a day with fluid.
Patches: Apply twice a week.

FORMS:

Tablets, patch.

PRECAUTIONS:

Not for use in pregnancy (D), breast feeding or children.
Use with caution in diabetes.
Do not take if:
- suffering from severe liver disease, jaundice or blood clots.
- male.

SIDE EFFECTS:

Common: Abnormal vaginal bleeding, headache.
Unusual: Sleeplessness, nervousness, dizziness, tremor, rash, sweating, nausea, breast tenderness, weight gain.
Severe but rare (stop medication, consult doctor): Blood clot, calf pain, chest pain, yellow skin (jaundice).

INTERACTIONS:

Other drugs:
- Other sex hormones.

Other substances:
- Smoking increases risk of serious side effects.

PRESCRIPTION:
Yes.

PBS:
Yes.

PERMITTED IN SPORT:
Yes.

OVERDOSE:
Unlikely to be serious. Vomiting and abnormal vaginal bleeding likely.

OTHER INFORMATION:

Widely used and safe medication. Useful for delaying menstrual period that may be due at an awkward time. Does not cause addiction or dependence. Often used as a contraceptive in women who are breast feeding, when they must be taken at the same time each day to be reliable.
See also ORAL CONTRACEPTIVES.

Norfloxacin

TRADE NAMES:

GenRx Norfloxacin, Insensye, Norflohexal, Noroxin, Roxin.

DRUG CLASS:

Quinolone antibiotic.

USES:

Urinary infections.

DOSAGE:

 One tablet twice a day.

FORMS:

Tablet (white) of 400mg.

PRECAUTIONS:

Not to be used in pregnancy (B3) and breast feeding unless medically essential.
Not for use in children.
Ensure adequate fluid intake.
Use with caution in epilepsy and kidney disease.
Avoid excessive sun exposure while taking medication.

SIDE EFFECTS:

Common: Nausea, headache, dizziness.
Unusual: Tiredness, rash, belly pain, depression, sleeplessness, constipation, excess wind, constipation.

Severe but rare (stop medication, consult doctor): Bloody diarrhoea, unusual bruising or bleeding, tender tendons.

INTERACTIONS:
Other drugs:
- Antacids, nitrofurantoin, theophylline, cyclosporin, probenecid, anticoagulants.

Other substances:
- Reacts with caffeine.

PRESCRIPTION:
Yes.

PBS:
Yes.

PERMITTED IN SPORT:
Yes.

OVERDOSE:
Exacerbation of side effects most likely result. Induce vomiting if medication taken recently. Maintain adequate fluid intake.

OTHER INFORMATION:
Introduced in late 1980s. Very effective in treating the more difficult infections of the bladder and kidneys.

See also Ciprofloxacin.

Normal Immunoglobulin
See Gamma globulin.

Nortriptyline
See TRICYCLIC ANTIDEPRESSANTS.

NSAIDs
(NONSTEROIDAL ANTI-INFLAMMATORY DRUGS)

DISCUSSION:
Despite their long name and unpronounceable acronym, the NSAIDs are some of the most widely used drugs in modern medicine. They are drugs that reduce inflammation in tissue, without being steroids (see separate entry), which are the most potent anti-inflammatory drugs available.

Inflammation is the redness, swelling, pain and heat that occurs in tissue that is subjected to some form of irritation or injury. NSAIDs not only reduce inflammation but also ease pain and lower fevers. Their main uses are in the treatment of rheumatoid and osteoarthritis, sporting injuries to joints, muscles and tendons, and to reduce the inflammation in the pelvis associated with menstrual period pain. They are all available as tablets or capsules, but some are also available as injections, and even as creams, gels and a rub-on lotion.

A subgroup of the NSAIDs are the salicylates, which are all derived from salicylic acid. The most commonly known member of this subgroup is aspirin which acts as a painkiller (analgesic), fever-reducing agent (antipyretic) and anti-inflammatory medication. It has the same side effects as the other NSAIDs.

The greatest problem with the use of NSAIDs is the possibility of causing peptic ulcers in the stomach or small intestine. Unfortunately, a significant proportion of the patients using these medications will develop some intestinal problem. This can be prevented to some extent by always taking the drugs after food, or in conjunction with an antacid or other ulcer-preventing medication. Any patient who develops stomach pains, vomits blood or passes black stools while on NSAIDs must cease them and see a doctor immediately.

Despite the problems associated with the use of NSAIDs, many patients with arthritis find that these drugs have improved their lives dramatically by controlling their previously painful and swollen joints. They can also enable sportsmen and women to overcome painful sprains and strains to enable them to return to competition as quickly as possible.

See **Aspirin, Bufexamac, Celecoxib, Diclofenac, Diflunisal, Flurbiprofen, Ibuprofen, Indomethacin, Ketoprofen, Ketorolac trometanol, Mefenamic Acid, Naproxen, Piroxicam, Rofecoxib, Sulindac, Tenoxicam, Tiaprofenic Acid.**

Nystatin

TRADE NAMES:
**Mycostatin, Nilstat.
Kenacomb, Otocomb** (with triamcinolone, neomycin and gramicidin).

DRUG CLASS:
Antifungal.

USES:
Treatment and prevention of fungal infections of skin (tinea), mouth, vagina (thrush) and intestine (candidiasis).

DOSAGE:

Tablets and capsules: One or two, three times a day.
Skin preparations: Apply three times a day.
Vaginal preparations: One pessary, tablet or applicator of cream at night for 14 days.

FORMS:
Cream, ointment, powder, tablets, capsules, drops, lozenges, vaginal cream, vaginal pessary, cream pessary.

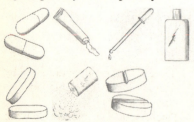

PRECAUTIONS:
Safe to use in pregnancy (A), breast feeding and children.
Applicator of vaginal preparations must be used with care in pregnancy.

SIDE EFFECTS:
Minimal.

INTERACTIONS:
None significant.

PRESCRIPTION:
Most forms: Yes.
Oral drops, Nilstat cream and vaginal cream: No.

PBS:
Most forms: Yes.
Oral drops, Nilstat cream and vaginal cream: No.

PERMITTED IN SPORT:
Yes.

OVERDOSE:
Diarrhoea, nausea and vomiting only likely effects.

OTHER INFORMATION:
Does not cause dependence or addiction. Available for over 30 years. Very safe. Use decreasing in recent years with introduction of more potent antifungals (eg. imidazoles).

See also **ANTIFUNGALS, Clotrimazole, Econazole, Fluconazole, Itraconazole, Ketoconazole, Miconazole.**

Medications

OBESITY DRUGS

See ANORECTICS, Diethylpropion hydrochloride, Orlistat, Phentermine, Silbutramine.

Octoxinol

See SPERMICIDES.

Octreotide

TRADE NAME:
Sandostatin.

USES:
Acromegaly (bone overgrowth caused by tumour of pituitary gland), relief of carcinoid tumour symptoms.

DOSAGE:
 One or more injections a day as determined by doctor.

FORMS:
Injection.

PRECAUTIONS:
Must not be used in pregnancy (C) or breast feeding. Use in children only when medically essential.
Use with caution in diabetes.
Regular checks on gall bladder and pituitary gland necessary.
Designed for short term or intermittent use.

SIDE EFFECTS:
Common: Pain at injection site, nausea, vomiting, loss of appetite, bloating, excess wind, diarrhoea.
Unusual: Headache, dizziness, fatigue, flushing.

INTERACTIONS:
Other drugs:
- Cyclosporin, cimetidine, bromocriptine.

PRESCRIPTION:
Yes.

PBS:
Yes (some forms only, and very restricted).

PERMITTED IN SPORT:
Yes.

Oestradiol
(Estradiol)

TRADE NAMES:
Climara, Dermestril, Estraderm, Estrofem, Femtran, Menorest, Natragen, Oestradiol Implants, Sandrena, Vagifem, Zumenon.
Aerodiol Spray (oestradiol hemihydrate).
Primogyn Depot, Progynova (oestradiol valerate).
Femoston (with dydrogesterone).
Climen (with cyproterone acetate).
Divina, Estrapak (with medroxyprogesterone acetate).
Estalis, Estracombi, Kliogest, Kliovance, Trisequens (with norethisterone).

DRUG CLASS:
Sex hormone.

USES:
Oestrogen (female hormone) replacement in menopause.

DOSAGE:
 Tablets: Dosage individualised by doctor. Usually one tablet once a day.
Patch: Apply once or twice a week.

399

Nose spray: One or two sprays in each nostril once a day. Do not inhale during spray, or blow nose for five minutes afterwards.
Gel: Apply daily to lower belly or thigh.
Cream: Insert into vagina with applicator once or twice a week.
Pessary: One pessary in vagina every night initially, reducing to twice a week.

FORMS:
Tablets, patches, gel, cream, nose spray, vaginal pessary, vaginal ring, injection, implant.

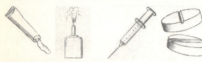

PRECAUTIONS:
Not to be used in pregnancy (B1), breast feeding or children. Accidental usage in these situations unlikely to be harmful. Not to be used by males.
Use with caution in epilepsy, migraine, heart failure, high blood pressure, kidney disease, diabetes, porphyria or uterine disease.

Do not take if:
☠ suffering from liver disease, breast or genital cancer, blood clots, sickle cell anaemia, undiagnosed bleeding from vagina, severe high blood pressure, or endometriosis.

SIDE EFFECTS:
Common: Abnormal uterine bleeding, vaginal thrush, nausea, fluid retention, weight gain, breast tenderness.
Unusual: Rash at site of patch application, blurred vision, vomiting, bloating, intestinal cramps, pigmentation of skin on face, nose bleeds with nasal spray use.
Severe but rare (stop medication, consult doctor): Blood clots, calf or chest pain, yellow skin (jaundice).

INTERACTIONS:
Other drugs:
- Other sex hormones, antibiotics, diabetes medications (hypoglycaemics), warfarin, epilepsy medications (anticonvulsants), imipramine, corticosteroids, thyroxine.
- Do not use oestradiol nose spray at same time as other nose sprays.

Herbs:
- Saw palmetto, alfalfa, dong quai, ginseng, liquorice, red clover.

Other substances:
- Smoking increases risk of serious side effects.

PRESCRIPTION:
Yes.

PBS:
Implants, vaginal ring, cream, nose spray: No.
Other forms: Yes.

PERMITTED IN SPORT:
Yes.

OVERDOSE:
Vomiting and abnormal vaginal bleeding only likely effects.

OTHER INFORMATION:
Does not cause addiction or dependence. Very useful in managing the effects of menopause, and reduces the risk of osteoporosis and heart disease after the menopause.

See Cyproterone acetate, Danazol, Dydrogesterone, Ethinyloestradiol, Etonogestrel, HORMONE REPLACEMENT THERAPY, Medroxyprogesterone acetate, Oestriol, Oestrogen, ORAL CONTRACEPTIVES, Piperazine oestrone sulfate, Testosterone.

Oestriol

TRADE NAME:
Ovestin.

DRUG CLASS:
Sex hormone.

USES:
Oestrogen (female hormone) replacement in menopause.

DOSAGE:
Tablets: Dosage individualised by doctor. Usually one tablet once a day.
Vaginal cream and pessaries: Use daily at bed time initially, reduce to twice a week long term.

FORMS:
Tablets (white) of 1mg,
vaginal cream,
vaginal pessaries.

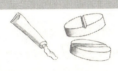

PRECAUTIONS:
Not to be used in pregnancy (B1), breast feeding or children. Accidental usage in these situations unlikely to be harmful. Use with caution in epilepsy, migraine, heart failure, high blood pressure, kidney disease, diabetes, porphyria or uterine disease.

Do not take if:
suffering from liver disease, breast or genital cancer, blood clots, undiagnosed vaginal bleeding, endometriosis, porphyria or otosclerosis.

SIDE EFFECTS:
Common: Abnormal uterine bleeding, vaginal thrush, nausea, fluid retention, weight gain, breast tenderness.
Unusual: Rash, blurred vision, vomiting, bloating, intestinal cramps, pigmentation of skin on face.
Severe but rare (stop medication, consult doctor): Blood clots, calf or chest pain, yellow skin (jaundice).

INTERACTIONS:
Other drugs:
- Other sex hormones.

Other substances:
- Smoking increases risk of serious side effects.

PRESCRIPTION:
Yes.

PBS:
Yes.

PERMITTED IN SPORT:
Yes.

OVERDOSE:
Vomiting and abnormal vaginal bleeding only likely effects.

OTHER INFORMATION:
Does not cause addiction or dependence. Very useful in managing the effects of menopause, and reduces the risk of osteoporosis and heart disease after the menopause.

See Cyproterone acetate, Danazol, Dydrogesterone, Ethinyloestradiol, Etonogestrel, HORMONE REPLACEMENT THERAPY, Medroxyprogesterone acetate, Oestradiol, Oestrogen, ORAL CONTRACEPTIVES, Oxandrolone, Piperazine oestrone sulfate, Testosterone.

Oestrogen

TRADE NAMES:
Premarin.
Menoprem (discontinued 2003), **Premia** (with medroxyprogesterone).
Provelle (with medroxyprogesterone).

DRUG CLASS:
Sex hormone.

USES:
Female hormone replacement in menopause.

DOSAGE:

Tablets: Dosage individualised by doctor. Usually one tablet once a day.
Vaginal cream: Insert daily, three weeks per month.

FORMS:
Tablets, vaginal cream, injection.

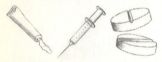

PRECAUTIONS:
Not to be used in pregnancy (B1), breast feeding or children. Accidental usage in these situations unlikely to be harmful. Not for use by males.
Use with caution in epilepsy, migraine, heart failure, high blood pressure, kidney disease, diabetes, porphyria, endometriosis or uterine disease.

Do not take if:
suffering from liver disease, breast or genital cancer, blood clots, undiagnosed vaginal bleeding.

SIDE EFFECTS:
Common: Abnormal uterine bleeding, vaginal thrush, nausea, fluid retention, weight gain, breast tenderness.
Unusual: Rash, blurred vision, vomiting, bloating, intestinal cramps, pigmentation of skin on face.
Severe but rare (stop medication, consult doctor): Blood clots, calf or chest pain, yellow skin (jaundice).

INTERACTIONS:
Other drugs:
- Other sex hormones, rifampicin.

Herbs:
- Saw palmetto, alfalfa, dong quai, ginseng, liquorice, red clover.

Other substances:
- Smoking increases risk of serious side effects.

PRESCRIPTION:
Yes.

PBS:
Yes.

PERMITTED IN SPORT:
Yes.

OVERDOSE:
Vomiting and abnormal vaginal bleeding only likely effects.

OTHER INFORMATION:
Does not cause addiction or dependence. Very useful in managing the effects of menopause, and reduces the risk of osteoporosis and heart disease after the menopause.

See Cyproterone acetate, Danazol, Dydrogesterone, Ethinyloestradiol, Etonogestrel, HORMONE REPLACEMENT THERAPY, Medroxyprogesterone acetate, Oestradiol, Oestriol, ORAL CONTRACEPTIVES, Oxandrolone, Piperazine oestrone sulfate.

Ofloxacin

TRADE NAME:
Ocuflox.

DRUG CLASS:
Quinolone antibiotic.

USES:
Severe bacterial infections of the eye.

DOSAGE:
 One drop in affected eye(s) every four to six hours for maximum of 10 days.

FORMS:
Eye drops.

PRECAUTIONS:
Use with caution in pregnancy (B3), breast feeding and children.
Use caution with contact lenses.
Not for prolonged use.

SIDE EFFECTS:
Common: Temporary eye pain and stinging, excess tear production.
Unusual: Red eye.

INTERACTIONS:
None significant.

PRESCRIPTION:
Yes.

PBS:
Yes.

PERMITTED IN SPORT:
Yes.

OTHER INFORMATION:
Introduced in 1997 for the treatment of serious infections unresponsive to other antibiotics.

Olanzapine

TRADE NAME:
Zyprexa.

DRUG CLASS:
Antipsychotic.

USES:
Schizophrenia, psychoses, dementia, other psychiatric conditions.

DOSAGE:
 2.5 to 20mg once a day. Increase dose slowly.

FORMS:
Tablets (white) of 2.5mg, 5mg, 7.5mg and 10mg, wafers (yellow) of 5mg and 10mg.

PRECAUTIONS:
Use with caution in pregnancy (B3), breast feeding and children.
Use with caution in enlarged prostate gland, glaucoma, diabetes, poor small bowel function, epilepsy, kidney and liver disease.
Use low doses in elderly.
Regular blood tests to check function of blood cells and bone marrow necessary.

Do not take if:
 suffering from leukaemia, bone marrow disease.

SIDE EFFECTS:
Common: Sleepiness, tiredness, weight gain, dizziness, low blood pressure, swelling of feet and hands, dry mouth.
Unusual: Liver damage, poor coordination, breast milk production.
Severe but rare (stop medication, consult doctor): Severe infection, jaundice (yellow skin).

INTERACTIONS:
Other drugs:
- Drugs affecting heart function, drugs acting on the brain, carbamazepine, fluoxetine, fluvoxamine.

Herbs:
- Evening primrose (linoleic acid).

Other substances:
- Alcohol, smoking.

PRESCRIPTION:
Yes.

PBS:
Yes (authority required).

PERMITTED IN SPORT:
Yes.

OVERDOSE:
Serious exacerbation of side effects likely. Induce vomiting or administer activated charcoal if taken recently. Seek urgent medical attention.

OTHER INFORMATION:
Introduced in 1997 for the treatment of the more difficult forms of schizophrenia. Now found to be very useful in the control of many forms of abnormal behaviour and dementia.

See also Amisulpride, Droperidol, Flupenthixol, Haloperidol, Lithium Carbonate, PHENOTHIAZINES, Pimozide, Quetiapine, Risperidone, Thiothixene, Zuclopenthixol.

Olopatadine

TRADE NAME:
Patanol.

USES:
Allergic conjunctivitis.

DOSAGE:

One or two drops into affected eye, once or twice a day.

FORMS:
Eye drops.

PRECAUTIONS:
Safe to use in pregnancy (B1), breast feeding and children.
Not for long term use over 14 weeks.
Use with caution if wearing soft contact lenses.

SIDE EFFECTS:
Common: Temporary blurred vision.
Unusual: Headaches, tiredness, eye burning and stinging, dry eye, irritated eye, red eye, swollen eyelid, abnormal taste.

INTERACTIONS:
None significant.

PRESCRIPTION:
Yes.

PBS:
No.

PERMITTED IN SPORT:
Yes.

See also Levocabastine.

Olsalazine

TRADE NAME:
Dipentum.

USES:
Treatment of complicated cases of ulcerative colitis.

DOSAGE:

250mg to 1000mg three times a day after meals.

FORMS:
Capsule of 250mg (beige), tablets of 500mg (yellow).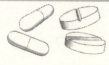

Medications

PRECAUTIONS:
Should be used with caution in pregnancy (B2) and breast feeding.
Should be used with caution in severe kidney disease.
Do not take if:
 sensitive to salicylates.
- suffering from a bleeding disorder or peptic ulcer.

SIDE EFFECTS:
Common: Diarrhoea (very common), nausea, belly pains.
Unusual: Rash, headache, joint pains.
Severe but rare (stop medication, consult doctor): Many rare and serious effects reported including blood cell abnormalities and liver damage.

INTERACTIONS:
Other drugs:
- Serious interaction with anticoagulants (eg. warfarin).

PRESCRIPTION:
Yes.

PBS:
Yes (authority required. Restricted to patients with colitis where hypersensitivity to other drugs exists).

PERMITTED IN SPORT:
Yes.

OTHER INFORMATION:
Used in only very special circumstances in the uncommon condition of ulcerative colitis.
See also Mesalazine

Omeprazole
See **PROTON PUMP INHIBITORS**.

Ondansetron

TRADE NAME:
Zofran.

USES:
Stops nausea and vomiting caused by cancer-treating drugs, radiotherapy or surgery.

DOSAGE:
 One to four tablets or wafers twice a day.

FORMS:
Tablets (yellow) of 4mg, injection, suppositories of 16mg, wafers of 4mg.

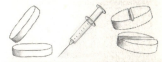

PRECAUTIONS:
May be used with caution in pregnancy (B1), breast feeding and children over 4 years.
Use with caution in liver and bowel disease.

SIDE EFFECTS:
Common: Hot flush, headache, upper belly discomfort.
Unusual: Dry mouth, constipation, hiccups.

INTERACTIONS:
Other drugs:
- Phenytoin, carbamazepine.

PRESCRIPTION:
Yes.

PBS:
Most forms: Yes (restricted to vomiting caused by anticancer drugs and radiotherapy).
Suppositories: No.

PERMITTED IN SPORT:
Yes.

OVERDOSE:
Exacerbation of side effects likely.

OTHER INFORMATION:
Introduced in 1993 to relieve the severe vomiting that may be caused by some anticancer drugs. More effective if given by injection.

See also Chlorpromazine, Metoclopramide, Prochlorperazine.

OPIATES

DISCUSSION:
Opiates (also known as narcotics) are strong, addictive and effective painkillers derived from the opium poppy. They are highly restricted in their use, and must be kept in safes by chemists and doctors. If they are used appropriately, they give relief from severe pain to patients with acute injuries, and pain from diseases such as cancer and kidney stones. They are often used before, during and after operations to ease the pain of the procedure. If used in this way, it is unlikely that addiction will occur. If used excessively, a psychological and physical addiction can rapidly develop. Heroin is an infamous illegal opiate that is broken down to morphine in the body. Opiates not only relieve severe pain, they also reduce anxiety, stop coughs, sedate and cause euphoria (a 'high' – artificial happiness). They should be used with caution in asthma and other lung diseases, liver disease and after head injuries.

See Alfentanil, Buprenorphine, Codeine Phosphate, Dextromoramide, Dextropropoxyphene, Fentanyl, Heroin, Hydromorphone, Methadone, Morphine, Oxycodone, Pentazocine, Pethidine.

ORAL CONTRACEPTIVES
(CONTRACEPTIVE PILLS)

TRADE and GENERIC NAMES:
In this section all oral contraceptive pills are divided into groups, depending on:
- whether the dosage:
  - does not vary (monophasic) during the month
  - varies twice (biphasic) during the month
  - varies three times (triphasic) during the month.
- whether they contain:
  - two hormones (combined oestrogen and progestogen).
  - one hormone (progestogen-only mini pill)

MONOPHASIC COMBINED OESTROGEN AND PROGESTOGEN PILLS:
Brevinor, Norimin (ethinyloestradiol, norethisterone).
Brenda, Diane, Juliet (cyproterone acetate, ethinyloestradiol).
Femoden, Minulet (gestodene, ethinyloestradiol).
Levlen, Loette, Microgynon, Microlevlen, Monofeme, Nordette (ethinyloestradiol, levonorgestrel).
Marvelon (desogestrel, ethinyloestradiol).
Norinyl (mestranol, norethisterone).
Yasmin (ethinyloestradiol, drospirenone).

BIPHASIC COMBINED OESTROGEN AND PROGESTOGEN PILLS:
Sequilar (ethinyloestradiol, levonorgestrel).
Synphasic (ethinyloestradiol, norethisterone).

TRIPHASIC COMBINED OESTROGEN AND PROGESTOGEN PILLS:
Improvil (ethinyloestradiol, norethisterone).
Logynon, Trifeme, Triphasil, Triquilar (ethinyloestradiol, levonorgestrel).
Tri-Minulet, Trioden (gestodene, ethinyloestradiol).

PROGESTOGEN ONLY (MINI) PILLS:
Microlut, Microval (levonorgestrel).
Locilan, Micronor, Noriday (norethisterone).

DRUG CLASS:
Sex hormones.

USES:
Prevention of pregnancy, control of irregular or painful menstrual cycle (combined forms only), control of acne in women (those containing cyproterone acetate).

DOSAGE:

One tablet a day on the day indicated on the pack for 21 or 28 days a month.
May fail as a contraceptive if progestogen-only pill missed by more than four hours of normal time of taking, or if low dose combined pill missed by more than eight hours of normal time. If a contraceptive pill is missed, take the missed pill with the next remembered pill, continue taking the pill, but use other forms of contraception (eg. condoms) for the next seven days, but if this seven-day period extends into the inactive (sugar) pill section of the pack or into the pill-free days of a 21-day pack, do not take the inactive pills or have a break, but continue with the next active pill in a new pack.

FORMS:
Tablets.

PRECAUTIONS:
Not for use in pregnancy (B3), but serious effects from taking oral contraceptive accidentally during pregnancy are unlikely. Progestogen only pills are recommended during breast feeding, but low dose combined pills may be used if necessary. Should be kept out of reach of children, and are obviously not for use in children, although accidental usage by children is unlikely to be serious.
Use with caution in heart disease, history of blood clots, epilepsy, migraine, diabetes, severe depression and sickle cell anaemia. Not to be used in pubertal girls until menstruation well established.

Before prescribing, a thorough history and physical check should be performed by a doctor.
Annual checks of blood pressure and breasts necessary.
Two yearly Pap smears and urine screening tests advisable.
Diarrhoea, vomiting or use of antibiotics may affect contraceptive action.

Do not take if:
suffering from high blood pressure, blood clots, stroke, very high cholesterol blood levels, severe liver disease, Dubin-Johnson syndrome, liver tumour, systemic lupus erythematosus, sex organ or breast cancer, jaundice, otosclerosis or severe skin irritation.
- male.

SIDE EFFECTS:
Common: Nausea, pigmentation of facial skin and nipples, headache, breast tenderness, weight change (up or down).
Unusual: Depression, increased sex drive, break through bleeding.
Severe but rare (stop medication, consult doctor): Severe headache, blood clot, calf or chest pain, severe shortness of breath, yellow skin (jaundice).

INTERACTIONS:
Other drugs:
- Antibiotics, phenytoin, primidone, barbiturates, rifampicin, anticoagulants (eg. warfarin), hypoglycaemics (medications that treat diabetes), imipramine.

Herbs:
- St John's wort, liquorice.

Other substances:
- Smoking increases risk of serious side effects.
- Vitamin C (ascorbic acid).

PRESCRIPTION:
Yes.

PBS:
Most forms: Yes.
Diane, Femoden, Improvil, Juliet, Marvelon, Minulet, Tri-Minulet, Trioden, Yasmin: No

PERMITTED IN SPORT:
Yes.

OVERDOSE:
Vomiting and abnormal vaginal bleeding only likely effects.

OTHER INFORMATION:
Sex hormones used as a contraceptive pill come in several different forms, but are mainly divided into the combined pill, which contains both oestrogen and progestogen, and the mini pill, which has only progestogen. Some of the combined pills have a two or three phase variation in their dosage during the month.

In 1961, a woman taking the first form of the oral contraceptive pill was taking more than 32 times the amount of hormone every month than the modern woman on the latest three-phase type of pill. Over the past few decades, the pill has been subjected to more clinical trials and more intensive investigation than any other medication used by womankind. There is no doubt that it is now much safer to take the contraceptive pill for many years than it is to have one pregnancy, and that is the realistic basis on which to judge the safety of any contraceptive.

Two different hormones (oestrogen and progestogen) control the menstrual cycle. At the time of ovulation, the levels of oestrogen drops, and progestogen rises, triggering the egg's release from the ovary. When the hormones revert to their previous level two weeks later, the lining of the womb is no longer able to survive and breaks away, giving the woman a period. The contraceptive pill maintains a more constant hormone level, and thus prevents the release of the egg. With the triphasic pills, the level of both hormones rises at the normal time of ovulation and then drops slightly thereafter to give a more natural hormonal cycle to the woman, while still preventing the release of an egg. When the pill is stopped (or the sugar pills started) at the end of the month, the sudden drop in hormone levels cause a menstrual period to start.

The so-called mini pill contains only one hormone (a progestogen), which is taken constantly without any sugar pills or break at the end of each month. This type of pill must be taken very carefully, as even missing it by four hours one day may drop the hormone levels sufficiently to allow ovulation and pregnancy. The failure rate of the mini pill is significantly higher than that of the combined pill.

The pill has several positive benefits besides almost perfect prevention of pregnancy. It regulates irregular periods, reduces menstrual pain and premenstrual tension, may increase the size of the breasts, reduces the severity of acne in some women, and libido (the desire for sex) is often increased. It even reduces the incidence of some types of gynaecological cancer. Women who have unwanted side effects from the pill can be assessed by a doctor, and a pill containing a different balance of hormones can be prescribed.

If taken correctly, the pill is very effective as a contraceptive, but missing a pill, or suffering from diarrhoea or vomiting can have a very pregnant result. Some antibiotics can also interfere with the pill, as can vitamin C. There is no need these days to take a break from the pill every year or so, as may have been the case in earlier years. On the other hand, many women find they can successfully skip a period by continuing to take the active pills of a monophasic combined contraceptive pill (does not work with biphasic, triphasic or progestogen only pills).

The effects of the pill are readily reversible. If a woman decides to become pregnant, she can find herself in that state in as little as two weeks after ceasing it, with no adverse effects on the mother or child.

Diane and Marvelon were introduced in 1994. Diane is particularly useful in women with acne.

Femoden, Minulet, Tri-Minulet and Trioden introduced in 1995, and are particularly useful in controlling heavy and irregular periods.

Yasmin was introduced in 2001 as a new combination of hormones that suits some women better than those used traditionally.

The 'morning after' pill is described under its active ingredient – Levonorgestrel.

The contraceptive implant is described under etonogestrel.

The contraceptive injection is described under medroxyprogesterone acetate.

See also Cyproterone acetate, Etonogestrel, HORMONE REPLACEMENT THERAPY, Levonorgestrel, Medroxyprogesterone acetate, SPERMICIDES.

Orciprenaline

TRADE NAME:
Alupent.

DRUG CLASS:
Bronchodilator.

USES:
Asthma, chronic bronchitis.

DOSAGE:

One or two inhalations three or four times a day.

FORMS:
Inhaler.

PRECAUTIONS:
Safe to use in pregnancy (A), breast feeding and older children.
Use with caution in high blood pressure, heart disease, diabetes and labour of pregnancy.
Tolerance may develop with overuse.
Not for prolonged use.
Never exceed prescribed dose.

Do not take if:

suffering from irregular or rapid heartbeat, aortic disease or overactive thyroid gland.

SIDE EFFECTS:
Common: Palpitations, tremor, restlessness, flush, headache.
Unusual: Nausea, giddiness, sleeplessness.
Severe but rare (stop medication, consult doctor): Chest pain (angina).

INTERACTIONS:
Other drugs:
- Sympathomimetics, beta blockers, MAOI, diuretics.

Other substances:
- Caffeine and alcohol.

PRESCRIPTION:
Yes.

PBS:
No.

PERMITTED IN SPORT:
No.

OVERDOSE:
Exacerbation of side effects likely. These may become distressing and may be serious in patients with heart disease or high blood pressure.

OTHER INFORMATION:
One of the early treatments for asthma that is no longer widely used.

See also Salbutamol.

Orlistat

TRADE NAME:
Xenical.

USES:
Treatment of obesity.

DOSAGE:

One tablet three times a day with meals.

FORMS:
Capsules of 120mg (turquoise).

PRECAUTIONS:
Use with caution in pregnancy (B1) and children.
Use with caution with peptic ulcers, psychiatric disturbances, adhesions in belly, kidney stones, serious heart, liver and kidney disease.
Do not take if:
 breast feeding
- suffering from pancreatitis, malabsorption, recent major surgery or some types of gall bladder disease.
- normal weight or underweight.

SIDE EFFECTS:
Common: Diarrhoea (worse if fat eaten), flatulence, liquid faeces, headache.
Unusual: Incontinence of faeces, nausea, indigestion, bowel noises, anal irritation, dizziness, muscle pains.
Severe but rare (stop medication, consult doctor): Liver damage.

INTERACTIONS:
Other drugs:
- Cyclosporin, pravastatin, other drugs for obesity.

Other substances:
- Vitamins within two hours.

PRESCRIPTION:
Yes.

PBS:
No.

PERMITTED IN SPORT:
Yes.

OVERDOSE:
Unlikely to be serious.

OTHER INFORMATION:
Introduced 2000 as a totally new type of anti-obesity drug that acts by preventing the absorption of fat from the intestine.
See also Diethylpropion hydrochloride, Phentermine, Silbutramine.

Orphenadrine

TRADE NAMES:
Norflex.
Norgesic (with paracetamol).

DRUG CLASS:
Antiparkinsonian, muscle relaxant.

USES:
Parkinsonism, severe dizziness, other movement disorders, muscle spasm.

DOSAGE:

One to three tablets, three times a day with food.

FORMS:
Tablets of 100mg (white).

PRECAUTIONS:
Should be used with caution in pregnancy (B2) and breast feeding. Not for use in children.
Use with caution with rapid heart rate and heart disease.
Use short term if possible.

Do not take if:

 suffering from glaucoma, myasthenia gravis, enlarged prostate gland.

SIDE EFFECTS:

Common: Dry mouth, blurred vision, light headedness, rash, drowsiness.
Unusual: Excitation.

INTERACTIONS:

None significant.

PRESCRIPTION:

Yes.

PBS:

No.

PERMITTED IN SPORT:

Yes.

OVERDOSE:

May cause excitement, confusion, convulsions, rapid heart rate, inability to pass urine and coma. Administer activated charcoal or induce vomiting if medication taken recently. Seek medical assistance.

OTHER INFORMATION:

Does not cause addiction or dependence.
See also Baclofen, LEVODOPA COMPOUNDS.

Oseltamivir

TRADE NAME:
Tamiflu.

DRUG CLASS:
Antiviral.

USES:
Treatment of influenza.

DOSAGE:

 One capsule twice a day for five days, starting within 48 hours of onset of symptoms.

FORMS:
Capsules of 75mg (cream/grey).

PRECAUTIONS:
Use with caution in pregnancy (B1) and breast feeding.
Not for use in children under 12 years.
Use with care with significant kidney disease.
Course not to be repeated immediately.

SIDE EFFECTS:
Common: Nausea, vomiting.
Unusual: Sleeplessness, diarrhoea, dizziness.

INTERACTIONS:
None significant.

PRESCRIPTION:
Yes.

PBS:
No.

PERMITTED IN SPORT:
Yes.

OVERDOSE:
Nausea and vomiting only likely effects.

OTHER INFORMATION:
Released in 2001 as a new way of combating influenza, but only if taken as soon as possible after symptoms first appear.
See also Zanamivir.

Oxandrolone

TRADE NAME:
Oxandrin.

DRUG CLASS:
Sex hormone.

USES:
Males: Short stature, small penis, underdeveloped sex organs.
Females: Turner's syndrome, breast cancer.
Both sexes: Aplastic anaemia, osteoporosis, myelosclerosis, some forms of severe kidney disease.

DOSAGE:

One to eight tablets a day in divided doses.

FORMS:
Tablets (white) of 2.5mg.

PRECAUTIONS:
Not to be used in pregnancy (D) or breast feeding. Use with caution in children. Use with caution in kidney and liver disease, heart disease, irregular menstrual periods, diabetes, and enlarged prostate gland.
Regular blood tests to check liver function and cholesterol levels recommended. Should be used short term only if possible.

Do not take if:
 suffering from prostate cancer, male breast cancer, severe kidney disease.

SIDE EFFECTS:
Common: Males – Enlargement of penis, frequent unwanted penis erections, infertility, shrinking of testes, breast enlargement.
Females – Increased body hair, baldness, deepening of voice, enlargement of clitoris.
Both sexes – Fluid retention, rash, nausea, loss of appetite, acne.
Severe but rare (stop medication, consult doctor): Yellow skin (jaundice).

INTERACTIONS:
Other drugs:
- Anticoagulants (eg. warfarin), hypoglycaemics (treat diabetes), anabolic steroids.

PRESCRIPTION:
Yes.

PBS:
No.

PERMITTED IN SPORT:
No.

OVERDOSE:
Vomiting and fluid retention only likely short term effects. Serious effects on sex organs if used long term in high doses.

OTHER INFORMATION:
Does not cause addiction or dependence.

Oxazepam

TRADE NAMES:
Alepam, Murelax, Serepax.

DRUG CLASS:
Benzodiazepine (anxiolytic).

USES:
Short term relief of anxiety.

DOSAGE:
 7.5mg to 60mg, one to four times a day.

FORMS:
Tablets of 15mg and 30mg.

PRECAUTIONS:
Should be used with caution in pregnancy (C), but not at all if delivery of infant imminent as it may decrease desire to breathe in newborn infant. Should be used with caution in breast feeding. Not for use in children.
Lower dose required in elderly.
Should be used intermittently and not constantly as dependency may develop. Use with caution in glaucoma, myasthenia gravis, heart disease, kidney or liver disease, psychiatric conditions, schizophrenia, depression and epilepsy.

Do not take if:
- suffering from severe lung disease, confusion.
- tendency to addiction or dependence.
- operating machinery, driving a vehicle or undertaking tasks that require concentration and alertness.

SIDE EFFECTS:
Common: Reduced alertness, dependence.
Unusual: Incoordination, tremor, confusion, increased risk of falls in elderly, rash, low blood pressure, nausea, muscle weakness.
Severe but rare (stop medication, consult doctor): Jaundice (yellow skin).

INTERACTIONS:
Other drugs:
- Sedatives, other anxiolytics, disulfiram, cimetidine, anticonvulsants (treat epilepsy), anticholinergics.

Herbs:
- Guarana, kava kava, passionflower, St John's wort, valerian.

Other substances:
- Reacts with alcohol to cause sedation and confusion.

PRESCRIPTION:
Yes.

PBS:
Yes.

PERMITTED IN SPORT:
Yes.

OVERDOSE:
Seldom life threatening. May cause drowsiness, confusion and coma. Induce vomiting if tablets taken recently. Seek medical assistance.

OTHER INFORMATION:
Widely used, and very safe if used correctly. Dependency becoming a significant problem, particularly in elderly, due to overuse. First introduced in 1970s.

See also Alprazolam, Bromazepam, Buspirone, Clobazam, Diazepam, Lorazepam.

Oxcarbazepine

TRADE NAME:
Trileptal.

DRUG CLASS:
Anticonvulsant.

USES:
Epileptic seizures.

DOSAGE:

300 to 1200mg twice a day.

FORMS:
Tablets of 300mg (yellow), suspension.
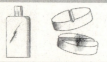

PRECAUTIONS:
Not to be used in pregnancy (D). Use with caution in breast feeding and children under 2 years.
Use with caution in heart failure and liver disease.
Lower dose in elderly.
Do not stop suddenly, but reduce dosage slowly.
Sodium levels in blood must be measured regularly.

SIDE EFFECTS:
Common: Biochemical abnormalities (low blood sodium levels), liver damage, tiredness, dizziness, headache.
Unusual: Acne, alopecia (hair loss), rash, nausea, diarrhoea.
Severe but rare (stop medication, consult doctor): Double vision, liver damage (jaundice).

INTERACTIONS:
Other drugs:
- NSAID (arthritis medication), oral contraceptives, phenobarbitone, phenytoin, citalopram, diazepam, imipramine, omeprazole, propranolol, clomipramine, amitriptyline, pantoprazole, lansoprazole, progesterone, cyclophosphamide.

Other substances:
- Alcohol, borage.

Herbs:
- St John's wort, evening primrose (linoleic acid), Gingko biloba.

PRESCRIPTION:
Yes.

PBS:
Yes (authority required).

PERMITTED IN SPORT:
Yes.

OVERDOSE:
Exacerbation of side effects likely. Seek medical advice.

OTHER INFORMATION:
Introduced in 2001.

See also BARBITURATES, BENZODIAZEPINES, Carbamazepine, Clonazepam, Ethosuximide, Gabapentin, Lamotrigine, Levetiracetam, Phenytoin, Primidone, Sodium valproate, Sulthiame, Tiagabine, Topiramate, Vigabatrin.

Oxethazine
See ANTACIDS.

Oxpentifylline

TRADE NAME:
Trental.

USES:
Poor arterial circulation to legs and arms.

DOSAGE:

One tablet three times a day with meals and liquid.

FORMS:
Tablet of 400mg.

PRECAUTIONS:
Should be used with caution in pregnancy (B1), breast feeding and in children.
Should be used with caution in low blood pressure, irregular heart rhythm, kidney and liver disease.
Lower dose may be required in elderly.

Do not take if:
 suffering from heart attack, peptic ulcer or excessive bleeding.

SIDE EFFECTS:
Common: Nausea, heartburn, burping, dizziness, headache, flushing, palpitations.
Unusual: Vomiting, tremor, shortness of breath, loss of appetite, anxiety, nose bleed, brittle finger nails, blurred vision, bad taste.
Severe but rare (stop medication, consult doctor): Unusual bleeding.

INTERACTIONS:
Other drugs:
- Warfarin, antihypertensives (treat high blood pressure), beta blockers, diuretics (fluid tablets), theophylline, hypoglycaemics (treat diabetes).

PRESCRIPTION:
Yes.

PBS:
No. Expensive.

PERMITTED IN SPORT:
Yes.

OVERDOSE:
Flushing, low blood pressure, convulsions, fever and coma may occur. No deaths reported. Seek medical assistance.

OTHER INFORMATION:
Unique drug that works by making cells slip more easily through the smallest capillaries. Introduced in the 1980s, it has had only limited use because of its cost, despite excellent clinical results.

Oxprenolol

TRADE NAME:
Corbeton.

DRUG CLASS:
Beta blocker.

USES:
High blood pressure, angina, rapid heart rate, irregular heartbeat, paroxysmal atrial tachycardia.

DOSAGE:

20 to 160mg a day in divided doses.

FORMS:
Tablets (white) of 20 and 40mg.

PRECAUTIONS:
Should be used in pregnancy (C) only if medically essential.
Safe to use in breast feeding.
May be used with caution in children.
Use with care if suffering from alcoholism, poor circulation to limbs, angina, over-active thyroid gland (hyperthyroidism), liver or kidney failure or about to have surgery.

Do not stop suddenly, but reduce dose slowly.

Do not take if:

 suffering from diabetes, asthma, or allergic conditions.
- suffering from heart failure, shock, slow heart rate, or enlarged right heart.
- if undertaking prolonged fast.

SIDE EFFECTS:

Common: Low blood pressure, slow heart rate, cold hands and feet, asthma.
Unusual: Loss of appetite, nausea, diarrhoea, impotence, tiredness, sleeplessness, nightmares, rash, loss of libido, hair loss, noises in ears, depression.
Severe but rare (stop medication, consult doctor): Severe asthma.

INTERACTIONS:

Other drugs:
- Calcium channel blockers, disopyramide, clonidine, adrenaline, other medications for irregular heartbeat, lignocaine, ergotamine, indomethacin, chlorpromazine.

PRESCRIPTION:
Yes.

PBS:
Yes.

PERMITTED IN SPORT:
Yes.

OVERDOSE:
Slow heart rate, low blood pressure, asthma and heart failure may result. Administer activated charcoal or induce vomiting if tablets taken recently. Use Salbutamol or other asthma sprays for difficulty in breathing. Seek medical assistance.

See also Atenolol, Carvedilol, Esmolol, Labetalol, Metoprolol, Pindolol, Propranolol, Sotalol.

Oxybuprocaine

See ANAESTHETICS, LOCAL.

Oxybutinin

TRADE NAME:
Ditropan.

DRUG CLASS:
Anticholinergic.

USES:
Relieves some forms of difficulty in passing urine caused by muscle spasm.

DOSAGE:
One tablet two or three times a day.

FORMS:
Tablet (light blue) of 5mg.

PRECAUTIONS:
Use with caution in pregnancy (B1), and children under 5 years. Not to be used in breast feeding, as breast milk production may be reduced.
Use with caution in hot climates.
Avoid vigorous exercise while using oxybutinin.
Use with caution in ulcerative colitis, reflux oesophagitis, over-active thyroid gland, heart disease, high blood pressure, enlarged prostate gland, liver and kidney disease.
Regular consultations with doctor necessary to monitor bladder function.

Do not take if:

 suffering from glaucoma, gut obstruction, megacolon, severe ulcerative colitis, myasthenia gravis, acute bleeding.

Oxycodone

SIDE EFFECTS:
Common: Palpitations, rapid heart rate, decreased sweating, constipation, dry mouth, nausea, dizziness.
Unusual: Impotence, rash, drowsiness, hallucinations, dry eyes.

INTERACTIONS:
Other drugs:
- Sedatives, other anticholinergics.

Other substances:
- Reacts adversely with alcohol.

PRESCRIPTION:
Yes.

PBS:
Yes.

PERMITTED IN SPORT:
Yes.

OVERDOSE:
Serious. Symptoms may include restlessness, irrational behaviour, flushing, low blood pressure, difficulty in breathing, paralysis, coma and death. Administer activated charcoal or induce vomiting if medication taken recently and patient alert. Seek urgent medical assistance.

OTHER INFORMATION:
Does not cause addiction or dependence. Released in Australia in 1994.

TRADE NAMES:
Endone, OxyContin, OxyNorm, Proladone.

DRUG CLASS:
Narcotic, Analgesic.

USES:
Moderate to severe pain.

DOSAGE:

Endone: One tablet every six to eight hours with food.
OxyContin, OxyNorm: One tablet every 12 hours.
Proladone suppository: One every six to eight hours.

FORMS:
Tablets, suppository.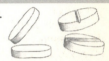

PRECAUTIONS:
Should be used in pregnancy (C) only if medically essential as use of oxycodone immediately before birth may cause difficulty in breathing for the infant. Use with caution in breast feeding. Not for use in children.
Not designed for prolonged use except in patients with terminal disease.
Do not stop suddenly, but reduce dosage slowly.
Use with caution in severe lung disease, myasthenia gravis, under-active thyroid gland, liver and kidney disease, enlarged prostate gland, shock or bowel obstruction.
Lower doses necessary in elderly and debilitated patients.

Do not take if:
suffering from severe asthma, severe lung disease, irregular heartbeat, brain tumour, alcoholism, head injury, convulsions, gut obstruction.
- operating machinery or driving a vehicle.

Medications

SIDE EFFECTS:
Common: Nausea, constipation, drowsiness, confusion.
Unusual: Vomiting, difficulty in passing urine, dry mouth, sweating, flushing, faintness, loss of appetite, dizziness, slow heart rate, mood changes.
Severe but rare (stop medication, consult doctor): Severe headache, convulsions, difficulty in breathing.

INTERACTIONS:
Other drugs:
- MAOI, amphetamines, chlorpromazine, sedatives, antihistamines, beta blockers, anticoagulants (eg. warfarin), anticholinergics, metoclopramide.

Other substances:
- Do not use alcohol with oxycodone.

PRESCRIPTION:
Yes.

PBS:
Yes.

PERMITTED IN SPORT:
No.

OVERDOSE:
Very serious. Symptoms may include drowsiness, difficulty in breathing, muscle weakness, coma, heart failure and death. Administer activated charcoal or induce vomiting if medication taken recently and patient alert. Seek urgent medical attention. Antidote available.

OTHER INFORMATION:
May cause addiction if taken inappropriately for long periods of time.
See also Alfentanil, Buprenorphine, Codeine Phosphate, Dextromoramide, Dextropropoxyphene, Fentanyl, Heroin, Hydromorphone, Methadone, Morphine, Pentazocine, Pethidine.

Oxymetazoline

TRADE NAMES:
Dimetapp 12 Hour Spray, Drixine Nasal, Logicin Rapid Relief Nasal Spray.
Nasex Nasal Decongestant, Vasylox (delisted 2002), **Vicks Sinex** (with menthol).
Locally produced and marketed brands also exist.

DRUG CLASS:
Vasoconstrictor.

USES:
Nose and ear congestion, sinusitis, colds.

DOSAGE:

One to three sprays in each nostril twice a day.

FORMS:
Nasal spray.

PRECAUTIONS:
Safe to use in pregnancy, breast feeding and children over six years.
Not to be used regularly for more than three days.
Use with caution in high blood pressure, heart disease, diabetes, prostate gland enlargement and over-active thyroid gland.
Do not share spray with others.
Do not exceed recommended dose.
Do not take if:
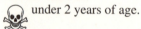 under 2 years of age.
- suffering from glaucoma.

SIDE EFFECTS:
Common: Burning and stinging of nose, sneezing, dry nose.
Unusual: Headache, lightheadedness, sleeplessness, palpitations, worsening congestion if over-used.

INTERACTIONS:
Other drugs:
- MAOI, tricyclic antidepressants, sympathomimetics.

Other substances:
- Reacts adversely with alcohol.

PRESCRIPTION:
No.

PBS:
No.

PERMITTED IN SPORT:
Yes.

OVERDOSE:
If used excessively, nasal congestion will worsen rather than improve.

OTHER INFORMATION:
Very useful and effective, but must not be used for more than three days on a regular basis.

See also Tramazoline, Xylometazoline.

Oxytocin

TRADE NAMES:
Syntocinon.
Syntometrine (with ergometrine).

USES:
Starting labour in pregnancy, stopping abnormal bleeding after delivery.

DOSAGE:
 As determined by doctor.

FORMS:
Injection.

PRECAUTIONS:
Safe to use for induction of labour in pregnancy (A), but should not otherwise be used in pregnancy. Safe for use in breast feeding. Not for use in children. Use with caution in heart disease.

Do not take injection if:
 previous Caesarean section, other obstetric complications.

SIDE EFFECTS:
Common: Rapid heart rate, retention of fluid.
Unusual: Low blood pressure.

PRESCRIPTION:
Yes.

PBS:
No.

PERMITTED IN SPORT:
Yes.

OVERDOSE:
Unlikely to have serious effects.

OTHER INFORMATION:
Injection commonly used to increase intensity of labour, and immediately after delivery to reduce bleeding.

See also Ergometrine.

Paclitaxel

TRADE NAMES:
Anzatax, Taxol.

DRUG CLASS:
Antimetabolite.

USES:
Cancer of the breast and ovaries.

DOSAGE:
 As determined by doctor for each patient.

FORMS:
Injection.

PRECAUTIONS:
Must not be used in pregnancy (D) or children. Use with caution in breast feeding.
Regular blood tests to check function of blood cells essential.
Use with caution in neuropathy (nerve disease).

SIDE EFFECTS:
Common: Flushes, rash, shortness of breath, chest pain, fainting, joint and muscle pain
Unusual: Low blood pressure, slow heart rate, damage to nerves (pins and needles sensation, numbness), damage to liver.
Severe but rare (stop medication, consult doctor): Jaundice (yellow skin).

INTERACTIONS:
Other drugs:
• Sex hormones.

PRESCRIPTION:
Yes.

PBS:
Yes (authority required. Restricted to metastatic cancer untreatable by other medication).

PERMITTED IN SPORT:
Yes.

OVERDOSE:
Serious damage to bone marrow and nerves likely.

Pamidronate

See Disodium pamidronate.

Pancrelipase

TRADE NAMES:
Cotazym-S Forte, Creon, Pancrease.
Panzytrat (with lipase and amylase).

USES:
Deficiency of pancreatic enzymes due to disease (eg. cystic fibrosis, chronic pancreatitis) or surgery.

DOSAGE:
 One or two taken with each meal in sufficient quantity to adequately digest food.
Dosage varies for each person.

FORMS:
Capsules.

PRECAUTIONS:
Use with caution in pregnancy (B3), breast feeding and children.
Do not use excessive dose.
Ensure adequate fluid intake.
Do not chew or crush contents of capsule.

Medications

Do not take if:
 suffering from acute pancreatitis.
- allergic to pork products.

SIDE EFFECTS:
Common: Minimal. Usually dose-related.
Unusual: Nausea, diarrhoea, passing excess wind, mouth soreness.

INTERACTIONS:
Other drugs: Antacids.
Other substances: Alkaline foods.

PRESCRIPTION:
No.

PBS:
Yes.

PERMITTED IN SPORT:
Yes.

OVERDOSE:
Diarrhoea only likely effect.

OTHER INFORMATION:
Totally natural products used to replace a missing digestive enzyme.
See also Tilactase.

Panthenol

TRADE NAMES:
An ingredient in numerous soothing creams.

USES:
Mild burns, nappy rash, sore nipples.

DOSAGE:
Apply several times a day as required.

FORMS:
Cream.

PRECAUTIONS:
Safe to use in pregnancy, breast feeding and children.

SIDE EFFECTS:
Nil.

INTERACTIONS:
None.

PRESCRIPTION:
No.

PBS:
No.

PERMITTED IN SPORT:
Yes.
See also Pantothenic acid.

Pantoprazole
See PROTON PUMP INHIBITORS.

Pantothenic acid
(Vitamin B5)

TRADE NAMES:
A large number of preparations include pantothenic acid (vitamin B5) or its derivative panthenol, alone or in combination with other vitamins and minerals.

DRUG CLASS:
Vitamin.

USES:
Vitamin B deficiency.
Cream used for mild burns, nappy rash and sore nipples.

DOSAGE:
 Recommended daily allowance: 4 to 7mg a day.
Apply creams several times a day as required.

Medications

FORMS:
Tablets, capsules, mixtures, drops, creams.

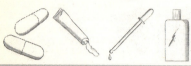

PRECAUTIONS:
Safe in pregnancy, breast feeding and children.
Do not take in high doses or for prolonged periods of time.

SIDE EFFECTS:
Minimal.

INTERACTIONS:
None significant.

PRESCRIPTION:
No.

PBS:
No.

PERMITTED IN SPORT:
Yes.

OVERDOSE:
Unlikely to have serious adverse effects.

OTHER INFORMATION:
Pantothenic acid is a water soluble vitamin. Remember, vitamins are merely chemicals that are essential for the functioning of the body, and if taken to excess, act as a drug.

See also Panthenol.

Papain

TRADE NAME:
Stop Itch. Also found in numerous other locally manufactured soothing creams and digestive aids.

USES:
Cream: Skin stinging and pain caused by rashes, sunburn, insect and jelly fish bites.
Tablets: Indigestion.

DOSAGE:
 Cream: Apply as often as necessary.
Tablets: Take with food.

FORMS:
Cream, tablets.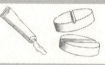

PRECAUTIONS:
Safe in pregnancy, breast feeding and children.
Avoid eye contact.

SIDE EFFECTS:
None significant.

INTERACTIONS:
None significant.

PRESCRIPTION:
No.

PBS:
No.

PERMITTED IN SPORT:
Yes.

Paracetamol
(Actaminophen)

TRADE NAMES:

Chemists' Own Paracetamol, Dymadon, Febridol, GenRx Paracetamol, Herron Paracetamol, Lemsip, Lemsip Headcold, Lemsip Max, Panadol, Panamax, Paracetamol, Parahexal, Paralgin, Setamol, Tylenol. **Biotech Cold & Flu Non-drowsy, Codral Cold and Flu, Codral Daytime, Nyal Plus Cold & Flu** (with pseudoephedrine, codeine).
Biotech Cold & Flu, Codral 4 Flu (with codeine, pseudoephedrine and chlorpheniramine).
Capadex, Digesic, Paradex (with dextropropoxyphene).
Codalgin Plus, Dolased Analgesic Relaxant, Dolased Night Pain Relief, Fiorinal, Mersyndol, Mersyndol Forte, Panadeine Plus, Panalgesic (with codeine and doxylamine).
Codalgin, Codalgin Forte, Codapane, Codral Pain Relief, Dolased Day Pain Relief, Dymadon Co, Dymadon Forte, Liquigesic Co, Mersyndol Day Strength, Panadeine, Panadeine Forte, Panamax Co, Prodeine 15 (with codeine).
Codral Cough Cold and Flu, Dimetapp Cold & Flu Liquid Caps, Logicin Flu, Orthoxicol Cold & Flu, Orthoxicol Day Cold & Flu, Panadol Cold & Flu, Pharma-Col Junior, Tylenol Cold & Flu Non-Drowsy (with pseudoephedrine and dextromethorphan).
Codral Daytime, Lemsip Pharmacy Flu Daytime, Nyal Plus Day Sinus Relief, Panadol Sinus, Sinutab Sinus & Pain, Sudafed Daytime Relief, Sudafed Sinus Pain Relief, Tylenol Sinus (with pseudoephedrine).
Codral Nightime, Sudafed Nightime Relief (with pseudoephedrine, triprolidine).
Demazin Cold & Flu, Logicin Flu Night, Logicin Hay Fever, Nyal Plus Night Cold & Flu, Nyal Plus Night Sinus Relief, Panadol Allergy Sinus, Panadol Sinus Night, Sinutab Sinus Allergy & Pain Relief, Tylenol Allergy Sinus (with chlorpheniramine and pseudoephedrine).
Dimetapp Cold Cough & Flu (with dextromethorphan, pseudoephedrine, guaiphenesin).
Dimetapp Cold Cough & Flu Day & Night Liquid Caps, Dimetapp Night Relief (with pseudoephedrine, dextromethorphan, doxylamine).
Lemsip Pharmacy Flu Nightime, Tylenol Cold & Flu (with chlorpheniramine, pseudoephedrine, dextromethorphan).
Norgesic (with orphenadrine).
Orthoxicol Night Cold & Flu (with chlorpheniramine and dextromethorphan).
Painstop (with codeine and promethazine).
Panadol Night (with diphenhydramine).
Sudafed Sinus Pain and Allergy Relief (with triprolidine and pseudoephedrine).
Also found in numerous other locally produced pain relievers and cold preparations.

DRUG CLASS:

Analgesic.

USES:

Mild to moderate pain relief, fever.

DOSAGE:

 One or two tablets every four to six hours. Maximum eight tablets a day.
Other forms as directed by directions on packaging, doctor or pharmacist.

FORMS:

Tablets, capsules, soluble tablets, chewable tablets, mixture, drops, suppository, powder.

Medications

PRECAUTIONS:
Safe in pregnancy (A), breast feeding, children and infants over one month of age.
Use with caution in severe liver and kidney disease.
Never exceed recommended dose.

SIDE EFFECTS:
Common: Minimal.
Unusual: Nausea, irritability, insomnia, rash, inability to pass urine.

INTERACTIONS:
Other drugs:
- Anticoagulants (eg. warfarin), metoclopramide, propantheline, chloramphenicol, antidepressants, narcotics, anticonvulsants (treat epilepsy).

PRESCRIPTION:
No.
Prescription required in some forms combined with narcotics.

PBS:
Most forms of paracetamol alone: Yes (some brands only).
Panadeine Forte, Panamax Co: Yes.
Most combinations with other medications: No.

PERMITTED IN SPORT:
Yes.

OVERDOSE:
Very serious, particularly in children. Symptoms may include vomiting, belly pain and sweating. Delayed effect can be serious liver damage that may cause liver failure, jaundice and death. Administer activated charcoal or induce vomiting if medication taken recently. Seek urgent medical attention. Effects of overdose can be treated with methionine (see separate entry).

OTHER INFORMATION:
The most widely used painkiller in the world. Very effective, and often underrated in its effectiveness. Extremely safe if taken according to directions. Up to eight tablets a day can be taken for years on end. Found in a wide variety of cold and flu preparations. Paracetamol is given the generic name acetaminophen in the United States.
See also Aspirin, Ibuprofen, NSAIDs.

Paraffin

TRADE NAMES:
Agarol, Cetaphil Moisturising Cream, Dermeze, Duratears, E45 Cream, Hamilton Dry Skin Treatment, Lacri-Lube, Oilatum Cleansing Bar, Oilatum Shower Gel, Parachoc, QV Bath Oil, Unitulle.
Alpha Keri, Poly Visc (with wool fat).
Egozite Baby Cream (with zinc oxide, dimethicone, glycerol).
Granugen (with zinc oxide and other ingredients).
Hamilton Cleansing Lotion (with glycerol, chlorhexidine).
Hamilton Skin Lotion, QV Skin Lotion (with glycerol).
Nutra D Cream (with dimethicone).
Oilatum Plus, QV Flare Up Oil (with triclosan, benzalkonium chloride).
QV Cream (with glycerol, dimethicone and other ingredients).
SOOV Prickly Heat Powder (with salicylic acid, zinc oxide and other ingredients).
Also used as a lubricant in many other skin and eye (see eye lubricants) preparations.

DRUG CLASS:
Laxative, lubricant.

USES:
Constipation, preventing straining at stool, vaginal dryness, skin dryness, eye dryness.

Medications

DOSAGE:

Liquid: 7.5 to 15mLs at bedtime. Always take with adequate liquid.
Creams: Apply three or more times a day.

FORMS:

Suspension, liquid, cream, oil, lotion, tulle (netting).

PRECAUTIONS:

Should be used orally with care in pregnancy (B2).
Should be used orally long term only under medical advice.

Do not take orally if:

 suffering from bowel obstruction.

- suffering from undiagnosed belly pains.

SIDE EFFECTS:

Common: Minimal.
Unusual: Oral preparations – Diarrhoea.
Severe but rare (stop medication, consult doctor): Oral preparations – Severe belly pain.

INTERACTIONS:

None significant.

PRESCRIPTION:

No.

PBS:

No.

PERMITTED IN SPORT:

Yes.

OVERDOSE:

Diarrhoea only effect.

OTHER INFORMATION:

Safe and widely used laxative that has been available for thousands of years. White soft paraffin and liquid paraffin are used in many creams as a vehicle for other medications.

See also EYE LUBRICANTS, LAXATIVES.

Paroxetine

TRADE NAMES:

Aropax, GenRx Paroxetine, Oxetine, Paxtine.

DRUG CLASS:

SSRI antidepressant.

USES:

Treatment and prevention of depression, anxiety, obsessive compulsive disorder, panic attacks, social anxiety disorder, and post-traumatic stress disorder.

DOSAGE:

One to three tablets a day in morning with food.

FORMS:

Tablet of 20mg (white).

PRECAUTIONS:

Should be used in pregnancy (C) and children with considerable caution.
Breast feeding should be ceased if paroxetine prescribed.
Should be used with caution in mania, epilepsy and heart disease.
Should not be stopped suddenly, but dose should be slowly reduced over several days.

Do not take if:

 taking MAOI antidepressants.

SIDE EFFECTS:

Common: Generally minimal and ease with continued use. Nausea, drowsiness, sweating, tremor, tiredness, dry mouth, sleeplessness, impotence.
Unusual: Headache, fever, poor libido, palpitations, sweating, rash, blurred vision, decreased appetite.
Severe but rare (stop medication, consult doctor): Seizures (fits).

Medications

INTERACTIONS:

Other drugs:
- Serious interaction with MAOI.
- Anticoagulants (eg. warfarin), thioridazine, phenytoin, tryptophan.

Herbs:
- St John's wort, ma huang.

Other substances:
- Use of alcohol with paroxetine is not advised.

PRESCRIPTION:
Yes.

PBS:
Yes.

PERMITTED IN SPORT:
Yes.

OVERDOSE:
Symptoms may include nausea, tremor, dilated pupils, dry mouth and irritability. Death or serious effects have not occurred. Seek medical attention.

OTHER INFORMATION:
One of the antidepressants released in Australia in the 1990s that has dramatically improved the treatment of depression because of its safety and lack of side effects. May take up to two weeks for patient to notice any improvement in symptoms.

See also Citalopram, Fluoxetine, Fluvoxamine, Sertraline, Venlafaxine.

Pectin

TRADE NAMES:

Bispectin (with kaolin, codeine, aluminium hydroxide, benzoic acid and other ingredients).
Diareze (Tablets – with aluminium hydrochloride, attapulgite; Suspension – with simethicone, attapulgite).
Donnagel (with kaolin, atropine, hyoscine and other ingredients).
Kaomagma with Pectin (with kaolin, aluminium hydroxide, benzoic acid and other ingredients).
Also found in some locally produced preparations.

DRUG CLASS:
Fibre.

USES:
Mild diarrhoea.

DOSAGE:
 As required to control diarrhoea.

FORMS:
Tablets, suspension.

PRECAUTIONS:
Safe in pregnancy (A), breast feeding and children over 5 years.
Use with caution in reduced intestinal absorption.
Ensure adequate fluid intake.

SIDE EFFECTS:
Minimal.

INTERACTIONS:

Other drugs:
- May affect absorption of some drugs (eg. digoxin).

PRESCRIPTION:
No.

PBS:
No.

PERMITTED IN SPORT:
Yes.

OVERDOSE:
Not likely to be harmful.

OTHER INFORMATION:
Derived from apple fibre.

See also Diphenoxylate hydrochloride, Frangula, Kaolin, Ispaghula, Loperamide, Methylcellulose, Psyllium, Sterculia.

Penicillamine

TRADE NAME:
D-Penamine.

USES:
Severe rheumatoid arthritis, Wilson's disease, cystinuria, heavy metal poisoning (eg. lead).

DOSAGE:
 Rheumatoid disease: One or two tablets, one to three times a day. Other conditions: Up to 2000mg a day depending upon severity and response.

FORMS:
Tablets (white) of 125mg and 250mg.

PRECAUTIONS:
Must not be used in pregnancy (D) unless essential for the life of the mother. Breast feeding should be ceased before use. May be used in children when medically indicated.
Use with caution in liver and kidney disease, brain disorders or feverish.
Avoid surgery if possible.
Regular blood tests essential.
Regular checks of skin, eyes and temperature necessary.

Ensure adequate vitamin B intake.
Patient must be made aware of the adverse effects of this medication before use.

Do not take if:
 using gold or chloroquine.

SIDE EFFECTS:
Common: Rash, fever, joint pains, enlarged glands, itch.
Unusual: Hair loss, ringing noise in ears, abnormal blood tests, nausea, loss of appetite, vomiting, diarrhoea, blood clots, taste changes.
Severe but rare (stop medication, consult doctor): Significant rash, severe belly pain, yellow skin (jaundice from liver damage), vision disturbances, unusual bleeding or bruising.

INTERACTIONS:
Other drugs:
- Gold, antimalarial drugs (eg. chloroquine), isoniazid.

PRESCRIPTION:
Yes.

PBS:
Yes.

PERMITTED IN SPORT:
Yes.

OVERDOSE:
May cause permanent organ damage. Administer activated charcoal or induce vomiting if medication taken recently. Seek medical attention.

OTHER INFORMATION:
Although it has serious side effects, Penicillamine may give great relief to sufferers of severe rheumatoid arthritis, and may be life saving in heavy metal poisoning. Risks minimal if taken under close supervision of a competent physician.

See also GOLD.

PENICILLINS

DISCUSSION:
Penicillins are the most widely used antibiotics in the world. There are many different types of penicillin now available. They are broad-spectrum antibiotics that kill a wide range of bacteria, and have been used for almost every conceivable type of infection at some time. Unfortunately, many bacteria are now becoming resistant to penicillins.

Allergies to penicillin are not more common than to other drugs, but appear to be so because it is so widely used. Patients who know they have a penicillin allergy should tell their doctors and wear a warning pendant or bracelet. Penicillins may cause a skin rash if given to a patient with glandular fever, and may start a vaginal thrush infection in some women.

See Amoxycillin, Ampicillin, Benzathine penicillin, Benzylpenicillin, Dicloxacillin, Flucloxacillin, Phenoxymethyl penicillin, Piperacillin, Procaine penicillin, Ticarcillin sodium.

Pentazocine
(Pentazocine hydrochloride and Pentazocine lactate)

TRADE NAME:
Fortral.

DRUG CLASS:
Narcotic, analgesic.

USES:
Moderate to severe pain.

DOSAGE:

One or two tablets every three or four hours after food.

FORMS:
Tablets (white) of 25 and 50mg, injection.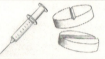

PRECAUTIONS:
Not for use in pregnancy (C) unless medically necessary. May cause difficulty in breathing for the newborn if given in the few hours before birth. Use with caution in breast feeding. May be used in children over one year.

Use with caution in severe kidney disease, severe lung disease, severe liver disease, asthma, thyroid disease, pituitary disease, epilepsy, heart attack or head injury.

Do not take if:
 Using machinery or driving a vehicle.

SIDE EFFECTS:
Common: Nausea, dizziness, sedation, mood changes, headache, sweating.
Unusual: Vomiting, contracted pupils, hallucinations, rapid heart rate.
Severe but rare (stop medication, consult doctor): Difficulty in breathing.

INTERACTIONS:
Other drugs:
- MAOI, sedatives, tetracycline, phenytoin.

Other substances:
- Do not use alcohol while taking pentazocine.

PRESCRIPTION:
Yes.

PBS:
No.

PERMITTED IN SPORT:
No.

OVERDOSE:
Serious. May cause convulsions, sedation, coma, difficulty in breathing and rarely death. Administer activated charcoal or induce vomiting if medication taken recently and patient alert. Seek urgent medical attention. Antidote available.

OTHER INFORMATION:
May cause dependence or addiction if used inappropriately. Available since the late 1960s.

See also Alfentanil, Buprenorphine, Codeine Phosphate, Dextromoramide, Dextropropoxyphene, Fentanyl, Heroin, Hydromorphone, Methadone, Morphine, Oxycodone, Pethidine.

Pentosan polysulfate

TRADE NAME:
Elmiron.

USES:
Bladder inflammation.

DOSAGE:

One capsule three times a day with water, but away from food intake.

FORMS:
Capsules of 100mg (white).

PRECAUTIONS:
May be used in pregnancy (B1) and breast feeding. Use with caution in children. Should be used with caution until diagnosis confirmed by cystoscopy. Regular blood tests to check bleeding tendency and liver function necessary.

Do not take if:
 suffering from haemophilia, recent or current bleeding.

SIDE EFFECTS:
Common: Swelling of hands and feet, headache, dizziness, diarrhoea, nausea.
Unusual: Vomiting, liver damage.
Severe but rare (stop medication, consult doctor): Jaundice (yellow skin).

INTERACTIONS:
Other drugs:
- Anticoagulants (heparin, warfarin).

PRESCRIPTION:
Yes.

PBS:
No (expensive).

PERMITTED IN SPORT:
Yes.

OVERDOSE:
Not likely to be serious. Induce vomiting or give activated charcoal if taken recently.

Medications

Pentoxyverine citrate

TRADE NAME:
Nyal Dry Cough.

DRUG CLASS:
Cough suppressant.

USES:
Cough.

DOSAGE:

10mLs every three to four hours as needed.

FORMS:
Syrup

PRECAUTIONS:
Use with caution in pregnancy and children.
Not to be used in breast feeding or under four years.
Use with caution with a fever and if symptoms persist.
Seek medical advice if cough persists.

Do not take if:
 suffering from glaucoma.

SIDE EFFECTS:
None significant.

INTERACTIONS:
Other drugs:
- MAOI.

Other substances:
- Alcohol.

PRESCRIPTION:
No.

PBS:
No.

PERMITTED IN SPORT:
Yes.

OVERDOSE:
Unlikely to have any serious adverse effects.

See also Ammonium chloride, Codeine Phosphate, Dextromethorphan, Dihydrocodeine, EXPECTORANTS, Pholcodine.

Peppermint oil

TRADE NAME:
Mintec.
Also found in numerous liniments, soothing creams and other medications for indigestion.

DRUG CLASS:
Antispasmodic.

USES:
Irritable bowel, excess bowel gas, passing excess wind.

DOSAGE:

Take three or four times a day 30 minutes before food as needed.

FORMS:
Capsules, creams, powders, salves, lotions.
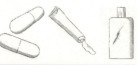

PRECAUTIONS:
Safe to use in pregnancy, breast feeding and children over six years.
Use with caution in heartburn.

SIDE EFFECTS:
Common: Minimal.
Unusual: Heartburn, anal irritation, rash.

INTERACTIONS:
None significant.

PRESCRIPTION:
No.

PBS:
No.

PERMITTED IN SPORT:
Yes.

OVERDOSE:
Exacerbation of side effects likely.

OTHER INFORMATION:
Very safe and effective ancient remedy.

Pergolide

TRADE NAME:
Permax.

DRUG CLASS:
Antiparkinsonian.

USES:
Parkinson's disease.

DOSAGE:

Gradually increasing dose taken three times a day until dose adequate to control condition.

FORMS:
Tablets of 0.05mg (white), 0.25mg (green) and 1mg (pink).

PRECAUTIONS:
Not to be used in pregnancy (C), breast feeding or children.
Use with care in irregular heartbeat, liver and kidney disease.
Should not be stopped suddenly, but dosage should be reduced slowly over some weeks.
Designed to be used only in combination with levodopa.

Do not take if:
 sensitive to ergot.

SIDE EFFECTS:
Common: Generalised pain, nausea, incoordination, runny nose, double vision, fainting.
Unusual: Belly pain, hallucinations, tiredness, sleeplessness, shortness of breath.
Severe but rare (stop medication, consult doctor): irregular heart rhythm.

INTERACTIONS:
Other drugs:
- Phenothiazines, metoclopramide, medications to lower blood pressure.

PRESCRIPTION:
Yes.

PBS:
Yes (restricted to use in combination with levodopa).

PERMITTED IN SPORT:
Yes.

OVERDOSE:
May cause vomiting, convulsions, fainting, agitation, hallucinations and twitching. Induce vomiting if medication taken recently. Seek medical assistance.

OTHER INFORMATION:
Not addictive. Released in Australia in 1993.

See also LEVODOPA COMPOUNDS.

Perhexiline

TRADE NAME:
Pexsig.

DRUG CLASS:
Antianginal.

USES:
Moderate to severe heart angina.

DOSAGE:
 100mg to 400mg a day

FORMS:
Tablets of 100mg (white).

PRECAUTIONS:
Use with caution in pregnancy (B2), breast feeding and children.
Regular blood tests to check liver function and drug levels essential.
Use with caution after recent heart attack.
Use with caution in diabetes and irregular heartbeat.

Do not take if:
 suffering from liver or kidney disease.

SIDE EFFECTS:
Common: Most patients suffer some side effects initially, but these may disappear. They may include dizziness, disturbed walking, unsteadiness, nausea, vomiting, headache, loss of appetite, weight loss.
Unusual: Weakness, nervousness, tiredness, sleeplessness, tremors, pins and needles sensation, fainting, poor libido, flushes, sweating, rash.
Severe but rare (stop medication, consult doctor): Pain in limbs, weakness in limbs.

INTERACTIONS:
Other drugs:
- Beta blockers, hypoglycaemics (lower blood sugar), doxorubicin, fluoxetine, quinidine, haloperidol.

Other substances:
- Alcohol.

PRESCRIPTION:
Yes.

PBS:
Yes (authority required. Restricted to angina untreatable by other medication).

PERMITTED IN SPORT:
Yes.

OVERDOSE:
Vomiting, headache, incoordination and liver damage possible. Induce vomiting or give activated charcoal if taken recently. Seek urgent medical attention.

OTHER INFORMATION:
Introduced in 1996 to control more resistant forms of angina.
See also Glyceryl trinitrate, Isosorbide nitrate, Nicorandil.

Pericyazine
See PHENOTHIAZINES.

Perindopril
See ACE INHIBITORS.

Permethrin

TRADE NAMES:
Lyclear, Pyrifoam, Quellada.

DRUG CLASS:
Antiparasitic.

USES:
Head lice, scabies.

DOSAGE:
 Varies depending on use and form. Follow directions on packaging.

FORMS:
Cream, liquid, foam.

PRECAUTIONS:
Use with caution in pregnancy (B2), breast feeding and children. Not for use under six months of age.
Avoid contact with vagina, anus, penis head, eyes, nostrils and mouth.
Use with caution in elderly.

SIDE EFFECTS:
Common: Skin stinging and burning, itch.

INTERACTIONS:
None significant.

PRESCRIPTION:
No.

PBS:
Lyclear: Yes.
Other forms: No.

PERMITTED IN SPORT:
Yes.

OVERDOSE:
If swallowed may cause alcohol intoxication, belly pain, nausea and vomiting. Seek medical attention.

OTHER INFORMATION:
Treat all members of family and other close contacts at same time. Use fine comb repeatedly on hair to remove egg cases. repeat treatment in one week if necessary.
See also Maldison, Piperonyl butoxide.

Pertussis Vaccine
See Whooping Cough Vaccine.

Pethidine

TRADE NAME:
Pethidine.

DRUG CLASS:
Narcotic, Analgesic.

USES:
Severe pain.

DOSAGE:
 As directed by doctor. One or two tablets every three to four hours.

FORMS:
Tablets of 50mg (white), injection.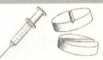

PRECAUTIONS:
Should only be used during the later stages of pregnancy (C) if medically essential as it may reduce the desire to breathe in newborn infants. Use with caution in breast feeding. May be used in children.
Use with caution in colic caused by gall stones, glaucoma, diabetes, pancreatitis, kidney and liver disease, heart disease, ulcerative colitis, underactive thyroid gland, enlarged prostate gland, head injury and shock.
Not designed for long term use. Use lowest dose possible for the shortest time possible.
Do not stop medication suddenly, but reduce dosage slowly.
Lower doses necessary in elderly.

Do not take if:
- suffering from heart failure, irregular heart rhythm, severe head injury, brain tumour, acute diabetes, severe liver disease, severe alcoholism, eclampsia of pregnancy, poor lung function or convulsions.
- operating machinery, driving a vehicle or undertaking tasks requiring concentration.

SIDE EFFECTS:
Common: Sedation, constipation, confusion, sweating, nausea, vomiting, loss of appetite, tolerance to effects if overused.
Unusual: Difficulty passing urine, flushing, dizziness, slow heart rate, irregular heart rate, fainting, mood changes.
Severe but rare (stop medication, consult doctor): Difficulty in breathing, convulsions.

INTERACTIONS:
Other drugs:
- Severe interaction with MAOI.
- Sedatives, pentazocine, phenytoin, paracetamol, barbiturates, phenothiazines, amphetamines, other narcotics.

Other substances:
- Should not be used with alcohol.

PRESCRIPTION:
Yes (tightly restricted).

PBS:
Injection: Yes.
Tablets: No.

PERMITTED IN SPORT:
No.

OVERDOSE:
Serious. Sedation, convulsions, coma and death may occur. Administer activated charcoal or induce vomiting if medication taken recently and patient alert. Seek emergency medical assistance. Antidote available.

OTHER INFORMATION:
Highly addictive if used inappropriately. Very effective and unlikely to cause addiction if used appropriately for severe pain. Derived from opium poppy and closely related to morphine and heroin, but not as addictive.

See also Alfentanil, Buprenorphine, Codeine Phosphates, Dextromoramide, Dextropropoxyphene, Fentanyl, Heroin, Hydromorphone, Methadone, Morphine, Oxycodone, Pentazocine.

Phenelzine
See MAOI.

Phenindione

TRADE NAME:
Dindevan.

DRUG CLASS:
Anticoagulant.

USES:
Prevention and treatment of blood clots (thromboses).

DOSAGE:

Very strictly as directed by doctor. Usually high dose on starting, then dose varies depending on results of regular blood tests.

FORMS:
Tablets of 10mg (white).

PRECAUTIONS:
Not to be used if pregnant (D) or breast feeding.
Care required in patients with high blood pressure, liver disease, kidney disease, peptic ulcer or bowel bleeding.
It is essential that all doctors in contact with the patient know that the patient is on phenindione.
No surgery can be performed unless phenindione has been ceased for some days.
Do not undertake any activity that may result in falls, bruising or extreme exertion.

Do not take:
Unless carefully monitored by a doctor.
- With recent eye, brain, spinal cord surgery or injury.
- With recent kidney or liver biopsy, or spinal anaesthetic.

SIDE EFFECTS:

Common: Bloating, passing wind.
Severe (consult doctor immediately): Blood in urine, blood in faeces, black sticky faeces, skin rash, diarrhoea, vomiting, fever, sore throat, mouth ulcers, bruising.

INTERACTIONS:

Other drugs:
- Interacts adversely with a wide range of medication. Do not take any other medication (including aspirin or cold mixtures) without medical permission.

Other substances:
- Alcohol may increase effect of medication.
- Avoid foods rich in vitamin K (eg. leafy greens, fish).

PRESCRIPTION:
Yes.

PBS:
No.

PERMITTED IN SPORT:
Yes, but not advised in vigorous sport.

OVERDOSE:
Life threatening! Will cause severe bleeding internally, bleeding gums, blood in urine and faeces. Urgent transport to hospital required. Antidote available.

OTHER INFORMATION:
Patients should read additional information provided by their doctor carefully. Wearing a bracelet or necklet with information about the medication is advised for anyone using phenindione long term. Very effective medication, but must be used with great care.

See also Warfarin.

Pheniramine
See ANTIHISTAMINES, SEDATING.

Phenobarbitone
See BARBITURATES.

PHENOTHIAZINES

TRADE and GENERIC NAMES:

Aldazine, Melleril (Thioridazine).
Anatensol, Fluphenazine, Modecate (Fluphenazine).
Largactil (Chlorpromazine).
Clopine, Clozaril (Clozapine).
Neulactil (Pericyazine).
Stelazine (Trifluoperazine).

DRUG CLASS:
Antipsychotics, Antiemetics (chlorpromazine).

USES:
Schizophrenia, mania, psychoses, senile agitation, severe agitation in children, intractable vomiting, intractable hiccups, severe anxiety, other psychiatric conditions, increasing the effect of painkillers.

DOSAGE:
One to three tablets or capsules, two or three times a day. Dosage varies widely from one form to another depending on length of action and potency. Follow doctor's instructions carefully.

FORMS:
Tablets, capsules, mixture, suppository, injection.

PRECAUTIONS:

Should only be used in pregnancy (C) if medically necessary. High doses should be avoided late in pregnancy. Should be used with caution in breast feeding. Most forms may be used in children.

Should be used with caution in epilepsy, under-active thyroid gland (hypothyroidism), enlarged prostate gland, glaucoma, Parkinsonism, hypoparathyroidism, myasthenia gravis, low blood pressure, liver and kidney diseases.

Use with caution if operating machinery or driving a vehicle.

Do not take if:

☠ suffering from depression, very poor circulation, uncontrolled epilepsy, phaeochromocytoma, liver disease or bone marrow disease.
- having a spinal anaesthetic.
- intoxicated with alcohol or marijuana.

SIDE EFFECTS:

Common: Drowsiness, reduced alertness, abnormal body temperature, low blood pressure, dermatitis, dry mouth, constipation, weight gain, blurred vision, stuffy nose.

Unusual: Itch, difficulty passing urine, confusion, dizziness, incoordination, tremor, slow breathing, irregular heartbeat, skin pigmentation.

Severe but rare (stop medication, consult doctor): Yellow skin (jaundice), convulsions, repetitive unwanted movements, muscle rigidity, fever, coma.

INTERACTIONS:

Other drugs:
- Adrenaline, tricyclic antidepressants, guanethidine, antacids, sedatives, barbiturates, phenytoin, lithium, levodopa, sedatives, amphetamines, beta blockers, hypoglycaemics (treat diabetes), MAOI, quinidine, suxamethonium.

Herbs:
- Evening primrose (linoleic acid), ginseng.

Other substances:
- Reacts adversely with alcohol and some foods.
- Marijuana.

PRESCRIPTION:
Yes.

PBS:
Yes (some forms very restricted).

PERMITTED IN SPORT:
Yes.

OVERDOSE:

Very serious. Symptoms include drowsiness, confusion, restlessness, rapid heart rate, tremor, convulsions, difficulty in breathing and swallowing, coma and death. Administer activated charcoal or induce vomiting if taken recently and patient alert. Seek urgent medical attention.

OTHER INFORMATION:

These drugs have revolutionised the lives of many psychiatric patients to the point where they can lead completely normal lives. First introduced in 1960s. Do not cause addiction or dependence.

See also Amisulpride, Droperidol, Flupenthixol, Haloperidol, Lithium Carbonate, Olanzapine, Pimozide, Prochlorperazine, Quetiapine, Risperidone, Thiothixene, Zuclopenthixol.

Phenoxybenzamine

TRADE NAME:
Dibenyline.

DRUG CLASS:
Vasodilator.

USES:
Severe high blood pressure, phaeochromocytoma, urinary retention.

DOSAGE:

One to three capsules twice a day.

FORMS:
Capsule of 10mg (red/white).

PRECAUTIONS:
Use in pregnancy only if medically essential. Not for use in breast feeding or children.
Use with caution in poor brain blood supply, poor heart blood supply, kidney disease, rapid heart rate, low blood pressure and chest infections.

Do not take if:
 suffering from recent heart attack or stroke.

SIDE EFFECTS:
Common: Nasal congestion, contracted eye pupil, low blood pressure, inhibited ejaculation, drowsiness, gut irritation.
Unusual: Dizziness, rapid heart rate, fatigue.

INTERACTIONS:
Other drugs:
• Adrenaline, stimulants.
Other substances:
• Reacts with alcohol.

PRESCRIPTION:
Yes.

PBS:
Yes.

PERMITTED IN SPORT:
Yes.

OVERDOSE:
Causes low blood pressure, dizziness, vomiting, rapid pulse and collapse. Administer activated charcoal or induce vomiting if tablets taken recently. Seek urgent medical assistance.

See also Betahistine, Diazoxide, Guanethidine, Nicotinic Acid.

Phenoxyisopropanol

TRADE NAMES:
Clearasil Medicated Face Wash.
SOOV Bite (with lignocaine and cetrimide).
SOOV Cream (with lignocaine, chlorhexidine and cetrimide).

DRUG CLASS:
Skin cleanser.

USES:
Prevents acne.
With other ingredients acts to ease skin irritations, insect bites, burns and grazes.

DOSAGE:

Liquid: Lather face once a day.
Cream, gel: Apply up to four times a day.

FORMS:
Liquid, cream, gel.

PRECAUTIONS:
Safe in pregnancy and breast feeding and children. Not for use on infants under 1 year.
Avoid eye contact.
Do not swallow.

SIDE EFFECTS:
Minimal.

INTERACTIONS:
None significant.

PRESCRIPTION:
No.

PBS:
No.

PERMITTED IN SPORT:
Yes.

OVERDOSE:
Diarrhoea and gut cramps likely if swallowed.

See also Adapalene, KERATOLYTICS.

Phenoxymethyl penicillin

TRADE NAMES:
Abbocillin V, Cilicaine V (phenoxymethyl penicillin benzathine).
Abbocillin VK, Cilicaine VK, Cilopen VK, Penhexal VK (phenoxymethyl penicillin potassium).
LPV (phenoxymethyl penicillin potassium and benzathine).

DRUG CLASS:
Penicillin antibiotic.

USES:
Treatment of infections caused by susceptible bacteria.

DOSAGE:

One or two capsules every four to six hours before food. Course (usually seven days) should be completed.

FORMS:
Tablets, capsules, mixture (store in door of refrigerator).

PRECAUTIONS:
Safe in pregnancy (A), children and breast feeding.
Use with caution in kidney failure and leukaemia.
Do not take if:
 allergic to penicillin.

- suffering from glandular fever.

SIDE EFFECTS:
Common: Mild diarrhoea, nausea, vomiting.
Unusual: Fever, headache, dizziness, hot flushes, tiredness, black tongue.
Severe but rare (stop medication, consult doctor): Itchy rash, hives, severe diarrhoea, yellow skin (jaundice), muscle pains, throat tightness.

INTERACTIONS:
Other drugs:
- Oral contraceptives, antacids.
Herbs:
- Guar gum.

PRESCRIPTION:
Yes.

PBS:
Yes.

PERMITTED IN SPORT:
Yes.

OVERDOSE:
Not life threatening unless allergic to penicillin. Vomiting and diarrhoea only likely effects.

OTHER INFORMATION:
One of the older types of penicillin. Does not cause dependence or addiction.

See also Amoxycillin, Ampicillin, Benzathine penicillin, Benzylpenicillin, Cloxacillin, Dicloxacillin, Flucloxacillin, Piperacillin, Procaine penicillin.

Phentermine

TRADE NAME:
Duromine.

DRUG CLASS:
Anorectic.

USES:
Reduction of appetite in obesity.

DOSAGE:

One capsule at breakfast time.

FORMS:
Capsules of
15mg (grey/green),
30mg (grey/maroon) and
40mg (grey/orange).

PRECAUTIONS:
Not for use in pregnancy (B3), breast feeding or children under 12 years.
Use with caution in high blood pressure, angina, diabetes and epilepsy.
Do not exceed recommended dosage.
Not for long term use.
Blood pressure should be checked regularly.
Always use in conjunction with appropriate diet and exercise program.

Do not take if:
suffering from uncontrolled high blood pressure, heart disease, over-active thyroid gland, recent stroke, glaucoma, hyperactive state, mania, schizophrenia, depression, anorexia nervosa, history of drug abuse.

SIDE EFFECTS:
Common: Palpitations, rapid heart rate, over stimulation, restlessness, sleeplessness, tremor, headache, dry mouth, bad taste, diarrhoea.
Unusual: High blood pressure, psychiatric disturbances, rash.

INTERACTIONS:
Other drugs:
- MAOI, sympathomimetics, sedatives, insulin, hypoglycaemics (treat diabetes), clomipramine, thyroxine, SSRI (treat depression).

Other substances:
- Reacts with caffeine and alcohol.

PRESCRIPTION:
Yes.

PBS:
No.

PERMITTED IN SPORT:
No.

OVERDOSE:
Serious. May cause restlessness, tremor, confusion, hallucinations, panic state, fatigue, irregular heartbeat, high blood pressure, vomiting, diarrhoea, heart attack, convulsions, coma and death. Administer activated charcoal or induce vomiting if medication taken recently. Seek urgent medical assistance.

OTHER INFORMATION:
Seldom used these days due to significant risk of dependence and addiction.

See also Diethylpropion hydrochloride, Orlistat, Silbutramine.

Phenylephrine

TRADE NAMES:
MIXTURES
Nyal Decongestant, Nyal Sinus Relief. Demazin Syrup, Duro-Tuss Cold and Allergy, Nyal Plus Decongestant (with chlorpheniramine).
Dimetapp (with brompheniramine).
Dimetapp DM (with brompheniramine, dextromethorphan and other ingredients).
Paedamin (with diphenhydramine).
TABLETS AND CAPSULES
Action (with chlorpheniramine and aspirin).
Dimetapp (with brompheniramine).
NOSE PREPARATIONS
Cophenylcaine Forte (with lignocaine).
Nasalate Cream (with chlorhexidine).
INJECTION
Neo-Synephrine.
EYE DROPS
Albalon Relief, Isopto Frin, Neo-Synephrine Ophthalmic, Prefrin, Visopt.
Minims Mydriatics (with atropine, cyclopentolate, homatropine, tropicamide).
Prednefrin Forte (with prednisolone).
Zincfrin (with zinc sulfate).
Also available in numerous other locally produced and marketed preparations.

DRUG CLASS:
Sympathomimetic, Decongestant.

USES:
Mixture, syrup, tablets and capsules: Nasal congestion.
Eye drops: Minor eye irritations.
Nose preparations: Nasal congestion.

DOSAGE:
 Mixture, syrup, tablets and capsules: Take recommended dose every four to six hours.
Eye drops: One or two drops every three or four hours.
Nose sprays: One or two sprays into each nostril two or three times a day.

FORMS:
Mixture, syrup, capsules, tablets, nasal spray, nose cream, nose drops, eye drops, injection.

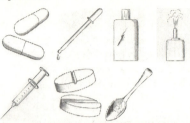

PRECAUTIONS:
Safe to use in pregnancy (B2 – preparations taken by mouth), breast feeding and children.
Use with caution in high blood pressure.
Do not use nasal sprays long term.
Do not use eye drops if:
 suffering from glaucoma.

SIDE EFFECTS:
Minimal.

INTERACTIONS:
Other drugs: Antidepressants, sedatives.
Other substances: Reacts with alcohol if taken by mouth.

PRESCRIPTION:
No.

PBS:
No.

PERMITTED IN SPORT:
If taken by mouth: No.
Eye and nose preparations: Yes.

OVERDOSE:
If taken by mouth may cause irritability, convulsions, palpitations, high blood pressure, angina and difficulty in passing urine. Administer activated charcoal or induce vomiting if medication taken recently. Seek urgent medical assistance. Nasal preparations if used excessively may cause rebound nasal stuffiness and congestion.

Medications

OTHER INFORMATION:

Used widely in cold mixtures, eye drops and nasal sprays to ease irritation and congestion. Safe and effective if taken as directed, but do not take more than recommended dose or over-use nose drops and sprays.

See also GLAUCOMA MEDICATIONS, MYDRIATICS, Oxymetazoline, Pseudoephedrine, Tramazoline.

Phenytoin

TRADE NAME:

Dilantin.

DRUG CLASS:

Anticonvulsant.

USES:

Epilepsy, some forms of irregular heartbeat.

DOSAGE:

One or two tablets, two or three times a day with water and food.

FORMS:

Capsules of 30mg (white) and 100mg (white/orange),
tablets of 50mg (yellow), mixture.

PRECAUTIONS:

Not for use in pregnancy (D) unless absolutely essential, as the risk of foetal deformity is increased.
Use with caution in breast feeding. May be used in children.
Lower doses required in elderly.
Use with caution in liver disease, heart disease, low blood pressure, porphyria. Do not stop suddenly, but reduce dosage slowly over several weeks.

Do not take if:

 suffering from some forms of heart disease.

SIDE EFFECTS:

Common: Most side effects eased by slight reduction in dose. Slurred speech, incoordination, jerky eye movements, confusion.
Unusual: Dizziness, sleeplessness, nervous twitching, headache.
Severe but rare (stop medication, consult doctor): Enlarged glands in neck, groin or armpits.

INTERACTIONS:

Other drugs:
- Wide range of medications can affect the blood levels of phenytoin. Do not take any prescription medication without checking possible interactions with a doctor or pharmacist.
- Non-prescription medications that interact with phenytoin include aspirin, antacids, calcium, vitamin D and folic acid.
- Oral contraceptive pill.

Herbs:
- St John's wort, evening primrose (linoleic acid), Gingko biloba, piperine (Ayurvedic Piper nigrum), shankhapushpl.

Other substances:
- Reacts adversely with alcohol.
- Borage.

PRESCRIPTION:

Yes.

PBS:

Yes.

PERMITTED IN SPORT:

Yes.

OVERDOSE:

Doses of over 2000mg to 5000mg (depending on size, sex etc.) may be fatal. Symptoms include incoordination, incoherent speech, tremor, tiredness, vomiting, slow heart rate, coma, dilated pupils and death. Administer activated charcoal or induce vomiting if tablets taken recently and patient alert. Seek urgent medical assistance.

OTHER INFORMATION:

For decades, Phenytoin has been the mainstay of epilepsy treatment worldwide. Does not cause addiction or dependence.

See also BARBITURATES, BENZODIAZEPINES, Carbamazepine, Clonazepam, Ethosuximide, Gabapentin, Lamotrigine, Levetiracetam, Oxcarbazepine, Primidone, Sodium valproate, Sulthiame, Tiagabine, Topiramate, Vigabatrin.

Pholcodine

TRADE NAMES:

**Actifed CC Dry Cough, Actuss, Duro-Tuss, Linctus Tussinol, Logicin Cough Suppressant, Nyal Plus Dry Cough.
Difflam Anti-inflammatory Cough Lozenges** (with benzydamine and cetylpyridinium).
Duro-Tuss Lozenges (with cetylpyridinium chloride).
Duro-Tuss Decongestant (with pseudoephedrine).
Duro-Tuss Expectorant (with bromhexine hydrochloride).
Phensedyl (with promethazine and pseudoephedrine).
Tixylix Nightime Linctus (with promethazine).
Numerous other locally produced brands also exist.

DRUG CLASS:
Cough suppressant.

USES:
Control of dry cough.

DOSAGE:
 Take every four to six hours.

FORMS:
Mixture, lozenges.

PRECAUTIONS:
Safe to use in pregnancy (A), breast feeding and children.
Not for long term use.

SIDE EFFECTS:
Common: Minimal.
Unusual: Nausea, drowsiness.

INTERACTIONS:
Other substances:
• Alcohol.

PRESCRIPTION:
No.

PBS:
No. Some forms available to Veteran Affairs pensioners.

PERMITTED IN SPORT:
Yes, unless combined with pseudoephedrine.

OVERDOSE:
Serious adverse effects unlikely.

OTHER INFORMATION:
Very old medication. Widely used and very safe.

See also Ammonium chloride, Codeine phosphate, Dextromethorphan, Dihydrocodeine, EXPECTORANTS, Pentoxyverine citrate.

Phosphorus

TRADE NAMES:
Phosphorus is added to numerous non-prescription vitamin and mineral supplements.

DRUG CLASS:
Mineral.

USES:
Nutritional deficiency, hyperparathyroidism, multiple myeloma, some form of rickets, bone cancer.

DOSAGE:
 Recommended daily dose 1000mg Higher doses used in treating diseases listed above.

FORMS:
Tablets, mixtures.

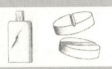

PRECAUTIONS:
Safe to use in pregnancy, breast feeding and children.
Use with caution in kidney disease.
If high doses used, regular blood tests to check balance of all minerals in blood necessary.

SIDE EFFECTS:
Common: Diarrhoea.
Unusual: Tissue calcium deposits, kidney stones.

INTERACTIONS:
None significant.

PRESCRIPTION:
No.

PBS:
No.

PERMITTED IN SPORT:
Yes.

OVERDOSE:
Unlikely to be serious.

OTHER INFORMATION:
Phosphorus is a mineral found naturally in many foods including dairy foods, meat, fish, nuts, eggs and cereals. A natural deficiency is very unusual.
See also **MINERALS**.

Phytomenadione

See **HAEMOSTATIC AGENTS**.

PILL, CONTRACEPTIVE

See **ORAL CONTRACEPTIVES**.

Pilocarpine

TRADE NAMES:
Isopto Carpine, Minims Pilocarpine, Pilocarpine, Pilopt, PV Carpine. Timpilo (with timolol).

USES:
Glaucoma.

DOSAGE:
 Two drops three or four times a day.

FORMS:
Eye drops.

PRECAUTIONS:
Safe to use in pregnancy, breast feeding and children.
Do not exceed prescribed dose.
Do not take if:
 suffering from acute iritis or retinal tear.

SIDE EFFECTS:
Common: Blurred vision.
Unusual: Red eye.

INTERACTIONS:
None significant.

PRESCRIPTION:
Yes.

PBS:
Most forms: Yes.
Minims Pilocarpine (individually packaged single doses): No.

PERMITTED IN SPORT:
Yes.

OVERDOSE:
Seek medical advice. Unlikely to be serious.

OTHER INFORMATION:
Commonly used medication for the treatment of glaucoma.
See also Betaxolol, Bimatroprost, Brimonidine, Brinzolamide, Timolol.

Pimozide

TRADE NAME:
Orap.

DRUG CLASS:
Antipsychotic.

USES:
Chronic psychotic disorders (eg. schizophrenia).

DOSAGE:

One or more tablets once a day to a maximum of 20mg a day.

FORMS:
Tablet of 2mg (white).

PRECAUTIONS:
Use with caution in pregnancy (B1), breast feeding and children.
Use with caution in heart disease, severe anxiety, epilepsy, aggressive behaviour, blood cell disorders, liver and kidney disease.
Do not take if:
suffering from active drug or alcohol abuse, depression, irregular or slow heartbeat, Parkinson's disease.

SIDE EFFECTS:
Common: Tremor, excess salivation, muscle stiffness, dizziness.
Unusual: Difficulty in swallowing, disorientation, sleeplessness, rapid heart rate, restlessness, constipation, loss of appetite, menstrual irregularities.
Severe but rare (stop medication, consult doctor): Unwanted and uncontrolled muscle movements particularly of face, rigid muscles, fever.

INTERACTIONS:
Other drugs:
- Severe interaction with ketoconazole, erythromycin, nefazodone, quinidine.

Medications

- Anticonvulsants, sedatives, stimulants, atropine, antihypertensives, antiarrhythmics, levodopa, phenothiazines, tricyclic antidepressants.

Herbs:
- Evening primrose (linoleic acid).

Other substances:
- Reacts adversely with alcohol.

PRESCRIPTION:
Yes.

PBS:
No.

PERMITTED IN SPORT:
Yes.

OVERDOSE:
Relatively safe. Confusion and drowsiness most likely symptoms. Administer activated charcoal or induce vomiting if taken recently. Seek medical assistance.

See also Amisulpride, Droperidol, Flupenthixol, Haloperidol, Lithium Carbonate, Olanzapine, PHENOTHIAZINES, Quetiapine, Risperidone, Thiothixene, Zuclopenthixol.

Pindolol

TRADE NAMES:
Barbloc, Visken.

DRUG CLASS:
Beta blocker.

USES:
High blood pressure, angina, rapid heart rate, irregular heartbeat, paroxysmal atrial tachycardia, heart attack.

DOSAGE:
 10 to 30mg a day.

FORMS:
Tablets of 5 and 15mg.

PRECAUTIONS:
Should be used in pregnancy (C) only if medically essential.
Safe to use in breast feeding.
May be used with caution in children.
Use with care if suffering from alcoholism, poor circulation, diabetes, hyperthyroidism (over-active thyroid gland), liver or kidney failure or about to have surgery.

Do not take if:

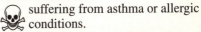 suffering from asthma or allergic conditions.
- suffering from heart failure, shock, slow heart rate, or enlarged right heart.
- if undertaking prolonged fast.

SIDE EFFECTS:
Common: Low blood pressure, slow heart rate, dizziness, headache, cold hands and feet, asthma.
Unusual: Loss of appetite, nausea, diarrhoea, impotence, tiredness, sleeplessness, nightmares, rash, loss of libido, hair loss, noises in ears.
Severe but rare (stop medication, consult doctor): Severe asthma.

INTERACTIONS:
Other drugs:
- Calcium channel blockers, disopyramide, clonidine, adrenaline, other medications for irregular heartbeat, lignocaine, ergotamine, indomethacin, chlorpromazine.

PRESCRIPTION:
Yes.

PBS:
Yes.

PERMITTED IN SPORT:
No.

OVERDOSE:
Slow heart rate, low blood pressure, asthma and heart failure may result. Administer activated charcoal or induce vomiting if tablets taken recently. Use Salbutamol or other asthma sprays for difficulty in breathing. Seek medical assistance.

OTHER INFORMATION:
Except for asthmatics, very safe and effective.

See also Atenolol, Carvedilol, Esmolol, Labetalol, Oxprenolol, Propranolol, Sotalol.

Pine tar
See TARS.

Pioglitazone

TRADE NAME:
Actos.

DRUG CLASS:
Hypoglycaemic.

USES:
Type 2 (non-insulin dependent) diabetes.

DOSAGE:

15mg to 45mg once a day. Low dose initially, then slowly increased.

FORMS:
Tablets of 15mg, 30mg and 45mg.

PRECAUTIONS:
Use with caution in pregnancy (B3), breast feeding and children.
Use with care in heart failure, liver and kidney disease.

SIDE EFFECTS:
Common: Oedema (swelling of tissue).
Unusual: Anaemia, liver damage, weight gain.

INTERACTIONS:
Other drugs: Oral contraceptives.

PRESCRIPTION:
Yes.

PBS:
No.

PERMITTED IN SPORT:
Yes.

OVERDOSE:
May be serious. Seek urgent medical attention.

OTHER INFORMATION:
Released in 2002 to treat more difficult cases of type 2 diabetes.

See also Acarbose, Glibenclamide, Gliclazide, Glimepride, Glipizide, INSULINS, Metformin, Repaglinide, Rosiglitazone, Tolbutamide.

Piperacillin

TRADE NAMES:
Pipril.
Tazocin (with tazobactam).

DRUG CLASS:
Penicillin antibiotic.

USES:
Treatment of infections caused by susceptible bacteria.

DOSAGE:
 One injection every three to six hours or by continuous drip infusion.

FORMS:
Injection.

PRECAUTIONS:
May be used in pregnancy (B1), children and breast feeding when medically appropriate.
Use with caution in kidney failure, liver disease, meningitis, and venereal disease. Not for prolonged use over three weeks. Blood tests to check liver and kidney function suggested.

Do not take if:
 allergic to penicillin.

- suffering from glandular fever.

SIDE EFFECTS:
Common: Pain at injection site, diarrhoea.
Unusual: Itch or rash, headache, nausea, dizziness, hot flushes, tiredness.
Severe but rare (stop medication, consult doctor): Itchy rash, hives, severe diarrhoea, yellow skin (jaundice), unusual bleeding or bruising.

INTERACTIONS:
Other drugs:
- Vercuronium, heparin, warfarin, methotrexate.

PRESCRIPTION:
Yes.

PBS:
No.

PERMITTED IN SPORT:
Yes.

OVERDOSE:
Vomiting and diarrhoea likely.

OTHER INFORMATION:
Used for more severe and unusual infections.

See also Amoxycillin, Ampicillin, Benzathine penicillin, Benzylpenicillin, Dicloxacillin, Flucloxacillin, Phenoxymethyl penicillin, Procaine penicillin, Ticarcillin.

Piperazine oestrone sulfate

TRADE NAMES:
Genoral, Ogen.

DRUG CLASS:
Sex hormone.

USES:
Oestrogen (female hormone) replacement in menopause, dry vagina after menopause.

DOSAGE:

Tablets: Dosage individualised by doctor. Usually one tablet once a day.

FORMS:
Tablet of 0.625mg (yellow), 1.25mg (peach) and 2.5mg (blue).

PRECAUTIONS:
Not to be used in pregnancy (D), breast feeding or children. Accidental usage in these situations unlikely to be harmful. Pre-treatment gynaecological and general examination essential.
Use with caution in epilepsy, migraine, heart failure, high blood pressure, kidney disease, diabetes, porphyria or uterine disease (eg. fibroids).
Use in conjunction with progestogen if still menstruating.

Do not take if:
suffering from liver disease, breast or genital cancer, blood clots or history thereof, otosclerosis, breast cancer, genital cancer, undiagnosed vaginal bleeding, sickle cell anaemia.

SIDE EFFECTS:
Common: Abnormal uterine bleeding, vaginal thrush, nausea, fluid retention, weight gain, breast tenderness.
Unusual: Rash, blurred vision, vomiting, bloating, intestinal cramps, pigmentation of skin on face.
Severe but rare (stop medication, consult doctor): Blood clots, calf or chest pain, yellow skin (jaundice).

INTERACTIONS:
Other drugs:
- Other sex hormones, warfarin, anticonvulsants (treat epilepsy), hypoglycaemics (treat diabetes), pethidine, theophylline, beta blockers, phenothiazines, thyroxine, tricyclic antidepressants, cyclosporin, bromocriptine.

Other substances:
- Smoking increases risk of serious side effects.
- Caffeine.

PRESCRIPTION:
Yes.

PBS:
Yes.

PERMITTED IN SPORT:
Yes.

OVERDOSE:
Vomiting and abnormal vaginal bleeding only likely effects.

OTHER INFORMATION:
Does not cause addiction or dependence. Very useful in managing the effects of menopause, and reduces the risk of osteoporosis and heart disease after the menopause.

See Cyproterone acetate, Danazol, Dydrogesterone, Ethinyloestradiol, Etonogestrel, HORMONE REPLACEMENT THERAPY, Medroxyprogesterone acetate, Oestradiol, Oestriol, Oestrogen, ORAL CONTRACEPTIVES, Oxandrolone, Testosterone.

Piperonyl butoxide

TRADE NAMES:
Only available in Australia in combination with other medications.
Banlice, Meditox (with pyrethrins and other ingredients).
Paralice (with bioallethrin).

DRUG CLASS:
Antiparasitic.

USES:
Head and pubic lice.

DOSAGE:

Apply to scalp or genital hair as directed by instructions on packaging. Repeat after two days if necessary.

FORMS:
Mousse, liquid.

PREΩCAUTIONS:
Safe to use in pregnancy (B3), breast feeding and children over six months. Avoid contact with eyes, nostrils and mouth.

SIDE EFFECTS:
Common: Skin irritation.

INTERACTIONS:
None significant.

PRESCRIPTION:
No.

PBS:
No.

PERMITTED IN SPORT:
Yes.

OTHER INFORMATION:
Treat all members of family and other close contacts at same time. Repeatedly use fine comb on hair to remove egg cases. Repeat in one week if necessary.
See also Maldison, Permethrin

Piprandrol

TRADE NAME:
Alertonic (with vitamin B group and minerals).

DRUG CLASS:
Tonic.

USES:
Fatigue, poor appetite.

DOSAGE:

15mLs three times a day before meals.

FORMS:
Mixture.

PRECAUTIONS:
May be used with caution in pregnancy. Safe to use in breast feeding and children. Use with caution in patients with drug dependency. Not for long term use.
Do not take if:
suffering from hyperactivity, agitation, psychiatric disturbances, chorea, depression, or obsessive compulsive state.

SIDE EFFECTS:
Common: Sleeplessness, nausea, diarrhoea, agitation, tremor.

INTERACTIONS:
Other drugs:
• None significant.
Other substances:
• Reacts with alcohol and caffeine.

PRESCRIPTION:
Yes.

PBS:
No.

PERMITTED IN SPORT:
Yes.

OVERDOSE:
Exacerbation of side effects likely.

OTHER INFORMATION:
Useful during convalescence from illness, and in patients with poor nutrition. May cause dependence.

Piroxicam

TRADE NAMES:
Feldene, GenRx Piroxicam, Mobilis, Pirohexal, Rosig.

DRUG CLASS:
NSAID (Nonsteroidal anti-inflammatory drug).

USES:
All forms of arthritis, inflammatory disorders, gout, back pain, ankylosing spondylitis.

DOSAGE:

Tablets and capsules: 10 to 20mg once a day with food.
Gel: Rub into affected area three or four times a day for up to two weeks.

FORMS:
Capsules, tablets, gel.

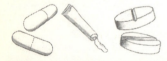

PRECAUTIONS:
Should not be used in pregnancy (C) unless medically essential. Breast feeding should be ceased if necessary to use NSAID. Not for use in children under 2 years. Gel safe in pregnancy.
Use tablets and capsules with caution in psychiatrically disturbed patients, epilepsy, severe infection, heart failure and kidney disease.
Lower doses required in elderly, who may suffer more side effects.

Do not take if:
 suffering from peptic ulcer at present or in recent past.
- due for surgery (including dental surgery).
- suffering from bleeding disorder or anaemia.

SIDE EFFECTS:
Common: Gel – Minimal.
Other forms – Stomach discomfort, diarrhoea, constipation, heartburn, nausea, headache, dizziness.
Unusual: Blurred vision, stomach ulcer, ringing noise in ears, retention of fluid, swelling of tissue, drowsiness, itch, rash, shortness of breath.
Severe but rare (stop medication, consult doctor): Vomiting blood, passing blood in faeces, other unusual bleeding, asthma induced by medication.

INTERACTIONS:
Other drugs:
- Must never be used with anticoagulants (eg. warfarin).
- Probenecid, diuretics, lithium, methotrexate, beta blockers, ACE inhibitors.
- Gel has minimal interactions.

Herbs:
- St John's wort.

PRESCRIPTION:
Gel: No.
Capsules and tablets: Yes.

PBS:
Gel: No.
Capsules and tablets: Yes.

PERMITTED IN SPORT:
Yes.

OVERDOSE:
Causes nausea, vomiting, severe headache, dizziness, confusion and convulsions. Administer activated charcoal or induce vomiting if taken recently. Seek medical assistance.

OTHER INFORMATION:

Used to give excellent relief to a wide variety of inflammatory conditions. Significant side effects (particularly on the stomach) in about 5% of patients limit their use. Specially coated forms reduce side effects. Minimal side effects with gels, but less effective.

See also Aspirin, Bufexamac, Celecoxib, Diclofenac, Diflunisal, Flurbiprofen, Ibuprofen, Indomethacin, Ketoprofen, Ketorolac trometanol, Mefenamic Acid, Naproxen, Rofecoxib, Salicylic acid, Sulindac, Tenoxicam, Tiaprofenic Acid.

Pizotifen

TRADE NAME:
Sandomigran.

DRUG CLASS:
Antimigraine.

USES:
Prevention of migraine.

DOSAGE:
 One to nine tablets a day in one or more doses.

FORMS:
Tablet of 0.5mg (white).

PRECAUTIONS:
Should be used with caution in pregnancy (B1), breast feeding and children. Pizotifen has no effect on acute migraine attacks.

Do not take if:
 suffering from glaucoma, difficulty in passing urine.

SIDE EFFECTS:
Common: Sedation, increased appetite.
Unusual: Dizziness, dry mouth, constipation, nervousness in children, swelling of tissues, headache, rash, muscle aches, tingling sensation, impotence.

INTERACTIONS:
Other drugs:
- Increased sedation with sedatives, hypnotics and antihistamines.

Other substances:
- Reacts with alcohol to cause drowsiness.

PRESCRIPTION:
Yes.

PBS:
Yes.

PERMITTED IN SPORT:
Yes.

OVERDOSE:
Serious. Administer activated charcoal or induce vomiting if taken recently. Symptoms include drowsiness, nausea, dizziness, reduced breathing, convulsions, coma. Seek urgent medical assistance.

OTHER INFORMATION:
Older, widely used medication. Large doses often necessary. Increase dosage slowly.

See also Clonidine, Methysergide, Propranolol.

Plague vaccine

See Yersinia pestis vaccine.

Medications

Pneumococcal vaccine

TRADE NAMES:
Pneumovax 23, Prevenar.

DRUG CLASS:
Vaccine.

USES:
Prevention of infections caused by Pneumococcal bacteria (usually a type of pneumonia).
Recommended for most people over 65 years, Aborigines over 55 years, those who have had a splenectomy (spleen removal) and anyone with poor immunity.

DOSAGE:
 Single injection. Repeat every five years.

FORMS:
Injection.

PRECAUTIONS:
Not designed for use in pregnancy (B2). May be used in breast feeding and children over 2 years.
Use with caution in heart and lung disease, fever, current antibiotic treatment.
Do not take if:
 receiving chemotherapy for Hodgkin's disease.
- previously vaccinated with this vaccine.

SIDE EFFECTS:
Common: Local soreness and redness at site of injection.
Unusual: Rash, joint pain, fever, joint pains, headache, tiredness, enlarged lymph nodes.

INTERACTIONS:
Other drugs:
- Immunosuppressives (used in cancer treatment).

PRESCRIPTION:
Yes.

PBS:
Yes.

PERMITTED IN SPORT:
Yes.

OVERDOSE:
Significant adverse reactions and allergy reactions may occur if a second vaccination is given to an adult. Children may require a second vaccination.

OTHER INFORMATION:
Now used routinely for most older people.

Podophyllotoxin
See PODOPHYLLUMS.

PODOPHYLLUMS

TRADE and GENERIC NAMES:
Condyline, Wartec (podophyllotoxin).
Posalfilin (podophyllum resin with salicylic acid).

USES:
Warts.

DOSAGE:
 Varies between brands and forms. Use as directed on packaging.

FORMS:
Ointment, cream, solution.

PRECAUTIONS:
Not to be used in pregnancy or breast feeding. Not for use in infants. Use with caution in children.
Use with caution in diabetes and poor circulation.

Do not use on moles, birthmarks or unusual warts, but seek medical advice.
Use on only a limited number of warts at one time.
Avoid use on normal and broken skin.
Be careful to avoid eyes, nose, vagina.

SIDE EFFECTS:
Common: Burning, redness of skin.
Unusual: Skin pain.

INTERACTIONS:
None significant.

PRESCRIPTION:
No.

PBS:
No. Posalfilin is available to some Veteran Affairs pensioners.

PERMITTED IN SPORT:
Yes.

OTHER INFORMATION:
Ancient and commonly used remedy for warts that is usually effective.

See also Glutaraldehyde, KERATOLYTICS, SALICYLATES.

Poliomyelitis vaccine

TRADE NAMES:
Ipol, Polio Sabin.

DRUG CLASS:
Vaccine.

USES:
Prevention of poliomyelitis.

DOSAGE:

Drops: Two drops on a spoon or lump of sugar given three times at two monthly intervals. Booster dose every five years.
Injection: Three doses at two month intervals, then a fourth dose after a year, then every five years.

FORMS:
Drops (must be carefully stored at 4°C), injection.
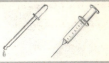

PRECAUTIONS:
Not designed to be used during pregnancy (B2), but inadvertent use unlikely to cause any serious effect. May be used during breast feeding, in children and infants.
Use with caution in diarrhoea, vomiting or infection.

Do not take if:
 suffering from fever or reduced immunity.

SIDE EFFECTS:
Common: Minimal.
Unusual: Headache, vomiting, diarrhoea, local reaction (injection).

INTERACTIONS:
Other drugs:
- Other live vaccines.

PRESCRIPTION:
Yes.

PBS:
No. Sabin supplied free to doctors by state governments.

PERMITTED IN SPORT:
Yes.

OVERDOSE:
Unintentional additional dose is unlikely to have any serious effect.

OTHER INFORMATION:
Poliomyelitis is a viral infection that causes muscle paralysis and sometimes death. It has been eradicated from Australia by vaccination, but is still widespread in many poorer countries. Last serious epidemic in Australia in 1956 created thousands of victims. Vaccination of children starts at two months of age, and Sabin vaccine is normally used.

Poloxamer
(Poloxalkol)

TRADE NAME:
Coloxyl Drops.

DRUG CLASS:
Laxative.

USES:
Constipation in infants and children. Softens faeces.

DOSAGE:

10 to 25 drops three times a day depending on age.

FORMS:
Drops (chocolate flavour).

PRECAUTIONS:
Safe in pregnancy (A), breast feeding and children.
Not for long term use. May cause intestinal dependence.
Do not take if:
 suffering from suspected appendicitis, bleeding from anus, belly pain, obstructed gut.

SIDE EFFECTS:
Common: Minimal.
Unusual: Colic, belly pain, diarrhoea.

INTERACTIONS:
Other drugs:
• Other laxatives.

PRESCRIPTION:
No.

PBS:
No.

PERMITTED IN SPORT:
Yes.

OVERDOSE:
Diarrhoea and belly cramps only likely effects.

See also Bisacodyl, Docusate sodium, FIBRE, Frangula, Glycerol, Lactulose, Paraffin, Psyllium, Sennosides, Sodium phosphate, Sodium picosulfate, Sorbitol, Sterculia.

Polymyxin B

TRADE NAME:
Only available in Australia in combination with other medications.
Neosporin (with neomycin and bacitracin).

DRUG CLASS:
Antibiotic.

USES:
Bacterial infections of skin and eyes.

DOSAGE:

Eye drops and ointment: Insert every three to six hours.
Skin ointment: Apply two or three times a day.

FORMS:
Eye drops,
eye ointment,
ointment.

PRECAUTIONS:
Use eye preparations with caution in pregnancy (D), breast feeding and children.
Not designed for long term regular use.
Do not use on large areas of skin or in ear with perforated ear drum.

SIDE EFFECTS:
Common: Minimal.
Severe but rare (stop medication, consult doctor): Skin or eye irritation, nerve deafness.

INTERACTIONS:
Other drugs:
• Aminoglycoside antibiotics.

PRESCRIPTION:
Yes.

PBS:
Eye preparations: Yes.
Skin ointment: No.

PERMITTED IN SPORT:
Yes.
See also Neomycin

Polyvinyl alcohol
See EYE LUBRICANTS.

Potassium aspartate
See ELECTROLYTES.

Potassium bicarbonate
See ELECTROLYTES.

Potassium carbonate
See ELECTROLYTES.

Potassium chloride
See ELECTROLYTES.

Potassium clavulanate
(Clavulanic acid)

TRADE NAMES:
Augmentin, Ausclav, Clamoxyl, Clavulin (with amoxycillin).
Timentin (with ticarcillin).

USES:
Only available as an additive to penicillin antibiotics to decrease bacterial resistance.

DOSAGE:

One or two capsules, two or three times a day.

FORMS:
Capsules, tablets, injection.

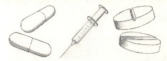

PRECAUTIONS:
Safe to use in pregnancy (B1), breast feeding and children.
Do not take if:
 suffering from jaundice (yellow skin from liver disease), allergic to penicillin.

SIDE EFFECTS:
Related to the form of penicillin with which it is combined. Diarrhoea very common.

INTERACTIONS:
See amoxycillin or ticarcillin.

PRESCRIPTION:
Yes.

PBS:
Yes.

PERMITTED IN SPORT:
Yes.

OVERDOSE:
Diarrhoea and vomiting only likely effects.

OTHER INFORMATION:
The combination of amoxycillin and potassium clavulanate is becoming very widely prescribed as very few bacteria are resistant to this potent combination.
See also Amoxycillin, Ticarcillin.

Povidone
See EYE LUBRICANTS.

Povidone-Iodine
See IODINE.

Pravastatin

TRADE NAME:
Pravachol.

DRUG CLASS:
Hypolipidaemic.

USES:
High blood levels of cholesterol.

DOSAGE:
 5mg to 40mg taken at bedtime on an empty stomach.

FORMS:
Tablets of 5, 10 and 20mg (white) and 40mg (yellow).

PRECAUTIONS:
Must not be taken in pregnancy (C) as pravastatin may cause miscarriage or foetal abnormalities. Adequate contraception must be used by all women of child-bearing potential who are taking this medication. Not to be used in breast feeding or children. Must be used with caution in elderly, with kidney and liver disease, and alcoholism. Regular blood tests to check cholesterol level and liver function necessary.

Do not take if:
 suffering from severe liver disease.

SIDE EFFECTS:
Common: Muscle pains, rash, headache, nausea, diarrhoea, constipation, excess wind.
Unusual: Chest pain, vomiting, belly pains, heartburn, fatigue, joint pain, muscle weakness.
Severe but rare (stop medication, consult doctor): Liver damage (yellow skin), severe muscle pain and weakness.

INTERACTIONS:
Other drugs:
- Gemfibrizol, nicotinic acid, cyclosporin, erythromycin, cimetidine, cholestyramine, colestipol.

Herbs:
- Alfalfa, fenugreek, garlic, ginger.

Other substances:
- Reacts with alcohol.

PRESCRIPTION:
Yes.

PBS:
Yes.

PERMITTED IN SPORT:
Yes.

OVERDOSE:
Unlikely to be serious.

OTHER INFORMATION:
Introduced in the early 1990s for treatment of more severe forms of excess blood cholesterol. Dangerous in pregnancy.

See also Atorvastatin, Cholestyramine, Colestipol, Fluvastatin, Gemfibrizol, Nicotinic acid, Probucol, Simvastatin.

Praziquantel

TRADE NAME:
Biltricide.

DRUG CLASS:
Anthelmintic.

USES:
Blood flukes (schistosomiasis).

DOSAGE:
 One to three tablets on three occasions four hours apart.

FORMS:
Tablets (white/yellow) of 600mg.

PRECAUTIONS:
May be used in pregnancy (B1), breast feeding and children if necessary.

Do not take if:

 suffering from cysticercosis of brain or eye.

SIDE EFFECTS:
Common: Nausea, headache.
Unusual: Belly pain, vomiting, dizziness, drowsiness, itch.

INTERACTIONS:
None significant.

PRESCRIPTION:
Yes.

PBS:
No.

PERMITTED IN SPORT:
Yes.

OTHER INFORMATION:
Rarely used in Australia as schistosomiasis (also known as bilharzia) is only contracted under normal circumstances in tropical developing countries (eg. Zimbabwe, Egypt).

Prazosin

TRADE NAMES:
GenRx Prazosin, Minipress, Prasig, Pratsiol, Prazohexal, Pressin.

DRUG CLASS:
Antihypertensive, alpha blocker.

USES:
High blood pressure, severe heart failure, Raynaud's phenomenon, enlargement of prostate gland.

DOSAGE:
 One or two tablets, two or three times a day to a maximum of 20mg per day.

FORMS:
Tablets of 1mg, 2mg and 5mg.

PRECAUTIONS:
Should be used with caution in pregnancy (B2) and breast feeding.
Not designed to be used in children.
Always start at a very low dose and increase slowly.
Use with caution in angina, heart valve narrowing causing heart failure, liver and kidney disease.

Do not take if:
suffering from phaeochromocytoma, low blood pressure on standing or poor liver function.

SIDE EFFECTS:
Common: Headache, drowsiness, palpitations, swelling of tissue, nausea, nasal congestion, blurred vision, low blood pressure on standing.
Unusual: Vomiting, itchy skin.
Severe but rare (stop medication, consult doctor): Fainting.

INTERACTIONS:
Other drugs:
- Additive effect from diuretics.
- Other antihypertensives.

PRESCRIPTION:
Yes.

PBS:
Yes.

PERMITTED IN SPORT:
Yes.

OVERDOSE:
Drowsiness and depressed reflexes only effects.

OTHER INFORMATION:
Very effective in high blood pressure. Also found to temporarily reduce the size of the prostate gland and make it easier to pass urine. Delays prostate surgery, but does not remove long term necessity for surgery.

See also ANTIHYPERTENSIVES.

Prednisolone and Prednisone

TRADE NAMES:

Minims Prednisolone, Panafcortelone, Predmix, Predsol, Redipred, Solone, Sterofrin (prednisolone).
Panafcort, Sone (prednisone).
Prednefrin Forte (prednisolone and phenylephrine).
Blephamide (prednisolone, sulfacetamide, phenylephrine).
Scheriproct (prednisolone, cinchocaine, clemizole).

DRUG CLASS:
Corticosteroid.

USES:
Severe inflammation of skin (eczema, dermatitis etc.), anus (piles), rectum (ulcerative colitis), eyes and other tissues. Severe asthma, rheumatoid and other forms of severe arthritis, autoimmune diseases (eg. Sjögren syndrome), severe allergy reactions, and other severe and chronic inflammatory diseases.

DOSAGE:

Enema: Insert once a day for up to four weeks.
Suppositories: Insert twice a day for up to three weeks.
Eye and ear drops: Insert every two to four hours.
Tablets and mixture: As directed by doctor.

FORMS:
Ear drops, enema, eye drops, mixture, suppository, tablets.

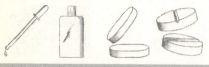

PRECAUTIONS:
Should be used in pregnancy (C), breast feeding and children only on specific medical advice.
Eye preparations safe in pregnancy, breast feeding and children over 3 years.
Use with caution if under stress, after recent surgery, and in patients with underactive thyroid gland, liver disease, diverticulitis, high blood pressure, myasthenia gravis or kidney disease.
Avoid eyes with all forms except eye drops.
Use for shortest period of time possible. Medication should not be ceased abruptly, but dosage should be slowly reduced.

Do not use if:
 suffering from any form of infection, peptic ulcer or osteoporosis.
- having a vaccination.

SIDE EFFECTS:
Most significant side effects occur only with prolonged use of tablets or rectal preparations.
Common: May cause bloating, weight gain, rashes and intestinal disturbances. Eye and ear drops – Rarely cause adverse reactions away from eyes and ears.
Unusual: Biochemical disturbances of blood, muscle weakness, bone weakness, impaired wound healing, skin thinning, tendon weakness, peptic ulcers, gullet ulcers, bruising, increased sweating, loss of fat under skin, premature ageing, excess facial hair growth in women, pigmentation of skin and nails, acne, convulsions, headaches, dizziness, growth suppression in children, aggravation of diabetes, worsening of infections, cataracts, aggravation of glaucoma, and sleeplessness.
Severe but rare (stop medication, consult doctor): Any significant side effect should be reported to a doctor immediately.

INTERACTIONS:
Other drugs:
- Tablets and rectal preparations may be affected by oral contraceptives, barbiturates, phenytoin and rifampicin.

Herbs:
- Liquorice, echinacea, ginseng, salbokuto, magnolia, Poria cocos.

Other substances:
- Zinc.

PRESCRIPTION:
Yes.

PBS:
Most forms: Yes.
Predmix, Scheriproct: No.

PERMITTED IN SPORT:
Most forms: No.
Eye and skin preparations: Yes.

OVERDOSE:
Medical treatment is required. Serious effects and death rare.

OTHER INFORMATION:
Extremely effective and useful medication if used correctly. Must be used with extreme care under strict medical supervision. Lowest dose and shortest possible course should be used.
Not addictive.

See also Cortisone acetate, Dexamethasone, Fludrocortisone, Flumethasone, Fluorometholone, Fluticasone propionate, Hydrocortisone, Methylprednisolone.

Prilocaine
See ANAESTHETICS, LOCAL.

Primaquine

TRADE NAME:
Primacin.

DRUG CLASS:
Antimalarial.

USES:
Treatment of malaria.

DOSAGE:
 15mg a day for two weeks.

FORMS:
Tablet of 7.5mg (pink/orange).

PRECAUTIONS:
Not for use in pregnancy (D). Use with caution in breast feeding. May be used in children.
Use with caution in rheumatoid arthritis, systemic lupus erythematosus, bone marrow disease and lactose intolerance.

Do not take if:
 suffering from G6PD deficiency (form of liver disease).

SIDE EFFECTS:
Common: Nausea, diarrhoea.
Unusual: Vomiting, headache, dizziness.
Severe but rare (stop medication, consult doctor): Abnormal bleeding.

INTERACTIONS:
Other drugs:
• Ketoconazole.

PRESCRIPTION:
Yes.

PBS:
No.

PERMITTED IN SPORT:
Yes.

OVERDOSE:
Serious. May cause heart and lung failure. Induce vomiting if taken recently, or give activated charcoal. Seek urgent medical attention.

See also Atovaquone, Chloroquine, Doxycycline, Hydroxychloroquine, Mefloquine, Proguanil, Pyrimethamine, Sulfadoxine.

Primidone

TRADE NAME:
Mysoline.

DRUG CLASS:
Anticonvulsant.

USES:
Epilepsy.

DOSAGE:

 Requires individual planning by a doctor, depending on nature and timing of convulsions.

FORMS:
Tablets of 250mg (white).

PRECAUTIONS:

Not to be used in pregnancy (D) unless absolutely necessary as it may cause bleeding problems in the newborn infant.
Use with caution in breast feeding. May be used in children.
Use with caution in kidney, liver and lung disease.
Lower doses necessary in elderly.
Do not stop suddenly, but reduce dosage slowly.
Use with caution if operating machinery, driving a vehicle or undertaking tasks that require coordination and alertness.

Do not take if:

 suffering from porphyria.

SIDE EFFECTS:

Common: Usually minimal and dose related. Drowsiness, vision disturbances.
Unusual: Nausea, headache, dizziness, vomiting, rash, poor coordination, personality changes, joint pains
Severe but rare (stop medication, consult doctor): Blood cell abnormalities, anaemia, liver damage (jaundice).

INTERACTIONS:
Other drugs:
- Anticonvulsants, anticoagulants (eg. warfarin), oral contraceptive pill, sedatives.

Herbs:
- Gingko biloba.

Other substances:
- Reacts adversely with alcohol.
- Borage.

PRESCRIPTION:
Yes.

PBS:
Yes.

PERMITTED IN SPORT:
Yes.

OVERDOSE:
Serious. Symptoms may include incoordination, reduced breathing and coma. Administer activated charcoal or induce vomiting if medication taken recently and patient alert. Seek urgent medical assistance.

See also BARBITURATES, BENZODIAZEPINES, Carbamazepine, Clonazepam, Ethosuximide, Gabapentin, Lamotrigine, Levetiracetam, Oxcarbazepine, Phenytoin, Sodium valproate, Sulthiame, Tiagabine, Topiramate, Vigabatrin.

Probenecid

TRADE NAME:
Pro-Cid.

DRUG CLASS:
Uricosuric.

USES:
Prevention of gout, prolonging the effectiveness of penicillins and cephalosporins, protects kidneys in conjunction with some other medications.

DOSAGE:
 One or two tablets twice a day.

FORMS:
Tablets of 500mg

PRECAUTIONS:
Use with caution in pregnancy (B2). Safe for use in breast feeding and children over two years.
Use with caution in kidney disease, peptic ulcer and acute gout.

Do not take if:
 suffering from kidney stones or blood cell abnormalities.

SIDE EFFECTS:
Common: Headache, nausea, frequent urination, rash, fever, sore gums.
Unusual: Vomiting, diarrhoea, flushing, hair loss, dizziness.

INTERACTIONS:
Other drugs:
- Aspirin, pyrazinamide, sulfonamides (antibiotics), paracetamol, thiazide diuretics, methotrexate.

Herbs:
- Willow bark.

Other substances:
- Alcohol may aggravate gout.

PRESCRIPTION:
Yes.

PBS:
Yes.

PERMITTED IN SPORT:
No.

OVERDOSE:
Exacerbation of side effects likely.

OTHER INFORMATION:
Does not cause addiction or dependence. Often used with penicillin in the treatment of gonorrhoea to extend effect of penicillin.
See also Allopurinol.

Probucol

TRADE NAME:
Lurselle

DRUG CLASS:
Hypoloidaemic

USES:
Inherited high blood cholesterol level that does not respond to other treatment.

DOSAGE:
 Two tablets twice a day with meals.

FORMS:
Tablet of 250mg (white).

PRECAUTIONS:
Should be used with caution in pregnancy (B1). Not for use in breast feeding. Use in children only if medically essential. Regular blood tests to check liver enzyme and blood cholesterol levels are necessary. Low cholesterol diet must be maintained.

Do not take if

☠ suffering from heart failure, heart electrical abnormalities, irregular heartbeat, recent heart attack.

SIDE EFFECTS:

Common: Diarrhoea, excess wind, nausea, belly pains.
Unusual: Pins and needles sensation, noises in ears, rash, heartburn, impotence, palpitations, headache, blurred vision.

INTERACTIONS:

Other drugs: Cholestyramine.

PRESCRIPTION:

Yes.

PBS:

Yes (authority required. Restricted to inherited high blood cholesterol levels not responding to other treatments).

PERMITTED IN SPORT:

Yes.

OVERDOSE:

Relatively safe. Diarrhoea likely.

OTHER INFORMATION:

Used in only the most difficult cases of high blood cholesterol levels.

Procainamide

TRADE NAME:

Pronestyl.

DRUG CLASS:

Antiarrhythmic.

USES:

Control and prevention of some types of heartbeat irregularities.

DOSAGE:

 One or two tablets, four to six times a day.

FORMS:

Capsules of 250mg (yellow), injection.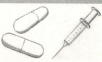

PRECAUTIONS:

Should be used with caution in pregnancy (B2). Should not be used in breast feeding. Should be used only if medically essential in children.

Should be used with caution in kidney and liver disease, after a recent heart attack, heart failure, heart structure abnormalities, blood chemistry abnormalities and in the elderly.

Routine blood tests may be required with long term treatment to check on cell types and numbers.

Do not take if:

 suffering from myasthenia gravis, SLE or atrio-ventricular heart conduction block.

SIDE EFFECTS:

Common: Generally well tolerated. Low blood pressure, stomach upsets.
Unusual: Depression, dizziness, hallucinations, fever, rash, flush, shivering, itchy skin, mild arthritis, bad taste.
Severe but rare (stop medication, consult doctor): Blood cell abnormalities.

Medications

INTERACTIONS:
Other drugs:
- Amiodarone, propranolol, other antiarrhythmics, cimetidine, anticholinergics, antihypertensives, captopril, sulphonamides, trimethoprim.

Other substances:
- Alcohol.

PRESCRIPTION:
Yes.

PBS:
Yes.

PERMITTED IN SPORT:
Yes.

OVERDOSE:
Rapid heart rate, vomiting and low blood pressure may occur. Administer activated charcoal or induce vomiting if tablets taken recently. Seek medical assistance.

See also Amiodarone, Disopyramide, Flecainide, Mexiletine, Quinidine bisulphinase, Sotalol, Verapamil.

Procaine penicillin

TRADE NAME:
Cilicaine.

DRUG CLASS:
Penicillin antibiotic.

USES:
Treatment of infections caused by susceptible bacteria (eg. throat, skin lung), gonorrhoea, syphilis, scarlet fever.

DOSAGE:
 One injection a day into muscle.

FORMS:
Injection.

PRECAUTIONS:
Safe in pregnancy (A), children and breast feeding.
Not to be injected into vein.

Do not take if:
 allergic to penicillin.

- suffering from glandular fever.

SIDE EFFECTS:
Common: Minimal.
Unusual: Genital itch or rash, tiredness.
Severe but rare (stop medication, consult doctor): Itchy rash, hives, yellow skin (jaundice).
Severe but rare (stop medication, consult doctor): Worsening infection, severe diarrhoea (pseudomembranous colitis).

INTERACTIONS:
Other drugs:
- Other antibiotics.

PRESCRIPTION:
Yes.

PBS:
Yes.

PERMITTED IN SPORT:
Yes.

OVERDOSE:
Adverse effects minimal.

OTHER INFORMATION:
The most basic and original form of penicillin. Widely used for acute infections in general practice.

See also Phenoxymethyl penicillin.

Procarbazine

TRADE NAME:
Natulan.

USES:
Hodgkin's disease, malignant lymphomas.

DOSAGE:
 One to six capsules a day to a total course dose of 120 tablets.

FORMS:
Capsules (pale yellow) of 50mg.

PRECAUTIONS:
Not to be used in pregnancy (D) unless mother's life at risk as damage to foetus probable.
Breast feeding must be ceased before use.
Use in children only if medically essential.
Women must use adequate contraception while using procarbazine.
Regular blood tests to check blood cells essential.

Do not take if:
 suffering from severe liver or kidney disease, bleeding disorders or blood cell abnormalities.

SIDE EFFECTS:
Common: Loss of appetite, nausea, reversible damage to bone marrow.
Unusual: Vomiting, unusual bleeding and bruising, rash.

INTERACTIONS:
Other drugs:
- Barbiturates, sympathomimetics, psychotropics.

Other substances:
- Reacts adversely with alcohol.

PRESCRIPTION:
Yes.

PBS:
No.

PERMITTED IN SPORT:
Yes.

OVERDOSE:
Exacerbation of side effects likely. Seek medical attention.

OTHER INFORMATION:
Despite significant side effects, procarbazine may be life saving in patients with some forms of gland tissue cancer.

Prochlorperazine

TRADE NAMES:
Stemetil, Stemzine.

DRUG CLASS:
Antiemetic, antihistamine.

USES:
Nausea, vomiting, dizziness, Ménière's disease.

DOSAGE:
 Tablets: One or two tablets at once, then one tablet in two hours, then one or two tablets every eight to 12 hours.
Suppository: One every six to eight hours as needed.

FORMS:
Tablets (white) of 5mg, suppositories, injection.

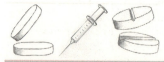

PRECAUTIONS:
Should be used in pregnancy (C) only if medically essential. Use with caution in breast feeding. Not for use in children under two years or less than 10kg.
Use with caution in epilepsy, Parkinson's

disease, under-active thyroid gland (hypothyroidism), myasthenia gravis, Reye syndrome, phaeochromocytoma, enlarged prostate gland, low calcium states, kidney or liver disease. Lower doses necessary in elderly.

Do not take if:

 suffering from shock, brain diseases, bone marrow disease.

SIDE EFFECTS:

Common: Constipation, dry mouth, drowsiness, tremor, blurred vision.
Unusual: Swelling of tissues (oedema), low blood pressure, irregular heartbeat, rash, difficulty in passing urine, headache, sleeplessness.
Severe but rare (stop medication, consult doctor): Yellow skin (jaundice), difficulty in breathing, convulsion.

INTERACTIONS:

Other drugs:
- Sedatives, desferrioxamine, anticholinergics, procarbazine, L-Dopa, anticoagulants, thiazides, propranolol, guanethidine, phenytoin, warfarin, tricyclic antidepressants.

Other substances:
- Reacts adversely with alcohol.

PRESCRIPTION:
Yes.

PBS:
Yes.

PERMITTED IN SPORT:
Yes.

OVERDOSE:
Serious, particularly in children. Symptoms include confusion, restlessness, rapid heart rate, tremor, twitching, convulsions, difficulty breathing, coma and rarely death. Administer activated charcoal or induce vomiting if medication taken recently and patient alert. Seek urgent medical assistance.

OTHER INFORMATION:
Widely used and effective. Available for over 30 years. Does not cause addiction or dependence. Related to the phenothiazines.
See also Domperidone, Metoclopramide, Promethazine.

Progesterone

TRADE NAMES:
Pro-Feme, Proluton.

DRUG CLASS:
Sex hormone.

USES:
Investigation of failure of menstrual periods.

DOSAGE:
 As determined by doctor.

FORMS:
Injection, cream.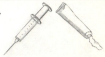

PRECAUTIONS:
Not to be used in pregnancy (D), breast feeding or children.
Use with caution in a history of blood clots in veins, eye disease, diabetes, depression, high blood pressure, heart failure.

Do not take if:

suffering from blood clot, stroke, liver disease, undiagnosed breast disease or genital herpes.

SIDE EFFECTS:
Common: Abnormal vaginal bleeding, headache.

INTERACTIONS:
Other drugs:
- Anticoagulants, hypoglycaemics, insulin.

PRESCRIPTION:
Yes.

PBS:
No.

PERMITTED IN SPORT:
Yes.

OVERDOSE:
Exacerbation of side effects likely.

Proguanil

TRADE NAMES:
Paludrine.
Malarone (with atovaquone).

DRUG CLASS:
Antimalarial.

USES:
Prevention (Paludrine) and treatment (Malarone) of malaria.

DOSAGE:

Prevention: Two tablets a day.
Treatment: Four tablets a day with food for three days.

FORMS:
Paludrine: Tablets of 100mg (white).
Malarone: Tablets (pink).

PRECAUTIONS:
Use with caution in pregnancy (B2) and breast feeding.
Use with caution in kidney disease.

SIDE EFFECTS:
Common: Loss of appetite, nausea, diarrhoea, headache.
Unusual: Vomiting, rash, dizziness, hair loss.

INTERACTIONS:
Other drugs:
- Magnesium salts (antacids).

PRESCRIPTION:
Yes.

PBS:
No.

PERMITTED IN SPORT:
Yes.

OVERDOSE:
Very serious. Administer activated charcoal or induce vomiting if taken recently. Seek urgent medical attention.

OTHER INFORMATION:
Not addictive or dependence forming.
See also Atovaquone, Chloroquine, Doxycycline, Hydroxychloroquine, Mefloquine, Primaquine, Pyrimethamine, Sulfadoxine.

PROKINETIC AGENTS

DISCUSSION:
Medications that increase the rate at which food is emptied from the stomach.
See Cisapride.

Promethazine

See ANTIHISTAMINES, SEDATING.

Propamidine isethionate and Dibromopropamide isethionate

TRADE NAMES:
Brolene (propamide isethionate and dibromopropamide isethionate).

DRUG CLASS:
Antiseptic.

USES:
Mild eye infections.

DOSAGE:

Drops: Two drops three or four times a day.
Ointment: Apply two or three times a day.

FORMS:
Eye drops, eye ointment.
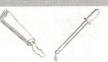

PRECAUTIONS:
Safe to use in pregnancy, breast feeding and children.
Not to be used regularly for longer than one week.
Use with caution if soft contact lenses used.

SIDE EFFECTS:
Minimal.

INTERACTIONS:
None significant.

PRESCRIPTION:
No.

PBS:
No.

PERMITTED IN SPORT:
Yes.

OTHER INFORMATION:
Commonly used as first-line treatment for conjunctivitis.

See also Chloramphenicol, Neomycin, Sulfacetamide.

Propantheline

TRADE NAME:
Pro-Banthine.

DRUG CLASS:
Anticholinergic.

USES:
Ulcers of the stomach and duodenum (upper small intestine), urinary incontinence, excessive sweating.

DOSAGE:

One to two tablets up to four times a day before meals.

FORMS:
Tablet of 15mg (pink).

PRECAUTIONS:
Use with caution in pregnancy (B2) and breast feeding.
Use with caution if suffering from heart disease, gut infection, fever, liver or kidney disease, chronic lung disease, ulcerative colitis, high blood pressure or difficulty in passing urine.
Use with care if ileostomy or colostomy present.

Do not take if:
suffering from bowel obstruction, megacolon, severe reflux oesophagitis from hiatus hernia, glaucoma, myasthenia gravis, severe kidney or liver disease.
- suffering from uncontrolled high blood pressure.
- suffering from an overactive thyroid gland (hyperthyroidism).
- rapid heart rate associated with heart disorder present.

SIDE EFFECTS:

Common: Drowsiness, blurred vision, difficulty in passing urine, reduced sweating, dry mouth.
Unusual: Nervousness, weakness, sleeplessness, headache, rapid heart rate, loss of taste, nausea, constipation, impotence, reduction of breast milk, allergic rash.
Severe but rare (stop medication, consult doctor): Fever, heat stroke, complete cessation of sweating.

INTERACTIONS:

Other drugs:
- Increases rate of digoxin absorption.
- Antacids, cisapride, L-dopa, metoclopramide, potassium chloride, corticosteroids.
- Delays absorption of many drugs (eg. pethidine, disopyramide, quinidine, procainamide, antihistamines, tricyclic antidepressants, phenothiazines).

PRESCRIPTION:
Yes.

PBS:
Yes.

PERMITTED IN SPORT:
Yes.

OVERDOSE:
Causes restlessness and psychotic behaviour, fall in blood pressure, paralysis and coma.

OTHER INFORMATION:
Relatively old-fashioned medication that is used usually as additional treatment for ulcers, but more commonly to reduce excessive sweating.

See also Dicyclomine, Hyoscine and Hyoscyamine.

Propranolol

TRADE NAMES:
Deralin, Inderal.

DRUG CLASS:
Beta blocker.

USES:
High blood pressure, angina, over-active thyroid gland, rapid heart rate, irregular heartbeat, paroxysmal atrial tachycardia, heart attack, prevention of migraine, tremors, phaeochromocytoma, prevention of anxiety-related symptoms (eg. stage fright, exam nerves).

DOSAGE:
 10 to 320mg a day.

FORMS:
Tablets of 10, 40 and 160mg.

PRECAUTIONS:
Should be used in pregnancy (C) only if medically essential.
Safe to use in breast feeding.
May be used with caution in children.
Use with care if suffering from alcoholism, liver or kidney failure, heart failure, diabetes or about to have surgery.

Do not take if:
 suffering from asthma or related allergic conditions.
- suffering from uncontrolled heart failure, shock, low blood pressure, slow heart rate, or enlarged right heart.
- if undertaking prolonged fast.

SIDE EFFECTS:
Common: Low blood pressure, slow heart rate, cold hands and feet, asthma.
Unusual: Loss of appetite, nausea, diarrhoea, impotence, tiredness, sleeplessness, nightmares, rash, loss of libido, hair loss, noises in ears.

Severe but rare (stop medication, consult doctor): Severe asthma.

INTERACTIONS:

Other drugs:
- Calcium channel blockers, disopyramide, clonidine, adrenaline, other medications for irregular heartbeat, lignocaine, ergotamine, indomethacin, chlorpromazine.

PRESCRIPTION:
Yes.

PBS:
Yes.

PERMITTED IN SPORT:
No.

OVERDOSE:
Slow heart rate, low blood pressure, asthma and heart failure may result. Administer activated charcoal or induce vomiting if tablets taken recently. Use Salbutamol or other asthma sprays for difficulty in breathing. Seek medical assistance.

OTHER INFORMATION:
An amazing drug that can help an extraordinarily wide range of problems. Except for asthmatics, very safe and effective. First developed in 1960s.

See also Atenolol, Carvedilol, Esmolol, Labetalol, Metoprolol, Oxprenolol, Pindolol, Sotalol.

Propylene glycol

TRADE NAMES:

Derma Tech, Intra Site Gel, Vosol.
Eulactol Heel balm (with urea, lanolin, dimethicone and other ingredients).
Solugel (with sodium chloride – common salt).

USES:
Leg ulcers, burns, pressure sores, persistent wounds, grazes, prevention and treatment of swimmer's ear.

DOSAGE:

Gel: Apply to wound daily and cover.
Ear drops: Five drops three or four times a day.

FORMS:
Gel, solution, ear drops.

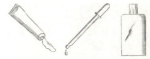

PRECAUTIONS:
Safe in pregnancy, breast feeding and children.

Do not use ear drops if:

 suffering from perforated ear drum, grommets inserted, ear discharge present.

SIDE EFFECTS:
Minimal.

INTERACTIONS:
None.

PRESCRIPTION:
No.

PBS:
No (subsidised for some products for Veteran Affairs pensioners).

PERMITTED IN SPORT:
Yes.

OVERDOSE:
Harmless.

OTHER INFORMATION:
Inert preparation that aids healing.

Propylthiouracil (PTU)

TRADE NAME:
Propylthiouracil.

DRUG CLASS:
Antithyroid.

USES:
Control of overactive thyroid gland.

DOSAGE:

One to 24 tablets a day in divided doses as directed by doctor.

FORMS:
Tablets (white) of 50mg.

PRECAUTIONS:
Not to be used in pregnancy (C) or breast feeding. To be used in children only if medically essential.
Use with caution in asthma.
Regular blood tests to check blood cells necessary if taken for a prolonged period.

SIDE EFFECTS:
Common: Dose related.
Unusual: Itchy skin.
Severe but rare (stop medication, consult doctor): Yellow skin (jaundice), unusual bleeding or bruising.

INTERACTIONS:
Other drugs:
- Anticoagulants (eg. warfarin, heparin).

PRESCRIPTION:
Yes.

PBS:
Yes.

PERMITTED IN SPORT:
Yes.

OVERDOSE:
Serious damage to blood cells possible. Administer activated charcoal or induce vomiting if tablets taken recently.

OTHER INFORMATION:
Commonly used to reduce activity of over-active thyroid gland before surgery to remove gland, or irradiation to destroy it.

Prostaglandin E1

See Alprostadil.

Protamine zinc insulin

See INSULINS.

PROTON PUMP INHIBITORS

GENERIC and TRADE NAMES:
Acimax, Losec, Maxor, Probitor (Omeprazole).
Nexium (Esomeprazole).
Pariet (Rabeprazole).
Somac (Pantoprazole).
Zoton (Lansoprazole).
Klacid HP7, Losec HP7 (Omeprazole with amoxycillin and clarithromycin).

DRUG CLASS:
Anti-ulcer.

USES:
Peptic ulcers of the stomach and duodenum, reflux oesophagitis, ulcers of the oesophagus, over production of acid in stomach (eg. Zollinger Ellison syndrome).

DOSAGE:
 One or two capsules or tablets once a day. Swallow whole.

FORMS:
Capsules, tablets, granules.

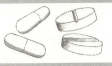

PRECAUTIONS:
May be used in pregnancy (B3), breast feeding and children with caution.
Cause of symptoms must be determined (eg. by gastroscopy) if they persist while on treatment.
Use with caution in liver disease.
Do not take if:
 suffering from severe liver disease.

SIDE EFFECTS:
Common: Minimal.
Unusual: Nausea, vomiting, diarrhoea, constipation, belly pains, passing wind, headache, dry mouth and throat, tiredness, joint pains.
Severe but rare (stop medication, consult doctor): Skin rash, breast enlargement in both sexes.

INTERACTIONS:
Other drugs:
- Diazepam (sedation), phenytoin (increases effect of phenytoin), warfarin (dosage of warfarin may need to be decreased), ketoconazole, theophylline, carbamazepine, low dose oral contraceptives, sucralfate, iron.

Herbs:
- Cranberry juice

PRESCRIPTION:
Yes.

PBS:
Yes.

PERMITTED IN SPORT:
Yes.

OVERDOSE:
Unlikely to be serious.

OTHER INFORMATION:
This very effective class of medications was introduced in 1991, and has revolutionised the treatment of more resistant peptic ulcers and persistent reflux oesophagitis. Newer agents (eg. Nexium, Pariet) were still being introduced in 2002. They act by inhibiting the activity of the enzyme in the stomach lining that is responsible for acid production.
See also ANTACIDS, Cimetidine, Famotidine, Nizatadine, Ranitidine.

Proxymetacaine

See ANAESTHETICS, LOCAL.

Pseudoephedrine

TRADE NAMES:

Demazin Sinus, Dimetapp Sinus, Logicin Sinus, Nyal Plus Decongestant, Sudafed Decongestant, Sudafed 12 Hour Relief.
Actifed (with triprolidine).
Actifed Chesty (with triprolidine and guaiphenesin).
Actifed Dry (with triprolidine and dextromethorphan).
Benadryl Chesty, Logicin Congested Chesty Cough, Nyal Plus Chesty Cough, Robitussin PS (with guaiphenesin).
Benadryl Dry (with dextromethorphan and diphenhydramine).
Biotech Cold & Flu (with chlorpheniramine, paracetamol and codeine phosphate).
Biotech Cold & Flu Non-Drowsy, Codral Cold & Flu, Codral Daytime, Nyal Plus Cold & Flu, Nyal Plus Day Cold & Flu (with paracetamol and codeine phosphate).
Bisolvon Sinus (with bromhexine).
Clarinase, Sinease Repetabs (with loratadine).
Codral 4 Flu, Demazin Cold & Flu, Logicin Flu Night, Logicin Hay Fever, Nyal Plus Night Cold & Flu, Nyal Plus Night Sinus Relief, Nyal Plus Sinus Relief with Antihistamine, Panadol Allergy Sinus, Panadol Children's Cold Elixir, Panadol Sinus Night, Sinutab Sinus Allergy and Pain Relief, Tylenol Allergy Sinus (with chlorpheniramine and paracetamol).
Codral Cough Cold & Flu Day, Dimetapp Cold & Flu, Dimetapp Day Cold Cough & Flu, Logicin Flu, Logicin Flu Day, Orthoxicol Cold & Flu, Orthoxicol Day Cold & Flu, Panadol Cold & Flu, Parke-Davis Day Cold & Flu, Pharma-Col Junior, Tylenol Cold & Flu Nondrowsy (with paracetamol and dextromethorphan).
Codral Cough Cold & Flu Night, Parke-Davis Night Cold & Flu (with dextromethorphan, chlorpheniramine).
Codral Dry Cough, Nucosef (with codeine phosphate).
Codral Nightime, Sudafed Sinus Pain and Allergy (with paracetamol and triprolidine).
Demazin Day/Night Relief (with dexchlorpheniramine).
Demazin Tablets (with chlorpheniramine).
Dimetapp Cold Cough & Flu (with dextromethorphan, doxylamine, paracetamol).
Dimetapp Cold Cough & Sinus (with dextromethorphan, guaiphenesin).
Dimetapp Cold Cough and Sinus Liquid Capsules, Sigma Relief, (with guaiphenesin and dextromethorphan).
Dimetapp Headcold & Flu, Nurofen Cold & Flu, Sudafed Congestion & Sinus Pain Relief, Tri-Profen Cold and Flu (with ibuprofen).
Dimetapp Night Cold Cough & Flu (with dextromethorphan, guaiphenesin, paracetamol).
Dimetapp Night Relief (with dextromethorphan and doxylamine).
Dur-Elix Plus (with bromhexine).
Duro-Tuss Decongestant (with pholcodine).
Lemsip Flu Day, Nyal Plus Day Sinus Relief, Nyal Plus Sinus Relief, Panadol Sinus, Panadol Sinus Day, Sinutab Sinus and Pain Relief, Sudafed Daytime Relief, Sudafed Sinus Pain Relief, Tylenol Sinus (with paracetamol).
Lemsip Flu Night, Tylenol Cold & Flu (with paracetamol, dextromethorphan, chlorpheniramine).
Logicin Dry Cough, Logicin Junior Children's Cough, Robitussin DM-P (with dextromethorphan).
Phensedyl Dry Family Cough (with pholcodine and promethazine).
Sudafed Nightime Relief (with triprolidine and paracetamol).
Telfast Decongestant (with fexofenadine).

Numerous locally produced and marketed brands also exist.

Medications

DRUG CLASS:
Decongestant.

USES:
Congestion of nose and sinuses.

DOSAGE:
 One tablet two to four times a day.

FORMS:
Tablets, capsules, mixture, syrup, drops, powder.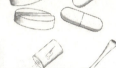

PRECAUTIONS:
Use with caution in pregnancy (B2) and breast feeding. May be used in children. Use with caution in treated high blood pressure, enlarged prostate gland and bladder problems.

Do not take if:
 suffering from uncontrolled blood pressure or angina.

SIDE EFFECTS:
Common: Sleeplessness, rapid heart rate.
Unusual: Hallucinations, palpitations, sweating, flushing, difficulty in passing urine.
Severe but rare (stop medication, consult doctor): Chest pain.

INTERACTIONS:
Other drugs:
- Severe interaction with MAOI.
- Other decongestants, medications used to treat high blood pressure.

PRESCRIPTION:
No.

PBS:
No.

PERMITTED IN SPORT:
No.

OVERDOSE:
Serious. May cause irritability, convulsions, palpitations, high blood pressure, angina and difficulty in passing urine. Administer activated charcoal or induce vomiting if medication taken recently. Seek urgent medical assistance.

OTHER INFORMATION:
One of the most widely used medications in the country. Safe and effective if taken in recommended dose. Should not be used to combat drowsiness.

See also Phenylephrine.

PSORALENS

See Methoxsalen.

PSYCHOTROPICS

DISCUSSION:
Medications that alter the functioning of the brain and can ease problems as widespread as depression and anxiety, but also include some illegally used drugs.

See ANTIDEPRESSANTS, ANTIPSYCHOTICS, ANXIOLYTICS, Marijuana.

Psyllium

TRADE NAMES:
Metamucil.
Nucolox (with starch).

DRUG CLASS:
Fibre, laxative.

USES:
Constipation.

DOSAGE:
 Take required amount with water two or three times a day.

FORMS:
Granules, powder.

PRECAUTIONS:
Safe in pregnancy and breast feeding.
Do not take if:
 on a salt, potassium or sugar-restricted diet
- suffering from severe constipation with impacted faeces.
- suffering from belly pain, nausea or vomiting.

SIDE EFFECTS:
Common: Minimal.
Unusual: Diarrhoea, belly discomfort, bloating.

INTERACTIONS:
Other drugs:
- Can affect the absorption of other drugs for up to two hours after use.

PRESCRIPTION:
No.

PBS:
No. Some forms available to Veterans Affairs pensioners.

PERMITTED IN SPORT:
Yes.

OVERDOSE:
Take additional water. Belly discomfort and passing excess wind only effects.

OTHER INFORMATION:
Widely used, natural fibre supplement.
See also **Bisacodyl, Docusate sodium, FIBRE, Frangula, Glycerol, Lactulose, Paraffin, Poloxamer, Senna, Sodium phosphate, Sodium picosulfate, Sorbitol, Sterculia.**

PTU
See **Propylthiouracil.**

Pyrantel embonate

TRADE NAMES:
Anthel, Combantrin, Early Bird.

DRUG CLASS:
Anthelmintic.

USES:
Treatment of threadworm, roundworm and hookworm infestations of gut.

DOSAGE:
 10mg of pyrantel per kilogram of weight as a single dose.

FORMS:
Tablets, syrup, suspension, chocolate squares.

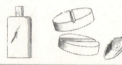

PRECAUTIONS:
Use in pregnancy (B2) only if medically necessary. May be used in breast feeding and children.
Use with care in children under 1 year.
If recurrence of infestation develops, another medication should be used.

Medications

Do not take if:

 suffering from liver disease.

SIDE EFFECTS:
Common: Minimal.
Unusual: Loss of appetite, nausea, belly discomfort, diarrhoea, vomiting, drowsiness, rash, tiredness.

INTERACTIONS:
None significant.

PRESCRIPTION:
No.

PBS:
Anthel: Yes.
Other forms: No.

PERMITTED IN SPORT:
Yes.

OVERDOSE:
Exacerbation of side effects only likely effect. Seek medical advice.

OTHER INFORMATION:
Widely used. Effective and safe.

See also Mebendazole.

Pyrazinamide

TRADE NAME:
Zinamide.

USES:
Tuberculosis.

DOSAGE:
 One tablet three or four times a day in combination with other medication for the treatment of tuberculosis.

FORMS:
Tablets (white) of 500mg.

PRECAUTIONS:
Should be used in pregnancy (B2) only if medically essential.
Breast feeding should be ceased before use.
Use with caution in children.
Use with caution with history of gout, diabetes and kidney disease.

Do not take if:

 suffering from liver disease, acute gout.

SIDE EFFECTS:
Common: Fever, loss of appetite.
Unusual: Liver tenderness and enlargement, gout, nausea, vomiting.
Severe but rare (stop medication, consult doctor): Yellow skin (jaundice), severe joint pain.

INTERACTIONS:
None significant.

PRESCRIPTION:
Yes.

PBS:
No.

PERMITTED IN SPORT:
Yes.

Medications

OVERDOSE:
Attacks the brain to cause convulsions and coma. Administer activated charcoal or induce vomiting if medication taken recently. Seek urgent medical attention.
See also Cycloserine, Ethambutol, Isoniazid, Rifampicin.

Pyrethrins

TRADE NAMES:
Only available in Australia in combination with other medications.
Banlice, Meditox (with piperonyl butoxide and other ingredients).

DRUG CLASS:
Antiparasitics.

USES:
Head and pubic lice.

DOSAGE:
 Apply to hair as directed on packaging. Repeat after seven to ten days if necessary. Wash hands after use.

FORMS:
Mousse, liquid.

PRECAUTIONS:
May be used with caution in pregnancy (B3), breast feeding and children over six months.
Avoid contact with eyes, nostrils and mouth.
Do not use if:
 suffering from ragweed allergy.

SIDE EFFECTS:
Common: Minimal.
Unusual: Skin irritation.

INTERACTIONS:
None significant.

PRESCRIPTION:
No.

PBS:
No.

PERMITTED IN SPORT:
Yes.

OTHER INFORMATION:
Treat all members of family and other close contacts at same time. Repeatedly use fine comb on hair to remove egg cases.
See also Benzyl benzoate, Maldison, Permethrin.

Pyridostigmine

TRADE NAME:
Mestinon.

DRUG CLASS:
Anticholinesterase.

USES:
Inability to pass urine, blockage of intestine.

DOSAGE:
 One to three tablets once or twice a day.

FORMS:
Tablets (10 & 60mg), slow release tablets (180mg).

PRECAUTIONS:
Should be used in pregnancy (C) only when medically essential. Safe for use in breast feeding. Use with caution in children.
Dosage must be carefully monitored by doctor.
Use with caution in epilepsy, slow heart rate, asthma, recent heart attack, irregular heartbeat, overactive thyroid gland, and peptic ulcer.

SIDE EFFECTS:
Common: Slow heart rate, headache, nausea, diarrhoea, excess salivation, cough, wheeze, bowel noises.
Unusual: Confusion, slurred speech, vomiting, belly cramps, desire to pass urine, muscle cramps, contracted pupils.
Severe but rare (stop medication, consult doctor): Difficulty breathing, chest pain.

INTERACTIONS:
Other drugs:
- Muscle relaxants, atropine, aminoglycosides, drugs used to treat irregular heartbeat, some anaesthetics.

PRESCRIPTION:
Yes.

PBS:
Yes.

PERMITTED IN SPORT:
Yes.

OVERDOSE:
Serious. May cause diarrhoea, vomiting, difficulty in breathing, weakness, low blood pressure, slow heart rate and heart attack. Seek urgent medical attention.

See also Donepezil, Neostigmine.

Pyridoxine
(Vitamin B6)

TRADE NAMES:
A large number of non-prescription preparations include pyridoxine (vitamin B6) alone or in combination with other vitamins and minerals.

DRUG CLASS:
Vitamin.

USES:
Vitamin B deficiency, nervous tension, mouth ulcers, premenstrual tension, hardening of arteries.

DOSAGE:

Recommended daily allowance: Females – 0.9 to 1.4mg a day; Males – 1.3 to 1.9mg a day.

FORMS:
Tablets, capsules, mixture, drops, injection.

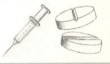

PRECAUTIONS:
Safe in pregnancy, breast feeding and children.
Do not take in high doses or for prolonged periods of time.
Ensure adequate protein intake in diet.

SIDE EFFECTS:
Common: Minimal.
Unusual: Sensory nerve damage.

INTERACTIONS:
Other drugs:
- Oral contraceptives, L-dopa.

PRESCRIPTION:
No.

PBS:
No.

Medications

PERMITTED IN SPORT:
Yes.

OVERDOSE:
May cause sensory nerve damage.

OTHER INFORMATION:
Pyridoxine is a water soluble vitamin. It is essential for the metabolism of protein. Remember, vitamins are merely chemicals that are essential for the functioning of the body, and if taken to excess, act as a drug.
See also **VITAMINS**.

Pyrimethamine

TRADE NAMES:
Daraprim.
Fansidar (with sulfadoxine).

DRUG CLASS:
Antimalarial.

USES:
Prevention and treatment of malaria, toxoplasmosis.

DOSAGE:
 Prevention: One tablet a week.
Treatment: Two tablets at once, then one tablet a day.

FORMS:
Tablets, injection.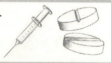

PRECAUTIONS:
Should not be used in pregnancy (B3) unless medically essential. May be used in breast feeding and children.
Use with caution in liver and kidney disease.
Ensure adequate fluid intake.
Do not take if:
 suffering from folate deficiency.

SIDE EFFECTS:
Common: Minimal.
Unusual: Rash, nausea, colic, vomiting, diarrhoea.
Severe but rare (stop medication, consult doctor): Blood cell abnormalities.

INTERACTIONS:
Other drugs:
• Co-trimoxazole, lorazepam, cytotoxics.

PRESCRIPTION:
Yes.

PBS:
Daraprim: Yes.
Fansidar: No.

PERMITTED IN SPORT:
Yes.

OVERDOSE:
Serious. Induce vomiting if taken recently. Give additional fluids. Seek urgent medical assistance.

OTHER INFORMATION:
Used in areas where chloroquine resistant malaria occurs (eg. New Guinea, Solomon Is, southeast Asia).

See also **Atovaquone, Artemether and Lumefantrine, Chloroquine, Doxycycline, Hydroxychloroquine, Mefloquine, Primaquine, Proguanil, Quinine.**

Pyrithione zinc

TRADE NAMES:
Dan-Gard.
Fongitar (with tar).

DRUG CLASS:
Antiseptic, antifungal.

USES:
Dandruff.

DOSAGE:
 Apply once every day or two.

FORMS:
Shampoo.

PRECAUTIONS:
Safe to use in pregnancy, breast feeding and children.
Avoid eye contact.

SIDE EFFECTS:
Common: Minimal.
Unusual: Skin irritation, sun sensitivity.

INTERACTIONS:
None.

PRESCRIPTION:
No.

PBS:
No. Dan-Gard available for some Veteran Affairs pensioners.

PERMITTED IN SPORT:
Yes.
See also TARS.

Quetiapine

TRADE NAME:
Seroquel.

DRUG CLASS:
Antipsychotic.

USES:
Treatment of schizophrenia.

DOSAGE:
 Gradually increased from 25mg twice a day to maximum dose of 350mg twice a day.

FORMS:
Tablets of 25mg (peach), 100mg (yellow) and 200mg (white).

PRECAUTIONS:
Use with caution in pregnancy (B3), breast feeding and children.
Use with caution in heart and liver disease, poor brain circulation, recent strokes, low blood pressure and epilepsy. Lower doses necessary in elderly.

SIDE EFFECTS:
Common: Dizziness and light headedness from low blood pressure, tiredness, dry mouth, runny nose, indigestion and constipation. Side effects often settle after two weeks.
Unusual: Rapid heart rate, fainting.
Severe but rare (stop medication, consult doctor): Seizures.

INTERACTIONS:
Other drugs:
- Sedatives, sleeping medication (benzodiazepines), thioridazine, phenytoin, barbiturates, rifampicin, carbamazepine, erythromycin, ketoconazole.

Herbs:
- Evening primrose (linoleic acid).

Other substances:
- Alcohol.

PRESCRIPTION:
Yes.

PBS:
Yes (authority required).

PERMITTED IN SPORT:
Yes.

OVERDOSE:
Unlikely to have serious consequences other than worsening of side effects. Seek medical attention.

OTHER INFORMATION:
Introduced in 2000 to treat previously uncontrolled patients with schizophrenia.

See also Amisulpride, Droperidol, Flupenthixol, Haloperidol, Lithium Carbonate, Olanzapine, PHENOTHIAZINES, Pimozide, Risperidone, Thiothixene, Zuclopenthixol.

Q Fever vaccine

See Coxiella burnetti vaccine.

Quinapril

See ACE INHIBITORS.

Quinidine bisulphate

TRADE NAME:
Kinidin Durules.

DRUG CLASS:
Antiarrhythmic.

USES:
Prevents some types of irregular heartbeats.

DOSAGE:
 Two to five tablets twice a day.

FORMS:
Tablets of 250mg (white).

PRECAUTIONS:
Should only be used in pregnancy (C) if medically essential. Should not be used in breast feeding or children.
Use with caution in atrial flutter, slow heartbeat, low blood potassium level, heart failure, and recent heart attack.

Do not take if:
suffering from heart block, thrombocytopenia, low blood pressure, bowel obstruction or kidney failure.

SIDE EFFECTS:
Common: Nausea, vomiting, loss of appetite, diarrhoea, dizziness, noises in ears, blurred vision, headache.
Unusual: Psychiatric disturbances, fever, rash, worsening of asthma, anaemia.
Severe but rare (stop medication, consult doctor): Unusual bleeding, yellow skin, asthma.

INTERACTIONS:
Other drugs:
- Digoxin (severe reaction), anticoagulants (eg. warfarin), cimetidine, phenytoin, barbiturates, rifampicin, procainamide, propranolol, verapamil, amiodarone, nifedipine.
- Absorption of quinidine slowed by antacids.

Herbs:
- Sparteine (Cytisus scoparius).

PRESCRIPTION:
Yes.

PBS:
Yes.

PERMITTED IN SPORT:
Yes.

OVERDOSE:
Very serious. Administer activated charcoal or induce vomiting if tablets taken recently. Seek urgent medical assistance. Symptoms include blurred vision, deafness, weakness, dizziness, headache, nausea, vomiting, low blood pressure, diarrhoea, irregular heart rate and death.

OTHER INFORMATION:
Old-fashioned but useful drug for specific types of heartbeat irregularities.

See also Adenosine, Amiodarone, Disopyramide, Flecainide, Lignocaine, Mexiletine, Procainamide, Sotalol, Verapamil.

Quinine

TRADE NAMES:
Biquinate, Myoquin, Quinbisul (quinine bisulfate).
Quinate, Quinoctal, Quinsul (quinine sulfate).

USES:
Night time muscle cramps, muscle spasms, prevention of malaria.

DOSAGE:

One or two tablets at night.

FORMS:
Tablets of 300mg.

PRECAUTIONS:
Not to be used in pregnancy (D) as foetal damage or miscarriage may occur. Use with caution in breast feeding and children.
Use with caution in heartbeat irregularities.
Do not take if:
suffering from tinnitus (noises in ears), G6PD deficiency, optic neuritis (eye nerve inflammation), blackwater fever (past or present), severe kidney disease or myasthenia gravis.

SIDE EFFECTS:
Common: Dose related. Tinnitus, headache, nausea, blurred vision.
Unusual: Rash, diarrhoea, dizziness, belly pain.
Severe but rare (stop medication, consult doctor): Unusual bleeding or bruising.

INTERACTIONS:
Other drugs:
- Anticoagulants (eg. warfarin), antacids, digoxin, mefloquine, cimetidine, urinary alkalinisers.

PRESCRIPTION:
Yes.

PBS:
Yes.

PERMITTED IN SPORT:
Yes.

OVERDOSE:
Very serious. Confusion, low blood pressure, blindness, low blood pressure, kidney failure and delayed death may occur. Induce vomiting if medication taken recently. Seek urgent medical attention. May be fatal despite intensive medical attention.

OTHER INFORMATION:
Very useful medication most commonly used to prevent night time cramps. Derived from the South American chincona bark that was first identified by the Spanish in the 16th century as having an effect on malaria.

QUINOLONES

DISCUSSION:
A group of widely used and very effective antibiotics.

See Ciprofloxacin, Enoxacin, Norfloxacin, Ofloxacin.

Medications

Rabeprazole
See PROTON PUMP INHIBITORS.

Rabies vaccine

TRADE NAME:
Merieux Inactivated Rabies Vaccine.

DRUG CLASS:
Vaccine.

USES:
Prevention of rabies.

DOSAGE:

Prevention: Two injections one month apart, repeat annually.
After suspect animal bite: Series of frequent injections as determined by doctor.

FORMS:
Injection.

PRECAUTIONS:
Not designed for use in pregnancy (B2), but must be used if mother exposed to bite from rabid animal. May be used in breast feeding and children.
Use with caution in immune deficiency and history of allergy.
Inject into muscle. Do not inject subcutaneously (under skin) or in to vein.

SIDE EFFECTS:
Common: Local redness, soreness and hardness at injection site.
Unusual: Fever, muscle pains, nausea, diarrhoea.

INTERACTIONS:
Other drugs:
- Corticosteroids, immunosupressants.

PRESCRIPTION:
Yes.

PBS:
No.

PERMITTED IN SPORT:
Yes.

OVERDOSE:
An inadvertent additional injection is unlikely to have any serious adverse effects.

OTHER INFORMATION:
Routinely given only to veterinarians and others working with animals in areas affected by rabies. Given after any bite by an animal in an area affected by rabies. Once symptoms of rabies occur, it is inevitably fatal. Rabies does not occur in Australia.

Radioactive iodine
See Sodium iodide.

Raloxifene

TRADE NAME:
Evista.

USES:
Prevention of osteoporosis after the menopause.

DOSAGE:
 One tablet a day.

FORMS:
Tablet (blue) of 60mg.

PRECAUTIONS:
Must never be used in pregnancy (X)(causes deformities of foetus), breast feeding or children.
Use with caution in liver disease and high triglyceride level.
Abnormal uterine bleeding must be diagnosed before use.

Do not take if:
still menstruating. For use in postmenopausal women only.
- medical history of blood clots.
- male.

SIDE EFFECTS:
Common: Hot flushes, leg cramps, sinus congestion.
Severe but rare (stop medication, consult doctor): Blood clots.

INTERACTIONS:
Other drugs:
- Oestrogen supplements, cholestyramine, ampicillin, warfarin.

PRESCRIPTION:
Yes.

PBS:
Yes (authority required. Restricted to women with osteoporosis after the menopause and who have suffered a fracture as a result).

PERMITTED IN SPORT:
Yes.

OVERDOSE:
Unlikely to result in serious consequences. Exacerbation of side effects likely. Seek medical assistance.

OTHER INFORMATION:
Released in 1999 to assist women who are unable to tolerate normal postmenopausal hormone replacement therapy.

See also Alendronate, Disodium etidronate, Salcatonin.

Ramipril

See ACE INHIBITORS.

Ranitidine

TRADE NAMES:
Ausran, GenRx Ranitidine, Hexal Ranitic, Rani 2, Ranihexal, Ranoxyl, Zantac.
Pylorid KA (with clarithromycin and amoxycillin).

DRUG CLASS:
Antiulcerant, H2 receptor antagonist.

USES:
Prevention and treatment of ulcers of the stomach, oesophagus (gullet) and duodenum (upper small intestine). Prevention of acid reflux into the oesophagus (heartburn).
Zollinger-Ellison syndrome (gastrinoma).

DOSAGE:
 Up to 600mg a day in one or two doses.

FORMS:
Tablets, soluble tablets, effervescent tablets, syrup, injection.

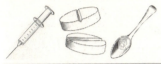

PRECAUTIONS:
Care should be taken with use in pregnancy (B1) and breast feeding. Children under 12 may be treated at the discretion of the doctor.
Cause of ulceration or pain must be determined (eg. by gastroscopy) if symptoms persist on treatment.
Use with caution in porphyria or on low salt diet.

Do not take if:
 suffering from severe kidney disease or phenylketonuria.

SIDE EFFECTS:
Common: Headache, diarrhoea, rash.
Unusual: Tiredness, dizziness, sleeplessness, speeding or slowing of heart rate, constipation, joint pains, breast tenderness (both sexes).
Severe but rare (stop medication, consult doctor): Hepatitis (jaundice), pancreatitis (severe stomach pain).

INTERACTIONS:
Other drugs:
- Sucralfate.

Herbs:
- Alfalfa, capsicum, eucalyptus, senega.

PRESCRIPTION:
Most forms: Yes.
Zantac 75mg: No.

PBS:
Most forms: Yes.
Zantac 75mg: No.

PERMITTED IN SPORT:
Yes.

OVERDOSE:
No serious effects reported.

OTHER INFORMATION:
Most widely used medication for the treatment of peptic ulcers. Available without prescription in some countries. Very safe and effective.
See also Cimetidine, Famotidine, Nizatadine.

Reboxetine

TRADE NAME:
Edronax.

DRUG CLASS:
Antidepressant.

USES:
Severe depression.

DOSAGE:
 One or two tablets twice a day.

FORMS:
Tablets of 4mg (white).

PRECAUTIONS:
May be used with care in pregnancy (B1), breast feeding and children.
Use with caution in epilepsy, bipolar disorders, heart disease, stroke, high blood pressure, dehydration, hyperthyroidism (over-active thyroid gland), liver and kidney disease, urine retention and enlarged prostate gland.

Do not take if:
 suffering from glaucoma.

SIDE EFFECTS:
Common: Headache, rapid heart rate, nausea, sleeplessness.
Unusual: Low blood pressure, sweating, dizziness, constipation, dry mouth.
Severe but rare (stop medication, consult doctor): Retention of urine.

INTERACTIONS:
Other drugs:
- Severe interaction with MAOI.
- Antihypertensives (lower blood pressure), ketoconazole, erythromycin, fluvoxamine, carbamazepine, lithium, thiazide diuretics (fluid tablets).

Other substances:
- Ergot.

PRESCRIPTION:
Yes.

PBS:
Yes.

PERMITTED IN SPORT:
Yes.

OVERDOSE:
May be serious. Induce vomiting or give activated charcoal if taken recently. Seek urgent medical attention.

OTHER INFORMATION:
Introduced in 2002 to treat depression that cannot be controlled by other medications.

See also Citalopram, Fluoxetine, Fluvoxamine, Paroxetine, Sertraline, Venlafaxine.

Repaglinide

TRADE NAME:
NovoNorm.

DRUG CLASS:
Hypoglycaemic.

USES:
Complicated type 2 (maturity onset, non-insulin dependent) diabetes.

DOSAGE:

0.5 to 4mg before meals three times a day.

FORMS:
Tablets of 0.5, 1 and 2mg.

PRECAUTIONS:
Not to be used in pregnancy (C), breast feeding or children.

Only to be used when other treatments for type 2 diabetes are not controlling disease. Use with caution in kidney and liver disease.

Do not take if:
suffering from type 1 (juvenile, insulin dependent) diabetes, severe liver disease or ketoacidosis.

SIDE EFFECTS:
Common: Nausea, dyspepsia, headache.
Unusual: Vomiting, pins and needles sensation, chest pain.
Severe but rare (stop medication, consult doctor): Jaundice (yellow skin from liver damage), low blood sugar (hypoglycaemia).

INTERACTIONS:
Other drugs:
- Oral contraceptives, metformin, insulin, thiazides, corticosteroids, danazol, thyroid hormones, MAOI, beta blockers, ACE inhibitors, salicylates, NSAID, octreotide, anabolic steroids.

Other substances:
- Alcohol.

Herbs:
- Alfalfa, celery, eucalyptus, fenugreek, garlic, ginger.

PRESCRIPTION:
Yes.

PBS:
No.

PERMITTED IN SPORT:
Yes.

OVERDOSE:
Low blood sugar with dizziness, headache, tremor, sweating and convulsions may occur. Give sweet drinks or injections of sugar. Seek medical assistance.

OTHER INFORMATION:
Introduced in 2000 as an additional treatment for severe forms of type 2 diabetes. Tolerance may gradually develop necessitating an increase in dosage.

See also Acarbose, Glibenclamide, Glicalazide, Glimepride, Glipizide, INSULINS, Metformin, Rosiglitazone, Tolbutamide.

Resorcinol

TRADE NAMES:
Acne and Pimple Gel (with sulphur, allantoin, zinc oxide and other ingredients).

USES:
Skin peeling agent, acne.
May be used alone for psoriasis.

DOSAGE:

Apply three times a day.

FORMS:
Gel.

PRECAUTIONS:
Safe in pregnancy and breast feeding.
Not for use in infants.
Use with caution in children.
Avoid contact with eyes, mouth, nose, anus and vagina.

Do not use on:
 inflamed or broken skin (cuts, grazes, burns etc.).

SIDE EFFECTS:
Common: Skin inflammation.

INTERACTIONS:
Other drugs:
- Other skin acne and psoriasis preparations.

PRESCRIPTION:
No.

PBS:
No.

PERMITTED IN SPORT:
Yes.

See also Adapalene, Benzoyl peroxide, Clindamycin, Isotretinoin, Phenoxyisopropanol, Triclosan.

Retinol
(Vitamin A)

TRADE NAMES:
A form of vitamin A found in numerous vitamin and mineral preparations, as well as soothing and healing creams and lotions.

DRUG CLASS:
Vitamin.

USES:
Vitamin A deficiency, malnutrition, poor diet, soothing agent in creams for minor burns.

DOSAGE:
 Recommended daily allowance: 2500 International Units a day.

FORMS:
Capsules, tablets, mixture, lotion, cream.

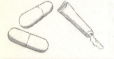

PRECAUTIONS:
Must not be used in pregnancy (D) as high doses may cause birth defects.
May be used in breast feeding and with caution in children.
Skin preparations safe in pregnancy.
Do not exceed recommended dose.
Use with caution in Vitamin K deficiency.

SIDE EFFECTS:
Common: Minimal.
Severe but rare (stop medication, consult doctor): Yellow skin, particularly of palms and soles.

INTERACTIONS:
None significant.

PRESCRIPTION:
No.

PBS:
No.

PERMITTED IN SPORT:
Yes.

OVERDOSE:
Chronic overdosage will lead to carotenaemia in which excess retinol is deposited in skin (causes it to turn yellow) and may cause damage to organs.

OTHER INFORMATION:
Fat soluble vitamin. Dangerous in pregnancy and overdose. Remember, vitamins are merely chemicals that are essential for the functioning of the body, and if taken to excess, act as a drug.

See also Betacarotene, Cod liver oil, VITAMINS.

REVERSIBLE INHIBITORS OF MONOAMINE OXIDASE
(RIMA)

See Moclobemide.

Ribavirin

TRADE NAMES:
Virazide.
Pegatron (with peginterferon).
Rebetron (with interferon).

DRUG CLASS:
Antiviral.

USES:
Some types of severe viral lung infections in children, hepatitis C.

DOSAGE:
 Virazide: Inhaled through special nebuliser for 12 to 18 hours a day.

Medications

FORMS:

Aerosol (Virazide), capsules (Rebetron), injection (Pegatron).

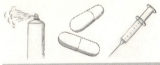

PRECAUTIONS:

Must not be used in pregnancy (X) or breast feeding.
Inhaler not to be used in children over 2 years of age.
Use with caution if on ventilator.
Use with caution in asthma.
Lung function and fluid balance must be carefully monitored.

Do not take if:

 adult woman unless on adequate contraception.

SIDE EFFECTS:

Common: Effects on lungs.
Unusual: Low blood pressure.
Severe but rare (stop medication, consult doctor): Heart attack.

INTERACTIONS:

Other drugs:
- Antibiotics.

PRESCRIPTION:

Yes.

PBS:

Virazide, Pegatron: No.
Rebetron: Yes (very restricted).

PERMITTED IN SPORT:

Yes.

OTHER INFORMATION:

Inhaler used only in hospital for life threatening lung infections caused by the respiratory syncitial virus.

Riboflavine
(Vitamin B2)

TRADE NAMES:

A large number of preparations include riboflavine (Vitamin B2) alone or in combination with other vitamins and minerals.

DRUG CLASS:

Vitamin.

USES:

Vitamin B deficiency, arabinoflavinosis.

DOSAGE:

 Recommended daily allowance: 1.0 to 1.7mg a day

FORMS:

Tablets, capsules, mixture, drops.

PRECAUTIONS:

Safe in pregnancy, breast feeding and children.

SIDE EFFECTS:

Minimal.

INTERACTIONS:

None significant.

PRESCRIPTION:

No.

PBS:

No.

PERMITTED IN SPORT:

Yes.

OVERDOSE:

Not harmful.

OTHER INFORMATION:

Riboflavine is a water soluble vitamin

found in dairy products, offal and green leafy vegetables. It is essential for the effective working of the lungs.
Remember, vitamins are merely chemicals that are essential for the functioning of the body, and if taken to excess, act as a drug.
See also VITAMINS.

Ricinoleic Acid
See Acetic Acid.

Rifabutin

TRADE NAME:
Mycobutin.

USES:
Tuberculosis (TB) and related infections.

DOSAGE:

One or two capsules once a day.

FORMS:
Capsule (red/brown) of 150mg.

PRECAUTIONS:
Not to be used in pregnancy (C) unless medically essential. Breast feeding should be ceased before use. Not to be used in children.
Use with caution in liver and kidney disease and eye inflammation.
Regular blood tests to check white cells, platelets and liver function essential.
Soft contact lenses may be stained.
Check eyes regularly for inflammation.

SIDE EFFECTS:
Common: Nausea, vomiting, yellow skin (jaundice), unusual bruising, anaemia, arthritis, muscle pains, orange urine, fever, rash.

Unusual: Eye inflammation, asthma.

INTERACTIONS:
Other drugs:
- Severe interaction with ritonavir and delavirdine.
- Dapsone, narcotics, anticoagulants (eg. warfarin), corticosteroids, quinidine, hypoglycaemics, clarithromycin, oral contraceptives.

PRESCRIPTION:
Yes.

PBS:
Yes (very restricted).

PERMITTED IN SPORT:
Yes.

OVERDOSE:
May be serious. Seek medical assistance.

OTHER INFORMATION:
Introduced in 1994 to treat resistant forms of tuberculosis.

See also Cycloserine, Pyrazinamide, Rifampicin.

Rifampicin

TRADE NAMES:
Rifadin, Rimycin.

USES:
Treatment of tuberculosis and leprosy, prevention of Meningococcal and Haemophilus bacterial infections.

DOSAGE:
 450mg to 600mg a day as a single daily dose in combination with other treatments on a regular basis for at least six months.

FORMS:
Capsules, tablets, syrup, infusion.

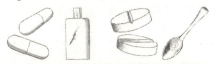

PRECAUTIONS:
Should not be used in pregnancy (C) unless medically essential. Not to be used in breast feeding or infants. May be used with caution in children.
Use with caution in liver disease, poor nutrition, porphyria, diabetes.
Designed to be used continuously long term.

Do not take if:
 suffering from jaundice (yellow skin).

SIDE EFFECTS:
Common: Heartburn, nausea, loss of appetite, intestinal cramps.
Unusual: Vomiting, headache, diarrhoea, drowsiness, fatigue, dizziness.
Severe but rare (stop medication, consult doctor): Yellow skin (jaundice).

INTERACTIONS:
Other drugs:
- Anticoagulants (eg. warfarin), corticosteroids, cyclosporin, digoxin, quinidine, hypoglycaemics (used to treat diabetes), dapsone, narcotics, oral contraceptives.

PRESCRIPTION:
Yes.

PBS:
Rimycin: Yes.
Rifadin: No.

PERMITTED IN SPORT:
Yes.

OVERDOSE:
Serious. Nausea, vomiting, drowsiness, brown stain to body fluids, convulsions, coma, jaundice and liver failure may occur. Administer activated charcoal or induce vomiting if medication taken recently. Seek urgent medical assistance.

See also Cycloserine, Ethambutol, Isoniazid, Pyrazinamide.

RIMA
(Reversible Inhibitor of Monoamine Oxidase Type A)
See Moclobemide.

Risedronate

TRADE NAME:
Actonel.

USES:
Osteoporosis, lose off calcium from bone, Paget's disease of bone.

DOSAGE:
 5 to 30mg a day. Must only be taken with plain water, 30 to 60 minutes before first food of day.
Patient must be upright when taking medication, and must not lie down for 30 minutes. Tablet must not be chewed, sucked or broken.

FORMS:
Tablets of 5 and 30mg.

PRECAUTIONS:
Not designed to be used in pregnancy (B3), breast feeding or children.
Food and beverages interfere with the absorption of Residronate.
Calcium and vitamin D supplements may be necessary.
Use with caution in kidney disease, oesophageal ulceration and peptic ulcers.

Do not take if:
- suffering from low blood calcium.
- unable to sit upright or stand for 30 minutes after taking tablet.

SIDE EFFECTS:
Common: Belly and muscle pain.
Unusual: Mouth inflammation, eye irritation, bowel inflammation.
Severe but rare (stop medication, consult doctor): Liver damage.

INTERACTIONS:
Other drugs:
- Antacids, aspirin, NSAIDs, other drugs used to treat osteoporosis.

Other substances:
- Minerals (eg. iron, magnesium).

PRESCRIPTION:
Yes.

PBS:
Yes (authority required).

PERMITTED IN SPORT:
Yes.

OVERDOSE:
Very low blood levels of calcium may occur. This may interfere with the function of nerves and other tissues. Other symptoms may include indigestion and vomiting. Induce vomiting if medication taken recently, or drink large amounts of milk.

OTHER INFORMATION:
Introduced in 2001 as a new way of preventing vertebral fractures and subsequent curvature of the spine in older women.
See also Alendronate.

Risperidone

TRADE NAME:
Risperdal.

DRUG CLASS:
Antipsychotic.

USES:
Schizophrenia and other psychoses, dementia, some behaviour disorders.

DOSAGE:
Start with low dose and gradually increase at direction of doctor. Maximum 8mg twice a day.

FORMS:
Tablets of 1mg (white), 2mg (orange), 3mg (yellow) and 4mg (green); solution.

PRECAUTIONS:
Use with caution and only when necessary in pregnancy (B3) and breast feeding. Not for use in children under 15.
Use with caution in heart disease, low blood pressure, dehydration, breast cancer, epilepsy or seizures, Parkinson's disease, liver or kidney disease.
Lower doses necessary in elderly.

SIDE EFFECTS:
Common: Low blood pressure, sleeplessness, agitation, anxiety, headache.
Unusual: Tiredness, dizziness, constipation, nausea, poor concentration, weight gain, blurred vision, belly pain, impotence.

INTERACTIONS:
Other drugs:
- Levodopa, antihypertensives (treat high blood pressure), carbamazepine, tricyclic antidepressants, quinidine, phenothiazines, beta blockers.

Herbs:
- Evening primrose (linoleic acid).

Medications

PRESCRIPTION:
Yes.

PBS:
Yes (authority required).

PERMITTED IN SPORT:
Yes.

OVERDOSE:
Drowsiness, sedation, rapid heart rate and low blood pressure may occur. Administer activated charcoal or induce vomiting if taken recently. Seek medical attention.

OTHER INFORMATION:
Often very effective, but expensive.

See also Amisulpride, Droperidol, Flupenthixol, Haloperidol, Lithium Carbonate, Olanzapine, PHENOTHIAZINES, Pimozide, Quetiapine, Thiothixene, Zuclopenthixol.

Ritonavir

TRADE NAMES:
Norvir.
Kaletra (with lopinavir).

DRUG CLASS:
Antiviral.

USES:
HIV infection, AIDS.

DOSAGE:
 Take twice a day.

FORMS:
Capsules, solution.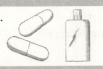

PRECAUTIONS:
Use with considerable caution in pregnancy (B3), breast feeding and children.
Use with caution in liver disease.

SIDE EFFECTS:
Common: Tiredness, raised triglyceride (fat) levels in blood, nausea, diarrhoea, abnormal pain, pins and needles sensation.
Unusual: Vomiting, dizziness, abnormal taste.

INTERACTIONS:
Other drugs:
- Do NOT use with amiodarone, benzodiazepines, cisapride, clonazepam, dextropropoxyphene, flecainide, quinidine, pethidine, piroxicam, rifabutin.
- Hypnotics, sedatives, oral contraceptives, other antivirals.

Herbs:
- St John's wort.

PRESCRIPTION:
Yes.

PBS:
Yes (authority required).

PERMITTED IN SPORT:
Yes.

OVERDOSE:
May be serious. Induce vomiting or administer activated charcoal if medication taken recently. Seek immediate medical attention.

OTHER INFORMATION:
Introduced in 1997. Treatment usually started only in hospital.

See Abacavir, Delavirdine, Didanosine, Efavirenz, Indinavir, Lamivudine, Nelfinavir, Nevirapine, Saquinavir, Stavudine, Tenofovir, Zidovudine.

Rivastigmine

TRADE NAME:
Exelon.

USES:
Alzheimer's disease.

DOSAGE:

1.5 to 6mg twice a day.

FORMS:
Capsules of
1.5, 3, 4.5 and 6mg.

PRECAUTIONS:
May be used with caution in pregnancy (B2). Not for use in breast feeding and children.
Use with care with history of peptic ulcer, irregular heartbeat, lung disease, difficulty in passing urine, epilepsy, and kidney disease.

Do not take if:
 suffering from severe liver disease.

SIDE EFFECTS:
Common: Nausea, diarrhoea, weight loss.

INTERACTIONS:
Other drugs:
- Anticholinergics.

Other substances:
- Smoking.

PRESCRIPTION:
Yes.

PBS:
Yes (authority required. Restricted to specialists only).

PERMITTED IN SPORT:
Yes.

OVERDOSE:
No information available.

OTHER INFORMATION:
Introduced in 2000 as a totally new treatment to slow the progress of Alzheimer's disease. Success rate relatively low, and success must be proved by serial tests on mental function for medication to be continued.

See also Donepezil, Galantamine, Tacrine.

Rofecoxib

TRADE NAME:
Vioxx.

DRUG CLASS:
COX-2 Inhibitor.

USES:
Osteoarthritis.

DOSAGE:

12.5 to 25mg once a day.

FORMS:
Tablets of 12.5mg (cream) and 25mg (yellow).

PRECAUTIONS:
Not for use in pregnancy (C). Use with caution in breast feeding and children.
Use with caution if history of peptic ulcer or intestinal bleeding.
Use with caution in smokers, alcoholics, dehydration, asthma, high blood pressure, heart failure, infection, liver or kidney disease.
Use lower doses in elderly.

Do not take if:
 suffering from active peptic ulcer, intestinal bleeding, active asthma, urticaria (hives).

SIDE EFFECTS:
Common: Minimal.
Unusual: Intestinal upsets, allergy, anaemia, fluid retention.
Severe but rare (stop medication, consult doctor): Peptic ulcer.

INTERACTIONS:
Other drugs:
- NSAID, aspirin, steroids, anticoagulants (eg. warfarin), rifampicin, methotrexate, ACE Inhibitors (treat high blood pressure and heart disorders), lithium, diuretics (fluid tablets), theophylline, amitriptyline, tacrine.

Other substances:
- Smoking increases risk of stomach ulcer.

PRESCRIPTION:
Yes.

PBS:
Yes.

PERMITTED IN SPORT:
Yes.

OVERDOSE:
Exacerbation of side effects likely. Induce vomiting or give activated charcoal if swallowed recently. Seek medical attention.

OTHER INFORMATION:
Introduced 2000. Far less likely than other treatments for arthritis (eg. NSAIDs) to cause intestinal bleeding.

See also Aspirin, Celecoxib, Diclofenac, Diflunisal, Flurbiprofen, Ibuprofen, Indomethacin, Ketoprofen, Mefenamic Acid, Naproxen, Piroxicam, Sulindac, Tenoxicam, Tiaprofenic Acid.

Ropivacaine
See ANAESTHETICS, LOCAL.

Rosiglitazone

TRADE NAME:
Avandia.

DRUG CLASS:
Hypoglycaemic.

USES:
Maturity onset (type 2) diabetes.

DOSAGE:
 4 to 8mg a day.

FORMS:
Tablets of 4mg (orange) and 8mg (reddish brown).

PRECAUTIONS:
Use with considerable caution in pregnancy (B3), breast feeding or children.
Use with caution in polycystic ovary disease, heart failure and severe liver disease.
Regular blood tests to check sugar levels and liver function necessary.

SIDE EFFECTS:
Common: Swelling of tissue.
Unusual: Liver damage, high cholesterol, weight gain, anaemia.

INTERACTIONS:
Other drugs:
- Troglitazone.

Herbs:
- Alfalfa, celery, eucalyptus, fenugreek, garlic, ginger.

PRESCRIPTION:
Yes.

PBS:
No.

PERMITTED IN SPORT:
Yes.

OVERDOSE:
Not likely to be very serious. Give glucose drinks and seek medical attention.

OTHER INFORMATION:
Introduced in 2000.
See also Acarbose, Glibenclamide, Glicalazide, Glimepride, Glipizide, INSULINS, Metformin, Repaglinide, Tolbutamide.

Roxithromycin

TRADE NAMES:
Biaxsig, Rulide.

DRUG CLASS:
Macrolide antibiotic.

USES:
Treatment of infections (eg. throat, sinuses, lung) caused by susceptible bacteria.

DOSAGE:
 One tablet twice a day.

FORMS:
Tablets (white) of 150 and 300mg.

PRECAUTIONS:
May be used in pregnancy (B1) and breast feeding if necessary. Not recommended for use in children.
Not designed for prolonged or repeated use.
Use with caution in liver and kidney disease.
Do not take if:
 suffering from severe liver disease, jaundice (yellow skin).

SIDE EFFECTS:
Common: Nausea, vomiting, diarrhoea, rash, headache.
Unusual: Belly pain, loss of appetite, excess wind, dizziness, ear noises.
Severe but rare (stop medication, consult doctor): Yellow skin (jaundice).

INTERACTIONS:
Other drugs:
- Disopyramide, theophylline, astemizole, cisapride, pimozide, digoxin, warfarin, midazolam.

PRESCRIPTION:
Yes.

PBS:
Yes.

PERMITTED IN SPORT:
Yes.

OVERDOSE:
Severe diarrhoea, stomach pains and deafness may occur.

OTHER INFORMATION:
Introduced in 1993. Widely used an effective antibiotic. Does not cause addiction or dependence.
See also Clarithromycin, Erythromycin.

RUBEFACIENTS

DISCUSSION:
Rubefacients are a type of liniment that causes redness of the skin.
See Capsaicin, Diethylamine salicylate, Menthol, Salicylic acid.

Rubella vaccine

TRADE NAMES:
Erevax, Meruvax II.
MMR II, Priorix (with measles and mumps vaccines).

DRUG CLASS:
Vaccine.

USES:
Prevention of rubella (German measles).

DOSAGE:

Two injections in childhood. Lifelong protection usual.

FORMS:
Injection.

PRECAUTIONS:
Not to be used in pregnancy (B2), but inadvertent use unlikely to have serious effects. May be used in breast feeding and children.
Use with caution if history of convulsions.

Do not take if:
 suffering from significant fever, immune system deficiency.
- blood transfusion within three months.
- allergic to neomycin.

SIDE EFFECTS:
Common: Pain, soreness, redness, firmness at site of injection.
Unusual: Fever, rash, headache, joint pains, sore throat, tender glands.

INTERACTIONS:
Other drugs:
- Immunoglobulin, other live vaccines at same site.

Other substances:
- Blood transfusion.

PRESCRIPTION:
Yes.

PBS:
No (MMR II and Priorix supplied free to doctors by state governments).

PERMITTED IN SPORT:
Yes.

OVERDOSE:
No adverse effects likely from an inadvertent additional dose.

OTHER INFORMATION:
Rubella (German measles) is usually a minor disease, although it may cause significant arthritis, headache and fever, but if caught by a mother during the first three months of pregnancy it may cause serious damage to the foetus.

Sabin vaccine

See Poliomyelitis vaccine.

Saint John's Wort
(Hypericum perforatum)

USES:

Mild depression and anxiety, skin inflammation, bruises and burns.

DOSAGE:

 Varies with form of preparation. Generally 300mg of standardised extract three times a day.
Apply topically three times a day.

FORMS:

Capsules, tablets, oils, creams, dried herb (for tea making).

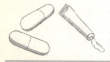

PRECAUTIONS:

None significant.

SIDE EFFECTS:

Common: Constipation, dry mouth, bloating, restlessness, tiredness.
Unusual: Diarrhoea, loss of appetite, nausea, belly pain, red skin, itchy skin, skin becomes sun sensitive (sunburn).
Severe but rare (stop medication, consult doctor): Sperm damage and infertility, nerve damage.

INTERACTIONS:

Other drugs:
- Severe interaction with MAOI.
- SSRI antidepressants, iron, oral contraceptive pill, theophylline, digoxin, sertraline, nefazadine, tetracyclines, sulfa antibiotics, quinolone antibiotics, thiazide diuretics, piroxicam, narcotics, barbiturates, cyclosporin, indinavir.

PRESCRIPTION:

No.

PBS:

No.

PERMITTED IN SPORT:

Yes.

OVERDOSE:

Exacerbation of side effects likely.

OTHER INFORMATION:

Not used in orthodox medical practice.

Salbutamol

TRADE NAMES:
Airomir, Asmol, Epaq, GenRx Salbutamol, Ventolin.
Combivent (with ipratropium bromide).

DRUG CLASS:
Bronchodilators (Beta-2 agonist).

USES:
Asthma, bronchitis, emphysema, spasm of airways in lung, prevention of labour in childbirth.

DOSAGE:

Inhalers and sprays: One or two inhalations every four hours.
Tablets: One three times a day.
Elixir: 5mLs to 10mLs three or four times a day.

FORMS:
Injection, spray, inhaler, nebuliser solution, dischaler, rotacaps.

PRECAUTIONS:
Safe to use in pregnancy (A), breast feeding and children.
Not designed for long term constant use. Use with care in high blood pressure, heart disease, overactive thyroid gland, diabetes, liver and kidney disease. Lower doses necessary in elderly. Seek urgent medical assistance if no response to medication.

SIDE EFFECTS:
Common: Tremor, rapid heart rate, palpitations, headache.
Unusual: Nausea, flush, mouth irritation.

INTERACTIONS:
Other drugs:
- Sympathomimetics, beta blockers, theophyllines, steroids, diuretics, digoxin, imipramine, chlordiazepoxide.

Other substances:
- Tablets and capsules may react with alcohol and caffeine.

PRESCRIPTION:
Nebuliser solution, injections: Yes.
Sprays, rotacaps: No.

PBS:
Most forms: Yes.
Discs: No.

PERMITTED IN SPORT:
Yes, but only under specific conditions set out by each sport. Must be declared by athlete to sport administrators.

OVERDOSE:
Exacerbation of side effects likely. May be dangerous in patients with heart disease or high blood pressure.

OTHER INFORMATION:
Designed for intermittent occasional use, and not to be taken regularly. Other medication should be used to prevent asthma if repeated doses of this medication are needed. Does not cause dependence or addiction. First introduced in the 1960s, beta-agonists have revolutionised life for asthmatics, but since deregulation in the mid 1980s, they have often been used excessively and inappropriately.

See also Fenoterol, Salmeterol, Terbutaline.

Salcatonin
(Calcitonin)

TRADE NAME:
Miacalcic.

USES:
Paget's disease of bone, excess blood calcium levels (hypercalcaemia).

DOSAGE:

By injection in a dose determined by doctor for each patient.

FORMS:
Injection.

PRECAUTIONS:
Not to be used in pregnancy (B2), or breast feeding. Use with great caution in children. Use long term with caution.

SIDE EFFECTS:
Common: Nausea, vomiting, injection site inflammation.
Unusual: Dizziness, pain.

INTERACTIONS:
Other drugs: Digoxin.

PRESCRIPTION:
Yes.

PBS:
Yes (restricted to specific diseases where treatment initiated in hospital).

PERMITTED IN SPORT:
Yes.

OTHER INFORMATION:
Derived from a natural hormone found in salmon.

SALICYLATES
See Aspirin, Choline salicylate, Diethylamine salicylate, Salicylic acid.

Salicylic acid

TRADE NAMES:
Clearasil, Clear Away, Duofilm Gel, Egozite Cradle Cap Lotion, Ionil.
Cornkil (with benzocaine, lactic acid).
Curaderm, Psor-Asist Scalp, Sunspot Cream (with urea).
Dermatech, Duofilm (with lactic acid).
Dermaveen Acne Bar, Movelat Sportz, Psor-Asist, Pyralvex, Seborrol,
SP Cream, Superfade (with other ingredients).
Egomycol (with undecylenamide, benzoic acid, chlorhexidine and other ingredients).
Goanna Analgesic Icel (with menthol).
Ionil T (with tar).
Mycoderm (with undecylenamide and other ingredients).
Posalfilin (with podophyllum).
Sebitar (with undecylenamide, tar).
Seborrol (with undecylenamide, resorcinol).
SM 33 Adult (with lignocaine and other ingredients).
SM 33 Gel (with menthol, lignocaine and other ingredients).
SOOV Prickly Heat Powder (with paraffin, zinc oxide and other ingredients).
Numerous other ointments, creams and liniments contain salicylic acid.

DRUG CLASS:
Rubefacient, Analgesic, Acid.

USES:
Temporary relief of pain (eg. muscular, arthritic).
Psoriasis, acne, skin irritation.
Wart removal.

DOSAGE:

Muscle and joint pain: Massage liniments into clean dry skin two or three times a day.
Psoriasis and acne: Apply to affected skin, leave for 10 minutes, then wash off.
Wart removal: Apply once or twice a day as directed by packaging instructions.

FORMS:

Lotion, gel, cream, ointment, paint, shampoo, soap, spray.

PRECAUTIONS:

Safe in pregnancy and breast feeding.
Use with caution in children under 5 years.
Avoid contact with eyes, mouth, nose, anus and vagina.
Use sparingly on face, skin folds and thin skin.
May stain clothing.

Do not use if:

 suffering from broken or infected skin.

SIDE EFFECTS:

Minimal.

INTERACTIONS:

None significant.

PRESCRIPTION:

No.

PBS:

No. Some forms available to Veterans Affairs pensioners.

PERMITTED IN SPORT:

Yes.

OVERDOSE:

May have serious effects in the unlikely event of the liniment being swallowed.

OTHER INFORMATION:

Widely used and very safe.

See also Diethylamine salicylate, KERATOLYTICS.

Salmeterol

TRADE NAMES:

Serevent.
Seretide (with fluticasone).

DRUG CLASS:

Bronchodilator.

USES:

Long term control of asthma.

DOSAGE:

 One or two inhalations twice a day.

FORMS:

Inhaler.

PRECAUTIONS:

Use with caution in pregnancy (B3), breast feeding and children over four years.
Do not exceed recommended dosage.
Use with caution in thyroid disease.
Not for treatment of acute asthma.
Regular checks of lung function advisable.

Do not use if:

 under four years.

SIDE EFFECTS:

Common: Tremor, rapid pulse, palpitations, headache.
Unusual: Temporary worsening of wheeze immediately after use.

INTERACTIONS:

None significant.

PRESCRIPTION:

Yes.

PBS:

Yes.

PERMITTED IN SPORT:

No (some exceptions apply, check with sport's governing body).

Medications

OVERDOSE:
Dramatic worsening of side effects may occur. Seek medical assistance.

OTHER INFORMATION:
Introduced in 1993 to assist in the control of chronic asthma that has been very successful. Does not cause addiction or dependence, but must be used under close medical supervision.
See also Eformoterol.

Salmonella typhi vaccine
(Typhoid vaccine)

TRADE NAMES:
Typherix, Typhim Vi (injection).
Typh-Vax Oral (capsules).
Vivaxim (injection with hepatitis A vaccine).

DRUG CLASS:
Vaccine.

USES:
Prevention of typhoid.

DOSAGE:
 Typherix, Typhim Vi: Single injection gives three years protection.
Typh-Vax Oral: One capsule one hour before food on three occasions two days apart. Gives six months protection.
Vivaxim: One injection two weeks before travel gives three years protection. Repeat hepatitis A vaccine after six to 12 months for long term protection against hepatitis A.

FORMS:
Injection,
capsule (pink/white).

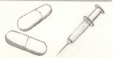

PRECAUTIONS:
Not designed for use in pregnancy (B2), but unintentional use in pregnancy is unlikely to have any serious effects. Use with caution in breast feeding. Not for use in children under 6 years.
Use with caution in immune diseases.
Do not take if:
☠ suffering from high fever, significant infection, diarrhoea (capsule only).

SIDE EFFECTS:
Common: Local pain, redness and swelling at injection site.
Unusual: Fever, nausea, diarrhoea, headache, tiredness.

INTERACTIONS:
Other drugs:
- Antibiotics (capsule only).
- Administer other injected vaccines at different site.

PRESCRIPTION:
Yes.

PBS:
No.

PERMITTED IN SPORT:
Yes.

OVERDOSE:
Inadvertent additional vaccination or capsules are unlikely to cause any serious adverse effects.

OTHER INFORMATION:
Not used routinely. Only given to persons travelling to or living in poorer countries where typhoid is widespread. Typhoid causes severe diarrhoea and vomiting and is caught from contaminated food or poor personal hygiene.
See also Hepatitis A vaccine.

Salt (Sodium chloride)
See ELECTROLYTES.

Saquinavir

TRADE NAMES:
Fortovase, Invirase.

DRUG CLASS:
Antiviral.

USES:
AIDS, HIV infection.

DOSAGE:

600 to 1200mg three times a day after a large meal and in combination with other antiviral agents.

FORMS:
Capsules of 200mg (light brown/green), gelcaps of 200mg (beige).

PRECAUTIONS:
Use with caution in pregnancy (B1), breast feeding and children.
Use with caution in diarrhoea, liver and kidney disease.
Use lower doses in elderly.
Should be used in combination with other medications for HIV infection.

SIDE EFFECTS:
Common: Tiredness, nausea, diarrhoea, abnormal pain, abnormal sensation.
Unusual: Vomiting, dizziness.

INTERACTIONS:
Other drugs:
- Severe interaction with astemizole, cisapride, pimozide, triazolam, midazolam, rifampicin, rifabutin, pentamidine.
- Nifedipine, clindamycin, nevirapine, efavirenz, indinavir, clarithromycin, ketoconazole, delavirdine, sildenafil, other drugs affecting liver function.

Herbs:
- St John's wort.

Other substances:
- Grapefruit juice

PRESCRIPTION:
Yes.

PBS:
Yes (authority required – very restricted).

PERMITTED IN SPORT:
Yes.

OVERDOSE:
No information available. Induce vomiting or administer activated charcoal if taken recently. Seek urgent medical attention.
See Abacavir, Delavirdine, Didanosine, Efavirenz, Indinavir, Lamivudine, Nelfinavir, Nevirapine, Ritonavir, Stavudine, Tenofovir, Zidovudine.

SEDATIVES AND HYPNOTICS

DISCUSSION:
Medications that sedate, relax and induce sleep.
See BARBITURATES, Chlormethiazole, Flunitrazepam, Midazolam, Nitrazepam, Temazepam, Triazolam, Zolpidem, Zopiclone.

SELECTIVE SEROTONIN REUPTAKE INHIBITORS

See Citalopram, Fluoxetine, Fluvoxamine, Paroxetine, Sertraline, Venlafaxine.

Selegiline

TRADE NAMES:
Eldepryl, Selgene.

DRUG CLASS:
MAOI. Antiparkinsonian.

USES:
Advanced forms of Parkinson's disease.

DOSAGE:
 One or two tablets once or twice a day.

FORMS:
Tablets of 5mg (white).

PRECAUTIONS:
Use with caution in pregnancy (B2), breast feeding and children.
Use with caution in heart disease, peptic ulcer, high blood pressure, angina and psychiatric conditions.
Normally used in conjunction with L-dopa (levodopa).
Do not take if:
 Other MAOI, pethidine or fluoxetine taken recently.

SIDE EFFECTS:
Common: Tremor, dry mouth, nausea, slow urination, sweating.
Unusual: Restlessness, hallucinations, headache, irregular heartbeat, vomiting, constipation, facial hair growth.

INTERACTIONS:
Other drugs:
- MAOI, pethidine, fluoxetine, moclobemide, SSRI, tricyclic antidepressants, tetracyclic antidepressants, clozapine, oral contraceptives, dopamine, tramadol, sympathomimetics.

Other substances:
- Ecstasy.

PRESCRIPTION:
Yes.

PBS:
Yes.

PERMITTED IN SPORT:
Yes.

OVERDOSE:
Very serious. Up to a 12 hour delay between taking overdose and onset of symptoms.
May cause drowsiness, dizziness, headache, hallucinations, convulsions, coma, irregular heartbeat and death. Administer activated charcoal or induce vomiting if medication taken recently. Seek urgent medical attention.

OTHER INFORMATION:
Does not cause addiction or dependence.
See also **LEVODOPA COMPOUNDS, MAOI**.

Selenium sulfide

TRADE NAME:
Selsun.

DRUG CLASS:
Antifungal.

USES:
Dandruff, mild fungal infections of skin and scalp.

DOSAGE:
 Apply to scalp for five minutes two or three times a week.

FORMS:
Lotion, shampoo.

PRECAUTIONS:
Safe to use in pregnancy, breast feeding and children.
Avoid eyes.
Do not use if:
 suffering from inflamed skin.
- permanent wave, tinting or bleaching of hair within two days.

SIDE EFFECTS:
Common: Minimal.
Severe but rare (stop medication, consult doctor): Skin irritation.

INTERACTIONS:
None significant.

PRESCRIPTION:
No.

PBS:
No.

PERMITTED IN SPORT:
Yes.

OVERDOSE:
Diarrhoea, nausea and vomiting may occur if swallowed.

OTHER INFORMATION:
Simple and effective treatment for dandruff and pityriasis versicolor (a common fungal skin condition that shows up as white patches).

Selenomethionine

TRADE NAME:
Selemite-B.
Also found in numerous other vitamin and mineral supplements.

DRUG CLASS:
Mineral.

USES:
Selenium deficiency.

DOSAGE:
 One to two tablets a day.

FORMS:
Tablet of 50µg (beige).

PRECAUTIONS:
Use with caution in pregnancy and breast feeding. Not for use under 15 years of age. Poisonous, do not exceed recommended dose.
Do not use if:
 suffering from significant kidney disease, yeast allergy.

SIDE EFFECTS:
Minimal.

INTERACTIONS:
Other substances: Heavy metals.

PRESCRIPTION:
Yes.

PBS:
No.

PERMITTED IN SPORT:
Yes.

OVERDOSE:
Poisonous. Induce vomiting or give activated charcoal if taken recently. Seek urgent medical attention.

Medications

Senega

TRADE NAME:
Marketed in Australia only in combination with other medications.
Senagar (with ammonium bicarbonate).

DRUG CLASS:
Expectorant.

USES:
Cough.

DOSAGE:
 10 to 20mLs every four hours.

FORMS:
Mixture.

PRECAUTIONS:
May be used in pregnancy, breast feeding and children over 1 year.
Do not take if:
 under one year of age.

SIDE EFFECTS:
Minimal.

INTERACTIONS:
Other drugs:
- Antacids, cimetidine, famotidine, nizatadine, ranitidine.

PRESCRIPTION:
No.

PBS:
No. Available to some Veteran Affairs pensioners.

PERMITTED IN SPORT:
Yes.

OVERDOSE:
Unlikely to cause any serious adverse effects.

OTHER INFORMATION:
Very old-fashioned remedy, but still effective.

Senna
See Sennosides.

Sennosides
(Senna)

TRADE NAMES:
Bekunis, Laxettes with Senna, Laxettes with Sennosides, Sennetabs, Senokot.
Agiolax (with fibre supplement).
Bioglan Prune and Senna (with prunes).
Coloxyl with Senna (with docusate sodium).

DRUG CLASS:
Laxative.

USES:
Constipation.

DOSAGE:
 Tablets: Two to four tablets once (before going to bed) or twice a day.
Granules: One or two teaspoonfuls a day.

FORMS:
Tablets, granules, chocolate squares.

PRECAUTIONS:
Safe in pregnancy (A) and breast feeding. May be used in children over 6 years. Do not use long term without medical advice.
Do not take if:
 suffering from stomach pain or gut obstruction, nausea, vomiting or diarrhoea.

SIDE EFFECTS:
Common: Minimal.
Unusual: Belly discomfort.
Severe but rare (stop medication, consult doctor): Severe belly pain.

INTERACTIONS:
None significant.

PRESCRIPTION:
No.

PBS:
No. Available in some forms for Veteran Affairs pensioners.

PERMITTED IN SPORT:
Yes.

OVERDOSE:
Diarrhoea and belly cramps only effects.

OTHER INFORMATION:
Safe and widely used.
See also Ispaghula.

Sertraline

TRADE NAME:
Zoloft.

DRUG CLASS:
SSRI antidepressant.

USES:
Depression.

DOSAGE:

One to four tablets a day in morning with or without food.

FORMS:
Tablet of 50 and 100mg (white)

PRECAUTIONS:
Should be used in pregnancy (B3) with considerable caution. Breastfeeding should be ceased if paroxetine prescribed. Not for use in children.
Should be used with caution in mania, epilepsy, liver and kidney disease.

Do not take if:
 taking MAOI antidepressants.

SIDE EFFECTS:
Common: Generally minimal. Nausea, drowsiness, sweating, tremor, tiredness, dry mouth, sleeplessness, impotence.
Unusual: Headache, fever, palpitations, sweating, rash, blurred vision.

INTERACTIONS:
Other drugs:
- Severe interaction with MAOI.
- Anticoagulants (eg. warfarin), phenytoin, tryptophan, lithium, tolbutamide, sumatriptan, fenfluramine.

Herbs:
- St John's wort, ma huang.

Other substances:
- Use of alcohol is not advised.

PRESCRIPTION:
Yes.

PBS:
Yes.

PERMITTED IN SPORT:
Yes.

OVERDOSE:
Symptoms may include nausea, tremor, dilated pupils, dry mouth and irritability. Death or serious effects unlikely. Seek medical attention.

OTHER INFORMATION:
One of the newer antidepressants released in Australia in the 1990s that has dramatically improved the treatment of depression because of its safety and lack of side effects. May take up to two weeks for patient to notice any improvement in depression.

See also Citalopram, Fluoxetine, Fluvoxamine, Paroxetine, Venlafaxine.

SEX HORMONES

DISCUSSION:

Sex hormones are produced by the ovaries in the woman and the testes in the man to give each sex its characteristic appearance. In men, they are responsible for the enlargement of the penis and scrotum at puberty, the development of facial hair and the ability to produce sperm and ejaculate. In women, the sex hormones that are produced for the first time at puberty cause breast enlargement, hair growth in the armpit and groin, ovulation, the start of menstrual periods, and later act to maintain a pregnancy.

If the sex hormones are reduced or lacking, these characteristics disappear. This happens naturally during the female menopause. During the transition from normal sex hormone production to no production in the menopause, there may be some irregular or inappropriate release of these hormones, causing the symptoms commonly associated with menopause such as irregular periods, irritability and hot flushes. After the menopause, the breasts sag, pubic and armpit hair becomes scanty, and the periods cease due to this lack of sex hormones. Men also go through a form of menopause, but more gradually, so the effects are far less obvious than in the female.

Sex hormones, and many synthesised drugs that act artificially as sex hormones, are used in medicine in two main areas – to correct natural deficiencies in sex hormone production; and to alter the balance between the two female hormones (oestrogen and progestogen) that cause ovulation, to prevent ovulation, and therefore act as a contraceptive.

It is now well recognised that hormone replacement therapy (HRT) in middle-aged women who have entered the menopause significantly improves their quality of life by not only controlling the symptoms of the menopause itself, but by preventing osteoporosis (bone weakening), reducing the apparent rate of ageing, reducing the risk of dementia, and reducing the risk of bowel cancer after the menopause. Women who have both their ovaries removed surgically at a time before their natural menopause will also require sex hormones to be given regularly by mouth, patch or injection.

Female sex hormones can also be used to control some forms of recurrent miscarriage and prolong a pregnancy until a baby is mature enough to deliver, to control endometriosis, and to treat certain types of cancer.

See Cyproterone acetate, Danazol, Dydrogesterone, Ethinyloestradiol, Etonogestrel, HORMONE REPLACEMENT THERAPY, Hydroxyprogesterone hexanoate, Medroxyprogesterone acetate, Oestradiol, Oestriol, Oestrogen, ORAL CONTRACEPTIVES, Oxandrolone, Piperazine oestrone sulfate, Testosterone.

Silbutramine

TRADE NAME:
Reductil.

DRUG CLASS:
Anorectic.

USES:
Obesity in conjunction with diet and exercise program.

DOSAGE:

One capsule a day.

FORMS:
Capsules of 10mg (blue/yellow) and 15mg (blue/white).

PRECAUTIONS:
Not for use in pregnancy (C), breast feeding and children.
Use with caution in liver and kidney disease, gallstones and epilepsy.

Regular checks of blood pressure and pulse necessary.
Not for long term use.

Do not take if:

 suffering from mental illness leading to excessive eating, Tourette syndrome, heart disease, recent stroke, uncontrolled high blood pressure, over-active thyroid gland (hyperthyroidism), enlarged prostate gland, glaucoma, history of drug abuse, severe liver or kidney disease.
- elderly.

SIDE EFFECTS:

Common: Rapid heart rate, dry mouth, sleeplessness.
Unusual: High blood pressure, nausea, diarrhoea.
Severe but rare (stop medication, consult doctor): Seizure.

INTERACTIONS:

Other drugs:
- Serious interactions with diethylpropion hydrochloride, orlistat, phentermine, MAOI.
- Sumatriptan, lithium, ketoconazole, macrolide antibiotics (eg. erythromycin), phenytoin, dexamethasone.

Other substances:
- Tryptophan.
- Excess alcohol.

PRESCRIPTION:
Yes.

PBS:
No.

PERMITTED IN SPORT:
No.

OVERDOSE:
Serious. May cause restlessness, tremor, rapid breathing, irregular heartbeat, high blood pressure, confusion, hallucinations, violence, panic state, vomiting, diarrhoea, coma, convulsions and death. Administer activated charcoal or induce vomiting if medication taken recently. Seek urgent medical attention.

OTHER INFORMATION:
Introduced in 2001. Must always be used in conjunction with an appropriate diet and exercise program. May be addictive.

See also Diethylpropion hydrochloride, Orlistat, Phentermine.

Sildenafil

TRADE NAME:
Viagra.

USES:
Impotence, inability to obtain erection of the penis with appropriate stimulation.

DOSAGE:
 25 to 100mg one to four hours before erection desired.

FORMS:
Tablets (blue) of 25, 50 and 100mg.

PRECAUTIONS:
No for use in pregnancy (B1), breast feeding or by children.
Not recommended for use by women.
Use with caution in all heart diseases, abnormal anatomy of the penis (eg. Peyronie's disease), bleeding disorders, peptic ulcer disease, untreated diabetes, multiple myeloma, leukaemia and all diseases of the retina in the eye.

Do not take if:

 taking medications containing nitrates (eg. antiangina medication such as glyceryl trinitrate).
- suffering from angina, untreated high blood pressure or recent stroke
- inherited disorders of the retina.
- suffering from significant liver disease.

SIDE EFFECTS:
Common: Headache, flush, indigestion.
Unusual: Blue halos in vision, blurred vision.
Severe but rare (stop medication, consult doctor): Serious adverse effects on the heart and circulation of blood, angina (chest pain).

INTERACTIONS:
Other drugs:
- Nitrate containing angina medications, other drugs for impotence, cimetidine, rifampicin, erythromycin, ketoconazole, saquinavir, ritonavir.

Herbs:
- Korean ginseng.

Other substances:
- Alcohol.

PRESCRIPTION:
Yes.

PBS:
No. Available on authority for some Veteran Affairs patients under very strict criteria.

PERMITTED IN SPORT:
Yes.

OVERDOSE:
May have adverse effects on the heart and circulation. Seek medical attention.

OTHER INFORMATION:
Introduced in 1998. Very effective, and generally very safe if precautions followed.
See also Alprostadil, Tadalafil.

Silver sulfadiazine (SSD)

TRADE NAME:
Silvazine (with chlorhexidine).

DRUG CLASS:
Antibiotic, Sulfonamide.

USES:
Burns, skin ulcers, sores.

DOSAGE:
 Apply very thickly once every day or two.

FORMS:
Cream.

PRECAUTIONS:
Not to be used in pregnancy (C) or newborn infants. May be used in breast feeding (but not on breast) and older children.
Use with caution in liver and kidney disease.

Do not use if:
 suffering from sulfur drug allergy.

SIDE EFFECTS:
Common: Minimal.
Unusual: Diarrhoea.
Severe but rare (stop medication, consult doctor): Damage to blood cells.

INTERACTIONS:
Other drugs:
- Oral hypoglycaemics (treat type 2 diabetes), phenytoin, cimetidine.

PRESCRIPTION:
Yes.

PBS:
Yes.

PERMITTED IN SPORT:
Yes.

Medications

OTHER INFORMATION:
Excellent cream for soothing serious burns and preventing or treating infection in burns and skin ulcers. Usually covered by a non-adhesive dressing over a thick (3 to 5mm) layer of cream.

Simethicone

TRADE NAMES:
De-Gas, De-Gas Infant, Infacol, Medefoam-2.
De-Gas Extra (with calcium carbonate, magnesium carbonate and other ingredients).
Gastrogel Tablets, Gelusil, Mucaine 2 in 1, Mylanta, Sigma Liquid Antacid (with aluminium hydroxide, magnesium hydroxide and other ingredients).
Imodium Advanced (with loperamide).
No Gas (with charcoal).
Titralac Sil (with calcium carbonate).

DRUG CLASS:
Antiflatulent.

USES:
Reduces the amount of gas produced in the gut, and therefore reduces burping, bubbling of gases in belly, and passage of wind.

DOSAGE:
 Taken as required for symptoms.

FORMS:
Capsules, drops and mixture.
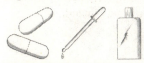

PRECAUTIONS:
Nil.
Safe in children, pregnancy (A) and breast feeding.

SIDE EFFECTS:
Minimal.

INTERACTIONS:
None reported.

PRESCRIPTION:
No.

PBS:
Yes – some forms only.

PERMITTED IN SPORT:
Yes.

OVERDOSE:
None significant.

OTHER INFORMATION:
Safe and widely used medication.
See also **ANTACIDS**.

Simvastatin

TRADE NAMES:
Lipex, Zocor.

DRUG CLASS:
Hypolipidaemic.

USES:
Excess blood levels of cholesterol.

DOSAGE:
 10 to 80mg a day at night.

FORMS:
Tablets of 5, 10, 20, 40 and 80mg.

PRECAUTIONS:
Should not be used in pregnancy (C) unless no alternative available. Not for use in breast feeding or children.
Regular blood tests to check blood fats and liver enzymes are necessary.
Use with caution in liver and kidney disease.

Do not take if:

 suffering from severe liver disease, myopathy.

SIDE EFFECTS:

Common: Constipation, diarrhoea, excess wind, nausea, headache.
Unusual: Vomiting, heartburn, back pain, muscle pain, dizziness, sleeplessness, cough, bronchitis, pins and needles sensation, rash, sinusitis, blurred vision, depression.
Severe but rare (stop medication, consult doctor): Yellow skin (jaundice), severe muscle pain and weakness.

INTERACTIONS:

Other drugs:
- Anticoagulants (eg. warfarin), niacin, nicotinic acid, digoxin, verapamil, gemfibrizol, cyclosporin, nefazodone, ketoconazole, itraconazole, macrolide antibiotics (eg. erythromycin, clarithromycin).

Other treatments:
- Immunosuppressive treatment.

Herbs:
- Alfalfa, fenugreek, garlic, ginger.

Other substances:
- Grapefruit juice.

PRESCRIPTION:
Yes.

PBS:
Yes.

PERMITTED IN SPORT:
Yes.

OVERDOSE:
Liver stress only likely effect.

OTHER INFORMATION:
Released in the late 1980s and has radically improved the treatment of excess cholesterol. Very safe and generally well tolerated.

See also Atorvastatin, Cholestyramine, Colestipol, Fluvastatin, Gemfibrizol, Nicotinic acid, Pravastatin, Probucol.

Sirolimus

TRADE NAME:
Rapamune.

DRUG CLASS:
Immunomodifier.

USES:
Prevents rejection of kidney transplants.

DOSAGE:
 2mg once a day initially, then adjust depending on results of blood tests. Take solution with orange juice.

FORMS:
Tablets of 1mg (white), solution.

PRECAUTIONS:
Use with significant caution in pregnancy (C), breast feeding and children under 13 years.
Use with caution in liver disease.
Avoid excess sunlight and UV rays.
Increased risk of cancers and infections.
Regular blood tests essential to monitor kidney function.

SIDE EFFECTS:
Common: Fever, tissue swelling, poor healing, belly pain, diarrhoea.
Unusual: High cholesterol levels, anaemia, abnormal blood chemistry, joint pains, acne.
Severe but rare (stop medication, consult doctor): Blood clots (thrombosis), lung damage, liver damage.

INTERACTIONS:
Other drugs:
- Cyclosporin, drugs that lower cholesterol, rifampicin, ketoconazole, diltiazem.
- Live vaccines (eg. polio).

Other substances:
- Grapefruit juice.

Medications

PRESCRIPTION:
Yes.

PBS:
No.

PERMITTED IN SPORT:
Yes.

OTHER INFORMATION:
Introduced in 2002. Must be taken regularly and consistently to be effective.

Sodium acid citrate
See ELECTROLYTES.

Sodium alginate
See ANTACIDS.

Sodium ascorbate
See Ascorbic acid.

Sodium aurothiomalate
(Gold)

TRADE NAME:
Myocrisin

DRUG CLASS:
Antirheumatic.

USES:
Rheumatoid arthritis.

DOSAGE:

Weekly injections until condition controlled, then reduce frequency slowly.

FORMS:
Injection.

PRECAUTIONS:
Should be used with caution in pregnancy (B2), breast feeding and children.
Use with caution in liver and kidney disease. Regular blood and urine tests required to assess kidney and liver function, blood cells and effectiveness of treatment.

Do not take if:
 suffering from severe liver or kidney disease, diabetes, severe eczema, some blood diseases.

SIDE EFFECTS:
Common: Dermatitis, itch, mouth ulcers, flushing, fainting.
Unusual: Sweating, dizziness, weakness, feeling unwell, eye damage, kidney damage.
Severe but rare (stop medication, consult doctor): Severe rash, unusual bleeding or bruising.

INTERACTIONS:
Other drugs:
- Phenylbutazone, penicillamine, ACE inhibitors.

PRESCRIPTION:
Yes.

PBS:
Yes.

PERMITTED IN SPORT:
Yes.

OTHER INFORMATION:
An unusual but remarkably effective treatment that has been used for over 30 years. Careful monitoring of blood tests and skin reactions essential. Gold is not addictive when swallowed or injected, only when collected!

See also Auranofin.

Sodium bicarbonate

See ANTACIDS, ELECTROLYTES.

Sodium carbonate

See ANTACIDS.

Sodium chloride
(Common Salt)

See ELECTROLYTES.

Sodium citrotartrate

See URINARY ALKALINISERS.

Sodium clodronate

TRADE NAME:

Bonefos.

USES:

High levels of calcium in blood and bone pain due to bone tumours.

DOSAGE:

 2400 to 3200mg once a day initially, reducing to 1600mg once a day. Do not take within two hours of food.

FORMS:

Capsules of 400mg (yellow), tablets of 800mg (white).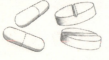

PRECAUTIONS:

Use with caution in pregnancy (B3), breast feeding and children.
Use with caution in dehydration and kidney disease.
Regular blood tests to check calcium levels necessary.
Maintain adequate fluid intake.

Do not take if:

 suffering from severe intestinal inflammation.

SIDE EFFECTS:

Common: Low blood calcium, stomach upsets.
Severe but rare (stop medication, consult doctor): Blood chemistry disorders, kidney failure, asthma.

INTERACTIONS:

Other drugs:
- Other medications affecting phosphorus or calcium levels.
- Estamustine, NSAIDs, antacids.

PRESCRIPTION:

Yes.

PBS:

Yes.

PERMITTED IN SPORT:

Yes.

OVERDOSE:

Serious blood chemistry disorders possible that may lead to major organ failure. Seek urgent medical attention. Induce vomiting or give activated charcoal if swallowed recently.

Sodium cromoglycate
(Cromolyn sodium, Disodium cromoglycate)

TRADE NAMES:
Cromese, Intal (for use in lungs).
Opticrom (for use in eyes).
Rynacrom (for use in nose).

USES:
Prevention (but not treatment) of asthma.
Prevention (but not treatment) of hay fever.
Prevention (but not treatment) of allergic reactions in the eye.

DOSAGE:

Inhaler: Two inhalations up to four times a day.
Nose spray: One spray two to four times a day.
Eye drops: One or two drops into eye, four to six times a day.

FORMS:
For use in eye: Drops (keep in door of refrigerator).
For use in lungs: Capsules for spinhaler (keep cool), metered aerosol, nebuliser solution.
For use in nose: Nose spray.

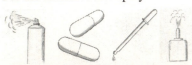

PRECAUTIONS:
Safe in pregnancy (A), children and breast feeding.

Do not stop suddenly from full dose, as recurrence of asthma or allergic condition may occur.

SIDE EFFECTS:
Common: Hoarse voice and bad taste with inhaled forms.
Unusual: Headache, stuffy nose, nosebleed, throat irritation.
Severe but rare (stop medication, consult doctor): Rash, hives, increased wheezing, joint pain, muscle pain, palpitations.

INTERACTIONS:
None significant.

PRESCRIPTION:
Yes.

PBS:
Most forms: Yes.
Nose spray: No (available to Veteran Affairs pensioners).

PERMITTED IN SPORT:
Yes.

OVERDOSE:
No problems encountered other than increased likelihood of side effects.

OTHER INFORMATION:
Excellent cheap and effective medication for prevention of many allergies and asthma. Minimal side effects. Very safe. In use for over 30 years and actions well understood. Newer presentation in pressurised inhaler and higher doses has increased use in recent years. Does not cause dependence or addiction. Cromoglycate is a preventative medication and cannot be used to treat asthma, hay fever or allergy reactions in the eye.

See also **Beclomethasone, Budesonide, Fluticasone propionate, Montelukast.**

Sodium fluoride
See **Fluoride.**

Sodium fusidate

TRADE NAMES:
Fucidin Topical.
Fucidin (with fusidic acid).

DRUG CLASS:
Antibiotic.

USES:
Infections caused by susceptible bacteria, particularly lung, heart and skin infections.

DOSAGE:

Tablets: Two tablets three times a day with meals.
Ointment: Apply two or three times a day for seven days.

FORMS:
Tablets, suspension, ointment, infusion.

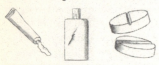

PRECAUTIONS:
Should not be used in pregnancy (C) unless medically essential. Should be used with caution in breast feeding and infants. Safe for use in children.
Ointment relatively safe in pregnancy except for last month.
Not designed for long term use.
Use with caution in liver disease.

SIDE EFFECTS:
Common: Ointment – Skin irritation, skin pain.
Swallowed forms – Nausea, loss of appetite, diarrhoea.
Unusual: Belly discomfort, vomiting, dizziness.
Severe but rare (stop medication, consult doctor): Yellow skin (jaundice).

INTERACTIONS:
Other drugs:
- Lincomycin, rifampicin.

PRESCRIPTION:
Yes.

PBS:
Tablets, suspension: Yes (restricted to certain severe infections).
Other forms: No.

PERMITTED IN SPORT:
Yes.

OVERDOSE:
Belly pain and diarrhoea likely. Long term overdosage may cause liver damage.

OTHER INFORMATION:
Used only for more severe and complex infections, particularly in cystic fibrosis.

Sodium hyaluronate

TRADE NAMES:
AMO Vitrax, Fermathron, Healon, ProVisc, Vismed.
Duo Visc, Viscoat (with sodium chondroitin sulfate).
Ophthalin (with other ingredients).

USES:
Dry eyes, osteoarthritic pain in the knee, protection of cornea during eye operations.

DOSAGE:
Eye drops: One or two drops in eye as often as needed.
Injection: One injection into knee every week for five weeks gives up to six month's relief of arthritis pain.

FORMS:
Injection, solution, eye drops.

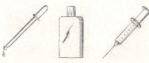

PRECAUTIONS:
Eye drops may be used safely in pregnancy and breast feeding.
Do not use other eye drops within five minutes.
Do not have injection if:
☠ suffering from skin disease or infection near knee.
• under 16 years.

SIDE EFFECTS:
Common: Eye drops – Short term blurred vision after use.
Injection – Temporary pain, swelling and inflammation of knee.
Severe but rare (stop medication, consult doctor): Injection – Infection of knee joint.

INTERACTIONS:
None significant.

PRESCRIPTION:
Eye drops: No.
Injection: Yes.

PBS:
Eye drops: Some brands available on PBS.
Injection: No.

PERMITTED IN SPORT:
Yes.

OTHER INFORMATION:
Injection introduced in 2000 as a radical new form of treatment for otherwise intractable arthritis. Used in eyes for many years.

Sodium iodide
(Iodine, radioactive; I131)

TRADE NAME:
Sodium iodide.

USES:
Over-active thyroid gland (hyperthyroidism), thyroid cancer.

DOSAGE:
 Very strictly as directed by doctor.

FORMS:
Capsules (yellow), injection.

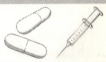

PRECAUTIONS:
Absolutely forbidden in pregnancy (X), breast feeding and children.
Ensure adequate contraception for at least two months before and after dosage.
Patient should avoid close contact with children for 10 days after dosage.
Ensure high fluid intake for 10 days after dosage.
Do not take if:
 suffering from kidney disease, vomiting or diarrhoea.

SIDE EFFECTS:
Common: Nausea, diarrhoea, itch, rapid heart rate.
Unusual: Vomiting, inflamed salivary glands, radiation sickness, lung damage, anaemia, bone marrow damage.
Severe but rare: Critical thyroid reaction, death.

INTERACTIONS:
Other drugs:
• Antithyroid drugs (eg. propylthiouracil), thyroxine, x-ray contract dye.
Other substances:
• Seafood, iodine containing foods.

PRESCRIPTION:
No.

PBS:
No.

OVERDOSE:
Significant overdose likely to be fatal.

OTHER INFORMATION:
Radioactive iodine is taken up specifically by the thyroid gland, and selectively destroys the most active cells in that gland. Very effective and commonly used treatment for both thyroid cancer and hyperthyroidism.

Sodium lauryl sulfoacetate

TRADE NAMES:
Fleet Microenema, Microlax (with sodium citrate).

DRUG CLASS:
Laxative.

USES:
Constipation. Used to prepare lower bowel before examination by doctor.

DOSAGE:
 One tube rectally at night.

FORMS:
Rectal enema in tube.

PRECAUTIONS:
Safe in pregnancy (A), breast feeding and children.
Insert only half nozzle length in children under 3 years.

SIDE EFFECTS:
Common: Minimal.
Unusual: Rectal burning sensation.

INTERACTIONS:
None significant.

PRESCRIPTION:
No.

PBS:
Yes.

PERMITTED IN SPORT:
Yes.

OVERDOSE:
Diarrhoea only effect.

OTHER INFORMATION:
Commonly used in elderly. Very safe and effective.
See Bisacodyl, Docusate sodium, Frangula, Glycerol, Lactulose, Paraffin, Psyllium, Sennosides, Sodium phosphate, Sodium picosulfate, Sorbitol, Sterculia.

Sodium perborate

TRADE NAME:
Amosan.

DRUG CLASS:
Antiseptic.

USES:
Mouth and gum inflammation and soreness.

DOSAGE:
 One sachet dissolved in water and used as mouthwash four times a day after meals.

FORMS:
Powder.

PRECAUTIONS:
Safe to use in pregnancy, breast feeding and children.
Do not swallow.

SIDE EFFECTS:
Minimal.

Medications

INTERACTIONS:
None significant.

PRESCRIPTION:
No.

PBS:
No.

PERMITTED IN SPORT:
Yes.

OVERDOSE:
Diarrhoea and nausea only likely effects if swallowed in large quantities.

Sodium phosphate

TRADE NAMES:
Fleet Phospho-Soda, Fleet Enema, Phosphoprep, Travad Phosphate Enema.

DRUG CLASS:
Laxative.

USES:
To clean bowel prior to surgery or colonoscopy, severe constipation.

DOSAGE:
 As directed by doctor for each patient, depending upon purpose.

FORMS:
Mixture, enema.

PRECAUTIONS:
Use with caution in pregnancy and breast feeding.
Use with caution in diabetes, kidney disease, electrolyte disturbances, colostomy, belly pain, vomiting, people prone to dehydration.
Reduce dose in elderly.
Not for repeated use.

Do not take if:
☠ suffering from bowel obstruction, bowel paralysis, impacted faeces, megacolon, ascites, poor kidney function, congestive heart failure, dehydration, ileostomy.
• under 12 years of age.

SIDE EFFECTS:
Common: Dehydration, nausea, electrolyte imbalances.
Unusual: Vomiting, allergic reactions.

INTERACTIONS:
Other drugs:
• Diuretics, lithium.
• Will affect absorption of all swallowed medications, including oral contraceptive pill.

PRESCRIPTION:
No.

PBS:
No.

PERMITTED IN SPORT:
Yes (guaranteed to cause failure in any sport!).

OVERDOSE:
Severe diarrhoea and dehydration with significant electrolyte disturbances that may lead to organ damage and heart attack. Vomiting likely after overdose as side effect of medication.

OTHER INFORMATION:
Normally only used as a preparation for a medical procedure on the large bowel in association with a strict diet, but may be used in cases of severe persistent constipation.

See Bisacodyl, Docusate sodium, FIBRE, Frangula, Glycerol, Lactulose, Paraffin, Poloxamer, Psyllium, Sennosides, Sodium lauryl sulfoacetate, Sodium picosulfate, Sorbitol, Sterculia.

Sodium picosulfate

TRADE NAMES:
Durolax SP, Picolax.
Picoprep (with other ingredients).

DRUG CLASS:
Laxative.

USES:
Preparation of bowel for surgery or colonoscopy, constipation.

DOSAGE:

Drops: 10 to 20 drops at night.
Powder: As determined for each patient by doctor, depending on reason for use.

FORMS:
Powder for solution, drops.

PRECAUTIONS:
Not to be used in pregnancy (C) or children under 20Kg.
Use with caution in breast feeding and children.
Use with caution in heart and kidney disease, phenylketonuria, dehydration, electrolyte disturbances, if prone to aspiration.
Reduce dose in elderly.

Do not take if:
 suffering from bowel obstruction, bowel paralysis, belly pain, colitis, bowel inflammation.

SIDE EFFECTS:
Common: Nausea, bloating, anal irritation, belly discomfort.
Unusual: Vomiting, recurrence of constipation.

INTERACTIONS:
Other drugs:
- Affects absorption of all swallowed medications, including oral contraceptive pill.

PRESCRIPTION:
No.

PBS:
No.

PERMITTED IN SPORT:
Yes.

OVERDOSE:
Severe diarrhoea and dehydration with significant electrolyte disturbances that may lead to organ damage and heart attack. Vomiting likely after overdose as side effect of medication.

See Bisacodyl, Docusate sodium, FIBRE, Frangula, Glycerol, Lactulose, Paraffin, Poloxamer, Psyllium, Sennosides, Sodium phosphate, Sorbitol, Sterculia.

Sodium polystyrene sulfonate

TRADE NAME:
Resonium A.

DRUG CLASS:
Detoxifying agent.

USES:
Reducing very high blood potassium levels.

DOSAGE:
 15g one to four times a day.

FORMS:
Powder.

Medications

PRECAUTIONS:
May be used in pregnancy, breast feeding and children over 1 year of age.
Use with caution in heart disease, high blood pressure and tissue swelling. Regular blood tests to monitor effect on blood chemistry essential.

Do not take if:

 suffering from bowel obstruction.

SIDE EFFECTS:
Common: Loss of appetite, bowel discomfort, constipation, nausea, vomiting.
Unusual: Impaction of faeces, stomach ulcer.

INTERACTIONS:
Other drugs:
- Digoxin, antacids, laxatives.

Other substances:
- Reacts with fruit juices.

PRESCRIPTION:
Yes.

PBS:
No. Available to Veteran Affairs pensioners.

PERMITTED IN SPORT:
Yes.

OVERDOSE:
Severe constipation possible.

OTHER INFORMATION:
Resonium A is not absorbed from the gut, but draws potassium out of the body to pass out in the faeces.

Sodium propionate

TRADE NAME:
Only available in Australia in combination with Salicylic acid.
Mycoderm (with salicylic acid).

DRUG CLASS:
Antifungal.

USES:
Fungal skin infections (eg. tinea, athlete's foot, ringworm).

DOSAGE:
 Apply two or three times a day.

FORMS:
Powder, cream.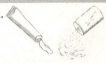

PRECAUTIONS:
Safe to use in pregnancy, breast feeding and children.

SIDE EFFECTS:
Minimal.

INTERACTIONS:
None.

PRESCRIPTION:
No.

PBS:
No.

PERMITTED IN SPORT:
Yes.

OTHER INFORMATION:
Often used on feet to prevent recurrence of tinea (athlete's foot).
See also IMIDAZOLES, Nystatin.

Sodium valproate

TRADE NAMES:
Epilim, Valpro.

DRUG CLASS:
Anticonvulsant.

USES:
Epilepsy.

DOSAGE:

Dosage increased slowly until desired control achieved, usually between 1000mg and 2000mg a day taken in one or more doses with or after food.

FORMS:
Tablets of 100mg, 200mg and 500mg; syrup, liquid.

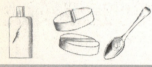

PRECAUTIONS:
Not to be taken in pregnancy (D) unless medically essential as the risk of foetal abnormality is significantly increased.
Use with caution in breast feeding. May be used in children.
Use with caution in in kidney disease and during surgery (may increase bleeding).
Use with care in bleeding disorders (eg. thrombocytopenia).
Do not stop medication suddenly, but reduce dosage slowly.
Syrup not for use in diabetes.

Do not take if:
 suffering from liver disease.
- family history of severe liver disease.

SIDE EFFECTS:
Common: Usually reduced by using slow release form or reducing dosage. Nausea, belly cramps, loss of appetite, diarrhoea.
Unusual: Drowsiness, hair loss, rash, irregular menstrual periods, swelling of tissues.

Severe but rare (stop medication, consult doctor): Unusual bleeding or bruising, yellow skin (jaundice), severe belly pain.

INTERACTIONS:
Other drugs:
- Other anticonvulsants (eg. ethosuximide), sedatives, lorazepam, midazolam, clozapine, diazepam, clonazepam, aspirin, anticoagulants (eg. warfarin), psychotropics (eg. chlorpromazine), fluoxetine, MAOI.

Herbs:
- Evening primrose (linoleic acid), Gingko biloba.

Other substances:
- Reacts adversely with alcohol.
- Borage.

PRESCRIPTION:
Yes.

PBS:
Yes.

PERMITTED IN SPORT:
Yes.

OVERDOSE:
Death possible but rare. Symptoms include drowsiness, slow breathing, incoordination, confusion and coma. Administer activated charcoal or induce vomiting if taken recently and patient alert. Seek urgent medical attention.

OTHER INFORMATION:
Very effective and relatively safe medication that has improved the life of many epileptics. Not addictive or dependence-forming.

See also BARBITURATES, BENZODIAZEPINES, Carbamazepine, Clonazepam, Ethosuximide, Gabapentin, Lamotrigine, Levetiracetam, Oxcarbazepine, Phenytoin, Primidone, Sulthiame, Tiagabine, Topiramate, Vigabatrin.

Somatropin
(Growth hormone)

TRADE NAMES:
Genotropin, Humatrope, Norditropin, Saizen, SciTropin.

DRUG CLASS:
Hormone.

USES:
Short stature due to growth hormone deficiency in children.

DOSAGE:
 Administered weekly by injection.

FORMS:
Injection.

PRECAUTIONS:
Not for use in pregnancy or breast feeding.
Use with caution in diabetes, ACTH deficiency, underactive thyroid gland, slipped epiphysis, increased pressure within brain.
Do not exceed recommended dose.

Do not take if:
 Suffering from active tumour, cancer, brain growths.
- Recent surgery or major injury.
- Adult.

SIDE EFFECTS:
Common: Irritation at injection site, allergy reaction, fluid retention, fat loss.
Unusual: Underactive thyroid gland, diabetes, slipped bony epiphysis.
Severe but rare (stop medication, consult doctor): Increased pressure of fluid within brain.

INTERACTIONS:
Other drugs:
- Steroids, sex hormones, cyclosporin.

PRESCRIPTION:
Yes.

PBS:
Yes (authority required for limited indications. Very strictly controlled).

PERMITTED IN SPORT:
No.

OVERDOSE:
Overgrowth of bones leading to pressure on nerves and brain (acromegaly), and imbalance in body's ability to deal with glucose.

OTHER INFORMATION:
Used illegally by some sportsmen to aid body building.

Sorbide Nitrate
See Isosorbide Nitrate.

Sorbitol

TRADE NAMES:
Sorbilax.
Aquae (with carmellose sodium).
Carbosorb S (with charcoal).
Fleet Micro-Enema, Microlax (with sodium citrate and sodium lauryl sulfoacetate).
Medevac (with arachis oil).

DRUG CLASS:
Laxative, softening agent.

USES:
Softening faeces in constipation, softening bile, lubricant.

DOSAGE:
 Liquid: 20mLs three times a day.
Enema: Once a day into rectum.
Mouth spray: Spray as often as required for dry mouth.

Home Guide to Medication

Medications

FORMS:
Mouth spray, suspension, enema, liquid.

PRECAUTIONS:
Usually safe to use in pregnancy, breast feeding and children.
Not for prolonged use.
Use with caution in diabetes.

Do not take if:
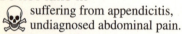 suffering from appendicitis, undiagnosed abdominal pain.
- intolerant to fructose.

SIDE EFFECTS:
Common: Passing excess wind, diarrhoea.
Severe but rare (stop medication, consult doctor): Disturbances to blood chemistry (electrolytes).

INTERACTIONS:
Other drugs:
- Other laxatives, may interfere with absorption of any medication taken by mouth, including oral contraceptives.
- Antacids, narcotics.

Other substances:
- Fructose-containing foods.

PRESCRIPTION:
No.

PBS:
No.

PERMITTED IN SPORT:
Yes.

OVERDOSE:
Exacerbation of side effects likely. May cause serious blood chemistry disorders.

OTHER INFORMATION:
Widely used and safe in correct dosage.
See Bisacodyl, Docusate sodium, Fibre, Frangula, Glycerol, Lactulose, Paraffin, Poloxamer, Psyllium, Sennosides, Sodium phosphate, Sodium picosulfate, Sterculia.

Sotalol

TRADE NAMES:
Cardol, GenRx Sotalol, Solavert, Sotab, Sotacor, Sotahexal.
Other locally produced brands also exist.

DRUG CLASS:
Beta blocker.

USES:
Irregular heartbeat, paroxysmal atrial tachycardia.

DOSAGE:
 160 to 320mg a day in divided doses.

FORMS:
Tablets of 80 and 160mg, injection.
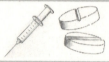

PRECAUTIONS:
Should be used in pregnancy (C) only if medically essential.
Safe to use in breast feeding.
May be used with caution in children.
Use with care if suffering from alcoholism, diabetes, psoriasis, hyperthyroidism (over-active thyroid gland), liver or kidney failure, or about to have surgery.
Regular checks on heart rhythm essential.
Do not stop suddenly, but reduce dose gradually.

Do not take if:
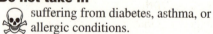 suffering from diabetes, asthma, or allergic conditions.
- suffering from heart failure, shock, slow heart rate, or enlarged right heart.
- if undertaking prolonged fast.

SIDE EFFECTS:
Common: Low blood pressure, slow heart rate, cold hands and feet, asthma.
Unusual: Loss of appetite, nausea, diarrhoea, impotence, tiredness, sleeplessness, nightmares, rash, loss of

libido, hair loss, noises in ears, dizziness.
Severe but rare (stop medication, consult doctor): Severe asthma.

INTERACTIONS:
Other drugs:
- Calcium channel blockers, disopyramide, clonidine, adrenaline, other medications for irregular heartbeat, lignocaine, ergotamine, indomethacin, chlorpromazine.

PRESCRIPTION:
Yes.

PBS:
Yes.

PERMITTED IN SPORT:
Restricted in some sports (eg. shooting, archery). Check with sport's governing body.

OVERDOSE:
Slow heart rate, low blood pressure, asthma and heart failure may result. Administer activated charcoal or induce vomiting if tablets taken recently. Use Salbutamol or other asthma sprays for difficulty in breathing. Seek medical assistance.

See also Atenolol, Carvedilol, Esmolol, Labetalol, Metoprolol, Oxprenolol, Pindolol, Propranolol.

SPASMOLYTICS

DISCUSSION:
Medications that ease spasms of the intestine to prevent colic.
See Dicyclomine, Hyoscine and Hyoscyamine.

Spectinomycin

TRADE NAME:
Trobicin.

DRUG CLASS:
Antibiotic.

USES:
Severe or resistant gonorrhoea (venereal disease).

DOSAGE:
 Single injection.

FORMS:
Injection.

PRECAUTIONS:
Use with caution in pregnancy (B1), breast feeding and infants. Safe to use in children.
Use with caution with syphilis and Chlamydia infections.

SIDE EFFECTS:
Common: Dizziness, nausea, chills, fever.
Unusual: Sleeplessness.

INTERACTIONS:
Other drugs:
- Muscle relaxants, anaesthetics.

PRESCRIPTION:
Yes.

PBS:
Yes.

PERMITTED IN SPORT:
Yes.

OTHER INFORMATION:
Very effective and safe medication.

SPERMICIDES

TRADE and GENERIC NAMES:
Ortho-Creme (nonoxynol 9).
Ortho-Gynol (octoxinol).

DRUG CLASS:
Contraceptive.

USES:
For use in combination with a diaphragm or condom to prevent pregnancy, kills sperm.

DOSAGE:
 Varies with form and product. Use strictly in accordance with directions on packaging.

FORMS:
Cream, gel.

PRECAUTIONS:
Safe if used accidentally in pregnancy (A). Safe in breast feeding. Not designed for use in children.
Wait six to eight hours after sex before removing diaphragm or using douche.
Do not retain diaphragm for more than 24 hours.
Ensure hands and diaphragm are completely clean before insertion.

SIDE EFFECTS:
Common: Minimal.
Unusual: Irritation of vagina or penis.

INTERACTIONS:
None.

PRESCRIPTION:
No.

PBS:
No.

PERMITTED IN SPORT:
Yes.

OTHER INFORMATION:
Not a reliable form of contraception if used alone. Even in combination with a diaphragm or condom, Spermicides have a failure rate of about 5% (ie: five out of 100 fertile women using this method of contraception for a year will fall pregnant).

Spironolactone

TRADE NAMES:
Aldactone, Spiractin.

DRUG CLASS:
Diuretic (aldosterone antagonist).

USES:
High blood pressure, congestive cardiac failure, excess fluid retention, cirrhosis of liver, nephrotic syndrome (kidney disease), prevents low blood potassium levels, excessive hairiness in women, primary hyperaldosteronism.

DOSAGE:
 Varies depending on usage from 25mg to 400mg a day in one or several doses.

FORMS:
Tablets of 25mg and 100mg.

PRECAUTIONS:
Should not be used in pregnancy (B3) unless medically essential. Should not be used in breast feeding or children. Regular blood tests for level of blood chemicals (electrolytes) may be necessary.

Do not take if:
 suffering from kidney failure, excess potassium in blood.

SIDE EFFECTS:
Common: Breast enlargement (both sexes), diarrhoea, gut cramps.
Unusual: Tiredness, headache, confusion, rash, fever, incoordination, impotence, irregular menstruation.
Severe but rare (stop medication, consult doctor): Unusual bleeding.

INTERACTIONS:
Other drugs:
- Do not take with potassium supplements, amiloride or triamterene.
- Reacts with carbenoxolone, digoxin.
- ACE inhibitors, NSAIDs.

Herbs:
- Celery, dandelion, liquorice, uva ursi.

PRESCRIPTION:
Yes.

PBS:
Yes.

PERMITTED IN SPORT:
No.

OVERDOSE:
Large doses required for adverse effects. Pins and needles sensation, weakness, muscle spasms and paralysis are possible symptoms. Induce vomiting if tablets taken recently. Give extra fluids. Seek medical assistance.

OTHER INFORMATION:
An old-fashioned medication for removal of excess fluid from the body that has recently been given a new life because of its ability to reduce excess facial hair (hirsutism) in women. Must be taken for many months for this purpose.
See also Amiloride, Bumetanide, Ethacrynic Acid, Frusemide, Indapamide, THIAZIDE DIURETICS.

SSD
See Silver sulfadiazine.

SSRI (SELECTIVE SEROTONIN REUPTAKE INHIBITORS)
See Citalopram, Fluoxetine, Fluvoxamine, Paroxetine, Sertraline, Venlafaxine.

Stavudine

TRADE NAME:
Zerit.

DRUG CLASS:
Antiviral.

USES:
HIV infection, AIDS.

DOSAGE:

Dosage as determined by doctor taken twice a day.

FORMS:
Capsules of 15mg (yellow/red), 20mg (light brown), 30mg (light orange/dark orange), 40mg (dark orange).

PRECAUTIONS:
Use with caution in pregnancy (B3), breast feeding and children under 12 years.
Use with caution in peripheral neuropathy (nerve inflammation), pancreatitis, liver and kidney disease.
Use with care if obese.
Use long term only on strict advice of doctor.

SIDE EFFECTS:
Common: Nerve pain and inflammation, inflammation of pancreas.
Unusual: Liver damage.

INTERACTIONS:
Other drugs:
- Zidovudine, didanosine, hydroxyurea, trimethoprim.

Medications

PRESCRIPTION:
Yes.

PBS:
Yes (restricted to specific patients with HIV infection on request to Commonwealth Government).

PERMITTED IN SPORT:
Yes.

OVERDOSE:
No information available. Seek urgent medical attention. Induce vomiting or administer activated charcoal if taken recently.

OTHER INFORMATION:
Introduced in 1997.
See Abacavir, Delavirdine, Didanosine, Efavirenz, Indinavir, Lamivudine, Nelfinavir, Nevirapine, Ritonavir, Saquinavir, Tenofovir, Zalcitabine, Zidovudine.

Sterculia

TRADE NAMES:
Normafibe.
Alvercol (with alverine citrate).
Granocol, Normacol Plus (with frangula).

DRUG CLASS:
Fibre, laxative.

USES:
Constipation.

DOSAGE:

Take one or two heaped teaspoons with water twice a day at least two hours before bed time.

FORMS:
Granules, powder.

PRECAUTIONS:
Safe in pregnancy and breast feeding.
Safe in children over 6 years.
Ensure adequate fluid intake.
Do not take if:
 about to go to bed.
- suffering from ulcerative colitis.

SIDE EFFECTS:
Common: Minimal.
Unusual: Diarrhoea, belly discomfort.

INTERACTIONS:
None significant.

PRESCRIPTION:
No.

PBS:
Some forms: Yes.

PERMITTED IN SPORT:
Yes.

OVERDOSE:
Take additional water. Belly discomfort and passing excess wind only effects.

OTHER INFORMATION:
Widely used, natural fibre supplement.
See Bisacodyl, Docusate sodium, FIBRE, Frangula, Glycerol, Lactulose, Paraffin, Poloxamer, Psyllium, Sennosides, Sorbitol.

STEROIDS
(CORTICOSTEROIDS)

DISCUSSION:

Cholesterol is the base substance from which the body produces natural steroids. There are many different types of steroids, including sex hormones, anabolic steroids (that are often abused by athletes) and trophic hormones (see separate entries). The type being described here are more correctly called corticosteroid hormones. They act as powerful reducers of inflammation in damaged tissue. Artificial steroids have been synthesised to control a wide range of diseases, including asthma, arthritis, dermatitis, eczema, and severe allergy reactions.

Steroids are available as tablets, mixtures, injections, creams, nasal sprays, inhaled sprays, eye drops, ear drops and suppositories. They are therefore an extremely useful group of drugs in a wide variety of conditions.

The actions of steroids include shrinking down inflamed tissue (eg. in allergies, injuries, piles) to normal, reducing itching (eg. in eczema and bites), and opening up airways by reducing mucus secretion and shrinking swollen tissue (eg. hay fever, asthma).

When used on the skin or on the surface of the airways (lungs, nose), side effects are uncommon. Overuse of sprays used for asthma is quite safe, but overuse in the nose can cause tissue damage. Creams and ointments that contain strong steroids should not be overused, particularly in children and on the face, as they can cause skin thinning and damage. Taken as injection into joints, steroids are very successful at controlling arthritis, but again, overuse may cause weakness and damage to the joint tissue instead of controlling the disease.

The greatest dangers occur when steroids are taken as tablets. Short courses, in which a high dose is given at the start and then reduced rapidly to zero over a couple of weeks, are quite safe. Low doses given for quite long periods of time are also relatively safe, but when high doses are given for months on end, damage can occur in the body.

Side effects of prolonged steroid tablet use include tissue swelling, an imbalance in blood chemicals, high blood pressure, weight gain, peptic ulcers, brittle bones (fracturing easily), heart failure, muscle weakness, delayed wound healing, headache, abnormal menstrual periods, fatty deposits under the skin, blood clots, cataracts, glaucoma and a host of rarer conditions. It is therefore obvious why doctors use these remarkably effective drugs with great caution. In some situations, the seriousness of the disease warrants taking the risk of using steroids to give a patient relief, or even saving a life.

If used judiciously, steroids can dramatically improve a patient's quality of life, but doctors must always be aware of the pros and cons of their use in every individual.

See Alclometasone, Beclomethasone dipropionate, Betamethasone, Budesonide, Cortisone acetate, Desonide, Dexamethasone, Fludrocortisone, Flumethasone, Fluorometholone, Fluticasone, Hydrocortisone, Medrysone, Methylprednisolone, Mometasone, Prednisolone and Prednisone, Triamcinolone.

STIMULANTS

DISCUSSION:
Stimulants are used in medicine to treat disorders of excessive sleep, some types of senility and (rather strangely) overactivity in children. They have been known to be abused by long-distance truck drivers and others who wish to stay awake for long periods of time. Dependence upon these drugs can develop rapidly.

See Caffeine, Cocaine, Dexamphetamine, Methylphenidate, Nicotine.

St John's Wort
See Saint John's Wort.

Streptodornase
See FIBRINOLYTICS.

Streptokinase
See FIBRINOLYTICS.

Sucralfate

TRADE NAMES:
Carafate, Ulcyte.

DRUG CLASS:
Antiulcerant.

USES:
Protects the lining of the stomach. Treats and prevents ulcers of the stomach and duodenum (upper small intestine).

DOSAGE:
One tablet three times a day one hour before meals, and a fourth tablet last thing at night before bed. Course usually limited to eight weeks.

FORMS:
Tablets of 1g (white).

PRECAUTIONS:
Use with caution in pregnancy (B1). Not recommended for use in children.
Cause of symptoms must be determined (eg. by gastroscopy) if symptoms persist or return after use.
Use with caution if swallowing difficult.

Do not take if:
 suffering from stomach cancer, bleeding ulcer or significant kidney disease.

SIDE EFFECTS:
Common: Constipation, headache, itchy rash, nausea.
Unusual: Indigestion, dry mouth, diarrhoea, back pain, sleepiness, dizziness.

INTERACTIONS:
Other drugs:
- Antacids should not be taken within half an hour.
- Tetracycline, phenytoin, digoxin, norfloxacin, ciprofloxacin, warfarin and cimetidine may have their effectiveness reduced while taking sucralfate.

PRESCRIPTION:
No.

PBS:
Yes.

PERMITTED IN SPORT:
Yes.

OVERDOSE:
Constipation and nausea only effects.

See also ANTACIDS, Cimetidine, Misoprostol, Nizatadine, PROTON PUMP INHIBITORS, Ranitidine.

SUGARS

See Fructose, Glucose.

Sulfacetamide

TRADE NAMES:
Acetopt, Bleph-10.

DRUG CLASS:
Antibiotic.

USES:
Conjunctivitis, ulcers on eye surface, trachoma.

DOSAGE:

Insert two drops every one or two hours.

FORMS:
Eye drops.

PRECAUTIONS:
May be used with care in pregnancy (C), breast feeding and children over 2 years. Use with caution in kidney disease. Remove contact lenses during use. Do not persist with treatment if symptoms persist for more than three days.

SIDE EFFECTS:
Common: Minimal
Unusual: Eye irritation and burning.

INTERACTIONS:
None significant.

PRESCRIPTION:
Yes.

PBS:
Yes.

PERMITTED IN SPORT:
Yes.

OTHER INFORMATION:
Sulfonamides were the first antibiotics in the 1930s. Used less frequently now due to resistant forms of bacteria developing. Allergy to Sulfonamides a problem in some patients.

See also drugs listed under SULFONAMIDES.

Sulfadoxine

TRADE NAME:
Fansidar (with pyrimethamine).

DRUG CLASS:
Antimalarial.

USES:
Prevention and treatment of malaria.

OTHER INFORMATION:
Only available in combination with pyrimethamine. See pyrimethamine entry for further information.

Sulfamethoxazole

TRADE NAMES:
Only available in Australia in combination with trimethoprim – this combination is known as co-trimoxazole.
Bactrim, Cosig, Resprim, Septrin, Trimoxazole-BC (with trimethoprim). Other locally produced brands also exist.

DRUG CLASS:
Sulfonamide antibiotic.

USES:
Infections caused by susceptible bacteria, particularly infections of sinuses, throat, lungs, urine and skin.

DOSAGE:
 One tablet twice a day.

FORMS:
Tablets, suspension.

PRECAUTIONS:
Should not be used in pregnancy (C) unless essential. Use with caution in breast feeding. May be used in children over three months.
Use with caution in AIDS, blood disorders, asthma, allergic conditions, kidney and liver disease.
Not designed for long term use.
Lower doses and caution necessary in elderly.
Give additional fluids to dilute.

Do not take if:
- suffering from severe liver disease, abnormal blood cells, bone marrow damage, severe kidney disease.
- under three months of age.

SIDE EFFECTS:
Common: Nausea, loss of appetite, rash.
Unusual: Vomiting, diarrhoea.
Severe but rare (stop medication, consult doctor): Unusual bleeding or bruising, yellow skin (jaundice), worsening infection, severe diarrhoea.

INTERACTIONS:
Other drugs:
- Hypoglycaemics, methotrexate, urinary acidifiers, anticoagulants (eg. warfarin), NSAID, salicylates, sulfinpyrazone, phenytoin, rifampicin, cyclosporin, thiazide diuretics, pyrimethamine, acetazolamide.

PRESCRIPTION:
Yes.

PBS:
Yes.

PERMITTED IN SPORT:
Yes.

OVERDOSE:
Exacerbation of side effects likely. Administer activated charcoal or induce vomiting if tablets taken recently. Take as much fluid as possible. Kidney damage possible. Seek medical assistance.

OTHER INFORMATION:
Widely used for two decades after its introduction in the mid 1960s, but now more effective and less toxic antibiotics tend to be used where possible.

See also SULFONAMIDES.

Sulfasalazine

TRADE NAMES:
Pyralin, Salazopyrin.

DRUG CLASS:
Sulfonamide antibiotic.

USES:
Ulcerative colitis, Crohn's disease, rheumatoid arthritis.

DOSAGE:
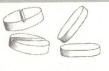
Tablets: 250mg to 2000mg up to four times a day with plenty of fluids.
Suppository: 500mg to 1000mg once or twice a day.

FORMS:
Tablets of 500mg, extended release tablets of 500mg, suppositories of 500mg.

PRECAUTIONS:
Safe in pregnancy (A). Use with caution in breast feeding.
Blood and urine tests must be taken regularly during treatment to detect any adverse effects.
Use with caution if suffering from a G6PD deficiency.
Ensure adequate fluids are drunk.

Do not take if:
 suffering from allergy conditions, porphyria, blood cell disorders, gut or urinary obstruction, significant liver or kidney disease, sensitivity to aspirin or sulfonamides.

SIDE EFFECTS:
Common: Nausea, vomiting, loss of appetite, fever, red skin, itchy skin, headache.
Unusual: Reversible infertility, belly pain, diarrhoea, pins and needles sensation, depression, dizziness, sleeplessness, cough.
Severe but rare (stop medication, consult doctor): Fever, bleeding, bruising, jaundice, sore throat. These symptoms may be signs of a severe blood disorder that may rarely occur with sulfasalazine.

INTERACTIONS:
Other drugs:
- Interacts with anticoagulants (eg. warfarin), methotrexate, sulfonylureas (used in diabetes), sulfonamides, penicillin, digoxin.
- Increased effect of sulfasalazine occurs if taken with indomethacin, phenylbutazone, urinary acidifiers or salicylates.

Other substances:
- Iron.

PRESCRIPTION:
Yes.

PBS:
Yes.

PERMITTED IN SPORT:
Yes.

OVERDOSE:
Diarrhoea, bloody urine and kidney damage may occur. Seek urgent medical attention.

OTHER INFORMATION:
Used for many years to successfully control intestinal inflammation. Found serendipitously to also control some forms of rheumatoid arthritis.

See also SULFONAMIDES.

SULFONAMIDES

DISCUSSION:
Sulfur (sulphur – the American spelling is now universal in pharmacology) containing antibiotics were the very first antibiotics developed, but the ones available in the late 1930s had severe side effects and were not very effective. Sulfonamides today are not as widely used as other antibiotics but still play a part in the treatment of some types of infections. The most commonly prescribed sulfa preparation is co-trimoxazole, which has a sulfa antibiotic (sulfasalazine) combined with a second type of antibiotic. They should be avoided in patients with liver disease and used with caution in the elderly.

See Silver sulfadiazine, Sulfacetamide, Sulfadoxine, Sulfamethoxazole, Sulfasalazine.

Sulfur
(Sulphur)

TRADE NAMES:
Clearasil Cream (with resorcinol, triclosan, aluminium hydroxide and other ingredients).
Curacel Acne and Pimple Gel (with allantoin, zinc oxide, resorcinol and other ingredients).
Egopsoryl TA (with phenol, tar).
Neo-Medrol Acne Lotion (with methylprednisolone, neomycin, aluminium chlorohydrate).
Psor-Asist (with tar, salicylic acid).
Also used in many other locally prepared medications.

USES:
Acne, psoriasis.

DOSAGE:

Varies. Apply medication as directed on label.

FORMS:
Cream, gel, lotion, shampoo.

PRECAUTIONS:
Most forms safe in pregnancy and breast feeding.
Use with caution in children.
For external use only – do not swallow.
Avoid eyes, nostrils, mouth, ears, anus, vagina.

Do not use if:
 skin broken, burnt or grazed.

- suffering from infected pustular acne or psoriasis.

SIDE EFFECTS:
Common: Skin inflammation.

INTERACTIONS:
Nil.

PRESCRIPTION:
Most forms: No.
Neo-Medrol: Yes.

PBS:
No.

PERMITTED IN SPORT:
Yes.

OTHER INFORMATION:
Normally only available in combination with other medications.

Sulindac

TRADE NAMES:
Aclin, Clinoril.

DRUG CLASS:
NSAID (Nonsteroidal anti-inflammatory drug).

USES:
All forms of arthritis, inflammatory disorders, gout, back pain, ankylosing spondylitis, bone pain.

DOSAGE:

One or two tablets, twice a day with food.

FORMS:
Tablets of 100mg.

PRECAUTIONS:
Should not be used in pregnancy (C) unless medically essential. Breast feeding should be ceased if necessary to use NSAID. Not for use in children under 2 years.
Use with caution in psychiatrically disturbed patients, epilepsy, severe infection, heart failure and kidney disease.
Lower doses required in elderly, who may suffer more side effects.

Do not take if:
 suffering from peptic ulcer at present or in recent past.
- due for surgery (including dental surgery).
- suffering from bleeding disorder or anaemia.

SIDE EFFECTS:
Common: Stomach discomfort, diarrhoea, constipation, heartburn, nausea, headache, dizziness.
Unusual: Blurred vision, stomach ulcer, ringing noise in ears, retention of fluid, swelling of tissue, drowsiness, itch, rash, shortness of breath.
Severe but rare (stop medication, consult doctor): Vomiting blood, passing blood in faeces, other unusual bleeding, asthma induced by medication.

INTERACTIONS:
Other drugs:
- Must never be used with anticoagulants (eg. warfarin).
- Probenecid, diuretics, lithium, methotrexate, beta blockers, ACE inhibitors.

PRESCRIPTION:
Yes.

PBS:
Yes.

PERMITTED IN SPORT:
Yes.

OVERDOSE:
Causes nausea, vomiting, severe headache, dizziness, confusion and convulsions. Administer activated charcoal or induce vomiting if taken recently. Seek medical assistance.

OTHER INFORMATION:
Significant side effects (particularly on the stomach) in about 5% of patients limit their use.

See also Aspirin, Bufexamac, Celecoxib, Diclofenac, Diflunisal, Flurbiprofen, Ibuprofen, Indomethacin, Ketoprofen, Ketorolac trometanol, Mefenamic Acid, Naproxen, Piroxicam, Rofecoxib, SALICYLATES, Tenoxicam, Tiaprofenic Acid.

SULPHONAMIDES

See SULFONAMIDES.

Sulthiame

TRADE NAME:
Ospolot.

DRUG CLASS:
Anticonvulsant.

USES:
Epilepsy, behavioural disorders, hyperactivity.

DOSAGE:

One or two tablets two or three times a day. Usually 200mg, three times a day.

FORMS:
Tablets of 50mg and 200mg (white).

PRECAUTIONS:
Not to be used in pregnancy (D) unless medically essential. Use with caution in breast feeding. May be used in children. Use with caution in kidney disease.

SIDE EFFECTS:
Common: Incoordination, pins and needles sensation (particularly of face), alterations in breathing, loss of appetite.
Unusual: Giddiness, rash, nausea, belly pain, weight loss, headache, depression.

INTERACTIONS:
Other drugs:
- Primidone, phenytoin, barbiturates.

Herbs:
- Evening primrose (linoleic acid), Gingko biloba.

Other substances:
- Reacts adversely with alcohol.
- Borage.

PRESCRIPTION:
Yes.

PBS:
Yes.

PERMITTED IN SPORT:
Yes.

OVERDOSE:
Symptoms may include vomiting, headache, dizziness, incoordination and inability to move muscles as desired. Induce vomiting if medication taken recently. Seek medical assistance.

OTHER INFORMATION:
Very useful and generally safe medication. Not addictive or dependence forming.
See also BARBITURATES, BENZODIAZEPINES, Carbamazepine, Clonazepam, Ethosuximide, Gabapentin, Lamotrigine, Levetiracetam, Oxcarbazepine, Phenytoin, Primidone, Sodium valproate, Tiagabine, Topiramate, Vigabatrin.

Sumatriptan

TRADE NAMES:
Imigran, Suvalan.

DRUG CLASS:
Antimigraine.

USES:
Treatment of acute migraine and cluster headache.

DOSAGE:

Tablets and nasal spray: One tablet or spray immediately symptoms of migraine appear. Repeat if necessary. Maximum of three a day.
Injection: Self-inject immediately symptoms of migraine appear. Repeat once in no less than one hour if necessary.

FORMS:
Tablets of 50mg and 100mg, nasal spray, injection (auto-injector kit available).

 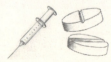

PRECAUTIONS:
Should not be used in pregnancy (B3) unless medically essential. Should be used with caution in breast feeding. Not for use in children under 12 years.
Should be used with caution in epilepsy, asthma, liver and kidney disease, heart disease and in elderly.
Not to be used for prevention of migraine, only treatment of acute attacks.
Must not be injected into a vein.

Do not take if:

☠ suffering from angina, poor circulation to heart or limbs, recent heart attack, severe high blood pressure, recent stroke, irregular heartbeat, significant liver disease.
- Ergotamine used in previous 24 hours.

SIDE EFFECTS:
Common: Chest pain, pain at injection site, tingling sensation, heat, heaviness, flushing, tightness, dizziness, weakness.
Unusual: Fatigue, drowsiness, nausea, vomiting.
Severe but rare (stop medication, consult doctor): Significant chest pain (angina), fitting.

INTERACTIONS:
Other drugs:
- Ergotamine, MAOI.

Herbs:
- St John's wort.

Other substances:
- Does not interact with alcohol.

PRESCRIPTION:
Yes.

PBS:
Tablets and nasal spray: Yes (authority required).
Injection: No.

PERMITTED IN SPORT:
Yes.

OVERDOSE:
Exacerbation of side effects only.

OTHER INFORMATION:
Considered a wonder drug when introduced in the early 1990s, Sumatriptan has given instant relief with minimal side effects to millions of migraine sufferers. It works far more effectively as an injection than if taken as tablets, but unfortunately, it is very expensive. Patients should use medication to prevent migraines in preference to treating migraines regularly.

See also Ergotamine, Naratriptan, Zolmitriptan.

SYMPATHOMIMETICS (DECONGESTANTS)

DISCUSSION:
Medications that clear blocked nose and sinuses in patients with a cold, flu or hay fever.

See Phenylephrine, Pseudoephedrine.

T3, T4

See **THYROID HORMONES**

Tacrine

TRADE NAME:
Cognex.

USES:
Treatment of dementia and Alzheimer's disease.

DOSAGE:
 40mg to 160mg a day in several doses

FORMS:
Capsules of
10mg (green/pink),
20mg (blue/pink),
30mg (red/pink) and
40mg (purple/pink).

PRECAUTIONS:
Not to be used in pregnancy (C), breast feeding or children.
Use with caution in irregular heartbeat, convulsions, Parkinson's disease and severe asthma.
Do not stop suddenly, but reduce dose slowly.
Regular blood tests of liver function and blood cells essential.

Do not take if:
suffering from liver disease, bleeding from intestine, peptic ulcer, gut obstruction or difficulty in passing urine.
• having a general anaesthetic.

SIDE EFFECTS:
Common: Nausea, diarrhoea, loss of appetite, dizziness, heartburn and belly pains.
Unusual: Vomiting, tiredness, weight loss, muscle pains, anxiety, runny nose, rash.
Severe but rare (stop medication, consult doctor): Yellow skin (jaundice).

INTERACTIONS:
Other drugs:
• Anticholinergics, NSAIDs, theophylline, cimetidine.

PRESCRIPTION:
Yes.

PBS:
No.

PERMITTED IN SPORT:
Yes.

OVERDOSE:
Serious. May cause vomiting, diarrhoea, sweating, excess saliva, slow heart rate, low blood pressure, collapse, convulsions and death. Administer activated charcoal or induce vomiting if medication taken recently. Seek urgent medical assistance.

OTHER INFORMATION:
Introduced in 1995 as one of the very few treatments for Alzheimer's disease. Results are very unpredictable, and the medication must be used for some months before effect can be assessed. Does not cause addiction or dependence. Also used in injection form to reverse paralysis induced during general anaesthesia. May be removed from market in 2003 due to lack of demand.

See also Donepezil, Galantamine, Rivastigmine.

Tacrolimus

TRADE NAME:
Prograf.

DRUG CLASS:
Immunosupressant.

USES:
Prevention of rejection of kidney and liver transplants.

DOSAGE:
 Complex. Must be determined individually for each patient by doctor.

FORMS:
Capsules of 0.5mg (yellow), 1mg (white) and 5mg (grey/red), injection.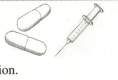

PRECAUTIONS:
Not to be used in pregnancy (C) except under exceptional circumstances.
Use with caution in breast feeding and children.
Careful monitoring of dosage and blood cells and body chemistry essential.
Usually commenced in hospital.

SIDE EFFECTS:
Common: Tremor, headache, pins and needles sensation, nausea, diarrhoea.
Unusual: High blood pressure, excess sugar in blood, excess calcium in blood, skin rashes, wheeze.
Severe but rare (stop medication, consult doctor): Heart damage, diabetes, kidney and liver damage.

INTERACTIONS:
Other drugs:
- Cyclosporin (serious interaction), aminoglycosides, NSAIDs, vancomycin, amphotericin B, co-trimoxazole, aciclovir, ganciclovir, potassium supplements, amiloride, some vaccines, oral contraceptives.

Herbs:
- St John's wort.

Other substances:
- Grapefruit juice.

PRESCRIPTION:
Yes.

PBS:
Capsules: Yes (very restricted).
Injection: No.

PERMITTED IN SPORT:
Yes.

OVERDOSE:
Likely to be very serious. Induce vomiting or give activated charcoal if swallowed recently. Seek urgent medical attention.

See also Mycophenolate mofetil, Sirolimus.

Tadalafil

TRADE NAME:
Cialis.

USES:
Impotence and erectile dysfunction in men.

DOSAGE:
 10mg or 20mg once a day. The lower dose is usually reserved for the elderly and those with and those with kidney disease.

FORMS:
Tablets of 10mg and 20mg (yellow).

PRECAUTIONS:
Not for use in women or children.
Use with caution in liver and kidney disease, and low blood pressure.

Do not take if:

 suffering from severe heart disease (eg. unstable angina, congestive heart failure).
- using nitrate medications (eg. glyceryl trinitrate for angina)

SIDE EFFECTS:

Common: Headache, indigestion.
Unusual: Muscle aches, flushing.
Severe but rare (stop medication, consult doctor): Chest pain.

INTERACTIONS:

Other drugs:
- Never use with glyceryl nitrate or other nitrate medications.
- Erythromycin, ritonavir, saquinavir, clarithromycin, itraconazole, rifampicin, phenobarb, phenytoin, angiotensin II receptor blockers (used for high blood pressure), warfarin.

PRESCRIPTION:
Yes.

PBS:
No.

PERMITTED IN SPORT:
Yes.

OVERDOSE:
Exacerbation of side effects likely.

OTHER INFORMATION:
Released in 2003 as a competitor to sildenafil (Viagra). Initial information indicates that it works faster, lasts longer, and has fewer side effects than its famous competitor.
See also Alprostadil, Sildenafil.

Tamoxifen

TRADE NAMES:
Genox, Nolvadex, Tamosin, Tamoxen.
Other generic brands exist.

USES:
Breast cancer.

DOSAGE:
 One or two tablets once a day.

FORMS:
Tablets of 10mg and 20mg.

PRECAUTIONS:
Must not be used in pregnancy (B3) unless mother's life is at risk.
Breast feeding must be ceased before use.
Not for use in children.
Adequate contraception must be used by all fertile women during use of tamoxifen.
Use with caution in bleeding disorders and blood cell abnormalities.
Regular gynaecological checks essential.

SIDE EFFECTS:
Common: Hot flushes, abnormal vaginal bleeding, itchy vulva, fluid retention, light headedness, nausea, vomiting, diarrhoea.
Unusual: Vaginal discharge, headache, blood clots (thrombosis), bone pain, vision changes.
Severe but rare (stop medication, consult doctor): Damage to uterus and ovary, blood cell changes.

INTERACTIONS:
Other drugs: Anticoagulants (eg. warfarin).
Herbs: Dong quai.

PRESCRIPTION:
Yes.

PBS:
Yes.

Medications

PERMITTED IN SPORT:
Yes.

OVERDOSE:
Exacerbation of side effects likely.

OTHER INFORMATION:
This medication has saved the lives of thousands of women with breast cancer, and has prevented recurrences in thousands more. Very useful and effective. Introduced in late 1980s.
See also Letrozole, Toremifene.

Tamsulosin

TRADE NAME:
Flomax.

DRUG CLASS:
Alpha 1 adrenergic blocker (alpha blocker).

USES:
Reduces size of enlarged prostate gland.

DOSAGE:
 One capsule a day, half hour before breakfast.

FORMS:
Capsule of 400μg.

PRECAUTIONS:
To be used only in males. If unintentionally taken during pregnancy (B2) or breast feeding, unlikely to be harmful.
Not for use in children.
Prostate cancer must be excluded before use.
Use with caution if heart attack within six previous months.
Do not take if:
 suffering from low blood pressure, severe liver or kidney disease.

SIDE EFFECTS:
Common: Palpitations, dizziness, low blood pressure, inability to ejaculate during sexual intercourse.
Unusual: Itch, urinary tract infection, sleeplessness, diarrhoea.
Severe but rare (stop medication, consult doctor): Sudden drop in blood pressure with changes in position resulting in falls.

INTERACTIONS:
Other drugs:
- Other alpha blockers, cimetidine, diclofenac, warfarin, frusemide.

PRESCRIPTION:
Yes.

PBS:
No. Available to Veteran Affairs pensioners.

PERMITTED IN SPORT:
Yes.

OVERDOSE:
Severe low blood pressure may occur. Give activated charcoal and seek medical attention.

OTHER INFORMATION:
Introduced in 2000 as a more specifically targeted drug against the prostate gland. Other alpha blockers lower blood pressure as well as shrinking the prostate.
See also Doxazosin, Labetalol, Prazosin.

TARS

TRADE and GENERIC NAMES:

Alphosyl Lotion (Coal tar with allantoin).
Egopsoryl TA, Fongitar, Polytar, Sebitar (Tar with other ingredients).
ER Cream (Coal tar with zinc oxide, allantoin, hydroxybenzoates and other ingredients).
Exorex Emulsion, Ionil T Plus, Linotar, Psorigel (Coal tar).
Ionil T, Psor-Asist (Coal tar with salicylic acid).
Pinetarsol (Pine tar).

USES:

Itchy skin, itchy anus, prickly heat, mild dermatitis, psoriasis, dandruff.

DOSAGE:

 Apply several times a day, or add to bath water.

FORMS:

Lotion, cream, ointment, solution, bar.

PRECAUTIONS:

Safe to use in pregnancy, breast feeding and children.

SIDE EFFECTS:

Common: Minimal.
Unusual: Skin irritation.

INTERACTIONS:

None significant.

PRESCRIPTION:

No.

PBS:

No. Some forms available to Veteran Affairs pensioners.

PERMITTED IN SPORT:

Yes.

OTHER INFORMATION:

The original dermatitis treatment, in use for thousands of years.

Tartaric acid

See ANTACIDS, URINARY ALKALINISERS.

Tazobactam

TRADE NAME:

Tazocin (with piperacillin).

DRUG CLASS:

Antibiotic.

USES:

Severe bacterial infections in hospital.

DOSAGE:

 4.5 grams every eight hours by injection into muscle or slow infusion by a drip into a vein.

FORMS:

Injection.

PRECAUTIONS:

May be used with care in pregnancy (B1), breast feeding and children.
Use with caution in syphilis, kidney and liver disease.
Not for prolonged use over three weeks.
Blood tests to check electrolyte balance, blood cells, kidney and liver function necessary.

SIDE EFFECTS:

Common: Nausea, diarrhoea, rash, vein inflammation.
Unusual: Vomiting, blood clots.
Severe but rare (stop medication, consult doctor): Bloody diarrhoea, other abnormal bleeding.

INTERACTIONS:
Other drugs:
- Heparin, anticoagulants (eg. warfarin), aminoglycoside antibiotics, methotrexate.

PRESCRIPTION:
Yes.

PBS:
No.

PERMITTED IN SPORT:
Yes.

See also Piperacillin.

TB vaccine
See BCG vaccine.

Tegaserod

TRADE NAME:
Zelmac.

DRUG CLASS:
Laxative.

USES:
Constipation associated with irritable bowel syndrome in women.

DOSAGE:

One tablet twice a day before meals.

FORMS:
Tablets of 6mg (cream).

PRECAUTIONS:
Use with caution in pregnancy (B3), breast feeding and children.
Use with caution in severe liver and kidney disease.

SIDE EFFECTS:
Common: Diarrhoea, headache.

INTERACTIONS:
None significant.

PRESCRIPTION:
Yes.

PBS:
No.

PERMITTED IN SPORT:
Yes.

OTHER INFORMATION:
Introduced in 2002 for use in a very small number of patients with a particular form of irritable bowel syndrome.

Medications

Telcoplanin

TRADE NAME:
Targocid.

DRUG CLASS:
Antibiotic.

USES:
Osteomyelitis (bone infection), septic arthritis (joint infection), septicaemia (blood infection).

DOSAGE:

Intravenous infusion as determined by doctor.

FORMS:
Injection.

PRECAUTIONS:
May be used with caution in pregnancy (B3), breast feeding and children.
Use with caution in kidney disease and elderly.
Blood tests to check liver, kidney and blood cell function necessary.
Not for prolonged use.

SIDE EFFECTS:
Common: Nausea, diarrhoea.
Unusual: Vomiting.
Severe but rare (stop medication, consult doctor): Liver and kidney damage, hearing or balance changes.

INTERACTIONS:
Other drugs: Aminoglycosides, amphotericin, cyclosporin, frusemide.

PRESCRIPTION:
Yes.

PBS:
No.

PERMITTED IN SPORT:
Yes.

Telmisartan

See ANGIOTENSIN II RECEPTOR ANTAGONISTS.

Temazepam

TRADE NAMES:
Euhypnos, Normison, Temaze, Temtabs.

DRUG CLASS:
Hypnotic/Sedative, Benzodiazepine.

USES:
Insomnia (sleeplessness).

DOSAGE:

One to three tablets or capsules 30 minutes before going to bed.

FORMS:
Capsules of 10mg and 20mg, tablets of 10mg.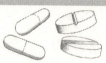

PRECAUTIONS:
Should be used with caution in pregnancy (C), but not at all if delivery of infant imminent as it may decrease desire to breathe in newborn infant.
Should be used with caution in breast feeding.
Not for use in children.
Lower dose required in elderly.
Should be used intermittently and not constantly as dependency may develop.
Use with caution in glaucoma, myasthenia gravis, heart disease, kidney or liver disease, psychiatric conditions, depression and epilepsy.

Do not take if:
- suffering from severe lung disease, confusion.
- tendency to addiction or dependence.
- operating machinery, driving a vehicle or undertaking tasks that require concentration and alertness.

Home Guide to Medication

SIDE EFFECTS:
Common: Confusion and falls in elderly, impaired alertness.
Unusual: Dizziness, incoordination, poor memory, headache, hangover in morning, slurred speech, nightmares.

INTERACTIONS:
Other drugs:
- Other medications that reduce alertness (eg. barbiturates, antihistamines, antianxiety drugs).
- Disulfiram, anticonvulsants, anticholinergics.

Herbs:
- Guarana, kava kava, passionflower, St John's wort, valerian, celery, camomile, goldenseal.

Other substances:
- Reacts with alcohol to cause excessive drowsiness.

PRESCRIPTION:
Yes.

PBS:
10mg: Yes.
20mg: No.

PERMITTED IN SPORT:
Yes.

OVERDOSE:
Seldom life threatening. May cause drowsiness, confusion and coma. Induce vomiting if tablets taken recently. Seek medical assistance.

OTHER INFORMATION:
Very widely used to help people get to sleep. Very safe, but dependency may develop. Often used to correct sleep pattern abnormalities induced by jet lag. Short half-life reduces morning hangover effect.
See also BARBITURATES, Chlormethiazole, Flunitrazepam, Midazolam, Nitrazepam, Triazolam, Zolpidem, Zopiclone.

Temozolomide

TRADE NAME:
Temodal.

DRUG CLASS:
Cytotoxic.

USES:
Brain cancers (glioma, astrocytoma).

DOSAGE:
 Complex. As determined for each patient by doctor.

FORMS:
Capsules (white) of 5, 20, 100 and 250mg.

PRECAUTIONS:
Not to be used in pregnancy (D) and breast feeding.
Use with caution in children.
Partners of males using medication must not fall pregnant.
Use with caution in liver and kidney disease.
Regular blood tests essential.
Use lower dose in elderly.
Do not take if:
 suffering from immunosupression (eg. AIDS).

SIDE EFFECTS:
Common: Nausea, diarrhoea, headache, tiredness.
Unusual: Vomiting, infertility.

INTERACTIONS:
Other drugs:
- Other cancer-treating drugs.

Other substances:
- Alcohol.

PRESCRIPTION:
Yes.

Medications

PBS:
Yes (authority required).

PERMITTED IN SPORT:
Yes.

OVERDOSE:
Likely to cause serious organ damage. Seek urgent medical attention. Induce vomiting or give activated charcoal if swallowed recently.

OTHER INFORMATION:
Introduced in 1998 for treatment of more resistant forms of brain cancer.

Tenofovir

TRADE NAME:
Viread.

DRUG CLASS:
Antiviral.

USES:
HIV (AIDS).

DOSAGE:
 One tablet a day.

FORMS:
Tablets of 300mg (light blue).

PRECAUTIONS:
Use with caution in pregnancy (B3), breast feeding and children under 18 years.
Use with caution in kidney disease and if used long term.
Always used in combination with other medications to treat HIV.
Regular blood tests recommended to assess kidney, liver and blood cell function.

SIDE EFFECTS:
Common: Nausea, diarrhoea, tiredness.
Unusual: Vomiting, dizziness, shortness of breath, rash.
Severe but rare (stop medication, consult doctor): Kidney damage, bone damage, pancreatitis (severe belly pain).

INTERACTIONS:
Other drugs:
• Didanosine.

PRESCRIPTION:
Yes.

PBS:
Yes (authority required).

PERMITTED IN SPORT:
Yes.

See also Didanosine, Nelfinavir, Nevirapine, Stavudine.

Tenoxicam

TRADE NAME:
Tilcotil.

DRUG CLASS:
NSAID (Nonsteroidal anti-inflammatory drug).

USES:
All forms of arthritis, inflammatory disorders, gout, back pain, ankylosing spondylitis.

DOSAGE:
 One or two tablets, once a day with food.

FORMS:
Tablets (yellow) of 10mg.

546　Home Guide to Medication

Medications

PRECAUTIONS:
Should not be used in pregnancy (C) unless medically essential. Breast feeding should be ceased if necessary to use NSAID. Not for use in children under 2 years.
Use tablets and capsules with caution in psychiatrically disturbed patients, epilepsy, severe infection, heart failure and kidney disease.
Lower doses required in elderly, who may suffer more side effects.

Do not take if:
- suffering from peptic ulcer at present or in recent past.
- due for surgery (including dental surgery).
- suffering from bleeding disorder or anaemia.

SIDE EFFECTS:
Common: Stomach discomfort, diarrhoea, constipation, heartburn, nausea, headache, dizziness.
Unusual: Blurred vision, stomach ulcer, ringing noise in ears, retention of fluid, swelling of tissue, drowsiness, itch, rash, shortness of breath.
Severe but rare (stop medication, consult doctor): Vomit blood, pass blood in faeces, other unusual bleeding, asthma induced by medication.

INTERACTIONS:
Other drugs:
- Must never be used with anticoagulants (eg. warfarin).
- Probenecid, diuretics, lithium, methotrexate, beta blockers, ACE inhibitors.

PRESCRIPTION:
Yes.

PBS:
No.

PERMITTED IN SPORT:
Yes.

OVERDOSE:
Causes nausea, vomiting, severe headache, dizziness, confusion and convulsions. Administer activated charcoal or induce vomiting if taken recently. Seek medical assistance.

OTHER INFORMATION:
Significant side effects (particularly on the stomach) in about 5% of patients limit their use.
See also Aspirin, Bufexamac, Celecoxib, Diclofenac, Diflunisal, Flurbiprofen, Ibuprofen, Indomethacin, Ketoprofen, Ketorolac trometanol, Mefenamic Acid, Naproxen, Piroxicam, Rofecoxib, SALICYLATES, Sulindac, Tiaprofenic Acid.

Terazosin hydrochloride

TRADE NAME:
Hytrin.

USES:
Benign enlargement of prostate gland, high blood pressure.

DOSAGE:
 Slowly increasing dosage for three weeks to a maintenance level of 5mg to 10mg once a day in the morning.

FORMS:
Tablets of 1mg (white), 2mg (pink), 5mg (grey) and 10mg (blue).

PRECAUTIONS:
Should be used with caution in pregnancy (B2), breast feeding and children.
Beware of sudden drop in blood pressure with first dose.

SIDE EFFECTS:
Common: Dizziness, light headedness, palpitations, blurred vision, tiredness.
Unusual: Low blood pressure, nasal congestion, faint, swelling of ankles, feet and hands.

Medications

INTERACTIONS:

Other drugs:
- Other antihypertensives, diuretics, beta blockers, NSAIDs.

PRESCRIPTION:
Yes.

PBS:
Yes (authority required).

PERMITTED IN SPORT:
Yes.

OVERDOSE:
Severe low blood pressure could result.

OTHER INFORMATION:
Does not cause addiction or dependence. Introduced to Australia in 1994.
See also Finasteride, Tamulosin

Terbinafine

TRADE NAME:
Lamisil.

DRUG CLASS:
Antifungal.

USES:
Fungal infections of skin (ringworm) and nails.

DOSAGE:

 Tablets: One tablet a day for several weeks.
Cream and gel: Apply once or twice a day to dry skin.

FORMS:
Tablet (white) of 200mg, cream, gel.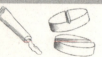

PRECAUTIONS:
Use tablets with caution in pregnancy (B1), breast feeding and children.
Use tablets with caution in liver and kidney disease.
Avoid eye contact with cream and gel.

Do not take tablets if:
 suffering from severe liver disease.

SIDE EFFECTS:
Common: Cream – Redness, itching, stinging.
Tablets – Nausea, diarrhoea, rash, itch, headache, dizziness.
Unusual: Tablets – Vomiting, red skin, tiredness, chest pain, light headedness.

INTERACTIONS:

Other drugs:
- Tablets – Oral contraceptives, cimetidine, rifampicin, tricyclic antidepressants, beta blockers, SSRI antidepressants, MAOI.

Other substances:
- Tablets react with alcohol.

PRESCRIPTION:
Tablets: Yes.
Cream and gel: No.

PBS:
Tablets: Yes (authority required).
Cream and gel: No. Available to Veteran Affairs pensioners.

PERMITTED IN SPORT:
Yes.

OVERDOSE:
Unlikely to have serious effects. Seek medical advice.

OTHER INFORMATION:
Introduced in 1993. Very effective and safe, but quite expensive.
See also Amphotericin, Fluconazole, Griseofulvin, Itraconazole, Ketoconazole.

Terbutaline

TRADE NAME:
Bricanyl

DRUG CLASS:
Bronchodilators (Beta-2 agonist).

USES:
Asthma, bronchitis, spasm of airways in lung.

DOSAGE:

Inhalers and sprays: One or two inhalations every four to six hours.
Mixture: 10 to 15mLs three times a day.

FORMS:
Spray, inhaler, nebuliser solution, mixture, injection.

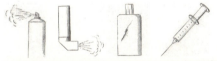

PRECAUTIONS:
Safe to use in pregnancy (A), breast feeding and children.
Not designed for long term constant use.
Use with care in high blood pressure, heart disease, over-active thyroid gland, diabetes, liver and kidney disease.
Lower doses necessary in elderly and children.
Seek urgent medical assistance if no response to medication.

SIDE EFFECTS:
Common: Tremor, rapid heart rate, palpitations, headache.
Unusual: Nausea, diarrhoea, flush, mouth irritation.
Severe but rare (stop medication, consult doctor): Irregular heart rhythm, low blood pressure.

INTERACTIONS:
Other drugs:
- Sympathomimetics, beta blockers, theophyllines, steroids, diuretics, digoxin.

Other substances:
- Mixture may react with alcohol and caffeine.

PRESCRIPTION:
Nebuliser solution, mixture, injection: Yes.
Sprays, inhaler: No.

PBS:
Inhaler, nebuliser solution: Yes.
Spray: No

PERMITTED IN SPORT:
Yes.

OVERDOSE:
Exacerbation of side effects likely. May be dangerous in patients with heart disease or high blood pressure.

OTHER INFORMATION:
Designed for intermittent occasional use, and not to be taken regularly. Other medication should be used to prevent asthma if repeated doses of this medication are needed. Does not cause dependence or addiction. First introduced in the 1960s, beta-agonists have revolutionised life for asthmatics, but since deregulation in the mid 1980s, they have often been used excessively and inappropriately.

See also Fenoterol, Salbutamol, Salmeterol.

Testosterone

TRADE NAMES:
Androderm, Andro-Feme, Andromen, Testosterone Implants.
Andriol (testosterone undecanoate).
Primoteston Depot (testosterone enenthate).
Sustanon (testosterone propionate, testosterone phenylpropionate, testosterone isocaproate).

DRUG CLASS:
Sex hormone.

USES:
Testosterone deficiency in males, male infertility, male osteoporosis, Klinefelter syndrome.
In combination with oestrogen used for menopause and after removal of ovaries in women.
Increasing libido in women.

DOSAGE:

Capsules: One or two capsules twice a day after food.
Patch: Apply one to three patches to soft smooth skin every night. Replace after 24 hours.

FORMS:
Capsules, injection, implant, patch, cream.

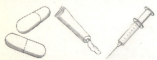

PRECAUTIONS:
Not to be used in pregnancy (D), breast feeding or children.
Used in postmenopausal women in combination with oestrogen.
Use with caution in heart disease, kidney disease, migraine, diabetes, epilepsy, high blood pressure.
Do not take if:
 suffering from prostate cancer, breast cancer.
- before puberty.

SIDE EFFECTS:
Common: Unwanted penile erections, retention of fluid, nausea, oily faeces.

INTERACTIONS:
Other drugs:
- Cyclosporin, hypoglycaemics (treat diabetes).

PRESCRIPTION:
Yes.

PBS:
Most forms: Yes (authority required).
Cream: No.

PERMITTED IN SPORT:
No.

OVERDOSE:
No specific problems short term. Long term inappropriate use may cause infertility, shrinking of testes, increased muscle bulk, high blood pressure, heart failure and increased risk of heart attack.

OTHER INFORMATION:
Does not cause addiction or dependence. Sometimes used illegally and inappropriately by athletes and body builders with potentially serious consequences.

See also SEX HORMONES.

Tetanus vaccine

TRADE NAMES:
Tet-Tox.
ADT, CDT (with diphtheria vaccine).
Boostrix, Infanrix, Tripacel (with diphtheria and whooping cough vaccines – triple antigen).
Infanrix HepB (with hepatitis B, diphtheria and whooping cough vaccines).

DRUG CLASS:
Vaccine.

USES:
Prevention of tetanus.

DOSAGE:
 Injections at two, four, six and 18 months, 5 years and then every 10 years throughout life.

FORMS:
Injection.

PRECAUTIONS:
Safe for use in pregnancy (A), breast feeding, children and infants.
Do not take if:
 suffering from significant chest, throat, ear, nose or sinus infection.
• having treatment for some types of cancer and leukaemia.

SIDE EFFECTS:
Common: Redness, swelling, soreness and lump at injection site.
Unusual: Fever, tiredness, allergic reaction.

INTERACTIONS:
Other drugs:
• Chloramphenicol.

PRESCRIPTION:
Yes.

PBS:
Yes. Some forms supplied free directly to doctors by government for use in specific immunisation schedules.

PERMITTED IN SPORT:
Yes.

OVERDOSE:
An unintentional additional vaccination is unlikely to have any significant adverse effect.

OTHER INFORMATION:
Tetanus is a worldwide disease that is caught from spores in the soil entering a wound. This disease kills about half its victims, but it can be completely prevented by vaccination.
See also Diphtheria vaccine, Whooping cough vaccine.

Tetrabenazine

TRADE NAME:
Tetrabenazine.

USES:
Chorea, muscle movement disorders.

DOSAGE:
 One to four tablets twice a day.

FORMS:
Tablets of 25mg (buff).

PRECAUTIONS:
Should be used with considerable caution in pregnancy (B2). Breast feeding should be ceased if prescribed.
Do not take if:
 suffering from Parkinsonism, depression.

SIDE EFFECTS:
Common: Drowsiness, muscle stiffness, tremor, depression, difficulty swallowing.
Unusual: Agitation, sleeplessness, confusion, fainting, tiredness.

INTERACTIONS:
Other drugs:
- Severe interaction with levodopa, reserpine and MAOI.
- Blood pressure medication, stimulants, tricyclic antidepressants.

Other substances:
- Reacts very adversely with alcohol.

PRESCRIPTION:
Yes.

PBS:
Yes (authority required).

PERMITTED IN SPORT:
Yes.

OVERDOSE:
May cause drowsiness, sweating and semi-comatose state. Administer activated charcoal or induce vomiting if medication taken recently and patient alert. Seek medical assistance.

OTHER INFORMATION:
Not addictive or dependence forming. Useful in a number of rare diseases affecting muscle action.

TETRACYCLIC ANTIDEPRESSANT
See Mianserin.

Tetracycline

TRADE NAMES:
Achromycin, Latycin Eye Ointment (tetracycline hydrochloride).
Tetrex (tetracycline phosphate).

DRUG CLASS:
Tetracycline antibiotic.

USES:
Infections caused by bacteria susceptible to tetracycline.

DOSAGE:

Capsules: One or two capsules, three or four times a day.
Eye ointment: Insert every two hours.

FORMS:
Capsules,
eye ointment.
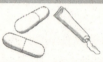

PRECAUTIONS:
Not to be used in pregnancy (D) or children under 8 years as tetracyclines may cause permanent staining of teeth of foetus or child. Use with caution in breast feeding.
Eye ointment safe to use in pregnancy, breast feeding and children.
Use capsules with caution in kidney disease.
Never use expired medication as it may become toxic.
Do not take capsules if:
suffering from severe kidney disease, systemic lupus erythematosus (SLE), Staphylococcal infection.

SIDE EFFECTS:
Common: Eye ointment – Minimal.
Capsules – Loss of appetite, nausea, sore mouth, diarrhoea, difficulty in swallowing, inflamed colon.
Unusual: Vomiting, inflamed pancreas, rash, secondary fungal infection (thrush).

Severe but rare (stop medication, consult doctor): Severe belly pain, severe diarrhoea, tooth discolouration, significant skin rash.

INTERACTIONS:
Other drugs:
- Anticoagulants (eg. warfarin), penicillin, antacids, iron, oral contraceptives.

Herbs:
- Dong quai, St John's wort.

Other substances:
- Milk may reduce absorption from gut.

PRESCRIPTION:
Yes.

PBS:
Yes.

PERMITTED IN SPORT:
Yes.

OVERDOSE:
Exacerbation of side effects only likely effect.

OTHER INFORMATION:
Used for a wide range of infections. Tetracycline has been superseded by more sophisticated antibiotics in the same group (eg. those listed below) in the last decade.
See also Demeclocycline, Doxycycline, Minocycline.

Tetrahydrozoline

TRADE NAMES:
Murine Sore Eyes, Optazine Fresh, Visine Original.
Visine Advanced Relief (with dextran, macrogol, povidone).

DRUG CLASS:
Vasoconstrictor.

USES:
Red, irritated eyes.

DOSAGE:

One or two drops in eye two or three times a day.

FORMS:
Eye drops.

PRECAUTIONS:
May be used in pregnancy, breast feeding and children.
Use with caution if wearing contact lenses.

Do not take if:
 suffering from glaucoma.

SIDE EFFECTS:
Minimal.

INTERACTIONS:
None significant.

PRESCRIPTION:
No.

PBS:
No.

PERMITTED IN SPORT:
Yes.

OTHER INFORMATION:
Common and simple, yet effective medication.
See also Naphazoline and Antazoline.

Tetrocosactrin

TRADE NAME:
Synacthen depot.

DRUG CLASS:
Trophic hormone.

USES:
Multiple sclerosis, some rare movement disorders.

DOSAGE:
 Initially injection twice a day, reducing to once or twice a week.

FORMS:
Injection.

PRECAUTIONS:
Not for use in pregnancy (D) and children under 1 year.
Use with caution in breast feeding, ulcerative colitis, diverticulitis, kidney disease, blood clots, osteoporosis, myasthenia gravis, under-active thyroid gland, liver disease (eg. cirrhosis), recent surgery, and unstable mental state.
Do not stop suddenly but reduce dose slowly.

Do not take if:
suffering from significant viral or bacterial infection, asthma, serious allergy, diabetes, untreated high blood pressure, severe psychiatric disturbance, peptic ulcer, Cushing syndrome, uncontrolled heart failure, or adrenogenital syndrome.
• after recent live vaccination (eg. polio).

SIDE EFFECTS:
Common: Fluid retention, muscle pains, joint pains, nausea, rash.
Unusual: Allergy reaction, vomiting, diarrhoea.

Severe but rare (stop medication, consult doctor): Psychological or mental disturbance, severe allergy, vision changes.

INTERACTIONS:
Other drugs:
• Hypoglycaemics (treat diabetes), antihypertensives (treat high blood pressure).

PRESCRIPTION:
Yes.

PBS:
Yes.

PERMITTED IN SPORT:
No.

THEOPHYLLINES

TRADE and GENERIC NAMES:
Aminophylline (aminophylline).
Nuelin (theophylline).
Brondecon Elixir (choline theophyllinate).
Brondecon Expectorant (choline theophyllinate with guaiphenesin).

DRUG CLASS:
Bronchodilator.

USES:
Asthma, emphysema, bronchitis.

DOSAGE:
 Mixture: 10mLs to 20mLs four times a day.
Tablets: One every six hours.
Sustained release tablets: One twice a day.

FORMS:
Tablets, sustained release tablets, mixture, injection.

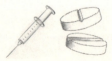

PRECAUTIONS:
Safe to use in pregnancy (A), breast feeding and children.
Use with caution in infants.
Use with caution in heart disease, irregular heart rhythm, angina, uncontrolled high blood pressure, stomach ulcers, heartburn, kidney disease and liver disease.
Lower doses necessary in elderly and lighter patients.
Higher doses may be necessary in smokers.
Blood tests to monitor blood level of theophylline may be necessary.
Use with caution in acute asthma.

SIDE EFFECTS:
Common: Nausea, vomiting, belly discomfort, rapid heart rate, tremor, palpitations.
Unusual: Irregular heart rate, convulsions, angina.

INTERACTIONS:
Other drugs:
- Cimetidine, allopurinol, propranolol, quinolone antibiotics, oral contraceptives, erythromycin, phenobarbitone, phenytoin, carbamazepine, rifampicin.

Herbs:
- St John's wort, piperine (Ayurvedic Piper nigrum).

Other substances:
- Reacts with alcohol, caffeine and nicotine.
- Marijuana.

PRESCRIPTION:
Yes.

PBS:
Aminophylline, theophylline: Yes.
Choline theophyllinate: No.

PERMITTED IN SPORT:
Yes.

OVERDOSE:
Serious. May cause vomiting, headache, irritability, rapid heart rate, confusion, fever, delirium and convulsions. Seek urgent medical assistance.

OTHER INFORMATION:
An early treatment for asthma that is still very useful.
Dose must be finely adjusted to give adequate clinical response while avoiding side effects.
See also Terbutaline.

Thiamine
(Vitamin B1)

TRADE NAMES:
Betamin, Beta-Sol.
A large number of other preparations include thiamine (Vitamin B1) alone or in combination with other vitamins and minerals.

DRUG CLASS:
Vitamin.

USES:
Vitamin B deficiency from fad diets, starvation and over-cooked foods.
Beriberi.

DOSAGE:
 Recommended daily allowance:
Females – 0.8mg;
Males – 1.1mg

FORMS:
Tablets, capsules, mixture, drops, injection.

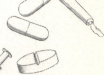

PRECAUTIONS:
Safe in pregnancy, breast feeding and children.

SIDE EFFECTS:
Minimal.

INTERACTIONS:

Other drugs:
- Diuretics, some laxatives.

PRESCRIPTION:
No.

PBS:
No.

PERMITTED IN SPORT:
Yes.

OVERDOSE:
No serious effects.

OTHER INFORMATION:
Thiamine is a water soluble vitamin found in liver, kidney, pork and whole grain. It is essential for the normal metabolism of carbohydrate foods. The symptoms of vitamin B deficiency include loss of appetite, muscle cramps, pins and needles sensation and ankle swelling. Remember, vitamins are merely chemicals that are essential for the functioning of the body, and if taken to excess, act as a drug.

THIAZIDE DIURETICS

TRADE and GENERIC NAMES:

Accuretic (hydrochlorothiazide, quinapril)
Amizide, Moduretic (hydrochlorothiazide, amiloride).
Aprinox (bendrofluazide).
Atacand Plus (hydrochlorothiazide, candesartan).
Avapro HCT, Karvezide (hydrochlorothiazide, irbesartan).
Dichlotride (hydrochlorothiazide).
Hydrene (hydrochlorothiazide, triamterene).
Hygroton (chlorthalidone – thiazide analogue diuretic).
Micardis Plus (hydrochlorothiazide, telmisartan).
Monoplus (hydrochlorothiazide, fosinopril).
Renitec Plus (hydrochlorothiazide, enalapril).
Teveten Plus (hydrochlorothiazide, eprosartan)
NB: Thiazides are underlined. Analogues are drugs that act like another drug.

DRUG CLASS:
Diuretic (increases urine production).

USES:
High blood pressure, tissue swelling, excess fluid in body.

DOSAGE:

One or two tablets in morning.

FORMS:
Tablets.

PRECAUTIONS:
Should not be used in pregnancy (C) unless medically essential. May reduce volume of milk in breast feeding, and is sometimes used for this purpose in women who wish to stop breast feeding.

Use with caution in children.
Use with caution in gout, kidney disease, liver disease, diabetes, SLE and asthma.

Do not take if:

 suffering from complete kidney failure.

SIDE EFFECTS:

Common: Increased urinary frequency.
Unusual: Nausea, vomiting, gut cramps, diarrhoea, dizziness, headache, rash.
Severe but rare (stop medication, consult doctor): Unusual bleeding, fainting.

INTERACTIONS:

Other drugs:
- Lithium, barbiturates, digoxin, insulin, steroids, lithium, NSAIDs.
- Tablets for controlling maturity onset diabetes.
- Beneficial interaction with most medications that lower blood pressure.

Herbs:
- Guarana, liquorice, celery, dandelion, uva ursi.

Other substances:
- Reacts with alcohol.

PRESCRIPTION:
Yes.

PBS:
Yes.

PERMITTED IN SPORT:
No (act as masking agents for other illegal drugs).

OVERDOSE:
Confusion, dizziness and gut spasms due to chemical (electrolyte) imbalances occur. Administer activated charcoal or induce vomiting if tablets taken recently, Give extra fluids. Seek medical assistance.

OTHER INFORMATION:
Widely used for fluid problems since the 1950s.

See also Amiloride, Bumetanide, Diazoxide, Frusemide, Indapamide, Spironolactone.

Thioguanine

TRADE NAME:
Lanvis.

USES:
Some types of acute leukaemia.

DOSAGE:

 Must be individually determined by doctor for each patient depending on severity of disease, age and weight of patient.

FORMS:
Tablets of 40mg (pale yellow).

PRECAUTIONS:
Must not be used in pregnancy (D) unless mother's life is at risk as damage to foetus may occur. Breast feeding must be ceased before use. May be used in children if medically essential.
Use with caution if infection present.
Regular blood tests to check blood cells and liver function essential.

Do not take if:

suffering from severe liver or kidney disease, significant viral infection, blood cell damage.

SIDE EFFECTS:
Common: Nausea, vomiting, diarrhoea, mouth soreness.
Severe but rare (stop medication, consult doctor): Yellow skin (jaundice), unusual bleeding or bruising.

INTERACTIONS:
Other drugs: Busulfan.

PRESCRIPTION:
Yes.

PBS:
Yes.

PERMITTED IN SPORT:
Yes.

Medications

OVERDOSE:
Serious. Induce vomiting if medication taken recently. Seek urgent medical assistance.

OTHER INFORMATION:
One of the original medications used to treat leukaemia, but still useful today.
See also **VINCA ALKALOIDS**.

Thioridazine
See PHENOTHIAZINES.

Thiothixene

TRADE NAME:
Navane.

DRUG CLASS:
Antipsychotic.

USES:
Schizophrenia, psychoses, other psychiatric conditions.

DOSAGE:
 Extremely variable, depending on patients condition. Tablets are taken two or three times a day. Follow doctors instructions carefully.

FORMS:
Tablets of 2mg (blue) and 10mg (cream).

PRECAUTIONS:
Should be used with caution in pregnancy (B1) and breast feeding.
Not for use in children under 12 years.
Use with caution in glaucoma, epilepsy, heart disease and high fevers.
Exposure to sunlight should be avoided, as a sun sensitive form of dermatitis may develop.
Should be used short term if possible.

Do not take if:
 suffering from depression or blood cell abnormalities.
- operating machinery, driving a vehicle or undertaking tasks that require concentration and alertness.

SIDE EFFECTS:
Common: Drowsiness, restlessness, agitation.
Unusual: Sleeplessness, rash, itch, breast enlargement, production of breast milk, dry mouth, blurred vision.
Severe but rare (stop medication, consult doctor): Unwanted and uncontrollable movements particularly of face, muscle rigidity, fever.

INTERACTIONS:
Other drugs:
- Atropine, barbiturates, narcotics, anaesthetics, other psychotropic drugs.

Herbs:
- Evening primrose (linoleic acid).

Other substances:
- Reacts adversely with alcohol.

PRESCRIPTION:
Yes.

PBS:
No.

PERMITTED IN SPORT:
Yes.

OVERDOSE:
May cause twitching, drowsiness, rigid muscles, weakness, incoordination and coma. Administer activated charcoal or induce vomiting it taken recently and patient alert. Seek urgent medical assistance.

OTHER INFORMATION:
Does not cause addiction or dependence.
See also **Amisulpride, Droperidol, Flupenthixol, Haloperidol, Lithium Carbonate, Olanzapine, PHENOTHIAZINES, Pimozide, Quetiapine, Risperidone, Zuclopenthixol.**

THYROID HORMONES
See Liothyronine, Thyroxine.

Thyroxine

TRADE NAMES:
Eutrosig, Oroxine (T4).

USES:
Under-active thyroid gland, thyroiditis.

DOSAGE:

One or two tablets a day on an empty stomach.
Start with low initial dose and slowly increase to a dose determined by doctor after regular blood tests.

FORMS:
Tablets (white) of 50μg, 100μg and 200μg.

PRECAUTIONS:
Safe to use in pregnancy (A), breast feeding and children.
Use with caution in heart disease, diabetes insipidus and high blood pressure.
Lower doses necessary in elderly.

Do not take if:
suffering from angina, over-active thyroid gland (hyperthyroidism), recent heart attack.

SIDE EFFECTS:
Only occur with overdosage.

INTERACTIONS:
Other drugs:
- Coumarin anticoagulants (eg. warfarin), barbiturates, narcotics, catecholamines, insulin, tricyclic antidepressants, digoxin, corticosteroids, colestipol, phenytoin.

Herbs:
- Horseradish, kelp, myrrh.

PRESCRIPTION:
Yes.

PBS:
Yes.

PERMITTED IN SPORT:
Yes.

OVERDOSE:
Serious. May cause rapid heart rate, irregular heartbeat, angina, restlessness, anxiety, tremor, headache, diarrhoea, vomiting, rapid breathing, fever, heart attack and death. Administer activated charcoal or induce vomiting if medication taken recently. Seek urgent medical assistance.

OTHER INFORMATION:
Widely used to counter the slowly progressive effects of thyroid underactivity, a problem that is common in middle-aged women. Does not cause addiction or dependence, but lifelong treatment usually necessary.

See also Liothyronine.

Tiagabine

TRADE NAME:
Gabitril.

DRUG CLASS:
Anticonvulsant.

USES:
Some types of epilepsy causing partial seizures.

DOSAGE:

7.5mg to 70mg a day in three divided doses with meals, usually in combination with other anticonvulsants.

FORMS:
Tablets of 5mg, 10mg and 15mg (white).

PRECAUTIONS:
Use with caution in pregnancy (B3) and breast feeding. May be used in children over 12 years of age.
Start with a very low dose and increase slowly.
Use with caution in anxiety states, liver disease and the elderly.
Do not stop suddenly, but reduce dose slowly.

Do not take if:
 suffering from severe liver disease.

SIDE EFFECTS:
Common: Dizziness, tiredness, nervousness, tremor, diarrhoea.
Unusual: Depression, temperamental.
Severe but rare (stop medication, consult doctor): Aggravation of epilepsy.

INTERACTIONS:
Other drugs:
- Phenytoin, carbamazepine, primidone, phenobarbitone.

Herbs:
- Evening primrose (linoleic acid), Gingko biloba.

Other substances:
- Alcohol, borage.

PRESCRIPTION:
Yes.

PBS:
Yes (authority required. Restricted to specific types of epilepsy not controlled by other medication).

PERMITTED IN SPORT:
Yes.

OVERDOSE:
Tiredness, dizziness, incoordination, dazed appearance and coma may occur. Induce vomiting or give activated charcoal if tablets taken recently. Seek medical assistance.

OTHER INFORMATION:
Introduced in 1998 for the management of more difficult and resistant cases of partial epilepsy.

See also **BARBITURATES, BENZODIAZEPINES, Carbamazepine, Clonazepam, Ethosuximide, Gabapentin, Lamotrigine, Levetiracetam, Oxcarbazepine, Phenytoin, Primidone, Sodium valproate, Sulthiame, Topiramate, Vigabatrin.**

Tiaprofenic acid

TRADE NAME:
Surgam.

DRUG CLASS:
NSAID (Nonsteroidal anti-inflammatory drug).

USES:
All forms of arthritis, inflammatory disorders, gout.

DOSAGE:

One tablet twice a day with food.

FORMS:
Tablets (white) of 200 and 300mg

PRECAUTIONS:
Should not be used in pregnancy (C) unless medically essential. Breast feeding should be ceased if necessary to use NSAID. Not for use in children under 3 years.
Use with caution in psychiatrically disturbed patients, epilepsy, severe infection, heart failure and kidney disease. Lower doses required in elderly, who may suffer more side effects.

Do not take if:

- suffering from peptic ulcer at present or in recent past.
- due for surgery (including dental surgery).
- suffering from bleeding disorder or anaemia.

SIDE EFFECTS:
Common: Stomach discomfort, diarrhoea, constipation, heartburn, nausea, headache, dizziness.
Unusual: Bladder irritation and inflammation, blurred vision, stomach ulcer, ringing noise in ears, retention of fluid, swelling of tissue, drowsiness, itch, rash, shortness of breath.

Severe but rare (stop medication, consult doctor): Vomit blood, pass blood in faeces, other unusual bleeding, asthma induced by medication.

INTERACTIONS:
Other drugs:
- Must never be used with anticoagulants (eg. warfarin).
- Probenecid, diuretics, lithium, methotrexate, beta blockers, ACE inhibitors.

PRESCRIPTION:
Yes.

PBS:
Yes.

PERMITTED IN SPORT:
Yes.

OVERDOSE:
Causes nausea, vomiting, severe headache, dizziness, confusion and convulsions. Administer activated charcoal or induce vomiting if taken recently. Seek medical assistance.

OTHER INFORMATION:
Used to give excellent relief to a wide variety of inflammatory conditions. Significant side effects (particularly on the stomach) in about 5% of patients limit their use.

See also Aspirin, Bufexamac, Celecoxib, Diclofenac, Diflunisal, Flurbiprofen, Ibuprofen, Indomethacin, Ketoprofen, Ketorolac trometanol, Mefenamic Acid, Naproxen, Piroxicam, Rofecoxib, SALICYLATES, Sulindac.

Tibolone

TRADE NAME:
Livial.

USES:
Symptoms of menopause, prevention of osteoporosis after menopause.

DOSAGE:
 One tablet a day.

FORMS:
Tablets of 2.5mg (white).

PRECAUTIONS:
Not to be used in pregnancy (D), breast feeding and children.
Use with caution in high cholesterol or triglycerides, liver disease or risk of blood clots (thromboses).
Do not commence in menopause until a year after last menstrual bleed.
Do not take if:
suffering from undiagnosed vaginal bleeding, hormone dependent tumours (eg. breast cancer), significant heart disease, recent stroke, blood clots or severe liver disorders.
• male.

SIDE EFFECTS:
Common: Weight gain, dizziness, headache, belly pain.
Unusual: Migraine, dermatitis, disturbed vision, skin irritation, nausea, constipation, breast pain, vaginal irritation.
Severe but rare (stop medication, consult doctor): Blood clots, liver damage, abnormal vaginal bleeding.

INTERACTIONS:
Other drugs:
• Hormone replacement therapies used in menopause, anticoagulants (eg. warfarin), barbiturates, carbamazepine, rifampicin.

PRESCRIPTION:
Yes.

PBS:
No.

PERMITTED IN SPORT:
Yes.

OVERDOSE:
Nausea and abnormal vaginal bleeding only likely effects.

OTHER INFORMATION:
Released in 2000 as a completely new method of managing symptoms of the menopause. Seems to suit many women very well, while others cannot tolerate it.
See also Norethisterone, Oestradiol, Oestriol, Piperazine oestrone sulphate.

Ticarcillin sodium

TRADE NAME:
Timentin (with potassium clavulanate).

DRUG CLASS:
Penicillin antibiotic.

USES:
Treatment of infections caused by susceptible bacteria (eg. septicaemia, pneumonia, bronchitis, osteomyelitis, septic arthritis, urinary infections, gynaecological infections and serious skin infections).

DOSAGE:
 Usually given by continuous drip infusion.

FORMS:
Injection.

PRECAUTIONS:
May be used in pregnancy (B2), children and breast feeding if clinically indicated. Use with caution in kidney failure and heart disease.

Do not take if:

 allergic to penicillin.

- suffering from glandular fever.

SIDE EFFECTS:
Common: Mild diarrhoea, nausea, vomiting.
Unusual: Itch, rash, headache, dizziness, hot flushes, tiredness.
Severe but rare (stop medication, consult doctor): Severe itchy rash, hives, severe diarrhoea, yellow skin (jaundice), unusual bruising or bleeding.

INTERACTIONS:
Other drugs:
- probenecid, aminoglycoside antibiotics.

PRESCRIPTION:
Yes.

PBS:
Yes.

PERMITTED IN SPORT:
Yes.

OVERDOSE:
Vomiting and diarrhoea likely.

OTHER INFORMATION:
Used only in more severe infections.

See also Amoxycillin, Ampicillin, Benzathine penicillin, Benzylpenicillin, Dicloxacillin, Flucloxacillin, Phenoxymethyl penicillin, Piperacillin, Procaine penicillin.

Ticlopidine

TRADE NAMES:
Ticlid, Ticlopidine Hexal, Tilodene.

DRUG CLASS:
Anticoagulant.

USES:
Prevention of blood clots (particularly in strokes) when other medications ineffective.

DOSAGE:
 One twice a day.

FORMS:
Tablets of 250mg.

PRECAUTIONS:
Should be used with caution in pregnancy (B1), breast feeding and children. Regular blood tests to monitor blood clotting time, liver function, blood cells and cholesterol required.

Do not take if:

suffering from severe liver or kidney disease, bleeding disorders, severe heart failure.
- due for surgery, including dental surgery and haemodialysis.

SIDE EFFECTS:
Common: Blood in faeces, black faeces, rash, headache, noises in ears.
Severe but rare (stop medication, consult doctor): Significant abnormal bleeding, blood cell abnormalities.

INTERACTIONS:
Other drugs:
- Must not be used with other anticoagulants (eg. warfarin) or aspirin.
- Theophylline, cimetidine, antacids, phenytoin, carbamazepine, NSAIDs.

PRESCRIPTION:
Yes.

PBS:
Yes (authority required. Restricted to patients at risk of stroke from blood clot who cannot tolerate aspirin, or who have had a brain blood vessel clot while on aspirin).

PERMITTED IN SPORT:
Yes.

OVERDOSE:
Serious. Seek urgent medical assistance.
See also Abciximab, Clopidrogel, Dipyridamole, Heparin, Phenindione, Warfarin.

Tilactase

TRADE NAMES:
Lactaid, Lact-Easy.

DRUG CLASS:
Pancreatic enzyme.

USES:
Deficiency of the enzyme lactase.

DOSAGE:
 One or two tablets with meal, or five to 20 drops mixed with milk feed.

FORMS:
Tablets, drops.

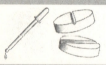

PRECAUTIONS:
Safe in pregnancy, breast feeding and children.
Drops must be mixed with milk and refrigerated for 24 hours before use. Use with caution in diabetes and galactosaemia.

SIDE EFFECTS:
None significant.

INTERACTIONS:
Nil.

PRESCRIPTION:
No.

PBS:
No.

PERMITTED IN SPORT:
Yes.

OVERDOSE:
Indigestion only likely effect.

OTHER INFORMATION:
Lactase is the enzyme that breaks down lactose, the sugar in milk. Some children are born without adequate amounts of this enzyme, and supplements must be given.
See also Pancrelipase.

Tiludronate disodium

TRADE NAME:
Skelid.

DRUG CLASS:
Bisphosphonate.

USES:
Paget's disease of bone.

DOSAGE:
 Two tablets once a day two hours before or after food, with water, for three months. Do not re-use for six months.

FORMS:
Tablets of 200mg.

PRECAUTIONS:
Use with caution in pregnancy (B2), breast feeding and children.
Ensure adequate calcium and vitamin D intake.
Use with caution in kidney disease.
Do not take if:
 suffering from severe kidney disease.

SIDE EFFECTS:
Common: Nausea, diarrhoea.
Unusual: Dizziness, giddiness, headache, tiredness, skin reaction.

INTERACTIONS:
Other drugs:
- Indomethacin, antacids, mineral supplements.

Other substances:
- Food containing calcium.

PRESCRIPTION:
Yes.

PBS:
Yes (authority required).

PERMITTED IN SPORT:
Yes.

OVERDOSE:
Serious. Symptoms include loss of appetite, tiredness, vomiting, diarrhoea, sweating, excess urine production, extreme thirst and headache. This may progress to high blood pressure and kidney failure. Administer activated charcoal or induce vomiting if taken recently. Seek medical assistance.

Timolol

TRADE NAMES:
Optimol, Tenopt, Timoptol, Timoptol-XE.
Cosopt (with dorzolamide).
Timpilo (with pilocarpine).
Xalacom (with latanoprost).

DRUG CLASS:
Beta blocker.

USES:
Glaucoma.

DOSAGE:
 One drop, once or twice a day.

FORMS:
Eye drops.

PRECAUTIONS:
Should be used with caution in pregnancy (C), but eye drops unlikely to cause problems.
Safe to use in breast feeding.
May be used with caution in children.
Use with care if suffering from alcoholism, liver or kidney failure or about to have surgery.
Use with caution in heart disease, shock or enlarged right heart.
Do not take if:
 suffering from diabetes, asthma, heart block, heart failure, slow heart rate, or allergic conditions.

SIDE EFFECTS:
Common: Low blood pressure, slow heart rate, burning eyes, stinging, asthma.
Severe but rare (stop medication, consult doctor): Severe asthma.

Medications

INTERACTIONS:
Other drugs:
- Calcium channel blockers, disopyramide, clonidine, adrenaline, other medications for irregular heartbeat, lignocaine, ergotamine, indomethacin, chlorpromazine, beta blocker tablets.

PRESCRIPTION:
Yes.

PBS:
Yes.

PERMITTED IN SPORT:
Yes.

OVERDOSE:
Unlikely to be serious effects if eye drops swallowed other than exacerbation of side effects.

See also Betaxolol, Bimatroprost, Brimonidine, Brinzolamide, Levobunolol, Pilocarpine, Travoprost.

Tinidazole

TRADE NAMES:
Fasigyn, Simplotan.

DRUG CLASS:
Antibiotic.

USES:
Infections caused by susceptible bacteria (particularly infections of gut and vagina), giardiasis, amoebic dysentery.

DOSAGE:
 Four tablets as a single dose.

FORMS:
Tablets of 500mg.

PRECAUTIONS:
Should not be used in pregnancy (B3) or breast feeding. Use with caution in children.
Use with caution in kidney disease.
Do not take if:
 suffering from brain disease, blood cell abnormalities.

SIDE EFFECTS:
Common: Bad taste, nausea, loss of appetite, diarrhoea.
Unusual: Vomiting, headache, constipation, dizziness, rash.

INTERACTIONS:
Other drugs:
- Anticoagulants (eg. warfarin).

Other substances:
- Reacts with alcohol.

PRESCRIPTION:
Yes.

PBS:
Yes.

PERMITTED IN SPORT:
Yes.

OVERDOSE:
Exacerbation of side effects only likely effect.

OTHER INFORMATION:
Introduced in the early 1980s as a rapid and effective form of treatment for Giardia of gut and Trichomonal infections of vagina.

See also Metronidazole.

Tiotropium

TRADE NAME:
Spiriva.

DRUG CLASS:
Anticholinergic.

USES:
Chronic obstructive airways disease, emphysema, chronic bronchitis.

DOSAGE:
 One capsule inhaled once a day.

FORMS:
Capsule (light green) of powder for inhalation through specific inhaler (Handihaler).

PRECAUTIONS:
Not designed for use in pregnancy (B1), breast feeding and children.
Not for acute treatment of wheeze or breathlessness.
Use with caution in severe kidney disease, glaucoma, or enlarged prostate.

SIDE EFFECTS:
Common: Dry mouth.
Unusual: Constipation, throat irritation, rapid heart rate.

INTERACTIONS:
None significant.

PRESCRIPTION:
Yes.

PBS:
Yes.

PERMITTED IN SPORT:
Yes.

OVERDOSE:
Excessive inhalation causes worsening of side effects. Swallowing capsules is harmless.

OTHER INFORMATION:
Introduced in 2003 as a new method of treating the very difficult to manage symptoms of lung damage caused by recurrent lung infections, smoking and other inhaled irritants.
See also Ipratropium bromide.

Tobramycin

TRADE NAMES:
Nebcin, Tobrex.
Generic brands also exist.

DRUG CLASS:
Aminoglycoside antibiotic.

USES:
Severe infections, particularly meningitis, blood, eye and belly infections.
Lung infections in cystic fibrosis.

DOSAGE:
 Injection: Every eight hours, or by continuous drip infusion.
Eye drops: Two drops every four hours.
Eye ointment: Insert two or three times a day.

FORMS:
Injection, eye drops, eye ointment.

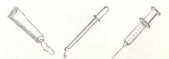

PRECAUTIONS:
Not to be used in pregnancy (D) unless absolutely essential for mother's well being. Breast feeding must be ceased before use. Use with caution and only when essential in children.
Use with caution in kidney disease and muscle disorders.
Blood tests to check that correct dose is being administered are recommended. Ensure adequate fluid intake during administration of medication.

SIDE EFFECTS:
Common: Rash, nausea, headache.
Unusual: Ear and kidney damage (dose related), vomiting, delayed wound healing (eye).
Severe but rare (stop medication, consult doctor): Ear noises or deafness, unusual bleeding or bruising.

INTERACTIONS:
Other drugs:
- Penicillin, cephalosporins, ethacrynic acid, frusemide, vitamin K.

PRESCRIPTION:
Yes.

PBS:
Yes (restricted to specific severe infections).

PERMITTED IN SPORT:
Yes.

OVERDOSE:
Ear and kidney damage possible. Give copious fluids to increase excretion through kidneys.

OTHER INFORMATION:
Very useful for the treatment of severe infections. Introduced in early 1980s.

See Amikacin, Gatifloxacin, Gentamicin, Neomycin.

Tocopherols
(Vitamin E)

TRADE NAMES:
A large number of preparations include tocopherols (Vitamin E) alone or in combination with other medications.

DRUG CLASS:
Vitamin.

USES:
Used in many soothing and healing creams, red blood cell disorders, fat absorption disorders.

DOSAGE:

Recommended daily allowance: 8 to 10mg a day.

FORMS:
Tablets, capsules, mixture, cream.

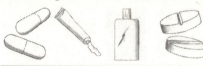

PRECAUTIONS:
Use with caution in pregnancy, breast feeding and children.
Do not take in high doses or for prolonged periods of time.

SIDE EFFECTS:
Minimal.

INTERACTIONS:
None significant.

PRESCRIPTION:
No.

PBS:
No.

PERMITTED IN SPORT:
Yes.

OVERDOSE:
Dangerous. May cause blood clots, high

blood pressure, breast lumps, headaches, vaginal bleeding, vision disturbances, muscle weakness and bowel disturbances if taken in high doses for a prolonged period of time.

OTHER INFORMATION:
Tocopherol is a fat soluble vitamin found in polyunsaturated fatty acids in a wide variety of foods. Remember, vitamins are merely chemicals that are essential for the functioning of the body, and if taken to excess, act as a drug.

Tolbutamide

TRADE NAME
Rastinon

DRUG CLASS
Hypoglycaemic

USES:
Diabetes not requiring insulin injections.

DOSAGE:
 One or two tablets twice a day after meals. Do not vary from prescribed dose without reference to a doctor.

FORMS:
Tablets (white) of 500mg and 1000mg.

PRECAUTIONS:
Not to be used in pregnancy (C), breastfeeding or children.
Illness, changes in diet, exercise and stress may change dosage requirements.
Lower doses required in elderley and dehabilitated patients.
Strict control of carbohydrates and sugars in diet essential.
Do not take if:
 severe liver or kidney disease, porphyria.

SIDE EFFECTS:
Common: Uncommon.
Unusual: Nausea, diarrhoea, belly discomfort, blurred vision.
Sever but rare (stop medication, consult doctor): Low blood sugar (see Overdose), yellow skin (jaundice), rash.

INTERACTIONS:
Other drugs: ACE inhibitors, beta blockers, other Hypoglycaemics, Chloramphenicol, Clofibrate, Clonidine, Coumarin, Pronenecid, MAOI, Miconazole, Salicylates, Tetracycline, Sulphonamides, Diazoxide, Corticosteroids, Nicotinic acid, Oestrogens, NSAIDs, Progestogens, Phenothiazines, Phenytoin, thyroid hormones, Laxatives.
Other substances: Reacts adversely with alcohol.

PRESCRIPTION:
Yes.

PBS:
Yes.

PERMITTED IN sport:
Yes.

OVERDOSE:
Serious. Symptoms of low blood sugar (hypoglycaemia) may include tiredness, confusion, chills, palpitations, sweating, vomiting, dizziness, hunger, blurred vision and fainting. Significant overdose can lead to coma and rarely death. Give sugary drinks or sweets if conscious. Seek urgent medical assistance.

OTHER INFORMATION:
Used mainly in elderly patients who develop maturity onset diabetes that is not severe enough to require insulin injections. Tolbutamide is less likely to cause hypoglycaemia (low blood sugar) than other Hypoglycaemics.

Tolnaftate

TRADE NAMES:
Curatin, Ringworm Ointment, Tinaderm, Tineafax.
Mycil Healthy Feet (with chlorhexidine).

DRUG CLASS:
Antifungal.

USES:
Fungal infections (tinea) of skin.

DOSAGE:
Apply two or three times a day.

FORMS:
Cream, powder, solution, spray.

PRECAUTIONS:
Safe to use in pregnancy, breast feeding and children.
Avoid eyes, nostrils, mouth, vagina and anus.
Seek medical advice if no improvement in 10 days.

SIDE EFFECTS:
Common: Skin irritation.

INTERACTIONS:
None significant.

PRESCRIPTION:
No.

PBS:
No.

PERMITTED IN SPORT:
Yes.

OTHER INFORMATION:
Old-fashioned, but very widely used, safe and generally effective.
See also IMIDAZOLES, Ketoconazole, Nystatin.

TONICS

See Piprandrol, Vitamins

Topiramate

TRADE NAME:
Topamax.

DRUG CLASS:
Anticonvulsant.

USES:
As additional treatment for some forms of partial epilepsy.

DOSAGE:
 25mg to 200mg twice a day. Increase dosage slowly.

FORMS:
Tablets of 25mg (white), 50mg (yellow), 100mg (yellow), 200mg (pink), sprinkle.

PRECAUTIONS:
Use with considerable caution in pregnancy (B3), breast feeding and children.
Use with caution in liver and kidney disease, psychiatric disorders.
Do not stop medication suddenly. Must be gradually withdrawn.

Do not take if:
 suffering from kidney stones.

SIDE EFFECTS:
Common: Drowsiness, dizziness, poor coordination, nausea, diarrhoea.
Unusual: Psychiatric disturbances, vomiting, low white blood cell count.
Severe but rare (stop medication, consult doctor): Kidney stones.

INTERACTIONS:

Other drugs:
- Phenytoin, carbamazepine, digoxin, sedatives, hypnotics, low dose oral contraceptives, phenobarbitone.

Herbs:
- Evening primrose (linoleic acid), Gingko biloba.

Other substances:
- Alcohol, borage.

PRESCRIPTION:
Yes.

PBS:
Yes (authority required. Restricted to use only when no other medication will control seizures).

PERMITTED IN SPORT:
Yes.

OVERDOSE:
No information available. Induce vomiting or administer activated charcoal if taken recently. Seek urgent medical attention.

OTHER INFORMATION:
Introduced in 1997. Not addictive.

See also BARBITURATES, BENZODIAZEPINES, Carbamazepine, Clonazepam, Ethosuximide, Gabapentin, Lamotrigine, Levetiracetam, Oxcarbazepine, Phenytoin, Primidone, Sodium valproate, Sulthiame, Tiagabine, Vigabatrin.

Toremifene

TRADE NAME:
Fareston.

DRUG CLASS:
Antineoplastic.

USES:
Some types of breast cancer in postmenopausal women.

DOSAGE:
 One tablet a day.

FORMS:
Tablets of 60mg (white).

PRECAUTIONS:
Not to be used in pregnancy (B3) unless essential for the health of the mother.
Not for use in breast feeding or children.
Use with caution in angina, heart disease, diabetes, liver disease or history of recent blood clots.
Not for prolonged use.

Do not take if:

 suffering severe liver disease or some conditions affecting the lining of the uterus.
- cancer of breast is oestrogen receptor negative.

SIDE EFFECTS:
Common: Excess calcium in blood, hot flushes, sweating, dizziness, diarrhoea, nausea, vaginal discharge.
Unusual: Vomiting, unusual bleeding from vagina, swelling of tissue, muscle pain.
Severe but rare (stop medication, consult doctor): Blood clots.

INTERACTIONS:

Other drugs:
- Phenytoin, carbamazepine, phenobarbitone, thiazide diuretics, warfarin, ketoconazole, macrolide antibiotics.

PRESCRIPTION:
Yes.

PBS:
Yes.

PERMITTED IN SPORT:
Yes.

OVERDOSE:
Exacerbation of side effects likely. Induce vomiting or administer activated charcoal if tablets taken recently. Seek medical assistance.

OTHER INFORMATION:
Released in 1998 as a new initial treatment for some types of breast cancer.
See also Letrozole, Tamoxifen.

Tramadol

TRADE NAMES:
Tramal, Zydol.

DRUG CLASS:
Analgesic.

USES:
Moderate to severe pain.

DOSAGE:
 One or two capsules, every four to six hours as needed. Maximum 600mg a day.

FORMS:
Capsules of 50mg (green/yellow), sustained release tablets of 100, 150 and 200mg, injection.

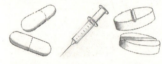

PRECAUTIONS:
Use with considerable caution in pregnancy, breast feeding and children. For short term use only.
Use with caution in undiagnosed abdominal pain, poor lung function, head injury, kidney and liver disease, and epilepsy.

Do not take if:

 suffering from alcoholism.

- addicted to narcotics (eg. heroin).

SIDE EFFECTS:
Common: Nausea, dizziness, constipation, sedation, sweating.
Unusual: Vomiting, convulsions, allergy reactions.

INTERACTIONS:

Other drugs:
- Hypnotics, other analgesics and narcotics, psychotropics, sedatives, general anaesthetics, buprenorphine, pentazocine, drugs used for depression (eg. SSRI, tricyclic antidepressants),

antipsychotics, MAOI, carbamazepine, quinidine, ketoconazole, erythromycin.
Other substances:
- Alcohol.

PRESCRIPTION:
Yes.

PBS:
Yes.

PERMITTED IN SPORT:
Yes.

OVERDOSE:
Symptoms may include drowsiness, confusion, difficulty in breathing, and coma. Induce vomiting if medication taken recently and patient alert. Seek urgent medical attention.

OTHER INFORMATION:
Very effective pain reliever, with small risk of dependency, introduced in 1999. Often prescribed or injected with a medication to reduce the risk of nausea and vomiting. Many doctors are using tramadol instead of narcotics as it is much safer.
See also Buprenorphine, Codeine Phosphate, Dextropropoxyphene, Methadone, Oxycodone.

Tramazoline

TRADE NAME:
Spray-Tish.

DRUG CLASS:
Vasoconstrictor.

USES:
Congestion of nose, hay fever.

DOSAGE:

One or two sprays to each nostril up to four times a day.

FORMS:
Nasal spray.

PRECAUTIONS:
Use in pregnancy only if medically essential. Use with caution in breast feeding and children. Not for use in children under 6 years.
Use with caution in high blood pressure or thyroid disease.
Avoid eye contact.
Not to be used regularly long term.
Do not take if:
 suffering from glaucoma.

SIDE EFFECTS:
Common: Tingling and burning of nose.
Unusual: Worsening of congestion in nose if used long term.

INTERACTIONS:
Other drugs:
- MAOI, tricyclic antidepressants.

Other substances:
- Reacts with alcohol.

PRESCRIPTION:
No.

PBS:
No.

PERMITTED IN SPORT:
Yes.

OVERDOSE:
Nasal congestion worsens if over used.

OTHER INFORMATION:
Very effective medication for stuffy noses from any cause.
See also Oxymetazoline, Xylometazoline.

Trandolapril
See ACE INHIBITORS.

Tranexamic acid

TRADE NAME:
Cyklokapron.

DRUG CLASS:
Haemostatic.

USES:
Hereditary angioedema, severe heavy periods (menorrhagia), hyphaemia, control of bleeding during surgery.

DOSAGE:
 As determined by doctor for each patient depending upon use.

FORMS:
Tablets of 500mg (white).

PRECAUTIONS:
May be used with caution in pregnancy (B1), breast feeding and children.
Use with caution in kidney disease, blood in urine due to kidney disease, bleeding into body cavities.

Do not take if:
 suffering from blood clots, recent history of blood clots, colour vision disturbances, bleeding around brain.

SIDE EFFECTS:
Common: Nausea, diarrhoea.
Unusual: Impaired colour vision, rash.
Severe but rare (stop medication, consult doctor): Blood clot in vein.

INTERACTIONS:
None significant.

PRESCRIPTION:
Yes.

PBS:
Yes.

PERMITTED IN SPORT:
Yes.

OVERDOSE:
Nausea and vomiting likely.
See also HAEMOSTATIC AGENTS.

Tranylcypromine
See MAOI.

Travoprost

TRADE NAME:
Travatan.

USES:
Glaucoma.

DOSAGE:

One drop in eye in evening. Use at least five minutes away from other eye drops.
Remove contact lenses before use, and do not replace for 15 minutes. Apply pressure to tear duct at inner corner of eye for two minutes after using drop.
May be used in conjunction with timolol drops.

FORMS:
Eye drops.

PRECAUTIONS:
Not for use in pregnancy (B3). Use with caution in breast feeding and children. Use with caution in dry eyes and inflammatory eye conditions.

SIDE EFFECTS:
Common: Red and itchy eye, eye discomfort.
Unusual: Changes in eyelash colour, dry eye.

INTERACTIONS:
None significant.

PRESCRIPTION:
Yes.

PBS:
Yes.

PERMITTED IN SPORT:
Yes.

OVERDOSE:
May have serious effects if eye drops swallowed. Seek urgent medical advice.

OTHER INFORMATION:
Introduced in 2002.
See Acetazolamide, Apraclonidine, Betaxolol, Bimatoprost, Brimonidine barbrate, Brinzolamide, Carbachol, Dipivefrine hydrochloride, Dorzolamide hydrochloride, Latanoprost, Levobunolol, Phenylephrine, Pilocarpine, Timolol.

Tretinoin
See KERATOLYTICS.

Triamcinolone

TRADE NAMES:
Aristocort, Kenacort-A, Kenalog in Orabase.
Kenacomb, Otocomb (with neomycin, gramicidin, nystatin).

DRUG CLASS:
Corticosteroid.

USES:
Severe inflammation of skin (eczema, dermatitis etc.), mouth and other tissues. Severe rheumatoid and other forms of severe arthritis, autoimmune diseases, and other severe and chronic inflammatory diseases.

DOSAGE:

Skin preparations: Apply two or three times a day.
Ear drops: Insert two drops twice a day.
Ear ointment: Insert once or twice a day.
Injection: Limited number of injections to affected site or joint once or twice a week.

FORMS:
Cream, ointment, paste, ear drops, injection.

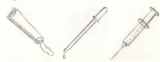

PRECAUTIONS:

Should be used in pregnancy (C), breast feeding and children only on specific medical advice.

Skin and ear preparations safe in pregnancy, breast feeding and children. Use injection with caution if under stress, and in patients with under-active thyroid gland, liver disease, diverticulitis, high blood pressure, myasthenia gravis or kidney disease.

Avoid eyes with all forms.

Use for shortest period of time, and in lowest concentration possible.

Do not use injection if:

 suffering from any form of infection, peptic ulcer, or osteoporosis.
- having a vaccination

Do not use cream if:

 suffering any form of fungal, viral or bacterial skin infection.

SIDE EFFECTS:

Most significant side effects occur only with prolonged use.

Common: Injection – May cause bloating, weight gain, rashes and intestinal disturbances.

Ear drops and skin preparations – Rarely cause adverse reactions.

Unusual: Injection – Dose related effects. Biochemical disturbances of blood, muscle weakness, bone weakness, impaired wound healing, skin thinning, tendon weakness, peptic ulcers, gullet ulcers, bruising, increased sweating, loss of fat under skin, premature ageing, excess facial hair growth in women, pigmentation of skin and nails, acne, convulsions, headaches, dizziness, growth suppression in children, aggravation of diabetes, worsening of infections, cataracts, aggravation of glaucoma, blood clots in veins and sleeplessness.

Skin preparations – thinning of skin, scarring of skin, premature ageing of skin.

Severe but rare (stop medication, consult doctor): Any significant side effect should be reported to a doctor immediately.

INTERACTIONS:
None significant.

PRESCRIPTION:
Yes.

PBS:
Most forms: Yes.
Kenalog in Orabase: No.

PERMITTED IN SPORT:
Yes.

OVERDOSE:
Exacerbation of side effects likely.

OTHER INFORMATION:
Extremely effective and useful medication if used correctly. Lowest dose and shortest possible course should be used. Not addictive.

See also Betamethasone, Desonide, Hydrocortisone, Methylprednisolone, Mometasone.

Triamterene
See THIAZIDE DIURETICS.

Triazolam

TRADE NAME:
Halcion.

DRUG CLASS:
Hypnotic/Sedative, Benzodiazepine.

USES:
Insomnia (sleeplessness).

DOSAGE:

One to four tablets 30 minutes before going to bed.

FORMS:
Tablet of 0.125mg (violet).

PRECAUTIONS:
Not for use in pregnancy (C), breast feeding and children.
Lower dose required in elderly.
Should be used intermittently and not constantly as dependency may develop. Use with caution in glaucoma, heart disease, low blood pressure, kidney or liver disease, psychiatric conditions, sleep apnoea, depression and epilepsy.

Do not take if:
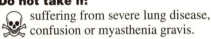 suffering from severe lung disease, confusion or myasthenia gravis.
- tendency to addiction or dependence.
- operating machinery, driving a vehicle or undertaking tasks that require concentration and alertness.

SIDE EFFECTS:
Common: Confusion and falls in elderly, impaired alertness.
Unusual: Dizziness, incoordination, poor memory, headache, hangover in morning, slurred speech, nightmares.

INTERACTIONS:
Other drugs:
- Severe interaction with ketoconazole, nefazodone, itraconazole.
- Other medications that reduce alertness (eg. barbiturates, antihistamines, antianxiety drugs).
- Disulfiram, anticonvulsants, anticholinergics, cimetidine, macrolide antibiotics (eg. erythromycin), verapamil, diltiazem, isoniazid, fluvoxamine, sertraline, paroxetine.

Herbs:
- Guarana, kava kava, passionflower, St John's wort, valerian, celery, camomile.

Other substances:
- Reacts with alcohol to cause excessive drowsiness.
- Grapefruit juice.

PRESCRIPTION:
Yes.

PBS:
No.

PERMITTED IN SPORT:
Yes.

OVERDOSE:
Seldom life threatening. May cause drowsiness, confusion and coma. Induce vomiting if tablets taken recently. Seek medical assistance.

OTHER INFORMATION:
Dependency may develop if used long term.

See also BARBITURATES, Chlormethiazole, Flunitrazepam, Midazolam, Nitrazepam, Temazepam, Zolpidem, Zopiclone.

Triclosan

TRADE NAMES:

Microshield T, Oxy Skin Wash, Phisohex, Sapoderm.
Clearasil Acne Cream (with sulfur and other ingredients).
Dettol (with chloroxylenol).
Oilatum Plus, QV Flare Up (with paraffin and benzalkonium chloride).

DRUG CLASS:

Antiseptic.

USES:

Acne, minor skin infections, skin cleansing.

DOSAGE:

 Depends on form. Usually once or twice a day.

FORMS:

Cream, solution, gel, dressing, soap.

PRECAUTIONS:

Safe to use in pregnancy, breast feeding and children.
Avoid eyes.
Not for long term use.

SIDE EFFECTS:

Common: Minimal.
Unusual: Reactive dermatitis.

INTERACTIONS:

None significant.

PRESCRIPTION:

No.

PBS:

No.

PERMITTED IN SPORT:

Yes.

OVERDOSE:

Diarrhoea and vomiting only likely effects if swallowed.

OTHER INFORMATION:

Very widely used and safe.
See also KERATOLYTICS.

TRICYCLIC ANTIDEPRESSANTS

TRADE and GENERIC NAMES:

Allegron (nortriptyline).
Anafranil, Clopram, GenRx Clomipramine, Placil (clomipramine).
Deptran, Sinequan (doxepin).
Dothep, Prothiaden (dothiepin).
Endep, Tryptanol (amitriptyline).
Melipramine, Tofranil (imipramine).
Surmontil (trimipramine).
Several locally marketed brands also produced.

DRUG CLASS:

Antidepressants.

USES:

Depression, sleeplessness (insomnia), bed wetting (amitriptyline and imipramine only).

DOSAGE:

One to four or more tablets or capsules usually taken in evening, but may be divided in equal or unequal doses through day when large amount of medication taken.

FORMS:

Tablets, capsules, mixture.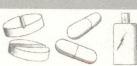

PRECAUTIONS:
Should not be used in pregnancy (C) or breast feeding unless medically essential. May be used with caution in children. Potentially suicidal patients should be watched carefully.
Use with caution in heart disease, psychotic and manic states, kidney and liver disease.
Lower doses required in elderly.
Do not stop medication suddenly, but gradually reduce dosage over some days or weeks.

Do not take if:

 suffering from glaucoma or difficulty in passing urine.

SIDE EFFECTS:
Common: Drowsiness, dry mouth, dizziness, tremor, nausea, constipation, rapid heart rate.
Unusual: Confusion, difficulty in passing urine, decreased libido, vomiting, blurred vision, poor concentration, hallucinations, breast enlargement, intestinal cramps, rash.
Severe but rare (stop medication, consult doctor): Yellow skin (jaundice).

INTERACTIONS:
Other drugs:
- Severe interaction with MAOI.
- Sedatives, anxiolytics, cimetidine, quinidine, barbiturates, guanethidine, antihistamines, phenytoin, carbamazepine, sympathomimetics, other antidepressants.

Herbs:
- Ma huang, yohimbine.

Other substances:
- Reacts with alcohol to cause drowsiness.

PRESCRIPTION:
Yes.

PBS:
Yes.

PERMITTED IN SPORT:
Yes.

OVERDOSE:
May be very serious. Symptoms include blurred vision, inability to pass urine, delirium, agitation, incoordination, convulsions, reduced breathing, coma and death. Administer activated charcoal or induce vomiting if taken recently and patient alert. Seek urgent medical assistance. Patients with Tricyclic overdose are often observed in intensive care.

OTHER INFORMATION:
Tricyclics are widely used and are the main medication for control of depression. They are slow acting and may take two or more weeks for any positive effect to occur. In use for over 40 years.

See also Citalopram, Fluoxetine, Fluvoxamine, MAOI, Mianserin, Mirtazapine, Moclobemide, Nefazodone, Paroxetine, Reboxetine, Sertraline, Venlafaxine.

Trifluoperazine
See PHENOTHIAZINES.

Triglycerides
See FATTY ACIDS.

Trigonella
See Fenugreek.

Trimeprazine
See ANTIHISTAMINES, SEDATING.

Trimethoprim

TRADE NAMES:
Alprim, Triprim.
Bactrim, Cosig Forte, Resprim, Septrin, Trimoxazole-BC (with sulfamethoxazole – this combination is known as co-trimoxazole).
Several locally marketed brands also produced.

DRUG CLASS:
Antibiotic.

USES:
Urinary tract (bladder and kidney) infections.
Co-trimoxazole used for a wide variety of infections.

DOSAGE:

One tablet a day at night with food.
Co-trimoxazole: One tablet twice a day.

FORMS:
Tablets, suspension, injection.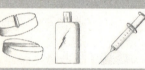

PRECAUTIONS:
Use in pregnancy (B3) only if medically essential. Not to be used in breast feeding, or in children under 6 years.
Use with caution in folate deficiency, liver and kidney disease.
Lower doses may be necessary in elderly. Normally not for constant long term use.
Do not take if:
 suffering from blood disorders, pernicious anaemia, severe liver and kidney disease.

SIDE EFFECTS:
Common: Itch, rash.
Unusual: Nausea, vomiting, fever.
Severe but rare (stop medication, consult doctor): Unusual bleeding or bruising.

INTERACTIONS:
Other drugs:
- Anticoagulants (eg. warfarin), methotrexate, pyrimethamine.

PRESCRIPTION:
Yes.

PBS:
Yes.

PERMITTED IN SPORT:
Yes.

OVERDOSE:
Nausea, vomiting, dizziness, headache, depression, confusion and damage to bone marrow may occur. Administer activated charcoal or induce vomiting if medication taken recently. Seek medical assistance.

OTHER INFORMATION:
Widely used for minor to moderate urinary infections. Synthetic antibiotic. Does not cause dependence or addiction.
See also ANTIBIOTICS.

Trimipramine
See **TRICYCLIC ANTIDEPRESSANTS**.

Triprolidine
See **ANTIHISTAMINES, SEDATING**.

TROPHIC HORMONES

DISCUSSION:

Trophic hormones are given as injections to aid infertility, prevent miscarriages, stimulate sperm production in men, control breast pain due to hormone imbalances, to start puberty in cases where it has been delayed, and to control some patients with asthma and arthritis. There are a number of rarer diseases in which they are also useful. Commonly used trophic hormones include menopausal gonadotrophin, chorionic gonadotrophin, and tetrocosactrin. Adverse reactions are uncommon but severe when they do occur. They include nausea, headaches, peptic ulcers, fluid retention, high blood pressure, inappropriate sexual development and skin markings.

See Chorionic gonadotrophin, Menopausal gonadotrophin.

Tropicamide

See MYDRIATICS.

Tropisetron

TRADE NAME:
Navoban.

USES:
Prevention of nausea and vomiting caused by surgery and cancer treatments.

DOSAGE:

One capsule in morning immediately on waking, one hour before food.

FORMS:
Capsule of 5mg (yellow/white), injection.
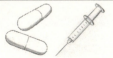

PRECAUTIONS:
Should not be used in pregnancy (B3) or children unless medically essential. Breast feeding should be ceased before use.
Use caution if operating machinery or driving a vehicle.
Use with caution in high blood pressure, irregular heart rhythm, kidney and liver disease.

SIDE EFFECTS:
Common: Tiredness, headache, dizziness, constipation.
Unusual: Diarrhoea, loss of appetite.

INTERACTIONS:
Other drugs:
• Rifampicin, barbiturates.
Other substances:
• Avoid food for one hour after taking capsule.

PRESCRIPTION:
Yes.

PBS:
Yes.

PERMITTED IN SPORT:
Yes.

OVERDOSE:
Hallucinations and high blood pressure may occur. Seek medical assistance.

OTHER INFORMATION:
Introduced in 1995.
See also Metoclopramide.

Tuberculosis vaccine
See BCG vaccine.

Typhoid vaccine
See Salmonella typhi vaccine.

Medications

Ultralente insulin

See INSULINS.

Undecenoic acid

TRADE NAME:
Pedoz (with zinc oxide and other ingredients).

DRUG CLASS:
Antifungal.

USES:
Tinea pedis (athlete's foot), smelly feet.

DOSAGE:
 Apply twice a day.

FORMS:
Dusting powder.

PRECAUTIONS:
Safe to use in pregnancy, breast feeding and children.
Avoid eyes, nose and mouth.
Use with caution on broken skin.

SIDE EFFECTS:
Minimal.

INTERACTIONS:
None significant.

PRESCRIPTION:
No.

PBS:
No.

PERMITTED IN SPORT:
Yes.

OVERDOSE:
Unlikely to have serious effects if swallowed.

Undecylenamide

TRADE NAMES:
Only available in Australia in combination with other medications.
Mycoderm (with salicylic acid, butyl hydroxybenzoate, sodium propionate).
Sebitar (with tar, salicylic acid).

DRUG CLASS:
Antifungal.

USES:
Mild fungal infections, dandruff.

DOSAGE:
 Powder: Apply to affected areas twice a day or more. May be sprinkled inside shoes.
Shampoo: Massage into wet hair and leave for five minutes before rinsing. Use at least once a week.

FORMS:
Shampoo, powder.

PRECAUTIONS:
Safe in pregnancy, breast feeding and children.
Avoid eye contact.

SIDE EFFECTS:
Minimal.

INTERACTIONS:
Nil.

PRESCRIPTION:
No.

PBS:
No. Sebitar available to Veterans Affairs pensioners.

PERMITTED IN SPORT:
Yes.

See also Clotrimazole, Econazole, Fluconazole, Itraconazole, Ketoconazole, Miconazole.

Urea

TRADE NAMES:
Aquacare, Hamilton Dry Skin Cream, Nutraplus, Urecare, Urederm.
Calmurid, Dermadrate (with lactic acid).
Curaderm (with salicylic acid, linoleic acid and other ingredients).
Eulactol Heel Balm (with lanolin and other ingredients).
SP cream (with salicylic acid and other ingredients).
Psor-Asist Scalp Lotion, Sunspot cream (with salicylic acid).
Found in numerous other creams in combination with other medications.

USES:
Skin moisturiser for dry skin, eczema, irritated skin.

DOSAGE:
 Apply as often as required.

FORMS:
Cream.

PRECAUTIONS:
Safe to use in pregnancy, breast feeding and children.

SIDE EFFECTS:
None.

INTERACTIONS:
None.

PRESCRIPTION:
No.

PBS:
Some forms: Yes.
Most forms: No.

PERMITTED IN SPORT:
Yes.

OTHER INFORMATION:
Safe, simple, cheap and effective. In use for hundreds of years as a moisturiser.

See also Icthammol, TARS, Zinc oxide.

URICOSURICS

DESCRIPTION:
Medications that reduce levels of uric acid in blood by increasing its loss in urine to prevent gout.

See Allopurinol, Probenecid.

URINARY ACIDIFIERS

DISCUSSION:
Medications that make urine more acid.
See Ammonium chloride.

URINARY ALKALINISERS

TRADE and GENERIC NAMES:
Citralite, Citravescent (citric acid, sodium bicarbonate, sodium citrotartrate, tartaric acid, and other ingredients).
Sodibic (sodium bicarbonate).
Ural (sodium citrotartrate).

USES:
Bladder and kidney infection, excess stomach acid.

DOSAGE:
 One or two sachets dissolved in water, three or four times a day.

FORMS:
Powder in sachet, granules in sachet, capsules.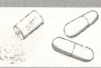

PRECAUTIONS:
Safe to use in pregnancy, breast feeding and children.
Use with caution in heart and kidney disease, high blood pressure.
Do not exceed prescribed dose.
Use long term with caution.
Do not take if:
 suffering from kidney failure, high blood sodium levels.

SIDE EFFECTS:
Common: Minimal.
Unusual: Diarrhoea.

INTERACTIONS:
Other drugs: Hexamine, quinolone antibiotics, antacids, laxatives, lithium.

PRESCRIPTION:
No.

PBS:
Most forms: Yes.
Sodibic: No (available to Veteran Affairs pensioners).

PERMITTED IN SPORT:
Yes.

OVERDOSE:
Severe diarrhoea likely.

OTHER INFORMATION:
Widely used to ease the symptoms of urinary infections and prevent recurrences. Does not cause addiction or dependence. Alkalinisers are designed to raise the pH (acidity) of the urine from a low value to a high value, making it more alkaline and less attractive to bacteria. They should not be used regularly in the long term.
See also Hexamine hippurate.

URINARY ANTISEPTICS

DISCUSSION:
Medications used to prevent urinary infections.
**See Hexamine hippurate,
URINARY ALKALINISERS.**

Ursodeoxycholic acid

TRADE NAME:
Ursofalk.

USES:
Cirrhosis of liver, dissolving some types of gall stones.

DOSAGE:

Complex. Must be determined individually for each patient by doctor.

FORMS:
Capsules of 250mg.

PRECAUTIONS:
Use with caution in pregnancy (B3), breast feeding and children.
Regular blood tests to check liver function necessary.
Do not take if:
 suffering from acute cholecystitis, bile duct inflammation, bile duct obstruction.

SIDE EFFECTS:
Common: Minimal.
Unusual: Diarrhoea, itchy skin, nausea, vomiting, sleep disturbances.
Severe but rare (stop medication, consult doctor): Worsening liver disease.

INTERACTIONS:
Other drugs:
- Ciprofloxacin, cyclosporin, cholestyramine, charcoal, colestipol, antacids, oral contraceptives, oestrogen.

PRESCRIPTION:
Yes.

PBS:
Yes (authority required).

PERMITTED IN SPORT:
Yes.

OVERDOSE:
No information available. Seek medical attention.

VACCINES

DISCUSSION:
Vaccines prevent diseases caused by viruses and bacteria by specifically stimulating the immune system to produce antibodies against the infecting agent.

See BCG (TB) vaccine, Chickenpox vaccine, Cholera vaccine, Coxiella burnetti (Q fever) vaccine, Diphtheria vaccine, Haemophilus influenzae B (HiB) vaccine, Hepatitis A vaccine, Hepatitis B vaccine, Influenza vaccine, Japanese encephalitis virus vaccine, Measles vaccine, Meningococcal Vaccine, Mumps vaccine, Poliomyelitis (Sabin) vaccine, Pneumococcal vaccine, Rabies vaccine, Rubella (German measles) vaccine, Salmonelli typhi (typhoid) vaccine, Tetanus vaccine, Whooping cough vaccine, Yellow fever vaccine, Yersinia (plague) vaccine.

Valaciclovir

TRADE NAME:
Valtrex.

DRUG CLASS:
Antiviral.

USES:
Shingles, genital herpes, herpes infection of eye.

DOSAGE:

Shingles: Two tablets three times a day for a week. Must be started within 72 hours of first sign of rash.
Herpes: One tablet twice a day.

FORMS:
Tablets of 500mg (white).

PRECAUTIONS:
Use with considerable caution in pregnancy (B3). Use with caution in breast feeding. Safe in children. Use with caution in dehydration, significant kidney and liver disease, immunosupression.

SIDE EFFECTS:
Common: Minimal.
Unusual: Headache, nausea.

INTERACTIONS:
Other drugs:
- Diuretics, probenecid, cimetidine, cyclosporin.

PRESCRIPTION:
Yes.

PBS:
Yes (authority required. Restricted to specific confirmed cases of shingles and herpes).

PERMITTED IN SPORT:
Yes.

OVERDOSE:
Exacerbation of side effects only likely problem.

OTHER INFORMATION:
Introduced in 1997 as a very effective antiviral.

See also Aciclovir, Famciclovir.

Valerian

USES:
Insomnia, anxiety.

DOSAGE:

100mg to 1800mg a day divided into several doses.

FORMS:
Capsules, liquid, tablets, tea bags.

PRECAUTIONS:
Do not use in pregnancy or breast feeding. Use care with driving or operating machinery after use.

SIDE EFFECTS:
Common: Nausea, diarrhoea.
Unusual: Headache, restlessness, insomnia, irregular heart rhythm.

INTERACTIONS:
Other drugs:
- Sedatives, barbiturates, benzodiazepines (eg. diazepam).

Other substances:
- Alcohol.

PRESCRIPTION:
No.

PBS:
No.

PERMITTED IN SPORT:
Yes.

OVERDOSE:
Exacerbation of side effects likely.

OTHER INFORMATION:
Not used in orthodox medical practice.

Valganciclovir

TRADE NAME:
Valcyte.

DRUG CLASS:
Antiviral.

USES:
CMV (cytomegalovirus) eye infection in patients with AIDS.

DOSAGE:

Two tablets twice a day for three weeks, then two tablets once a day.

FORMS:
Tablets of 450mg.

PRECAUTIONS:
Not for use in pregnancy (D) and breast feeding.
Use with caution in children.
Regular blood tests to check blood cells essential.

Do not take if:

suffering from low haemoglobin, white cell or platelet count.

SIDE EFFECTS:
Common: Nausea, diarrhoea, anaemia, fever, tiredness, headache, cough, rash.
Unusual: Blood cell abnormalities, decreased fertility, reduced alertness, poor coordination, dizziness.
Severe but rare (stop medication, consult doctor): Bone marrow damage, convulsions, psychotic episodes, eye damage.

INTERACTIONS:
Other drugs:
- Severe interaction with ganciclovir, aciclovir, valaciclovir.
- Probenecid, zidovudine, didanosine, zalcitabine.

PRESCRIPTION:
Yes.

PBS:
Yes (very restricted, authority required).

PERMITTED IN SPORT:
Yes.

OVERDOSE:
Very serious. Seek urgent medical attention.

OTHER INFORMATION:
introduced in 2002 for the treatment of an uncommon complication of AIDS.

Valproate

See Sodium valproate.

Vancomycin

TRADE NAME:
Vancocin.

DRUG CLASS:
Antibiotic.

USES:
Capsules: Severe intestinal infections.
Injection, infusion: Very severe infections of heart, bone, lungs, blood and soft tissue.

DOSAGE:
 One capsule every six hours.

FORMS:
Capsules of 125mg (peach/blue) and 250mg (grey/blue), injection, infusion.

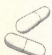 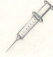

PRECAUTIONS:
Use with caution in pregnancy (B2) and breast feeding. May be used when appropriate in children.
Use with caution in kidney disease, bowel inflammation and hearing loss.
Lower doses necessary in elderly.
Not designed for long term use.

SIDE EFFECTS:
Common: Indigestion, nausea, chills, diarrhoea.
Unusual: Vomiting, hearing loss, rash, muscle pain.
Severe but rare (stop medication, consult doctor): Noises in ears or reduced hearing.

INTERACTIONS:
Other drugs:
• Aspirin, some other antibiotics.

PRESCRIPTION:
Yes.

PBS:
Yes (restricted to complicated infections).

PERMITTED IN SPORT:
Yes.

OVERDOSE:
May cause kidney damage. Seek medical assistance.

OTHER INFORMATION:
Very potent and effective antibiotic when used appropriately.

Varicella zoster vaccine

See Chickenpox vaccine.

VASOCONSTRICTORS

DISCUSSION:

Vasoconstrictors are drugs that constrict (reduce in size) blood vessels (arteries in particular) and raise blood pressure. When a patient collapses with a heart attack, severe allergy or shock, it is often due to the sudden overdilation of all the arteries in the body, which causes a very low blood pressure. This can be corrected by a doctor giving an injection of a vasoconstrictor such as adrenaline. Otherwise, vasoconstrictors are used mainly as drops in the eye and nose, and as additives (eg. pseudoephedrine) to some cold and hay fever remedies. Vasoconstrictor eye drops constrict any dilated arteries criss-crossing the white of the eye to leave it looking and feeling much better. Nose drops and sprays containing phenylephrine shrink down the dilated arteries in the nose that develop with hay fever. They can therefore ease the congestion and stuffiness in the nose and allow victims to breathe more easily. Overuse can cause a rebound effect, and the nose becomes inflamed because the drops cause it to swell again. All swallowed or injected vasoconstrictors should be used with caution in patients with high blood pressure, diabetes, thyroid disease or heart disease.

See Adrenaline, Naphazoline and Antazoline, Oxymetazoline, Phenylephrine, Pseudoephedrine, Tetrahydrozoline, Tramazoline, Xylometazoline.

VASODILATORS

DISCUSSION:

Arteries, and to a lesser extent veins, are surrounded by tiny muscles that control the diameter of the blood vessel tube by contracting and relaxing it. If arteries in the arms and legs are excessively contracted or blocked by plaques of cholesterol (atherosclerosis), the amount of blood reaching the distant parts of the body may be insufficient for them to work properly. The earliest sign of a poor blood supply is pallor of the skin. This is followed by muscle weakness and pain. Vasodilators will relax the tiny muscles around the artery, enabling it to dilate to its maximum extent and allowing the greatest possible amount of blood to reach the affected areas. Vasodilators can also be used in the emergency treatment of very high blood pressure.

See Betahistine, Diazoxide, Guanethidine, Nicorandil, Nicotinic Acid, Phenoxybenzamine.

Vasopressin

TRADE NAME:

Pitressin.

DRUG CLASS:

Antidiuretic.

USES:

Diabetes insipidus, some investigations.

DOSAGE:

 May be given by injection, or soaked onto cotton buds that are inserted into nose.

FORMS:

Injection.

PRECAUTIONS:

Use with caution in pregnancy (B2), breast feeding and children.
Must not be given by intravenous injection.
Use with caution in artery disease, heart disease, angina, kidney disease, epilepsy, migraine, asthma, goitre, heart attack, blood clots, hardening of arteries.

SIDE EFFECTS:
Common: Minimal.
Unusual: Sweating, tremor, dizziness, fainting, headache, nausea, gut cramps.

INTERACTIONS:
None significant.

PRESCRIPTION:
Yes.

PBS:
No.

PERMITTED IN SPORT:
Yes.

OVERDOSE:
Unlikely to cause serious effects.

OTHER INFORMATION:
One of the few effective treatments for the rare disease diabetes insipidus, which is completely unrelated to sugar diabetes (diabetes mellitus).
See also Desmopressin acetate.

Venlafaxine

TRADE NAME:
Efexor.

DRUG CLASS:
Antidepressant.

USES:
Depression.

DOSAGE:

37.5mg to 225mg a day. May be given in one or more doses. Increase dose slowly.

FORMS:
Tablets (peach) of 37.5mg and 75mg, capsules of 75mg (peach), and 150mg (orange).
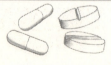

PRECAUTIONS:
Use with caution in pregnancy (B2), breast feeding and children.
Use with caution in higher doses.
Check blood pressure regularly.
Use with caution in epilepsy, other psychiatric conditions, recent heart attack, rapid heart rate, bleeding tendency, glaucoma, liver and kidney diseases.
Watch patient carefully if suicidal.
Lower doses necessary in elderly.
Do not stop suddenly, but reduce dose slowly.

Do not take if:
 taking MAOI.

SIDE EFFECTS:
Common: Dizziness, sleeplessness, nervousness, nausea, diarrhoea, dry mouth.
Unusual: Tiredness, vomiting, excess sweating, impotence, general tiredness.
Severe but rare (stop medication, consult doctor): High blood pressure.

INTERACTIONS:
Other drugs:
- MAOI may cause very serious effects.
- Other antidepressants.
- Haloperidol, clozapine, imipramine, desipramine, warfarin, amiodarone, erythromycin, fluconazole, quinidine.

Herbs:
- St John's wort, ma huang.

Other substances:
- Grapefruit.

PRESCRIPTION:
Yes.

PBS:
Yes.

PERMITTED IN SPORT:
Yes.

OVERDOSE:
May be serious. Induce vomiting or give activated charcoal if taken recently. Seek urgent medical attention.

OTHER INFORMATION:
Introduced in 1997 for the management of more difficult cases of depression.

See also Citalopram, Fluoxetine, Fluvoxamine, Paroxetine, Reboxetine, Sertraline.

Verapamil

TRADE NAMES:
Anpec, Cordilox, Isoptin, Veracaps, Verahexal.

DRUG CLASS:
Calcium channel blocker (calcium antagonist).

USES:
High blood pressure, angina, rapid heart rate.

DOSAGE:

180 to 240mg once a day. maximum dose 240mg twice a day.

FORMS:
Tablets of 180 and 240mg, injection.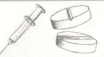

PRECAUTIONS:
Should only be used in pregnancy (C) and breast feeding if medically essential. Not designed for use in children.

Do not take if:

 suffering from severe heart failure, low blood pressure, atrial flutter or fibrillation.

SIDE EFFECTS:
Common: Constipation, tiredness, headache, dizziness, indigestion, swelling of feet and ankles.
Unusual: Flushing, palpitations, slow heart rate, scalp irritation, depression, flushes, nightmares, excess wind.
Severe but rare (stop medication, consult doctor): Fainting.

INTERACTIONS:
Other drugs:
- Beta blockers (eg. propranolol), cyclosporin, digoxin, cimetidine, diazepam, amiodarone, quinidine, rifampicin, phenytoin, cisapride, theophylline, terbutaline, salbutamol, diltiazem.
- Additive effect with other medications for high blood pressure.

Herbs:
- Goldenseal, guarana, hawthorn, Korean ginseng, liquorice.

Other substances:
- Smoking may aggravate conditions that these medications are treating.
- Grapefruit juice.

PRESCRIPTION:
Yes.

PBS:
Yes.

PERMITTED IN SPORT:
Yes.

OVERDOSE:
May continue to be absorbed for up to 48 hours after overdose. Administer activated charcoal or induce vomiting. Purging should be encouraged to eliminate drug from gut. Overdose may cause low blood pressure, irregular heart rhythm, difficulty in breathing, heart attack and death. Obtain urgent medical attention.

OTHER INFORMATION:
Commonly used as a first line medication in high blood pressure and to prevent angina.

See also Amlodipine, Diltiazem, Felodipine, Nifedipine, Nimodipine.

Vibrio Cholera vaccine

See Cholera vaccine.

Vigabatrin

TRADE NAME:
Sabril.

DRUG CLASS:
Anticonvulsant.

USES:
Epilepsy, particularly difficult to control epilepsy.

DOSAGE:

Tablets: One or two tablets twice a day.
Powder: Dissolve in water immediately before use. Use 250mg to 2g twice a day.

FORMS:
Tablets (white) of 500mg, powder.

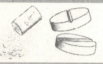

PRECAUTIONS:
Not to be used in pregnancy (D) or breast feeding.
Use with care in psychiatric conditions and kidney disease.
Response to medication must be checked regularly by a doctor.
Use with caution in elderly.
Medication should not be stopped suddenly.
Interferes with some laboratory blood tests.

SIDE EFFECTS:
Common: Drowsiness, weight gain, nausea, diarrhoea.
Unusual: Disturbed brain function, disturbed bowel function, vomiting, reduced alertness.

INTERACTIONS:
Other drugs:
- Phenytoin.

Herbs:
- Evening primrose (linoleic acid), Gingko biloba.

Other substances:
- Borage.

PRESCRIPTION:
Yes.

PBS:
Yes (authority required. Restricted to patients whose epilepsy cannot be controlled by other medication).

PERMITTED IN SPORT:
Yes.

OTHER INFORMATION:
Released in 1994. Not addictive or dependence forming.
See also BARBITURATES, BENZODIAZEPINES, Carbamazepine, Clonazepam, Ethosuximide, Gabapentin, Lamotrigine, Levetiracetam, Oxcarbazepine, Phenytoin, Primidone, Sodium valproate, Sulthiame, Tiagabine, Topiramate.

Vinblastine

See VINCA ALKALOIDS.

VINCA ALKALOIDS

TRADE and GENERIC NAMES:
Eldisine (vindesine sulfate).
Navelbine (vinorelbine).
Oncovin, Vincristine (vincristine sulfate).
Velbe, Vinblastine (vinblastine sulfate).

USES:
Leukaemia, some lung cancers, advanced breast cancer (Vinorelbine), blood disorders, Hodgkin's disease, some other forms of cancer.

DOSAGE:

Must be individualised for each patient by doctor depending on disease, severity, response and weight of patient.

FORMS:
Injection, infusion.

PRECAUTIONS:
Must not be used in pregnancy (D) unless mother's life is at risk as foetus may be damaged. Breast feeding must be ceased before use. May be used with caution in children.
Adequate contraception must be used by all women during treatment.
Regular blood and marrow tests to check blood and marrow cells and liver function essential.
Use with caution in nerve, muscle and lung disease.

Do not take if:
suffering from serious infection, nerve damage, thrombocytopenia (bleeding disorder due to low blood platelet count).

SIDE EFFECTS:
Common: Loss of all body hair, pins and needles, nerve pain, muscle weakness, nausea, vomiting.
Unusual: Paralysis of some muscles, convulsions, constipation or diarrhoea, depression, headache, rash, fever.
Severe but rare (stop medication, consult doctor): Unusual bleeding or bruising, yellow skin (jaundice).

INTERACTIONS:
Other drugs:
- Phenytoin, mitomycin, cisplatin.
- Live virus vaccines (eg. Sabin polio).

Other substances:
- Alcohol should be avoided during treatment.

PRESCRIPTION:
Yes.

PBS:
Eldesine: No.
Other forms: Yes.

OVERDOSE:
Frequently fatal.

OTHER INFORMATION:
Despite significant side effects, these drugs may save the life of patients with leukaemia and other cancers.

See also Amsacrine, Busulfan, Chlorambucil, Cyclophosphamide, Cytarabine, Daunorubicin, Mercaptopurine, Thioguanine

Vincristine
See VINCA ALKALOIDS.

Vindesine
See VINCA ALKALOIDS.

Vinorelbine
See VINCA ALKALOIDS.

VITAMINS

DISCUSSION:

Vitamins are a group of totally unrelated chemicals that have only one thing in common: they are essential (usually in tiny amounts) for the normal functioning of the body. All vitamins have been given letter codes, sometimes with an additional number to differentiate vitamins within a group. The missing letters and numbers in the series are due to substances initially having been identified as vitamins but later being found to lack the essentials for the classification.

See Ascorbic acid (Vitamin C), Biotin (Vitamin H), Cholecalciferol, Calcitriol, Ergocalciferol (Vitamin D), Cyanocobalamin, Hydroxocobalamin (Vitamin B12), Folic acid, Nicotinic Acid (Vitamin B3), Pantothenic acid (Vitamin B5), Phytomenadione (Vitamin K), Pyridoxine (Vitamin B6), Retinol (Vitamin A), Riboflavine (Vitamin B2), Thiamine (Vitamin B1), Tocopherols (Vitamin E).

Vitamin A
See Betacarotene, Retinol.

Vitamin B1
See Thiamine.

Vitamin B2
See Riboflavine.

Vitamin B3
See Nicotinic acid.

Vitamin B5
See Panthenol (Pantothenic acid).

Vitamin B6
See Pyridoxine.

Vitamin B12
See Cyanocobalamin, Hydroxocobalamin.

Vitamin C
See Ascorbic acid.

Vitamin D
See Cholecalciferol, Calcitriol, Ergocalciferol.

Vitamin E
See Tocopherols.

Vitamin H
See Biotin.

Vitamin K
See HAEMOSTATIC AGENTS (Phytomenadione).

Medications

Warfarin

TRADE NAMES:
Coumadin, Marevan.

DRUG CLASS:
Anticoagulant.

USES:
Prevention and treatment of blood clots (eg. lung clots, heart clots).

DOSAGE:
Precise dose as directed by doctor once a day at the same time.

FORMS:
Tablets of 1mg (tan or brown), 2mg (lavender), 3mg (blue) and 5mg (green or pink).

PRECAUTIONS:
Must not be used in pregnancy (D) as it may cause foetal damage and death.
Breast feeding should be ceased if use is medically necessary. May be used with caution in children.
Regular blood tests to check blood clotting time essential.
Other illnesses (eg. infection) may require an adjustment of warfarin dosage.
Read literature accompanying medication very carefully. Ask questions of doctor about anything you do not understand.
Do not undertake any activity that may result in falls, bruising or extreme exertion.
Coumadin and Marevan are not interchangeable at the same doses.

Do not take if:
 suffering from bleeding tendency, peptic ulcer, dementia, mental diseases, severe high blood pressure, blood cell abnormalities, alcoholism.
- due to have essential surgery, including dental surgery.

SIDE EFFECTS:
Common: Bruising, nose bleeds.
Unusual: Hair loss, itch, rash, fever, nausea, diarrhoea, belly pains.
Severe but rare (stop medication, consult doctor): Significant bleeding, blood in urine, blood in faeces, vomiting blood, black patch of skin.

INTERACTIONS:
Other drugs:
- Interacts with a very wide range of medications. Do not take any medication (including cold mixtures, vitamins, and other chemist and supermarket lines) without checking with a doctor.
- Never take aspirin or arthritis (NSAID) drugs with warfarin.

Herbs:
- Alfalfa, bilberry, celery, camomile, clove, devil's claw, dong quai, fenugreek, feverfew, garlic, ginger, ginkgo biloba, ginseng, guarana, Korean ginseng, liquorice, papaya, pau d'arco, red clover, slippery elm bark, St John's wort, tumeric, willow bark.

Other substances:
- Reacts with alcohol and caffeine.
- Reacts with many foods. Do not alter diet without discussing with a doctor.
- Eat a constant amount of green leafy vegetables, meat and dairy products as a variation may affect the effect of warfarin.
- Do not diet or binge eat without discussing with a doctor.

PRESCRIPTION:
Yes.

PBS:
Yes.

PERMITTED IN SPORT:
Yes, but not recommended in active sport. Body contact sport forbidden.

Medications

OVERDOSE:
Extremely serious. Administer activated charcoal or induce vomiting only if tablets taken very recently. Seek emergency medical assistance. Massive internal bleeding may cause sudden death. Antidote (vitamin K) available. Blood transfusion may be necessary.

OTHER INFORMATION:
Warfarin is the active ingredient of many rat poisons. If used correctly and carefully, warfarin can save and prolong life with minimal or no side effects. Slightest variation of dose may cause adverse effects. Wearing a bracelet or necklet with information about the medication is advised for anyone using warfarin long term.

See also Heparin, Phenindione.

WEIGHT LOSS DRUGS
See ANORECTICS, Diethylpropion hydrochloride, Orlistat, Phentermine, Silbutramine.

Whooping cough vaccine
(Pertussis vaccine)

TRADE NAMES:
Only available in Australia in combination with other vaccines.
Boostrix, Infanrix, Tripacel (with tetanus and diphtheria vaccines – previously called the triple antigen).
Infanrix HepB (with hepatitis B, diphtheria and tetanus vaccines).

DRUG CLASS:
Vaccine.

USES:
Prevention of whooping cough.

DOSAGE:

Injection given at two, four, six and eighteen months.

FORMS:
Injection.

PRECAUTIONS:
Not designed for use over 2 years of age. Use with caution if history of brain disease or convulsions.

Do not take if:
- suffering from acute illness, significant fever or epilepsy.
- previously infected with whooping cough.

SIDE EFFECTS:
Common: Local redness and tenderness at injection site, persistent lump, fever.
Unusual: Tiredness, irritability, faint.
Severe but rare: Convulsion, brain inflammation.

INTERACTIONS:
None significant.

PRESCRIPTION:
Yes.

PBS:
No, but supplied free to doctors by state health departments.

PERMITTED IN SPORT:
Yes.

OVERDOSE:
An unintentional additional dose is unlikely to have any serious effect.

OTHER INFORMATION:
A vaccination that should be given to all infants. Whooping cough still occurs in Australia and may cause brain damage and death.

See also Diphtheria vaccine, Hepatitis B vaccine, Tetanus vaccine.

Medications

Xylometazoline

TRADE NAMES:
Otrivin.
Murine Allergy (with antazoline).

DRUG CLASS:
Vasoconstrictor.

USES:
Nasal congestion, hay fever, eye inflammation, eye allergy.

DOSAGE:
 Nose: Use in each nostril one to four times a day.
Eye: One or two drops two or three times a day.

FORMS:
Nose drops and spray, eye drops.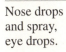

PRECAUTIONS:
Safe to use in pregnancy, breast feeding and children.
Ensure children's strength and not adult strength nose preparations used in children.
Use eye drops with caution in children.
Not to be used in nose long term.

Do not take any form if:
 suffering from glaucoma or serious eye disease.

Do not use eye drops if:
 using contact lenses.

Do not use nose drops if:
 recent brain surgery performed through nose.

SIDE EFFECTS:
Common: Eye drops – temporary blurred vision, stinging.
Nose drops – burning, stinging, sneezing, dry nose.
Unusual: Nose drops – worsening nasal congestion if over-used, sleeplessness, lightheadedness, palpitations, headache.

INTERACTIONS:
Other drugs:
• MAOI.
Other substances:
• Reacts with alcohol.

PRESCRIPTION:
No.

PBS:
No.

PERMITTED IN SPORT:
Yes.

OVERDOSE:
If used excessively, nasal congestion rather than relief may occur.
If swallowed, sedation, high blood pressure, rapid irregular heart rate and coma may occur. Seek medical assistance.

OTHER INFORMATION:
Ensure instructions are followed and medication is not over-used.
See also Oxymetazoline, Tramazoline.

Medications

Yellow fever vaccine

TRADE NAME:
Stamaril.

DRUG CLASS:
Vaccine.

USES:
Prevention of yellow fever.

DOSAGE:
 Single injection gives 10 years protection.

FORMS:
Injection.

PRECAUTIONS:
Use with caution in pregnancy, breast feeding and children over 1 year.
Not for use in children under six months, and with great caution between six and 12 months.
Given as an injection into muscle.

Do not take if:
 suffering from significant illness, cancer or immune disease.
• allergic to poultry or eggs.

SIDE EFFECTS:
Common: Fever, tiredness, joint pains, redness at injection site.
Unusual: Headache, muscle pains, bruise at injection site.

INTERACTIONS:
None significant.

PRESCRIPTION:
Yes.

PBS:
No. Only available from state government clinics, major hospitals or authorised travel medicine centres.

PERMITTED IN SPORT:
Yes.

OVERDOSE:
An inadvertent additional vaccination is unlikely to have any serious consequences.

OTHER INFORMATION:
Not routinely used. Only given to persons travelling to, or resident in, countries of tropical Africa and South America where yellow fever occurs. The disease is spread by mosquitoes.

Yersinia pestis vaccine
(Plague vaccine)

TRADE NAME:
Plague vaccine.

DRUG CLASS:
Vaccine.

USES:
Prevention of plague (black death).

DOSAGE:

Two injections at an interval of one to four weeks. Third injection necessary for children under 12. Additional booster doses required every six months.

FORMS:
Injection.

PRECAUTIONS:
Use with caution in pregnancy.
May be used in breast feeding and children.
Use with caution in fever from infection or current respiratory tract infection.

SIDE EFFECTS:
Common: Minimal.
Unusual: Fever, muscle spasms, loss of appetite.
Severe but rare: Brain inflammation, speech disorders, muscle wasting.

INTERACTIONS:
Other drugs:
- Other vaccines.

PRESCRIPTION:
Yes.

PBS:
No.

PERMITTED IN SPORT:
Yes.

OVERDOSE:
Additional inadvertent vaccination unlikely to have any serious consequences.

OTHER INFORMATION:
Not routine in Australia. Only given to residents and visitors to an area where plague occurs.

Medications

Zafirlukast

TRADE NAME:
Accolate.

DRUG CLASS:
Leukotrene receptor antagonist.

USES:
Prevention and treatment of asthma.

DOSAGE:

One or two tablets twice a day.

FORMS:
Tablets (white) of 20mg.

PRECAUTIONS:
May be used with caution in pregnancy (B1) and breast feeding. Use with caution in children under 12 years.
Use with caution in unstable and sudden onset asthma.
Do not stop medication suddenly.
Use with caution if withdrawing from steroids.
Use with caution in liver disease.

SIDE EFFECTS:
Common: Chest infection.
Unusual: Abnormal bleeding.
Severe but rare (stop medication, consult doctor): Liver and white blood cell damage.

INTERACTIONS:
Other drugs:
- Warfarin, theophylline, erythromycin, aspirin.

PRESCRIPTION:
Yes.

PBS:
No.

PERMITTED IN SPORT:
Yes.

OVERDOSE:
May cause damage to liver and blood cells. Induce vomiting or give activated charcoal if taken recently. Seek urgent medical attention.

OTHER INFORMATION:
Expensive medication introduced in 1999 to assist asthmatics who are not adequately controlled by other medications.
See Montelukast.

Zalcitabine

TRADE NAME:
Hivid.

DRUG CLASS:
Antiviral.

USES:
AIDS, HIV infection.

DOSAGE:

One or two tablets three times a day. Often used in combination with zidovudine.

FORMS:
Tablets of 0.375mg (beige) and 0.75mg (grey).

PRECAUTIONS:
Must not be used in pregnancy (D). Use with caution in breast feeding and children.
Use with caution in peripheral neuropathy, pancreatitis, kidney and liver disease.

Regular blood tests to check liver and kidney function, and blood cells, are necessary.

SIDE EFFECTS:
Common: Mouth ulcers, nausea, rash, itch, headache, muscle pain, tiredness.
Unusual: Pain on swallowing, loss of appetite, vomiting, dizziness, throat inflammation.
Severe but rare (stop medication, consult doctor): Belly pain (pancreatitis), numbness and burning in hands and feet (neuropathy).

INTERACTIONS:
Other drugs:
- Aminoglycosides, amphotericin, foscarnet, chloramphenicol, cisplatin, dapsone, didanosine, disulfiram, glutethamide, hydralazine, iodoquinol, isoniazid, nitrofurantoin, phenytoin, ribavirin, vincristine.

PRESCRIPTION:
Yes.

PBS:
Yes (authority required).

PERMITTED IN SPORT:
Yes.

OVERDOSE:
No information available. Induce vomiting or administer activated charcoal if taken recently. Seek urgent medical attention.

OTHER INFORMATION:
Usually combined with other medications used to treat HIV infections.

See Abacavir, Delavirdine, Didanosine, Efavirenz, Indinavir, Lamivudine, Nelfinavir, Nevirapine, Ritonavir, Saquinavir, Stavudine, Tenofovir, Zidovudine.

Zanamivir

TRADE NAME:
Relenza.

DRUG CLASS:
Antiviral.

USES:
Treatment of influenza. Must be started within 48 hours of first symptoms of influenza appearing.

DOSAGE:

Two inhalations twice daily for five days.

FORMS:
Disc inhaler.

PRECAUTIONS:
Use with caution in pregnancy (B1) and breast feeding.
Use with caution in severe asthma.
Not for prevention of influenza.

SIDE EFFECTS:
Common: Minimal.
Unusual: Dizziness, diarrhoea, wheeze, headache.

INTERACTIONS:
None significant.

PRESCRIPTION:
Yes.

PBS:
No.

PERMITTED IN SPORT:
Yes.

OVERDOSE:
Unlikely to have any serious effects.

OTHER INFORMATION:
Released in 1999 as the first medication for the treatment of influenza. Developed in Australia.

See also Oseltamivir.

Zidovudine
(Azidothymidine, AZT)

TRADE NAMES:
Retrovir.
Combivir (with lamivudine).
Trivizir (with abacavir, lamivudine).

DRUG CLASS:
Antiviral.

USES:
AIDS (Acquired Immune Deficiency Syndrome), HIV (Human Immunodeficiency Virus) positive patients.

DOSAGE:

As determined by doctor, depending on medication combinations and severity of disease.

FORMS:
Capsules, syrup.

PRECAUTIONS:
Use with caution in pregnancy (B3), breast feeding and children.
Use with caution if infection present, and in liver and kidney disease.
Regular blood tests to assess effectiveness and side effects of medication essential.
Do not take if:
 low red or white blood cell count present.

SIDE EFFECTS:
Many side effects of zidovudine may be caused by the disease (AIDS) it is treating.
Common: Tiredness, fever, headache, loss of appetite, nausea, vomiting, muscle aches, sleeplessness, rash, blood cell damage.
Unusual: Belly discomfort, dizziness, pins and needles, shortness of breath.
Severe but rare: Impairs fertility, may cause cancer.

INTERACTIONS:
Other drugs:
- Codeine, methadone, morphine, paracetamol, NSAIDs, oxazepam, lorazepam,
  cimetidine, probenecid, phenytoin, ribavirin, clofibrate, dapsone, stavudine.

PRESCRIPTION:
Yes.

PBS:
Yes (authority required).

PERMITTED IN SPORT:
Yes.

OVERDOSE:
Causes vomiting. Uneventful recovery likely.

OTHER INFORMATION:
Introduced in early 1990s as the first drug to slow the progress of HIV/AIDS, but does not cure the disease. Almost invariably used in combination with other antiviral drugs.

See Abacavir, Delavirdine, Didanosine, Efavirenz, Indinavir, Lamivudine, Nelfinavir, Nevirapine, Ritonavir, Saquinavir, Stavudine, Tenofovir, Zalcitabine.

Zinc

TRADE NAMES:
Included in many mineral and vitamin supplements, as well as cold and flu medications.

DRUG CLASS:
Mineral.

USES:
Zinc deficiency, treatment of common cold, aid to wound healing.

DOSAGE:

Recommended daily intake 12mg.
Tablets: One or two a day.
Lozenges: Up to eight a day dissolved in mouth.
Injection: By infusion into a vein as determined by doctor.

FORMS:
Tablets, mixture, lozenges, injection.

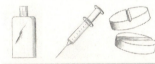

PRECAUTIONS:
Use with caution in pregnancy and breast feeding. May be used when clinically necessary in children.
Must not be directly injected into muscle.
Regular blood tests to check levels of zinc and other minerals necessary if taken regularly.
Use with caution in kidney disease.
Not for long term use.

SIDE EFFECTS:
Common: May alter blood test results.
Unusual: Nausea, chest pain, anaemia.

INTERACTIONS:
None significant.

PRESCRIPTION:
No.

PBS:
No.

PERMITTED IN SPORT:
Yes.

Zinc oxide

TRADE NAMES:
Curash Powders, Destin Nappy Rash, Prickly Heat Powder, Zinc Cream.
Acne and Pimple Gel (with sulfur, allantoin, resorcinol and other ingredients).
Anusol (with benzyl benzoate).
Caltrate Plus, Citracal Plus (with other minerals).
Daktozin (with miconazole).
Eczema Cream (with coal tar, dimethicone and other ingredients).
Egoderm, Hemocane, Pedoz, Rapaid Powder, ZSC Powder (with multiple other ingredients).
Egozite Baby Cream (with dimethicone, paraffin).
ER Cream (with coal tar, allantoin, hydroxybenzoates and other ingredients).
Granugen (with paraffin and other ingredients).
Rectinol (with adrenaline and local anaesthetic).
SOOV Prickly Heat Powder (with paraffin, salicylic acid and other ingredients).
Vitaline (with lysine).
VR Gel (with allantoin and other ingredients).
Xyloproct (with hydrocortisone, aluminium acetate, lignocaine).
Also included in many other soothing and sunscreen preparations.

DRUG CLASS:
Mineral.

USES:
Skin protection, skin inflammation, piles, skin ulcers, aid to healing.

DOSAGE:
 Applied to affected area as needed.

FORMS:
Cream, ointment, suppository, powder, tablets, impregnated dressing.

PRECAUTIONS:
Safe in pregnancy, breast feeding and children of all ages.

SIDE EFFECTS:
Common: Minimal.
Unusual: Sensitivity reactions.

INTERACTIONS:
Other drugs:
- May prevent other creams from reaching and acting on skin if zinc oxide is applied first.

PRESCRIPTION:
No.

PBS:
No.
Anusol and Egoderm are available to Veteran Affairs pensioners.

PERMITTED IN SPORT:
Yes.

OTHER INFORMATION:
Zinc oxide has been used for centuries to protect skin from injury, and to soothe irritation.
See also Urea.

Zinc pyrithione
See Pyrithione zinc

Zinc sulfate

TRADE NAMES:
Zincaps.
Zincfrin (with phenylephrine).
Zinvit (with magnesium, vitamin B1).
Zinvit C-250 (with magnesium, vitamin C).
Zinvit G (with magnesium, vitamin B1, vitamin B2, folic acid).
Zinc sulfate is also found in numerous mineral and vitamin supplements.

DRUG CLASS:
Mineral.

USES:
Mineral supplement, astringent (contracts blood vessels and dries secretions), acne.

DOSAGE:
 Mineral supplement: Recommended daily intake 12mg per day.

FORMS:
Tablets, capsules, mixture.

PRECAUTIONS:
May be used in pregnancy and breast feeding. use with caution in children.
Do not exceed recommended dose.
Do not take tablets constantly, but suspend medication intermittently.
Ensure adequate intake of fibre while taking tablets.

SIDE EFFECTS:
Minimal.

INTERACTIONS:
None significant.

PRESCRIPTION:
No.

Medications

PBS:
No

PERMITTED IN SPORT:
Yes.

OVERDOSE:
Constipation only likely serious effect.

OTHER INFORMATION:
Low levels of zinc in the blood may reduce the body's ability to repair damage.

Zolmitriptan

TRADE NAME:
Zomig.

DRUG CLASS:
Antimigraine.

USES:
Treatment of acute migraine.

DOSAGE:

One tablet at onset of migraine. Repeat after two hours if necessary.

FORMS:
Tablets of 2.5mg (yellow).

PRECAUTIONS:
Use with considerable caution in pregnancy (B3), breast feeding and children.
Use with caution in irregular heart rhythm and liver disease.
Do not take if:
 ☠ suffering from angina, serious heart disease, poor circulation, significant high blood pressure, poor kidney function.
• history of recent heart attack, stroke or transient ischaemic attack.

SIDE EFFECTS:
Common: Tiredness, nausea, dizziness, warm sensation, pins and needles sensation.
Unusual: Dry mouth, throat pressure, muscle aches.
Severe but rare (stop medication, consult doctor): Chest pain.

INTERACTIONS:
Other drugs:
• Ergotamine, MAOI, cimetidine, fluvoxamine, quinolone antibiotics.
Herbs:
• St John's wort.

PRESCRIPTION:
Yes.

PBS:
Yes (authority required. Restricted to patients who have uncontrolled migraine).

PERMITTED IN SPORT:
Yes.

OVERDOSE:
Sedation only likely effect.

OTHER INFORMATION:
Very effective medication, particularly if taken immediately migraine starts.
See also Ergotamine, Naratriptan, Sumatriptan.

Zolpidem

TRADE NAME:
Stilnox.

DRUG CLASS:
Sedative.

USES:
Insomnia (sleeplessness).

DOSAGE:
 Half to one tablet before going to bed.

FORMS:
Tablets of 10mg (white).

PRECAUTIONS:
Use with caution in pregnancy (B3) and breast feeding. Not for use in children. Use with caution in liver or kidney disease, schizophrenia, epilepsy and depression.
Not for long term use.
Use lower doses in elderly.

Do not take if:
 suffering from sleep apnoea, myasthenia gravis, severe liver or lung disease.

SIDE EFFECTS:
Common: Tolerance to dose, dependence, rebound inability to sleep when drug ceased, nausea.
Unusual: Daytime drowsiness, loss of memory, dizziness, headache, vomiting.

INTERACTIONS:
Other drugs:
- Other sedatives, rifampicin, ketoconazole.

Herbs:
- Celery, camomile.

Other substances:
- Alcohol.

PRESCRIPTION:
Yes.

PBS:
No.

PERMITTED IN SPORT:
Yes.

OVERDOSE:
Prolonged drowsiness, sleep or coma may occur. Death unlikely unless mixed with other drugs. Induce vomiting or give activated charcoal if swallowed recently. Seek medical assistance.

OTHER INFORMATION:
Introduced in 2000. May cause dependence if used regularly.

See also BARBITURATES, Chlormethiazole, Flunitrazepam, Midazolam, Nitrazepam, Temazepam, Triazolam, Zopiclone.

Zopiclone

TRADE NAME:
Imovane.

DRUG CLASS:
Sedative/Hypnotic.

USES:
Insomnia (sleeplessness).

DOSAGE:

One tablet 30 minutes before bedtime.

FORMS:
Tablet of 7.5mg (white).

PRECAUTIONS:
Should not be used in pregnancy (C), breast feeding or children.
Designed for short term use only.
Use with caution in severe kidney and liver disease, poor thyroid function, depression and epilepsy.
Lower doses needed in elderly.
Dependence possible.

Do not take if:

- suffering from myasthenia gravis, severe lung disease, sleep apnoea, recent stroke.
- operating machinery, driving a vehicle or undertaking tasks that require concentration and alertness.

SIDE EFFECTS:
Common: Drowsiness, headache, fatigue, taste disturbances, dry mouth.
Unusual: Dependency on medication.

INTERACTIONS:
Other drugs:
- Other sedatives, erythromycin.

Other substances:
- Reacts with alcohol to increase sedation.

PRESCRIPTION:
Yes.

PBS:
No. Available to Veteran Affairs pensioners.

PERMITTED IN SPORT:
Yes.

OVERDOSE:
Seldom life threatening. May cause drowsiness, confusion and coma. Induce vomiting if tablets taken recently. Seek medical assistance.

OTHER INFORMATION:
Introduced in 1993 as an alternative to temazepam. Very safe and effective. May cause dependence.

See also BARBITURATES, Chlormethiazole, Flunitrazepam, Midazolam, Nitrazepam, Temazepam, Triazolam, Zolpidem.

Zuclopenthixol

TRADE NAME:
Clopixol.

DRUG CLASS:
Antipsychotic.

USES:
Schizophrenia, severe psychoses, mania.

DOSAGE:

Depot injection: One injection every two to four weeks.
Injection: One injection every two to four days.

FORMS:
Injection, depot injection.

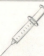

PRECAUTIONS:
Use only as a last resort in pregnancy (C).
Use with caution in breast feeding and children.
Use with caution in Parkinsonism, epilepsy, glaucoma, poor blood supply to brain, severe hardening of arteries and heart disease, kidney and liver disease.
Use with caution in climates with high temperatures.
Regular blood tests to check liver and blood cell function recommended.
Consider options carefully before using for prolonged period.
Avoid contact with organophosphate insecticides.

Do not take if:
- suffering from coma, brain injury, abnormal blood cells in past or present, phaeochromocytoma.
- alcohol, narcotics or barbiturates recently consumed.

SIDE EFFECTS:
Common: Drowsiness, twitching, dry mouth, constipation.
Unusual: Uncontrolled movements, liver damage, blood cell damage, inability to vomit.
Severe but rare (stop medication, consult doctor): High fever, jaundice (yellow skin).

INTERACTIONS:
Other drugs:
- Anticholinergics, sedatives, hypnotics, tricyclic antidepressants, metoclopramide, piperazine.

Herbs:
- Celery, camomile, evening primrose (linoleic acid).

Other substances:
- Alcohol.
- Organophosphate insecticides.

PRESCRIPTION:
Yes.

PBS:
Depot injection: Yes.
Other forms: No.

PERMITTED IN SPORT:
Yes.

OVERDOSE:
Tiredness, convulsions, coma, low blood pressure and altered temperature may occur. Induce vomiting or give activated charcoal if capsules taken recently. Seek urgent medical attention.

OTHER INFORMATION:
Introduced in 1996 to control more difficult cases of schizophrenia and other psychiatric conditions. Does not cause addiction or dependence.

See also Amisulpride, Droperidol, Flupenthixol, Haloperidol, Lithium Carbonate, Olanzapine, PHENOTHIAZINES, Pimozide, Quetiapine, Risperidone, Thiothixene.

INDEX

All trade (brand) names, generic names and drug classes in this book are listed. Drug classes are shown in CAPITAL LETTERS.

3TC 315

A

Abacavir..21
Abbocillin V 438
Abbocillin VK 438
Abbott Cold Sore Balm 53, 394
Abciximab..21
Abelcet...50
Acamprosate......................................22
Acarbose..22
Accolate...600
Accupril...23
Accure...304
Accuretic..................................23, 556
ACE INHIBITORS............................23
Acenorm..23
Acetaminophen...............................423
Acetazolamide...................................24
Acetic acid..25
Acetopt...531
Acetylcholine chloride......................26
Acetylcysteine..................................26
Acetylsalicylic Acid..........................72
Achromycin....................................552
Aci-Jel......................................25, 262
Aciclovir...27
Acihexal..27
Acimax...471
Acitretin..28
Aclin...535
Acne and Pimple Gel.............487, 603
Acnederm.......................................127
Acnederm Foaming Wash..............131
Acnederm Lotion...........................309
Acnederm Ointment.......................190
Acriflavine..28
Act-3...288
Actacode.................................152, 472
Actifed..63
Actifed CC Dry Cough..................442
Actifed CC Junior..........................175
Actifed Chesty.......................266, 472
Actifed Dry............................175, 472

Actilax 315
Actilyse...229
Action...440
Action Cold & Flu Effervescent......72
Action Cold and Flu........................63
Actiprofen......................................288
Actonel...491
Actos..446
Actrapid..296
Actrapid Novolet............................296
Actrapid Penfill..............................296
Actuss..442
Acular...312
Acyclo-V...27
Ad-Sorb..128
Adalat...390
Adalat Oros....................................390
Adapalene..29
Adenocor..29
Adenoscan.......................................29
Adenosine..29
Adrenaline..30
ADT......................................192, 551
Advantan..357
Aerodiol Spray...............................399
Agarol...424
Agiolax...506
Agon SR...225
Agrylin...54
Airomir..499
Akamin..365
Akineton..97
Albalon...379
Albalon Relief................................440
Albalon-A.......................................379
Albay...35
Albendazole.....................................31
Alcaine..53
Alclometasone.................................32
Alcohol..218
Aldactone......................................526
Aldara..291
Aldazine...435
Aldecin..84

Index

Aldioxa	32
Aldomet	355
Alendronate	33
Alepam	413
Alertonic	449
Aleve	380
Alfare	224
Alfentanil	33
Algicon	114
Alka-Seltzer	72, 208
Alkeran	343
Alkylaters	118
Allantoin	34
Allegron	578
ALLERGEN EXTRACTS	35
Allermax	370
Allohexal	35
Allopurinol	35
Allorin	35
Allypral	35
Alodorm	393
ALPHA BLOCKERS	36
Alpha Keri	424
Alphacin	50
Alphagan	101
Alphamox	49
Alphapress	277
Alphapril	23
Alphosyl	34
Alphosyl Lotion	542
Alprax	36
Alprazolam	36
Alprim	580
Alprostadil	37
Alteplase	229
Altretamine	38
Alu-Tab	57
Aluminium chloride	38
Aluminium hydroxide	57
Aluminium oxide	39
Aluminium salts	57
Aluminium sulfate	40
Alupent	409
Alvercol	40, 528
Alverine Citrate	40
Amantadine	41
Amaryl	259
AmBisome	50
Amethocaine	53
Amfamox	223
Amfebutamone	108
Amicar	44
Amifostine	42
Amikacin	42
Amikin	42
Amiloride	43
Aminacrine hydrochloride	43
Aminocaproic Acid	44
Aminoglutethamide	44
AMINOGLYCOSIDES	45
Aminophylline	554
Amiodarone	45
Amisulpride	46
Amitriptyline	578
Amizide	43
Amizide	556
Amlodipine	47
Ammonium bicarbonate	47
Ammonium chloride	48
AMO Vitrax	516
Amohexal	49
Amorolfine	48
Amosan	518
Amoxil	49
Amoxil Duo	49
Amoxycillin	49
Ampexin	49
Amphocil	50
Amphotericin	50
Ampicillin	50
Ampicyn	50
Amprace	23
Amsacrine	51
Amsidyl	51
Amylmetacresol	52
Amylobarbitone	82
Amytal Sodium	82
ANABOLIC STEROIDS	52
ANAESTHETICS, LOCAL	53
Anafranil	578
Anagrelide	54
ANALGESICS	55
Anamorph	372
Anandron	391
Anaprox	380
Anastrozole	55
Anatensol	435
Ancotil	232
Andrews Antacids	114
Andrews Tums	57, 114
Andriol	550
Andro-Feme	550
Androcur	162
Androderm	550
Andromen	550
ANGINA MEDICATIONS	56

Anginine	263
Angiotensin Converting Enzyme Inhibitors	23
ANGIOTENSIN II RECEPTOR ANTAGONISTS	56
ANORECTICS	57
Anpec	591
Anselol	73
Antabuse	197
ANTACIDS	57
Antazoline	379
Antehexal	73
Antenex	178
Anthel	474
ANTHELMINTICS	58
Anthistine-Privine	379
Anthralin	197
ANTIALLERGEN	59
ANTIANDROGEN	59
ANTIANGINALS	59
ANTIARRHYTHMICS	59
ANTIBIOTICS	59
ANTICHOLINERGICS	60
ANTICHOLINESTERASES	60
ANTICOAGULANTS	60
ANTICONVULSANTS	60
ANTIDEPRESSANTS	61
ANTIDIARRHOEALS	61
ANTIDIURETICS	61
ANTIDOTES	61
ANTIEMETICS	61
ANTIFUNGALS	61
ANTIHISTAMINES, NON-SEDATING	62
ANTIHISTAMINES, SEDATING	63
ANTIHYPERTENSIVES	65
ANTIMALARIALS	65
Antimetabolites	118
ANTIMIGRAINE	65
Antineoplastics	118
ANTIPARASITICS	66
ANTIPARKINSONIANS	66
ANTIPSYCHOTICS	66
ANTIPYRETICS	66
ANTIRHEUMATICS	66
ANTISEPTIC, URINARY	67
ANTISEPTICS	66
ANTISPASMODICS	67
ANTITHYROIDS	67
ANTIVENOMS	67
ANTIVIRALS	68
Antroquoril	92
Anusol	603
Anusol Wipes	262
ANXIOLYTICS	68
Anzatax	420
Anzemet	199
Apatef	125
Apomine	68
Apormorphine hydrochloride	68
Apoven	299
Applicaine	138
Applicaine Drops	53, 126, 128
Applicaine Gel	126, 128
APR Cream	345
Apraclonidine	69
Apresoline	277
Aprinox	556
Aprotinin	69
Aquacare	583
Aquae	523
Aquae	222
Aquaear	25, 302
Arachis Oil	70
Aratac	45
Arava	318
Aredia	195
Aricept	200
Arima	369
Arimidex	55
Aristocort	575
Aromasin	221
Aropax	425
Artane	86
Artemether	70
Arthrexin	294
Arthrotec	180
Arthrotec	368
Asasantin SR	72, 194
Ascabiol	88
Ascorbic acid	71
Asig	23
Asmol	499
Aspalgin	152
Aspalgin	72
ASPART INSULIN	296
Aspirin	72
Aspro	72
Astrix	72
Atacand	56
Atacand Plus	56, 556
Atenolol	73
Ativan	332
Atorvastatin	74
Atovaquone	75
Atrobel	75, 286
Atropine	75, 375
Atropt	75

Index

Atrovent	299
Attapulgite	76
Attenta	356
Augmentin	49, 455
Auralgan Otic	53
Auranofin	77
Aurorix	369
Auscap	239
Auscard	188
Ausclav	49, 455
Ausgem	253
Auspril	23
Ausran	484
Austrapen	50
Avandia	495
Avanza	367
Avapro	56
Avapro HCT	56, 556
Avaxim	273
Avil	63
Avil Decongestant	48, 63, 345
Avonex	297
Azactam	80
Azahexal	78
Azamun	78
Azatadine	64
Azathioprine	78
Azelaic acid	309
Azelastine	78
Azep	78
Azidothymidine	602
Azithromycin	79
Azol	167
Azopt	102
AZT	78, 602
Aztreonam	80

B

Bacitracin	81
Baclo	81
Baclofen	81
Baclohexal	81
Bactigras	131
Bactrim	532, 580
Bactroban	374
Banlice	449
Banlice	476
BARBITURATES	82
Barbloc	445
Bayer Aspirin	72
BCG vaccine	83
Becloforte	84
Beclomethasone dipropionate	84
Beconase	84
Beconase Allergy	242
Becotide	84
Bekunis	506
Benadryl Dry	472
Benadryl Family Original	48, 63
Benadryl for the Family – Dry	63, 175
Benadryl for the Family Chesty	266, 472
Benadryl for the Family Dry Forte	175
Bendrofluazide	556
BenPen	89
Benzac	309
Benzalkonium chloride	85
Benzathine penicillin	85
Benzemul	88
Benzhexol	86
Benzocaine	53
Benzocaine	53
BENZODIAZEPINES	86
Benzoic acid	309
Benzoyl peroxide	309
Benztrop	87
Benztropine	87
Benzydamine hydrochloride	87
Benzyl benzoate	88
Benzylpenicillin	89
Bepanthen	85
Berberine hydrochloride	89
Berotec	226
BETA-2 AGONISTS	90
BETA ADRENERGIC BLOCKING AGENTS	90
BETA BLOCKERS	90
Beta-Sol	555
Betacarotene	90
Betadine	298
Betaferon	297
Betagan	322
Betahistine	91
Betaine	91
Betaloc	360
Betamethasone	92
Betamin	555
Betaxolol	93
Bethanechol	94
Betnovate	92
Betoptic	93
Betoquin	93
Bex	72
Bgramin	49
Biaxsig	496
Bicalutamide	94
Bicarbonates	57

Index

Bicillin L-A	85
Bicnu	123
Bicor	98
Bifonazole	95
Biltricide	457
Bimatoprost	95
Bioallethrin	96
Biodone Forte	350
Bioglan B Complex	114
Bioglan Evening Primrose Oil	224
Bioglan Junior	114
Bioglan Maxepa	208, 224
Bioglan Primrose Micelle	224
Bioglan Prune and Senna	506
Bioglan Synergy B	114
Bion Tears	222
Biosal	345
Biotech Cold & Flu	63, 152, 423, 472
Biotech Cold & Flu Non-Drowsy	152, 423, 472
Biotin	96
Biperiden	97
BIPHASIC INSULIN	296
BIPHASIC PILLS	406
Biquinate	482
Bis-Pectin	152
Bisacodyl	97
Bisalax	97
Bisolvon Chesty	103
Bisolvon Dry	175
Bisolvon Dry Junior	175
Bisolvon Sinus	103, 472
Bisoprolol	98
Bispectin	308, 426
BISPHOSPHONATES	99
Blackmores B12	159
Blackmores Bio Calcium	115
Blackmores Bio Magnesium	115
Blackmores Evening Primrose Oil	224
Blackmores Fish Oil	224
Blackmores For Women Folic Acid	244
Blackmores for Women Total Calcium	115
Blackmores Iron Compound	300
Blenamax	99
Blenoxane	99
Bleomycin Injection	99
Bleomycin sulfate	99
Bleph-10	531
Blephamide	458
Blistex Balm	34
Blistex Lip Ointment	34
Bonefos	514
Bonjela	126, 138
Bonnington's Irish Moss	345
Boostrix	192, 551, 596
Bosentan	100
Botox	100
Botulinum toxin	100
Box jellyfish antivenom	67
Brasivol	39
Brenda	162, 406
Brevibloc	216
Brevinor	406
Brevoxyl	309
Bricanyl	549
Brimonidine tartrate	101
Brinzolamide	102
Brolene	467
Bromazepam	102
Bromhexine	103
Bromocriptine	104
Bromohexal	104
Bromolactin	104
Brompheniramine	63
BRONCHODILATORS	105
Brondecon Elixir	554
Brondecon Expectorant	266, 554
Brufen	288
Budamax	105
Budesonide	105
Bufexamac	106
Bugesic	288
Bumetanide	106
Bupivacaine	53
Buprenorphine	107
Bupropion	108
Burinex	106
Buscopan	286
Buspar	109
Buspirone	109
Busulfan	109
Butesin Pictrate With Metaphen	110, 394
Butyl aminobenzoate pictrate	110

C

C-Flox	140
Cabaser	111
Cabergoline	111
Cadexomer Iodine	111
Cafergot	112, 214
Caffeine	112
Cal-Sup	114
Calamine	113
Calcijex	114
Calciparine	271
Calcipotriol	113
Calcitonin	500

Index

Calcitriol 114
Calcium 114
Calcium alginate 116
CALCIUM ANTAGONISTS 116
Calcium ascorbate 115
Calcium carbonate 57, 114
CALCIUM CHANNEL BLOCKERS 116
Calcium citrate 115
Calcium folinate 116
Calcium gluconate 115
calcium hydrogen phosphate 115
Calcium pantothenate 114
Calcium phosphate 115
Calmurid 309, 583
Calogen 224
Caltrate 114
Caltrate + D 115
Caltrate Plus 115, 155, 603
Calvita 300
Camphor 117
Campral 22
CANCER TREATING DRUGS 118
Candesartan 56
Canesten 151
Canesten Once Daily Bifonazole 95
Cannabis 336
Capadex 177, 423
Capecitabine 118
Capoten 23
Capsaicin 119
Captohexal 23
Captopril 23
Capurate 35
Carafate 530
Carbachol 120
Carbamazepine 120
Carbimazole 121
Carbocaine 53
Carbomer 940 222
Carbomer 974 222
Carbomer 980 222
Carboplatin 122
Carbosorb 128
Carbosorb S 128, 523
CARDIAC GLYCOSIDE 123
Cardinorm 45
Cardiprin 72
Cardizem 188
Cardol 524
Carmellose sodium 222
Carmustine 123
Cartia 72
Carvedilol 123

Catapres 149
Caverject 37
CDT 192, 551
Ceclor 125
CeeNU 330
Cefaclor 125
Cefalexin-BC 125
Cefazolin 125
Cefepime 125
Cefkor 125
Cefotaxime 125
Cefotaxime-BC 125
Cefotetan 125
Cefoxitin 125
Cefpiromine 125
Cefrom 125
Ceftazidime 125
Ceftriaxone 125
Cefuroxime 125
Celapram 143
Celebrex 124
Celecoxib 124
Celestone Chronodose 92
Celestone-M 92
Celestone-V 92
Celestone-VG 92, 254
Cellcept 374
Cellufresh 222
Celluvisc 222
Cenovis B Complex 114
Cepacaine 53, 128
Cepacol Cough 128, 175
Cepacol Lozenges 53
Cephalexin 125
CEPHALOSPORINS 125
Cephalothin 125
Cephamandole 125
Cephazolin 125
Cerumol Ear Drops 70
Cetalkonium chloride 126
Cetaphil Moisturising Cream 424
Cetirizine 64
Cetomacrogol 127
Cetrimide 127
Cetylpyridinium 128
Charcoal 128
Charcocaps 128
Chemists' Own Chesty Cough 103
Chemists' Own Chesty Mucus Cough 103
Chemists' Own Cold & Flu Night 63
Chemists' Own Coldeze 63
Chemists' Own Difenacol Cough 63
Chemists' Own Dry Raspy Cough 63, 175

Index

Chemists' Own Hayfever Sinus Relief 63
Chemists' Own Infant's Cold &
   Allergy Drops...63
Chemists' Own Kiddicol 63
Chemists' Own Paracetamol.........................423
Chemists' Own Peetalix....................................63
Chemists' Own Promethazine 63
Chemists' Own Soothing Lotion 34
Chickenpox vaccine.......................................129
Chlorambucil 130
Chloramphenicol 130
Chlorhexidine 131
Chlormethiazole 132
Chloromycetin 130
Chloroquine 133
Chloroxylenol 134
Chlorphenesin 135
Chlorpheniramine 63
Chlorpromazine 435
Chlorquin 133
Chlorsig 130
Chlorthalidone 556
Chlorvescent 208
Cholecalciferol 135
Cholera vaccine 136
Cholestyramine 137
Choline salicylate 138
Choline theophyllinate..................................554
Chorionic gonadotrophin, human................138
Cialis 539
Cicatrin 81, 384
Cilamox 49
Cilastatin 139
Cilex 125
Cilicaine..463
Cilicaine V 438
Cilicaine VK 438
Cilopen VK..438
CiloQuin 140
Ciloxan 140
Cimehexal 139
Cimetidine 139
Cinchocaine 53
Cipramil 143
Cipro 140
Ciprofloxacin 140
Ciproxin 140
Ciproxin HC 140, 278
Cisapride 141
Cisplatin 142
Citalopram 143
Citanest 53
Citanest Dental 30

Citracal 115
Citracal + D 115
Citracal Plus..115, 155, 603
Citralite 584
Citravescent 208, 584
Citrihexal 114
Claforan 125
Clamoxyl 49, 455
Claratyne..62
Clarinase 62, 472
Clarithromycin 144
Clavulanic acid 455
Clavulin 49, 455
Clear Away..500
Clear Eyes...379
Clearasil 500
Clearasil Acne Cream 578
Clearasil Cream 534
Clearasil Medicated Face Wash. 437
Clearasil Medicated Foam 309
Clearasil Medicated Wipes 309
Clearasil Ultra...309
Clearaway Wart Remover 309
Cleocin...145
Clerz 222
Clexane..209
Climara 399
Climen 162, 399
Clindamycin 145
Clindatech 145
Clinoril 535
Clioquinol 145
Clobazam 146
Clobemix 369
Clofazime 147
Clofeme 151
Clofen..81
Clomhexal...147
Clomid 147
Clomiphene...147
Clomipramine 578
Clonazepam 148
Clonea 151
Clonidine 149
Clopidogrel 150
Clopine 435
Clopixol 608
Clopram 578
Clotreme 151
Clotrimazole 151
Clozapine 435
Clozaril 435
Clozole 151

Coal tar	542
Cocaine	151
Cod liver oil	153
Codalgin	152, 423
Codalgin Forte	152
Codalgin Forte	423
Codalgin Plus	63, 152, 423
Codapane	152, 423
Codeine Phosphate	152
Codiphen	72, 152
Codis	72, 152
Codox	72, 187
Codral 4 Flu	63, 152, 423, 472
Codral Cold & Flu	152, 423, 472
Codral Cough Cold & Flu Day	472
Codral Cough Cold & Flu Night	63, 472
Codral Cough Cold & Flu	175, 423
Codral Daytime	152, 423, 472
Codral Dry Cough	152, 472
Codral Forte	72, 152
Codral Night Time	63, 423, 472
Codral Pain Relief	152, 423
Cogentin	87
Cognex	538
Coke	151
Colchicine	154
Colese	338
Colestid	155
Colestipol	155
Colgout	154
Colifoam	278
Colofac	338
Coloxyl Drops	454
Coloxyl Enema	198
Coloxyl Suppositories	97, 198
Coloxyl Tablets	198
Coloxyl with Senna	198, 506
Combantrin	474
Combantrin Mebendazole	338
Combivent	299, 499
Combivir	315, 602
Comtan	210
Comvax	269, 273
Condyline	452
CONTRACEPTIVE PILLS	406
Cophenylcaine Forte	53, 440
Copper	155
Coras	188
Corbeton	415
Cordarone X	45
Cordilox	591
Cornkil	53, 309, 500
Cortaid	278
Cortate	156
Cortef	278
Cortic	278
CORTICOSTEROIDS	156, 529
Cortisol	278
Cortisone Acetate	156
Cosig	532
Cosig Forte	580
Cosmegen	165
Cosopt	201, 565
Cosudex	94
Cotazym-S Forte	420
COUGH SUPPRESSANTS	157
Coumadin	595
Coversyl	23
Coversyl Plus	23, 293
COX-2 INHIBITORS	157
Coxiella burnetti vaccine	158
Cozaar	56
Crack	151
Creon	420
Crixivan	293
Cromese	515
Cromolyn sodium	515
Crotamiton	158
Crysanal	380
CRYSTALLINE INSULIN ZINC SUSPENSION	296
Curacel Acne and Pimple Gel	34, 208, 534
Curacleanse Antiseptic Gel	127
Curacleanse Gel	131
Curaderm	309, 500, 583
Curash Powders	603
Curatin	570
Cyanocobalamin	159
Cycloblastin	160
Cyclogyl	375
Cyclopentolate	375
Cyclophosphamide	160
Cycloserine	161
Cyclosporin	161
Cyklokapron	574
Cymevene	252
Cyproheptadine	64
Cyprone	162
Cyprostat	162
Cyproterone Acetate	162, 406
Cysporin	161
Cystadane	91
Cystagon	163
Cysteamine	163
Cytadren	44

Index

Cytamen 159
Cytarabine 164
Cytotec 368
Cytotoxics 118

D

D-Penamine 427
Dactinomycin 165
Daivonex 113
Daktagold 310
Daktarin 364
Daktozin 603
Daktozin 364
Dalacin C 145
Dalacin T 145
Dalacin V 145
Dalteparin 165
Dan-Gard 479
Danaparoid 166
Danazol 167
Danocrine 167
Dantrium 168
Dantrolene 168
Daonil 257
Dapa-Tabs 293
Daraprim 478
Daunorubicin 168
Daunoxome 168
Day & Night Cold & Flu 175
DBL Aspirin 72
DBL Baclofen 81
De Witt's Antacid 114
De-Gas 511
De-Gas Extra 511
De-Gas Infant 511
Deca Durabolin 378
DECONGESTANTS 169, 537
Deep Heat 345
Degas Extra 57
Degas Extra Chewable 114
Delavirdine 169
Demazin Cold & Flu 63, 423, 472
Demazin Day/Night Relief 63, 472
Demazin Repetabs 63
Demazin Sinus 472
Demazin Syrup 63, 440
Demazin Tablets 63, 472
Demeclocycline 170
Dencorub Arthritis Ice 345
Dencorub Pain Cream 345
Depo Provera 339
Depo Ralovera 339
Depo-Medrol 357

Depo-Nisolone 357
Deptran 578
Deralin 468
Derm-Aid 278
Derma Tech 469
Derma Drate 309, 583
Dermatech 309
Dermatech 500
Dermaveen Acne Bar 309, 500
Dermazole 205
Dermestril 399
Dermeze 424
Deseril 358
Desferal 171
Desferrioxamine 171
Desmopressin acetate 171
Desogestrel 406
Desonide 172
Desowen 172
Destin Nappy Rash 603
Dettol 578
Dettol Antiseptic Spray 85
Dettol Cream 134
Dettol Liquid 134
DeWitt's Antacid 57, 308
DeWorm 338
Dexamethasone 173
Dexamphetamine 174
Dexchlorpheniramine 63, 64
Dexi-Tuss 175
Dexmethsone 173
Dexsal 57, 261
Dextromethorphan 175
Dextromoramide 176
Dextropropoxyphene 177
Diabex 349
Diaformin 349
Diamicron 258
Diamox 24
Diane 162
Diane 406
Diareze 76, 426
Diazepam 178
Diazoxide 179
Dibenyline 437
Dibromopropamide isethionate 467
Dichlotride 556
Diclocil 181
Diclofenac 180
Diclohexal 180
Dicloxacillin 181
Dicloxsig 181
Dicyclomine 182

Index

Didanosine 182
Didrocal 115, 194
Didronel 194
Diethylamine salicylate 183
Diethylpropion hydrochloride 184
Differin 29
Difflam Anti-inflammatory
  Cough Lozenges 87, 128, 442
Difflam Anti-inflammatory Lozenges 87
Difflam Anti-inflammatory Throat Spray 87
Difflam C Anti-inflammatory Antiseptic 131
Difflam Cream 87
Difflam Gel 87
Difflam Lozenges 128
Difflam Mouth Gel 87
Difflam Solution 87
Difflam Sugar-free Lozenges 87
Difflam-C Anti-inflammatory
  Antiseptic Solution 87
Diflucan 232
Diflunisal 185
Digesic 177, 423
Digoxin 186
Dihydergot 187
Dihydrocodeine 187
Dihydroergotamine 187
Dihydroxyacetone 188
Dilantin 441
Dilatrend 123
Dilaudid 280
Dilosyn 63
Diltahexal 188
Diltiazem 188
Dilzem 188
Dimenhydrinate 189
Dimetapp 440
Dimetapp 440
Dimetapp 12 Hour Spray 418
Dimetapp Cold & Flu 175, 423, 472
Dimetapp Cold Cough & Flu 175, 423, 472
Dimetapp Cold Cough & Flu Day & Night . 175
Dimetapp Cold Cough & Flu Day & Night
  Liquid Caps 423
Dimetapp Cold Cough & Flu Night 63
Dimetapp Cold Cough & Sinus 175, 472
Dimetapp Cold Cough & Flu
  Liquid Capsules 266
Dimetapp Cold Cough & Sinus
  Liquid Capsules 266, 472
Dimetapp Day Cold Cough & Flu 472
Dimetapp DM 63, 175, 440
Dimetapp Drops 63
Dimetapp Elixir 63
Dimetapp Headcold & Flu 288, 472
Dimetapp Night Cold Cough & Flu 472
Dimetapp Night Relief 423, 472
Dimetapp Sinus 472
Dimethicone 190
Dimethicream 190
Dimetriose 255
Dinac 180
Dindevan 434
Dinoprost F2 Alpha 191
Dinoprostone 191
Dipentum 404
Diphemanil methylsulfate 191
Diphenhydramine 63, 64
Diphenoxylate hydrochloride 192
Diphtheria vaccine 192
Dipivefrine hydrochloride 193
Dipoquin 193
Diprosone 92
Dipyridamole 194
Disodium cromoglycate 515
Disodium etidronate 194
Disodium pamidronate 195
Disopyramide 196
Disprin 72
Disprin Forte 72, 152
Distaph 181
Disulfiram 197
Diswart 262
Dithranol 197
Dithrasal 197
Dithrocream 197
Ditropan 416
DIURETICS 198
Divina 399
Docosahexaenoic acid 224
Docusate sodium 198
Dolased Analgesic Relaxant 63, 152, 423
Dolased Day Pain Relief 423
Dolased Day Relief 152
Dolased Night Pain 63
Dolased Night Pain Relief 423
Dolased Night Relief 152
Dolasetron 199
Dolobid 185
Doloxene 177
Domperidone 200
Donepezil 200
Donnagel 75, 286, 308, 426
Donnalix 75, 286
Donnatab 75, 286
Doryx 202
Dorzolamide hydrochloride 201

Index

Dostinex 111
Dothep 578
Dothiepin 578
Doxepin 578
Doxsig 202
Doxy 202
Doxycycline 202
Doxyhexal 202
Doxylamine 63
Doxylin 202
Dozile 63
Dramamine 189
Driclor 38
Drixine Nasal 418
Droleptan 203
Droperidol 203
Drospirenone 406
Ducene 178
Duo Visc 516
Duocal 224
Duofilm 309, 500
Duofilm Gel 309, 500
Duphalac 315
Duphaston 204
Dur-Elix Plus 103, 472
Duratears 222, 424
Duride 303
Duro-Tuss 442
Duro-Tuss Cold & Allergy 63, 440
Duro-Tuss Decongestant 442, 472
Duro-Tuss Expectorant 103, 442
Duro-Tuss Lozenges 128, 442
Duro-Tuss Mucolytic 103
Durogesic 227
Durolax 97
Durolax SP 520
Duromine 439
Dydrogesterone 204
Dymadon 423
Dymadon Co 152, 423
Dymadon Forte 152, 423
Dynamo 112, 261, 389
Dysport 100

E

E-Mycin 215
E45 Cream 424
Ear Clear for Swimmers Ear 25, 302
Early Bird 474
Echinacea 205
Econazole 205
Ecotrin 72
Eczema Cream 603

Edecril 216
EDP 298
Edronax 485
EES 215
Efacal 224
Efavirenz 206
Efexor 590
Eformoterol 207
Efudix 238
Egocort 278
Egoderm 603
Egoderm Cream 289
Egoderm Ointment 289
Egomycol 500
Egopsoryl TA 534, 542
Egozite 262
Egozite Baby Cream 190, 424, 603
Egozite Cradle Cap Lotion 309, 500
Egozite Protective Baby Lotion 190
Eicosapentaenoic acid 208
Eldepryl 504
Eldisine 593
ELECTROLYTES 208
Eleuphrat 92
Elmiron 429
Elocon 370
Emetrol 248, 261
EMLA 53
Enahexal 23
Enalapril 23
Endep 578
Endone 417
Endoxan 160
Engerix-B 273
Enidin 101
Eno 57
Enoxaparin 209
Entacapone 210
Entocort 105
Enzace 23
Epaq 499
Ephedrine 211
Epilim 522
Epipen 30
Epoeitin 212
Eprosartan 56
ER Cream 34, 208, 542, 603
Erevax 497
Ergamisol 321
Ergocalciferol 212
Ergodryl 63, 112, 214
Ergodryl Mono 214
Ergometrine 213

Entry	Page
Ergotamine	214
Eryacne	215
Eryc	215
Erythrocin	215
Erythromycin	215
Erythropoietin	212
Eskazole	31
Esmolol	216
Esomeprazole	471
Estalis	395, 399
Estracombi	395, 399
Estraderm	399
Estradiol	399
Estrapak	399
Estrofem	399
Ethacrynic Acid	216
Ethambutol	217
Ethanol	218
Ethinyloestradiol	406
Ethosuximide	219
Ethyl alcohol	218
Ethyol	42
Etonogestrel	219
Etopophos	220
Etoposide	220
Euhypnos	544
Euky Bear Cough Syrup	63
Eulactol	364
Eulactol Heel balm	190, 469, 583
Eulexin	241
Eurax	158
Eutrosig	559
Evening Primrose Oil	224
Evista	484
Exelon	494
Exemestane	221
Exorex Emulsion	542
EXPECTORANTS	221
EYE LUBRICANTS	222

F

Entry	Page
FAB Iron and B	300
FAB Trical	115
Famciclovir	223
Famotidine	223
Famvir	223
Fansidar	478, 531
Fareston	571
Fasigyn	566
FATTY ACIDS	224
Faverin	243
Febridol	423
Fefol	244, 300
Feldene	450
Felodipine	225
Felodur ER	225
Femara	320
Femoden	406
Femoston	204, 399
Femtran	399
Fenac	180
Fenamine	63
Fenoterol	226
Fentanyl	227
Fentanyl Injection	227
Fenugreek	228
Fergon	300
Fermathron	516
Ferro-Gradumet	300
Ferrograd C	300
Ferrosig	300
Ferrous gluconate	300
Ferrous phosphate	300
Ferrous sulfate	300
Ferrum H	300
Feverfew	228
Fexofenadine	62
FGF	244, 300
FIBRE	229
FIBRINOLYTICS	229
Fibsol	23
Finasteride	229
Fiorinal	63, 152, 423
Fisamox	49
Fishaphos	208, 224
Flagyl	361
Flarex	237
Flecainide	230
Flecatab	230
Fleet	97
Fleet Enema	519
Fleet Micro-Enema	523
Fleet Microenema	518
Fleet Phospho-Soda	519
Flixotide	242
Flomax	541
Flopen	231
Florinef	233
Floxapen	231
Floxsig	231
Fluanxol	239
Fluarix	295
Flucil	231
Flucloxacillin	231
Flucon	237
Fluconazole	232

Index

Flucytosine 232
Fludrocortisone 233
Flumethasone 234
Flunitrazepam 235
Fluocortolone 236
Fluohexal 239
Fluoride 236
Fluorometholone 237
Fluorouracil 238
Fluoxetine 239
Flupenthixol 239
Fluphenazine 435
Flurbiprofen 240
Flutamide 241
Flutamin 241
Fluticasone propionate 242
Fluvastatin 242
Fluvax 295
Fluvirin 295
Fluvoxamine 243
FML 237
Folic acid 244
Follicle stimulating
hormone 245
Follitropin 245
Fongitar 479, 542
Foradile 207
Fortovase 503
Fortral 428
Fortum 125
Fosamax 33
Fosfestrol 246
Fosinopril 23
Fragmin 165
Framycetin 246
Frangula 247
Frisium 146
Fructose 248
Frusehexal 248
Frusemide 248
Frusid 248
FSH 245
Fucidin 516
Fucidin Topical 516
Fugerel 241
Fungilin 50
Fungizone 50
Fungo Cream 190, 364
Fungo Powder 364
Fungo Solution 364
Fungo Soothing Balm 106, 190, 364
Fungo Vaginal 190, 364
Fungocort 278, 364
Funnel web spider antivenom 67
Furadantin 394
Furosemide 248
Fybogel 305

G

Gabapentin 250
Gabitril 560
Galantamine 250
Gamma Globulin 251
Gammalinoleic acid 224
Ganciclovir 252
Gantin 250
Gastro Stop 331
Gastrogel Suspension 57
Gastrogel Tablets 57, 511
Gastrolyte 208, 261
Gastrolyte-R 208
Gatifloxacin 252
Gaviscon 57, 114
Gaviscon Double Strength 57
Gel Tears 222
Gelusil 57, 511
Gemfibrizol 253
Gemhexal 253
Genlac 315
Genoptic 254
Genoral 448
Genotropin 523
Genox 540
GenRx Aciclovir 27
GenRx Atenolol 73
GenRx Azathioprine 78
GenRx Baclofen 81
GenRx Cefaclor 125
GenRx Cephalexin 125
GenRx Cimetidine 139
GenRx Clomiphene 147
GenRx Clomipramine 578
GenRx Diclofenac 180
GenRx Diltiazem 188
GenRx Doxycycline 202
GenRx Enalapril 23
GenRx Fluoxetine 239
GenRx Frusemide 248
GenRx Gabapentin 250
GenRx Gemfibrizol 253
GenRx Gliclazide 258
GenRx Indapamide 293
GenRx Lisinopril 23
GenRx Metformin 349
GenRx Nifedipine 390
GenRx Norfloxacin 396

Index

GenRx Paracetamol 423
GenRx Paroxetine 425
GenRx Piroxicam 450
GenRx Prazosin 457
GenRx Ranitidine 484
GenRx Salbutamol 499
GenRx Sotalol 524
Gentamicin 254
Genteal Eye Drops 222
Genteal Moisturising Eye Gel 222
Gentlees 128, 262
Gestodene 406
Gestodene 406
Gestrinone 255
Ginkgo biloba 256
Ginseng 256
GLAUCOMA MEDICATIONS 257
Gliadel 123
Glibenclamide 257
Gliclazide 258
Glimel 257
Glimepride 259
Glipizide 260
Glivec 290
Glucagen 261
Glucagon 261
Gluco-lyte 261
Glucobay 22
Glucohexal 349
Glucomet 349
Glucophage 349
Glucose 261
Glutaraldehyde 262
Glyade 258
Glycerin Suppositories 262
Glycerol 262
Glycerol Suppositories 262
Glyceryl Trinitrate 263
Glycyrrhizin 328
Go Kit 97
Goanna Analgesic Icel 500
Gold 77, 513
Gold Cross Antihistamine 63
Gonal-F 245
Gopten 23
Goserelin acetate 264
Gramicidin 265
Granocol 247, 528
Granugen 424, 603
Griseofulvin 266
Griseostatin 266
Grisovin 266
Growth hormone 523

GTN 263
Guaiphenesin 266
Guanethidine 267
Guarana 268
Gyne-Lotremin 151

H

H-B-Vax II 273
H2 RECEPTOR ANTAGONISTS 269
Haemophilus influenzae B vaccine 269
HAEMOSTATIC AGENTS 270
Halcion 577
Haldol 270
Haloperidol 270
Hamilton Body Lotion 262
Hamilton Cleansing Lotion 131, 262, 424
Hamilton Dry Skin Cream 583
Hamilton Dry Skin Treatment 424
Hamilton Eczema Cream 190
Hamilton Skin Lotion 424
Hamilton Skin Repair 190
Harmonise 331
Hash 336
Havrix 1440 273
Havrix Junior 273
HCG 138
Healon 516
Healthsense Fluoxetine 239
Hemineurin M 132
Hemocane 34, 53, 131, 603
Heparin 271
Heparinoid 272
Hepatitis A vaccine 273
Hepatitis B vaccine 273
Heroin 274
Herron Aspirin 72
Herron Baby Teething Gel 138
Herron Paracetamol 423
Hexal Diclac 180
Hexal PI 298
Hexal Ranitic 484
Hexamethylmelamine 38
Hexamine hippurate 275
Hexol 131
Hexylresorcinol 275
HiB vaccine 269
Hiberix 269
Himega 208, 224
Hiprex 275
Hirudoid 272
Hivid 600
Homatropine hydrobromide 375
Honvan 246

Index

HORMONE REPLACEMENT THERAPY 276
HRT 276
Humalog 296
Humatrope 523
Humegon 344
Humulin 296
Humulin L 296
Humulin NPH 296
Humulin R 296
Humulin UL 296
Hyalase 277
Hyaluronidase 277
Hycor Eye Drops 278
Hydopa 355
Hydraderm 127
Hydralazine 277
Hydrea 284
Hydrene 556
Hydrochlorothiazide 556
Hydrocortisone 278
Hydroform 145, 278
Hydrogen peroxide 280
Hydromorphone 280
Hydroquinone 281
Hydroxocobalamin 282
Hydroxychloroquine 283
Hydroxyethylcellulose 222
Hydroxyethylrutosides 284
Hydroxypropylcellulose 222
Hydroxyurea 284
Hydrozole 151, 278
Hygroton 556
Hylan 285
Hyoscine 286
Hyoscyamine 286
Hypericum perforatum 498
Hypnodorm 235
HYPNOTICS 287
Hypnovel 365
HYPOGLYCAEMICS 287
Hypol 208
HYPOLIPIDAEMIC 287
Hypromellose 222
Hypurin Isophane 296
Hypurin Neutral 296
Hysone 278
Hytrin 547

I

I131 517
Ibilex 125
Ibuprofen 288

Ice Gel 345
Ichthammol 289
Ichthammol Ointment 289
Idarubicin 289
Idoxuridine 290
Ikorel 387
Imatinib 290
Imdur Durules 303
Imigran 536
Imipenem 139
Imipramine 578
Imiquimod 291
Immucyst 83
Immunoglobulin 251
IMMUNOGLOBULINS 292
IMMUNOMODIFIERS 292
Imodium Advanced 331, 511
Imodium 331
Imovane 607
Implanon 219
Improvil 406
Imtrate SR 303
Imukin 297
Imuran 78
In a Wink Moisturising Drops 222
Indahexal 293
Indapamide 293
Inderal 468
Indinavir 293
Indocid 294
Indomethacin 294
Infacol 511
Infanrix 192, 551, 596
Infanrix HepB 192, 273, 551, 596
Infant Gaviscon 57
Influenza virus vaccine 295
Influvac 295
Insensye 396
Insig 293
Insta Glucose 261
INSULIN ZINC SUSPENSION 296
INSULINS 296
Intal 515
Interferon 297
Intra Site Gel 469
Intraglobulin 251
Intragram 251
Intron A 297
Invirase 503
Inza 380
IODINE 298
Iodine, radioactive 517
Iodoflex 111

Index

Iodosorb 111
Ionil 309, 500
Ionil Rinse 85
Ionil T 309, 500, 542
Ionil T Plus 542
Iopidine 69
Ipol 453
Ipratrin 299
Ipratropium bromide 299
Ipravent 299
Irbesartan 56
IRON 300
Iron amino acid chelate. 300
Iron polymaltose 300
Iscover 150
Ismelin 267
Isohexal 304
Isoniazid 301
ISOPHANE INSULIN 296
Isophyl 309
Isoprenaline 301
Isopropyl alcohol 302
Isoptin 591
Isopto Carbachol 120
Isopto Carpine 443
Isopto Frin 440
Isopto Homatropine 375
Isopto Tears 222
Isordil 303
Isosorbide nitrate 303
Isotretinoin 304
Isotrex 304
Ispaghula 305
Isuprel 301
Itraconazole 305
Ivermectin 306

J

Japanese encephalitis virus vaccine 307
Je-Vax 307
Jezil 253
Juliet 162, 406

K

K-Mag 208
K-Thrombin 270
Kaletra 493
Kalma 36
Kaltostat 116
Kaluril 43
Kaolin 308
Kaomagma with Pectin 308, 426
Kapanol 372

Karvea 56
Karvezide 56, 556
Karvol 345
Keflex 125
Keflin 125
Keflor 125
Kefzol 125
Kenacomb 265, 384, 398, 575
Kenacort-A 575
Kenalog in Orabase 575
Keppra 322
KERATOLYTICS 309
Ketoconazole 310
Ketoprofen 311
Ketorolac trometanol 312
Kinidin Durules 481
Kinson 324
Klacid 144
Klacid HP7 ....49, 144, 471
Kliogest 395, 399
Kliovance 395, 399
Konakion 270
Kosteo 114
Kredex 123
Kripton 104
KSR 208
Kwells 286

L

L-dopa 324
Labetalol 314
Lac-Dol 315
Lacri Lube 222, 424
Lacrisert 222
Lact-Easy 564
Lactaid 564
Lactic acid 309
Lactulose 315
Lamictal 316
Lamisil 548
Lamivudine 315
Lamotrigine 316
Lamprene 147
Lanoxin 186
Lansoprazole 471
Lanvis 557
Largactil 435
Lariam 341
Lasix 248
Lasonil 272, 277
Latanoprost 317
Latycin Eye Ointment 552
LAXATIVES 317

Index

Laxettes with Senna	506
Laxettes with Sennosides	506
Ledermycin	170
Ledertrexate	353
Leflunomide	318
Lemsip	423
Lemsip Chesty Cough	266
Lemsip Flu	175
Lemsip Flu Day	472
Lemsip Flu Night	472
Lemsip Headcold	423
Lemsip Lozenges	128
Lemsip Max	423
Lemsip Pharmacy Flu Daytime	423
Lemsip Pharmacy Flu Nightime	423
Lemsip Pharmacy Flu Strength Nightime	63
LENTE INSULIN	296
Lercanidipine	319
Lescol	242
Letrozole	320
Leucovorin	116
Leukeran	130
Leuko Fungex	364
LEUKOTRENE RECEPTOR ANTAGONISTS	320
Leuprorelin	320
Levamisole	321
Levetiracetam	322
Levlen	406
Levobunolol	322
Levocabastine	323
LEVODOPA COMPOUNDS	324
Levonorgestrel	325, 406
Lexotan	102
Lice Rid	334
Lignocaine	53
Lignocaine Gel	53
Lignocaine Gel with Chlorhexidine	53, 131
Lignospan	30
Lignospan Special	53
Lincocin	326
Lincomycin	326
Linctus Tussinol	442
Linezolid	326
LINIMENTS	327
Linoleic acid	224, 309
Linotar	542
Lioresal	81
Liothyronine	327
Lipazil	253
Lipex	511
Lipitor	74
Liprace	23
Liquifilm	222
Liquigen	224
Liquigesic Co	152, 423
Liquorice	328
Lisinopril	23
Lisodur	23
LISPRO INSULIN	296
Lithicarb	328
Lithium carbonate	328
Livial	562
Livostin	323
Locacorten Vioform	145, 234
Loceryl	48
Locilan	395, 406
Lodoxamide	329
Loette	406
Lofenoxal	75, 192
Logicin Chest Rub	345
Logicin Congested Chesty Cough	266, 472
Logicin Cough Suppressant	442
Logicin Dry Cough	175, 472
Logicin Expectorant	103, 267
Logicin Flu	175, 423, 472
Logicin Flu Day	472
Logicin Flu Day & Night	175
Logicin Flu Night	63, 423, 472
Logicin Flu Strength Night	63
Logicin Hay Fever	63, 423, 472
Logicin Junior Children's Cough	175, 472
Logicin Rapid Relief	53
Logicin Rapid Relief Lozenges	87
Logicin Rapid Relief Nasal Spray	418
Logicin Sinus	472
Logoderm	32
Logynon	406
Lomide	329
Lomotil	75, 192
Lomustine	330
Loniten	366
LOOP DIURETICS	330
Loperamide	331
Lopid	253
Lopresor	360
Lorastyne	62
Loratadine	62
Lorazepam	332
Losartan	56
Losec	471
Losec HP7	49, 144, 471
Lovan	239
Lovir	27
LPV	438
Lucrin	320

Index

Lumefantrine 70
Lumigan 95
Lumin 363
Lurselle 461
Luvox 243
Lyclear 432

M

Macro Mega B 114
Macro Natural Vitamin E Cream 34
Macrodantin 394
Macrogol 400 222
MACROLIDES 333
Madopar..324
Magicul...139
Magnesium 333
Magnesium alginate....................................57
Magnesium aspartate 208
Magnesium carbonate.................................57
Magnesium hydroxide 57
Magnesium Plus 208
Magnesium salts 57
Magnesium sulfate....................................334
Magnoplasm 334
Malarone 75, 466
Maldison 334
Mandol..125
MAOI..335
Maosig 369
Marcain 30, 53
Marevan 595
Marijuana 336
Marvelon 406
Maxamox 49
Maxepa 224
Maxepa & EPO 224
Maxidex 173
Maxipime 125
Maxolon 359
Maxor 471
MCT Oil 224
Measles vaccine 337
Mebendazole 338
Mebeverine 338
Medefizz 208
Medefoam-2 511
Medevac 523
Medevac Solution 70
Medi Creme 34, 131
Medi Pulv 34, 131
Medijel 43, 53
Meditox 449, 476
Medroxyhexal 339

Medroxyprogesterone acetate 339
Mefenamic Acid 340
Mefic 340
Mefloquine 341
Mefoxin 125
Megace 342
Megafol 244
Megestrol 342
Melipramine 578
Melizide 260
Melleril 435
Meloxicam 342
Melphalan 343
Menadione 270
Mencevax ACWY 344
Meningitec 344
Meningococcal vaccine 344
Menjugate 344
Menomune 344
Menopausal gonadotrophin, human 344
Menoprem 339, 402
Menorest 399
Menotrophin 344
Menthol 345
Mepivacaine 53
Mepyramine 64
Meracote 57
Merbentyl 182
Mercaptopurine 346
Merieux Inactivated Rabies Vaccine 483
Meropenem 347
Merrem 347
Mersyndol 63, 152, 423
Mersyndol Day 152, 423
Mersyndol Forte 63, 152, 423
Meruvax II 497
Mesalazine 347
Mesasal 347
Mesna 348
Mesterolone 349
Mestinon 476
Mestranol 406
Metamucil 474
Metformin 349
Methadone 350
Methdilazine 63
Methenolone 351
Methionine 352
Methnine 352
Methoblastin 353
Methopt 222
Methotrexate 353
Methoxsalen 354

Index

Methylcellulose	354
Methyldopa	355
Methylphenidate	356
Methylphenobarbitone	82
Methylprednisolone	357
Methysergide	358
Metoclopramide	359
Metohexal	360
Metolol	360
Metopirone	362
Metoprolol	360
Metrogyl	361
Metronidazole	361
Metronide	361
Metsal	345
Metyrapone	362
Mexiletine	362
Mexitil	362
Miacalcic	500
Mianserin	363
Micanol	197
Micardis	56
Micardis Plus	56, 556
Miconazole	364
Microgynon	406
Microlax	518, 523
Microlevlen	406
Microlut	406
Micronor	395, 406
Microshield Antiseptic Concentrate	131
Microshield Preparations	131
Microshield PVP	298
Microshield T	578
Microval	406
Midamor	43
Midazolam	365
Minax	360
MINERALS	365
Minidiab	260
Minidine	298
Minims Artificial Tears	222
Minims Atropine	75
Minims Chloramphenicol	130
Minims Gentamicin	254
Minims Local Anaesthetic	53
Minims Mydriatics	375, 440
Minims Neomycin	384
Minims Pilocarpine	443
Minims Prednisolone	458
Minipress	457
Minirin	171
Minitran	263
Minocycline	365
Minomycin	365
Minoxidil	366
Mintec	430
Minulet	406
Miochol	26
Miostat	120
MIOTICS	367
Mirena	325
Mirtazapine	367
Mirtazon	367
Misoprostol	368
Mixtard	296
MMR II	337, 373, 497
Mobic	342
Mobilis	450
Moclobemide	369
Modafinil	370
Modavigil	370
Modecate	435
Moduretic	43, 556
Mogadon	393
Mohexal	369
Mometasone	370
Monistat	364
Monoamine oxidase inhibitors	335
Monodur	303
Monofeme	406
MONOPHASIC PILLS	406
Monoplus	23, 556
Monopril	23
Monotard	296
Montelukast	371
Morning-after pill	325
Morphalgin	72, 372
Morphine	372
Motilium	200
Movelat Sportz	272, 309, 500
Movox	243
Moxacin	49
MPA	339
MS Mono	372
MS-Contin	372
Mucaine	57
Mucaine 2 in 1	57, 511
MUCOLYTICS	373
Mucomyst	26
Mumps vaccine	373
Mupirocin	374
Murelax	413
Murine	89
Murine Allergy	379, 597
Murine Contact	222
Murine Revital	222

Index

Murine Sore Eyes 553
Murine Tears..222
MUSCLE RELAXANTS 374
Muse 37
Myambutol...217
Mycil Healthy Feet 85, 131, 570
Mycobutin..490
Mycoderm...........................309, 500, 521, 582
Mycophenolate mofetil............................374
Mycospor...95
Mycostatin...398
Mycozol...309
Mydriacyl..375
MYDRIATICS..375
Mylanta...511
Mylanta Double Strength 57
Mylanta Heartburn Relief...................57, 114
Mylanta Original 57
Mylanta Rolltabs 57, 115
Myleran...109
Myocrisin...513
Myoquin..482
Mysoline..460

N

Nafarelin...376
Naloxone...376
Naltrexone...377
Nandrolone decanoate 378
Napamide..293
Naphazoline..379
Naphcon A 63, 379
Naphcon Forte 379
Naprogesic..380
Naprosyn...380
Naproxen..380
Naramig..381
Naratriptan..381
Narcan..376
NARCOTICS..382
Nardil...335
Naropin..53
Naropin with Fentanyl......................53, 227
Nasalate..131
Nasalate Cream.....................................440
Nasex Nasal Decongestant 418
Nasonex..370
Natragen...399
Natrilix...293
Natulan...464
Nature's Own Folic Acid 244
Naudicelle...224
Navane..558

Navelbine..593
Navoban..581
Nebcin...567
Nedocromil sodium 382
Nefazodone..383
NeisVac-C..344
Nelfinavir..384
Nemdyn..81, 384
Neo-Cytamen...282
Neo-Diophen...175
Neo-Medrol Acne Lotion 357, 384, 534
Neo-Mercazole.......................................121
Neo-Synephrine Ophthalmic 440
Neo-Synephrine.....................................440
Neomycin..384
Neoral..161
Neosporin 81, 265, 384, 454
Neostigmine..385
Neosulf...384
Neotigason..28
Netilmicin..386
Netromycin...386
Neulactil...435
Neur-Amyl..82
Neurontin...250
NeutraFluor..236
NEUTRAL INSULIN 296
Nevirapine..387
Nexium...471
Niacin...389
Nicabate...388
Nicorandil...387
Nicorette..388
Nicotinamide...389
Nicotine...388
Nicotinell..388
Nicotinic Acid.......................................389
Nidem..258
Nifecard...390
Nifedipine...390
Nifehexal..390
Nilstat..398
Nilutamide..391
Nimodipine...392
Nimotop..392
Nitrazepam...393
Nitro-Dur..263
Nitrofurantoin.......................................394
Nitroglycerine.......................................263
Nitrolingual Spray 263
Nitromersol..394
Nizatadine..395
Nizoral...310

Index

No Gas 128, 511
NoDoz 112
NoDoz Plus 112, 389
Nolvadex 540
Nonoxynol 9 526
NONSTEROIDAL
   ANTI-INFLAMMATORY DRUGS 397
Nordette 406
Norditropin 523
Norethindrone 395
Norethisterone 395, 406
Norflex 410
Norflohexal 396
Norfloxacin 396
Norgesic 410, 423
Noriday 395, 406
Norimin 406
Norinyl 406
Normacol Plus 247, 528
Normafibe 528
Normal Human Immunoglobulin 251
Normal Immunoglobulin 251
Normison 544
Noroxin 396
Nortriptyline 578
Norvasc 47
Norvir 493
Noten 73
Novasone 370
NovoMix 30 296
NovoNorm 486
NovoRapid 296
NSAIDs 397
Nucolox 474
Nucosef 152, 472
Nucosef DM 175
Nuelin 554
Nurocain 53
Nurofen 288
Nurofen Cold & Flu 288, 472
Nurofen Plus 152
Nurolasts 380
Nutra D Cream 190, 424
Nutraplus 583
Nyal Chesty Cough 267
Nyal Cold Sore Cream 345
Nyal Decongestant 440
Nyal Dry Cough 430
Nyal Plus Chesty Cough 266, 472
Nyal Plus Cold & Flu 152, 423, 472
Nyal Plus Day Cold & Flu 472
Nyal Plus Day Sinus Relief 423, 472
Nyal Plus Decongestant 440, 472
Nyal Plus Dry Cough 442
Nyal Plus Night Cold & Flu 423, 472
Nyal Plus Night Sinus Relief 423, 472
Nyal Plus Sinus Relief 472
Nyal Plus Sinus Relief with Antihistamine .472
Nyal Sinus Relief 440
Nyefax 390
Nystatin 398

O

OBESITY DRUGS 399
Octostim 171
Octoxinol 526
Octreotide 399
Ocufen 240
Ocuflox 403
Odrik 23
Oestradiol 399
Oestradiol Implants 399
Oestriol 401
Oestrogen 402
Ofloxacin 403
Ogen 448
Oilatum Cleansing Bar 424
Oilatum Plus 85, 424, 578
Oilatum Shower Gel 424
Olanzapine 403
Olopatadine 404
Olsalazine 404
Omeprazole 471
Oncotice 83
Oncovin 593
Ondansetron 405
Ophthalin 516
Ophthetic 53
OPIATES 406
Optazine 379
Optazine Fresh 553
Opticrom 515
Optimol 565
Optrex 379
Ora-Sed Jel 85, 138
ORAL CONTRACEPTIVES 406
Orap 444
Oratane 304
Orciprenaline 409
Ordine 372
Organan 166
Orlistat 410
Orochol 136
Oroxine 559
Orphenadrine 410
ORS 208

Ortho-Creme 526
Ortho-Gynol 526
Orthoxicol Cold & Flu 175, 423, 472
Orthoxicol Day & Night Cold & Flu 175
Orthoxicol Day Cold & Flu 423, 472
Orthoxicol Night Cold & Flu 63, 175, 423
Orudis 311
Oruvail 311
Oseltamivir 411
Ospolot 536
Ostelin 212
Otocomb 265, 384, 398, 575
Otodex 173, 246, 265
Otrivin 597
Ovestin 401
Oxandrin 412
Oxandrolone 412
Oxazepam 413
Oxcarbazepine 414
Oxetine 425
Oxis 207
Oxpentifylline 415
Oxprenolol 415
Oxsoralen 354
Oxy 309
Oxy Skin Wash 578
Oxybutinin 416
Oxycodone 417
OxyContin 417
Oxymetazoline 418
OxyNorm 417
Oxytocin 419

P

Paclitaxel 420
Paedamin 63, 440
Painstop 63, 152, 423
Palfium 176
Paludrine 466
Pamisol 195
Panadeine 152, 423
Panadeine Forte 152, 423
Panadeine Plus 423
Panadol 423
Panadol Allergy Sinus 63, 423, 472
Panadol Children's Cold Elixir 63, 472
Panadol Children's Cold Relief Elixir 63
Panadol Cold & Flu 175, 423, 472
Panadol Night 63, 423
Panadol Sinus 423, 472
Panadol Sinus Day 472
Panadol Sinus Night 63, 423, 472
Panafcort 458

Panafcortelone 458
Panalgesic 63, 152, 423
Panamax Co 152, 423
Panamax 423
Parahexal 423
Pancrease 420
Pancrelipase 420
Panoxyl 309
Panquil 64
Panthenol 421
Pantoprazole 471
Pantothenic acid 422
Panzytrat 420
Papain 422
Paracetamol 423
Parachoc 424
Paracodin 187
Paraderm 106
Paraderm Plus 53, 106, 131
Paradex 177, 423
Paraffin 222
Paraffin 424
Paralgin 423
Paralice 96, 449
Pariet 471
Parke-Davis Cold and Flu 175
Parke-Davis Day Cold & Flu 472
Parke-Davis Night Cold & Flu 63, 472
Parlodel 104
Parnate 335
Paroven 284
Paroxetine 425
Parvolex 26
Patanol 404
Paullinia cupana 268
Paxam 148
Paxtine 425
Paxyl 34, 53, 85
Pectin 426
Pedialyte 208, 261
Pedoz 582, 603
Pedvax HiB 269
Pegatron 488
Pendine 250
Penhexal VK 438
Penicillamine 427
PENICILLINS 428
Pentazocine hydrochloride 428
Pentazocine lactate 428
Pentosan polysulfate 429
Pentoxyverine citrate 430
Pepcid 223
Pepcidine 223

Index

Peppermint oil	430
Pepti-Junior	224
Pergolide	431
Perhexiline	432
Periactin	64
Pericyazine	435
Perindopril	23
Permax	431
Permethrin	432
Persantin	194
Persantin SR	194
Pertussis vaccine	596
Pethidine	433
Pevaryl	205
Pexsig	432
Pharma-Col Junior	175, 423, 472
Pharmacia Chlorhexidine and Cetrimide	131
Phenelzine	335
Phenergan	63
Phenindione	434
Pheniramine	63
Pheniramine	63
Phenobarb	82
Phenobarbitone	82
PHENOTHIAZINES	435
Phenoxybenzamine	437
Phenoxyisopropanol	437
Phenoxymethyl penicillin	438
Phensedyl	442
Phensedyl Dry Family Cough	64, 472
Phentermine	439
Phenylephrine	375, 440
Phenytoin	441
Phisohex	578
Pholcodine	442
Phosphoprep	519
Phosphorus	443
Physeptone	350
Phytomenadione	270
Picolax	520
Picoprep	520
Pilocarpine	443
Pilopt	443
Pimozide	444
Pindolol	445
Pine tar	542
Pine Tar Lotion with Menthol	127
Pinetarsol	542
Pioglitazone	446
Piperacillin	447
Piperazine oestrone sulfate	448
Piperonyl butoxide	449
Piprandrol	449
Pipril	447
Pirohexal	450
Piroxicam	450
Pitressin	589
Pizotifen	451
Placil	578
Plague vaccine	599
Plaqacide	131
Plaquenil	283
Plavix	150
Plendil ER	225
Pneumococcal vaccine	452
Pneumovax 23	452
Podophyllotoxin	452
Podophyllum resin	452
PODOPHYLLUMS	452
Polaramine	64
Polio Sabin	453
Poliomyelitis vaccine	453
Poloxalkol	454
Poloxamer	454
Poly Gel Lubricant	222
Poly Visc	222, 424
Poly-Tears	222
Polymyxin B	454
Polytar	542
Polytar Medicated Bar	70
Polyvinyl alcohol	222
Ponstan	340
Portagen	224
Posalfilin	309, 452, 500
Postinor	325
Pot	336
Potassium aspartate	208
Potassium bicarbonate	57, 208
Potassium chloride	208
Potassium clavulanate	455
Povidone	222
Pramin	359
Prantal	191
Prasig	457
Pratsiol	457
Pravachol	456
Pravastatin	456
Praziquantel	457
Prazohexal	457
Prazosin	457
Predmix	458
Prednefrin Forte	440, 458
Prednisolone	458
Prednisone	458
Predsol	458
Prefrin	440

Pregestimil	224
Pregnyl	138
Premarin	402
Premia	339, 402
Prepulsid	141
Presolol	314
Pressin	457
Prevenar	452
Prickly Heat Powder	603
Prilocaine	53
Primacin	459
Primaquine	459
Primaxin	139
Primidone	460
Primobolan	351
Primogyn Depot	399
Primolut-N	395
Primoteston Depot	550
Prinivil	23
Priorix	337, 373, 497
Pritor	56
Pro-Banthine	467
Pro-Cid	461
Pro-Feme	465
Probenecid	461
Probitor	471
Probucol	461
Procainamide	462
Procaine penicillin	463
Procarbazine	464
Prochlorperazine	464
Proctosedyl	53, 278
Procur	162
Prodeine-15	152, 423
Profasi	138
Progesterone	465
PROGESTOGEN PILLS	406
Progout	35
Prograf	539
Proguanil	466
Progynova	399
PROKINETIC AGENTS	466
Proladone	417
Proluton	465
Promethazine	63
Prominal	82
Pronestyl	462
Propamidine isethionate	467
Propantheline	467
Propecia	229
Propine	193
Propranolol	468
Propylene glycol	469
Propylthiouracil	470
Proquin	140
Proscar	229
Prostaglandin E1	37
Prostin E2	191
Prostin VR	37
Protaphane	296
Prothiaden	578
PROTON PUMP INHIBITORS	471
Provelle	339, 402
Provera	339
Proviron	349
ProVisc	516
Proxen	380
Prozac	239
Pseudoephedrine	472
Psor-Asist	500, 534, 542
Psor-Asist Cream	309
Psor-Asist Scalp Lotion	309, 500, 583
Psorigel	542
PSYCHOTROPICS	473
Psyllium	471
PTU	470
Pulmicort	105
Puregon	245
Puri-Nethol	346
PV Carpine	443
PVA Forte	222
PVA Tears	222
Pylorid KA	49, 144, 484
Pyralin	533
Pyralvex	309, 500
Pyrantel embonate	474
Pyrazinamide	475
Pyrethrins	476
Pyridostigmine	476
Pyridoxine	477
Pyrifoam	432
Pyrimethamine	478
Pyrithione zinc	479

Q

Q fever vaccine	158
Q-Vax	158
Quellada	432
Questran Lite	137
Quetiapine	480
Quilonum SR	328
Quinapril	23
Quinate	482
Quinbisul	482
Quinidine bisulphate	481
Quinine	482

Index

Quinoctal 482
QUINOLONES 482
Quinsul 482
QuitX 388
QV Bar 190
QV Bath Oil 424
QV Cream 262, 424
QV Flare Up 85, 424, 578
QV Lip Balm 190
QV Skin Lotion 424
QV Wash 262
Qvar 84

R

Rabeprazole 471
Rabies vaccine 483
Radian B 345
Rafen 288
Ralodantin 394
Ralovera 339
Raloxifene 484
Ramace 23
Ramipril 23
Rani 2 484
Ranihexal 484
Ranitidine 484
Ranoxyl 484
Rapaid Powder 603
Rapamune 512
Rapifen 33
Rastinon 569
Rebetron 297, 488
Rebif 297
Reboxetine 485
Rectinol 30, 53, 603
Rectinol HC 53, 278
Rectogesic 263
Red back spider antivenom 67
Redipred 458
Reductil 508
Refresh 222
Refresh Liquigel 222
Refresh Tears Plus 222
Regaine Topical 366
Relaxa-Tabs 64
Relenza 601
Remeron 367
Reminyl 250
Renitec 23
Renitec Plus 23, 556
Rennie 57
Rennie 21, 115
Repaglinide 486
Repalyte 208, 261
Replens 262
Rescriptor 169
Resonium A 520
Resorcinol 487
Respocort 84
Resprim 532, 580
Restavit 63
Retin-A 309
Retinol 488
Retrieve 309
Retrovir 602
Revia 377
Rhinocort 105
Rhoto Zi Contact Eye Drops 222
Rhoto Zi Fresh Eye Drops 222
Riamet 70
Ribavirin 488
Riboflavine 489
Ridaura 77
Rifabutin 490
Rifadin 491
Rifampicin 491
Rikodeine 187
Rimycin 491
Ringworm Ointment 570
Risedronate 491
Risperdal 492
Risperidone 492
Ritalin 356
Ritonavir 493
Rivastigmine 494
Rivotril 148
Roaccutane 304
Robitussin DM 175, 267
Robitussin DM-P 175, 472
Robitussin DX 175
Robitussin EX 266
Robitussin Honey Cough 175
Robitussin ME 103, 267
Robitussin PS 266, 472
Rocaltrol 114
Rocephin 125
Rofecoxib 494
Roferon A 297
Rohypnol 235
Ropivacaine 53
Rosig 450
Rosiglitazone 495
Rosken Skin Repair 190
Roxin 396
Roxithromycin 496
Rozex 361

Home Guide to Medication   **633**

Index

RUBEFACIENTS 496
Rubella vaccine 497
Rubesal 183, 345
Rulide 496
Rynacrom 515
Rythmodan 196

S

Sabin vaccine 453
Sabril 592
Saint John's Wort 498
Saizen 523
Salazopyrin 533
Salbutamol 499
Salcatonin 500
Salicylic acid 309, 500
Salmeterol 501
Salmonella typhi vaccine 502
Salofalk 347
Salt 208
Salvital 57
Sandimmun 161
Sandocal 1000 115
Sandoglobulin 251
Sandomigran 451
Sandostatin 399
Sandrena 399
Sapoderm 578
Saquinavir 503
Sarna Lotion 345
Savacol 131
Savlon 131
Savlon Antiseptic 127
Savlon Antiseptic Powder 298
Scandonest 30, 53
Scheriproct 53, 458
SciTropin 523
Sea snake antivenom 67, 309
Sebitar 309, 500, 542, 582
Sebizole 310
Seborrol 309, 500
Seda-Gel 138, 345
Seda-Gel Gel 126
Seda-Gel Lotion 53, 128, 131
SEDATIVES 287
SEDATIVES AND HYPNOTICS 503
Selegiline 504
Selemite-B 505
Selenium sulfide 504
Selenomethionine 505
Selgene 504
Selsun 504
Senagar 47, 506
Senega 506
Senna 506
Sennesoft 198
Sennetabs 506
Sennosides 506
Senokot 506
Septopal 254
Septrin 532, 580
Sequilar 406
Serc 91
Serenace 270
Serepax 413
Seretide 242, 501
Serevent 501
Serophene 147
Seroquel 480
Sertraline 507
Serzone 383
Setacol 286
Setamol 423
SEX HORMONES 508
Sigma Liquid Antacid 511
Sigma Liquid Antacid 57
Sigma Relief 175, 266, 472
Sigmacort 278
Sigmaxin 186
Sigmetadine 139
Siguent Hycor Eye Ointment 278
Siguent Neomycin 384
Silbutramine 508
Silcon Cream 190
Sildenafil 509
Silic 15 190
Silvazine 131, 510
Silver sulfadiazine 510
Simethicone 57, 511
Simplotan 566
Simvastatin 511
Sinease Repetabs 62, 472
Sinemet 324
Sinequan 578
Singulair 371
Sinutab Sinus & Pain 423
Sinutab Sinus Allergy &
   Pain Relief 63, 423, 472
Sinutab Sinus and Pain Relief 472
Sirolimus 512
Sitriol 114
Skelid 564
Skinoren 309
Slow Sodium 208
Slow-K 208
SM-33 .... 53, 309

Index

SM-33 Adult 500
SM-33 Gel 345, 500
Snakes antivenom 67
Sodibic 57, 208, 584
Sodium acid citrate 208
Sodium alginate 57
Sodium ascorbate 71
Sodium aurothiomalate 513
Sodium bicarbonate 57, 208
Sodium carbonate 57
Sodium chloride 208
Sodium citrotartrate 57
Sodium clodronate 514
Sodium cromoglycate 515
Sodium fluoride 236
Sodium fusidate 516
Sodium hyaluronate 516
Sodium iodide 517
Sodium lauryl sulfoacetate 518
Sodium perborate 518
Sodium phosphate 519
Sodium picosulfate 520
Sodium polystyrene sulfonate 520
Sodium propionate 521
Sodium valproate 522
Sofra-Tulle 246
Sofradex 173, 246, 265
Soframycin 246, 265
Solavert 524
Solian 46
Solone 458
SoloSite 34
Solosite Wound Gel 262
Solprin 72
Solu-Cortef 278
Solu-Medrol 357
Solugel 469
Solyptol 134
Solyptol Cream 34, 85
Somac 471
Somatropin 523
Sone 458
SOOV 127, 131
SOOV Bite 53, 345, 437
SOOV Burn 53
SOOV Cream 53, 437
SOOV Prickly Heat
 Powder 309, 424, 500, 603
Sorbidin 303
Sorbilax 523
Sorbitol 523
Sorbolene 127
Sorbsan 116

Sotab 524
Sotacor 524
Sotahexal 524
Sotalol 524
SP Cream 309, 500, 583
Span-K 208
SPASMOLYTICS 525
Spectinomycin 525
SPERMICIDES 526
Spiractin 526
Spiriva 567
Spironolactone 526
Sporahexal 125
Sporanox 305
Spray-Tish 573
Spren 72
SSD 510
St.John's Wort 498
Stamaril 598
Staphylex 231
Stavudine 527
Stelazine 435
Stemetil 464
Stemzine 464
Sterculia 528
Sterofrin 458
STEROIDS 529
Stieva-A 309
Stilnox 606
STIMULANTS 530
Stingose 40
Stocrin 206
Stonefish antivenom 67
Stop Itch 422
Stoxil 290
Strepfen 240
Strepsils 52
Strepsils Cough Relief 175
Strepsils Extra 275
Strepsils Plus 52, 53
Strepsils Sugar-Free 52
Streptase 229
Streptodornase 229
Streptokinase 229
Stromectol 306
Stud 100 Spray 53
Sublimaze 227
Subutex 107
Sucralfate 530
Sudafed 12 Hour Relief 472
Sudafed Congestion & Sinus
 Pain Relief 288, 472
Sudafed Daytime Relief 423, 472

Sudafed Decongestant 472
Sudafed Nightime Relief 63, 423, 472
Sudafed Sinus Pain and Allergy 63, 423, 472
Sudafed Sinus Pain Relief 423, 472
Sulfacetamide 531
Sulfadoxine 531
Sulfamethoxazole 532
Sulfasalazine 533
SULFONAMIDES 534
Sulfur 534
Sulindac 535
Sulphur 534
Sulthiame 536
Sumatriptan 536
Sunspot Cream 500, 583
Superfade 281, 309, 500
Surgam 561
Surmontil 578
Sustanon 550
Suvalan 536
Symbicort 105, 207
Symmetrel 41
SYMPATHOMIMETICS 169, 537
Synarel 376
Synphasic 406
Syntocinon 419
Syntometrine 213, 419
Synvisc 285

T

T3 327
T4 559
Tacrine 538
Tacrolimus 539
Tadalafil 539
Tagamet 139
Talohexal 143
Tambocor 230
Tamiflu 411
Tamosin 540
Tamoxen 540
Tamoxifen 540
Tamsulosin 541
Tanacetum parthenium 228
Targocid 544
TARS 542
Tartaric acid 57
Taxo 420
Tazac 395
Tazobactam 542
Tazocin 447, 542
Teardrops 222
Tears Naturale 222

Tears Plus 222
Tegaserod 543
Tegretol 120
Telcoplanin 544
Telfast 62
Telfast Decongestant 62, 472
Telmisartan 56
Temaze 544
Temazepam 544
Temgesic 107
Temodal 545
Temozolomide 545
Temtabs 544
Tenofovir 546
Tenopt 565
Tenormin 73
Tenoxicam 546
Tensig 73
Tenuate 184
Tenuate Dospan 184
Tequin 252
Terazosin hydrochloride 547
Terbinafine 548
Terbutaline 549
Teril 120
Tertroxin 327
Testosterone 550
Testosterone Implants 550
Tet-Tox 551
Tetanus vaccine 551
Tetrabenazine 551
Tetracycline 552
Tetrahydrocannabinol 336
Tetrahydrozoline 553
Tetrex 552
Teveten 56
Teveten Plus 56, 556
THC 336
Theophylline 554
THEOPHYLLINES 554
Thiamine 555
THIAZIDE DIURETICS 556
Thioguanine 557
Thioprine 78
Thioridazine 435
Thiothixene 558
Thyroxine 559
Tiagabine 560
Tiaprofenic acid 561
Tibolone 562
Ticarcillin sodium 562
Tick antivenom 67
Ticlid 563

Ticlopidine	563
Ticlopidine Hexal	563
Tilactase	564
Tilade	382
Tilcotil	546
Tilodene	563
Tiludronate disodium	564
Timentin	455, 562
Timolol	565
Timoptol	565
Timoptol-XE	565
Timpilo	443, 565
Tinaderm	570
Tinaderm Extra	151
Tineafax	570
Tinidazole	566
Tiotropium	567
Titralac	57, 114
Titralac SIL	57, 511
Tixylix Nightime Linctus	64, 442
Tobramycin	567
Tobrex	567
Tocopherols	568
Tofranil	578
Tolbutamide	569
Tolnaftate	570
Tolvon	363
TONICS	570
Topamax	570
Topiramate	570
Toradol	312
Toremifene	571
Tracleer	100
Tramadol	572
Tramal	572
Tramazoline	573
Trandate	314
Trandolapril	23
Tranexamic acid	574
Transiderm Nitro	263
Tranylcypromine	335
Trasylol	69
Travacalm	112, 189, 286
Travacalm HO	286
Travad Phosphate Enema	519
Travatan	575
Travoprost	575
Trental	415
Tri-Minulet	406
Tri-Profen	288
Tri-Profen Cold and Flu	472
Triamcinolone	575
Triazolam	577
Triclosan	578
TRICYCLIC ANTIDEPRESSANTS	578
Trifeme	406
Trifluoperazine	435
Triglycerides	224
Trigonella	228
Trileptal	414
Trimeprazine	63
Trimethoprim	580
Trimipramine	578
Trimoxazole-BC	532, 580
Trioden	406
Tripacel	192, 551, 596
TRIPHASIC PILLS	406
Triphasil	406
Triple Antigen	192
Triprim	580
Triprofen Cold and Flu	288
Triprolidine	63
Triquilar	406
Trisequens	395, 399
Tritace	23
Trivizir	21, 315, 602
Trobicin	525
TROPHIC HORMONES	581
Tropicamide	375
Tropisetron	581
Trusopt	201
Tryptanol	578
Tuberculosis vaccine	83
Tussinol Actifed Dry Cough and Nasal Congestion	175
Tussinol Cough & Cold Infant	64, 175
Tussinol Expectorant	103, 267
Tussinol for Dry Coughs	175
Tussinol Night Time Cough & Cold	64, 175
Twinrix	273
Tylenol	423
Tylenol Allergy Sinus	63, 423, 472
Tylenol Cold & Flu	63, 175, 423, 472
Tylenol Cold & Flu Non-Drowsy	175, 423, 472
Tylenol Sinus	423, 472
Typh-Vax Oral	502
Typherix	502
Typhim Vi	502
Typhoid vaccine	502

U

Ulcyte	530
Ultracal	224
ULTRALENTE INSULIN	296
Ultraproct	53, 236

Index

Ultratard..296
Undecenoic acid 582
Undecylenamide 582
Unisom Sleepgels 64
Unitulle 424
Ural 584
Urea 583
Urecare 583
Ureder 583
Uremide 248
Urex 248
URICOSURICS..583
URINARY ACIDIFIERS............................583
URINARY ALKALINISERS 584
URINARY ANTISEPTICS 584
Urocarb 94
Uromitexan 348
Ursodeoxycholic acid 585
Ursofalk 585

V

VACCINES 586
Vagifem..399
Valaciclovir 586
Valcyte 587
Valerian 587
Valganciclovir 587
Valium 178
Vallergan 63
Valpam 178
Valpro 522
Valtrex 586
Vancocin 588
Vancomycin 588
VAQTA 273
Varicella zoster vaccine 129
Varidase 229
Varilix 129
Varivax II 129
Vasocardol CD 188
VASOCONSTRICTORS............................589
VASODILATORS 589
Vasopressin 589
Vastin 242
Vasylox 345, 418
Vaxigrip 295
Veganin 72, 152
Velbe 593
Venlafaxine 590
Ventolin..499
Vepesid 220
Veracaps 591
Verahexal 591

Verapamil..591
Vermox 338
Vesanoid 309
Viagra 509
Vibra-Tabs 202
Vibramycin..202
Vibrio cholera vaccine 136
Vicks Chesty Cough 266
Vicks Inhaler 345
Vicks Sinex 345, 418
Vicks Vaporub 345
Videx 182
Vigabatrin 592
Vinblastine 593
VINCA ALKALOIDS 593
Vincents 72
Vincristine..593
Vindesine sulfate 593
Vinorelbine 593
Viodine 298
Vioxx 494
Viracept..384
Viramune 387
Virasolve 53, 85, 290
Virazide..488
Viread 546
Viscoat..516
Viscotears 222
Visine Advanced Relief 222, 553
Visine Allergy with Antihistamine 63, 379
Visine Original..553
Visine True Tears 222
Visken 445
Vismed 516
Visopt 440
Vitadye 188
Vitaline 603
Vitamin A..90, 488
Vitamin B1 555
Vitamin B2 489
Vitamin B3 389
Vitamin B5 422
Vitamin B6 477
Vitamin B12 ....159, 282
Vitamin C..71
Vitamin D 135
Vitamin E..568
Vitamin H 96
Vitamin K..270
VITAMINS 594
Vitrasert Implant 252
Vivaxim..273, 502
Voltaren..180

Index

Vosol 469
VR Gel 34, 603

W

Warfarin 595
Wartec 452
Waxsol 198
WEIGHT LOSS DRUGS 596
Wellvone 75
Whooping cough vaccine 596

X

Xalacom 317, 565
Xalantan 317
Xanax 36
Xeloda 118
Xenical 410
Xylocaine 30, 53
Xylocaine Jelly with hlorhexidine 53
Xylocard 53
Xylometazoline 597
Xyloproct 53, 278, 603

Y

Yasmin 406
Yellow fever vaccine 598
Yersinia pestis vaccine 599

Z

Zactin 239
Zadine 64
Zafirlukast 600
Zalcitabine 600
Zanamivir 601
Zanidip 319
Zantac 484
Zarontin 219
Zavedos 289
Zeasorb 32, 134
Zeffix 315

Zelmac 543
Zentel 31
Zerit 527
Zestril 23
Ziagen 21
Zidovudine 602
Zinamide 475
Zinc 603
Zinc Cream 603
Zinc oxide 603
Zinc sulfate 604
Zincaps 604
Zincfrin 440, 604
Zinnat 125
Zinvit 604
Zinvit C-250 604
Zinvit G 604
Zithromax 79
Zocor 511
Zofran 405
Zoladex 264
Zolaten 27
Zolmitriptan 605
Zoloft 507
Zolpidem 606
Zomig 605
Zopiclone 607
Zostrix 119
Zoton 471
Zovirax 27
ZSC Powder 135, 603
Zuclopenthixol 608
Zumenon 399
Zyban 108
Zyclir 27
Zydol 572
Zyloprim 35
Zyprexa 403
Zyrtec 64
Zyvox 326

Index